# PDR for all of your drug information needs.

### Physicians' Desk Reference®
Physicians have turned to the PDR for the latest word on prescription drugs for more than 55 years. Today, PDR is still considered the standard prescription drug reference and can be found in virtually every physician's office, hospital and pharmacy in the United States. You can search the more than 4,000 drugs by using one of many indices and look at more than 2,100 full-color photos of drugs cross-referenced to the label information. More than 3,000 pages—our largest ever!

### PDR® Companion Guide
This unique 1,900-page all-in-one clinical companion to the PDR assures safe, appropriate drug selection with ten critical checkpoint indices including *Indications, Side Effects, Interactions, Off-Label Treatment* and much more.

### PDR® Pharmacopoeia Pocket Dosing Guide – Second Edition 2002
This pocket dosing guide brings important dispensing information to the practitioner's fingertips. Organized in tabular format, this small, 280-page quick reference is easy to navigate and gives important FDA approved dosing information, black box warning summaries and much more, whenever it is needed. Based on the PDR information, this guide proves that other Dosing Guides just don't measure up!

### PDR® for Nutritional Supplements™ – 1st Edition
The definitive information source for more than 300 nutritional supplements. This first, comprehensive, unbiased source of solid, evidence based information about nutritional and dietary supplements provides practitioners with more than 700 pages of the most current and reliable information available.

### PDR for Nonprescription Drugs and Dietary Supplements™
This acknowledged authority offers full FDA-approved descriptions of the most commonly used OTC medicines in four separate indices within more than 400 pages. Plus, it includes a section on supplements, vitamins and Herbal remedies.

### PDR® for Herbal Medicines™ – 2nd Edition
This guide, the most comprehensive reference on Herbal remedies, is based upon the work by Germany's Commission E and Jöerg Grüenwald, Ph. D. a botanist and renowned expert on herbal medicines. This detailed guide provides more than 1,100 pages of thorough descriptions on over 600 botanical remedies; the plant and the derived compounds.

### PDR for Ophthalmic Medicines™
The definitive reference for the eye-care professional offers 230 pages of detailed information on drugs and equipment used in the fields of ophthalmology and optometry. With five full indices and information on specialized instruments, lenses and much more, this guide is the most comprehensive of its kind.

### PDR® Medical Dictionary™ – 2nd Edition
This fully updated second edition with more than 2,100 pages, includes a complete medical etymology section on medical/scientific word formation as well as a complete cross-reference table of generic and brand name pharmaceuticals and manufacturers and much more!

## Complete Your 2002 PDR® Library NOW! Enclose payment and save shipping costs.

| Item | Product | Price |
|---|---|---|
| 101501 | ____ copies **2002 Physicians' Desk Reference®** | $89.95 ea. $_____ |
| 101519 | ____ copies **2002 PDR® Companion Guide** | $64.95 ea. $_____ |
| 101584 | ____ copies **PDR Pharmacopoeia Pocket Dosing Guide*** | $9.95 ea. $_____ |
| 101568 | ____ copies **PDR® for Nutritional Supplements™, 1st EDITION!** | $59.95 ea. $_____ |
| 101527 | ____ copies **2002 PDR for Nonprescription Drugs and Dietary Supplements™** | $55.95 ea. $_____ |
| 101550 | ____ copies **PDR® for Herbal Medicines™, 2nd EDITION!** | $59.95 ea. $_____ |
| 101535 | ____ copies **2002 PDR for Ophthalmic Medicines™** | $61.95 ea. $_____ |
| 101543 | ____ copies **PDR® Medical Dictionary™, 2nd EDITION!** | $49.95 ea. $_____ |

Shipping & Handling (Add $9.95 S&H per book if paying later*) $_____

Sales Tax (FL, GA, IA, & NJ) $_____

Total Amount of Order $_____

(*Shipping and handling is $1.95 for PDR Pharmacopoeia)

Mail this order form to: **PDR**, P.O. Box 10689, Des Moines, IA 50336-0689
e-mail: customer.service@ medec.com

### For Faster Service—FAX YOUR ORDER (515) 284-6714 or CALL TOLL-FREE (888) 859-8053
*Do not mail a confirmation order in addition to this fax.*

*Valid for 2002 editions only, prices and shipping & handling higher outside U.S.*

**PLEASE INDICATE METHOD OF PAYMENT:**
**Payment Enclosed** (shipping & handling FREE)
☐ Check payable to PDR
☐ VISA ☐ MasterCard
☐ Discover ☐ American Express

Account No. _____

Exp. Date _____

Telephone No. _____

Signature _____

Name _____

Address _____

City _____

State/Zip _____

### SAVE TIME AND MONEY EVERY YEAR AS A STANDING ORDER SUBSCRIBER
☐ Check here to enter your standing order for future editions of publications ordered. They will be shipped to you automatically, after advance notice. As a standing order subscriber, you are **guaranteed** our lowest price offer, earliest delivery and FREE shipping and handling. **756403**

☐ **Bill me later**
(Add $9.95 per book for shipping and handling*)

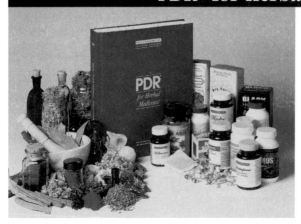
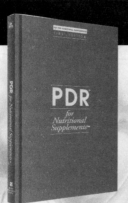

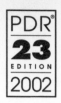

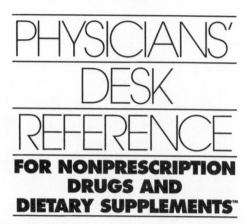

# FOR NONPRESCRIPTION DRUGS AND DIETARY SUPPLEMENTS™

**Executive Vice President, Directory Services:** Paul Walsh

**Vice President, Sales and Marketing:**
Dikran N. Barsamian

**National Sales Manager:** John A. Schmidt

**National Sales Manager, Custom Sales:**
Anthony Sorce

**Senior Account Managers:** Marion Gray, RPh,
Frank Karkowsky, Elaine Musco

**Account Managers:** Lawrence C. Keary, Lois Smith,
Eileen Sullivan, Suzanne E. Yarrow, RN

**Director of Trade Sales:** Bill Gaffney

**Associate Product Manager:** Jason Springer

**Director of Financial Planning and Analysis:**
Mark S. Ritchin

**Director of Direct Marketing:** Michael Bennett

**Direct Mail Managers:** Jennifer M. Fronzaglia,
Lorraine M. Loening

**Senior Marketing Analyst:** Dina A. Maeder

**Promotion Manager:** Linda Levine

**Vice President, Clinical Communications and New
Business Development:** Mukesh Mehta, RPh

**New Business Development Manager:**
Jeffrey D. Dubin

**Manager, Professional Data Services:**
Thomas Fleming, PharmD

**Manager, Concise Data Content:**
Christine Wyble, PharmD

**Drug Information Specialists:** Maria Deutsch, MS,
PharmD, CDE; Anu Gupta, PharmD

**Editor, Directory Services:** David W. Sifton

**Project Manager:** Edward P. Connor

**Senior Associate Editor:** Lori Murray

**Assistant Editor:** Gwynned L. Kelly

**Director of Production:** Brian Holland

**Senior Data Manager:** Jeffrey D. Schaefer

**Production Manager:** Amy B. Brooks

**Senior Production Coordinator:** Gianna Caradonna

**Production Coordinators:** Dee Ann DeRuvo,
Melissa Johnson, Christina Klinger

**Index Editors:** Noel Deloughery, Shannon Reilly

**Format Editor:** Stu W. Lehrer

**Art Associate:** Joan K. Akerlind

**Digital Imaging Supervisor:** Shawn W. Cahill

**Digital Imaging Coordinator:** Frank J. McElroy, III

**Production Design Supervisor:** Adeline Rich

**Electronic Publishing Designers:** Rosalia Sberna,
Livio Udina

**Fulfillment Managers:** Louis J. Bolcik,
Stephanie Struble

# FOREWORD

Two important additions to the *PDR* library of references deserve your attention this year. Both can supply you with a quick synopsis of the facts you need most for routine prescribing.

For complicated cases and special patient problems, there is of course no substitute for the in-depth data contained in *Physicians' Desk Reference*. But on other occasions, you may find that the new **PDR® Monthly Prescribing Guide™** provides a handy alternative. Distilled from the pages of *PDR*, this 360-page digest-sized reference presents the key facts on over 1,000 drugs, including the form, strength, and route; therapeutic class; approved indications; dosage; contraindications; warnings; precautions; pregnancy rating; drug interactions; and adverse reactions. Each entry alerts you to the significant precautions you need to take, spells out the most common or dangerous adverse effects, summarizes the recommended adult and pediatric dosages, and supplies you with the *PDR* page number to turn to for further information.

Issued monthly, the guide is continuously updated with the latest FDA-approved revisions to existing product information, augmented with detailed descriptions of newly released medications. In addition, you'll receive bulletins about major new developments on the pharmaceutical scene, an overview of important new agents nearing approval, a heads-up on the latest pharmaceutical issues to hit the consumer media, in-depth analysis of the common nutritional supplements that patients are taking, and a handy reminder of upcoming medical meetings.

In fact, in one neat package you'll find just about everything you need to make a routine prescribing decision—secure in the knowledge that you're acting on the latest FDA-approved data. To order your personal subscription to this important new monthly publication, simply call 1-800-232-7379.

If you prefer to keep information such as this on a handheld device like a Palm® or Pocket PC, our other new reference may be just what you're looking for. Called **mobilePDR™**, this easy-to-use software allows you to instantly retrieve the basic facts you need on any drug, lets you run automatic interaction checks on multidrug regimens, and even alerts you to significant changes in updated drug entries. Covering a total of 1,500 drugs, this portable electronic reference is updated as often as daily with the latest FDA-approved revisions to existing product information, plus the essential facts you need to safely prescribe newly approved agents; and it's available for downloading from www.PDR.net whenever you want to bring your data up to date. It works with both the Palm and Windows CE operating systems, and it's free to U.S.-based MDs, DOs, NPs, and PAs in full-time patient practice. Check it out today.

## Other Prescribing Aids from PDR

For those times when all you need is quick confirmation of a particular dosage, you may also want to order a copy of the *PDR Pharmacopoeia™ Pocket Dosing Guide*. This handy little book can accompany you wherever you need to go, around the office or on rounds. Only slightly larger than an index card and a quarter of an inch thick, it fits easily into any pocket, while providing you with FDA-approved dosing recommendations for over 1,500 drugs. Unlike other condensed drug references, it's drawn almost exclusively from the FDA-approved drug labeling published in *Physicians' Desk Reference*. And its tabular presentation makes lookups a breeze. At $9.95 a copy, it's a tool you really can't afford to be without.

Recently, the use of over-the-counter nutritional supplements has sky-rocketed, and *PDR* has responded with a brand new medical reference covering this unfamiliar—even exotic—set of agents. Entitled *PDR® for Nutritional Supplements™*, it offers the latest scientific consensus on hundreds of popular supplement products, including an array of amino acids, co-factors, fatty acids, probiotics, phytoestrogens, phytosterols, over-the-counter hormones, hormonal precursors, and much more. Focused on the scientific evidence for each supplement's claims, this unique new reference offers you today's most detailed, informed, and objective overview of a burgeoning new area in the field of self-treatment. To protect your patients from bogus remedies and steer them towards truly beneficial products, this book is a must.

For counseling patients who favor herbal remedies, another *PDR* reference may prove equally valuable. Now in its second edition, *PDR® for Herbal Medicines™* provides you with the latest science-based assessment of some 700 botanicals. Indexed by scientific, common, and brand names (as well as Western, Asian, and homeopathic indications) this volume also includes a Side Effects Index, a Drug/Herb Interactions Guide, an Herb Identification Guide with nearly 400 color photos, and a Safety Guide that lists herbs to be avoided during pregnancy and herbs to be used only under professional supervision. Although botanical products are not officially regulated or monitored in the United States, *PDR for Herbal Medicines* provides you with the closest analog to FDA-approved labeling—the findings of the German Regulatory Authority's herbal watchdog agency, Commission E.

To maximize the value of *PDR* itself, you'll also need a copy of the 2002 edition of the *PDR Companion Guide™*, an 1,800-page reference that augments *PDR* with a total of nine unique decision-making tools:

- **Interactions Index** identifies all pharmaceuticals and foods capable of interacting with a chosen medication.

- **Food Interactions Cross-Reference** lists the drugs that may interact with a given dietary item.

- **Side Effects Index** pinpoints the pharmaceuticals associated with each of 3,600 distinct adverse reactions.

- **Indications Index** presents the full range of therapeutic options for any given diagnosis.

- **Off-Label Treatment Guide** lists medications routinely used—but never officially approved—for treatment of nearly 1,000 specific disorders.

- **Contraindications Index** lists all drugs to avoid in the presence of any given medical condition.

- **International Drug Name Index** names the U.S. equivalents of some 15,000 foreign medications.

- **Generic Availability Guide** shows which forms and strengths of a brand-name drug are also available generically.

- **Imprint Identification Guide** enables you to establish the nature of any unknown tablet or capsule by matching its imprint against an exhaustive catalog of identifying codes.

The *PDR Companion Guide* includes all drugs described in *PDR*, *PDR for Nonprescription Drugs and Dietary Supplements*™, and *PDR for Ophthalmic Medicines*™. We're certain that you'll find it makes safe, appropriate selection of drugs faster and easier than ever before.

*PDR* and its major companion volumes are also found in the *PDR® Electronic Library*™ on CD-ROM, now used in over 100,000 practices. This Windows-compatible disc provides users with a complete database of *PDR* prescribing information, electronically searchable for instant retrieval. A standard subscription includes *PDR's* sophisticated search software and an extensive file of chemical structures, illustrations, and full-color product photographs. Optional enhancements include the complete contents of *The Merck Manual Seventeenth Edition*, *Stedman's Medical Dictionary*, and *Stedman's Spellchecker*. For anyone who wants to run a fast double check on a proposed prescription, there's also the *PDR® Drug Interactions and Side Effects System*™ — sophisticated software capable of automatically screening a 20-drug regimen for conflicts, then proposing alternatives for any problematic medication. This unique decision-making tool now comes free with the *PDR Electronic Library*.

For more information on these or any other members of the growing family of *PDR* products, please call, toll-free, 1-800-232-7379 or fax 201-722-2680.

## How to Use This Book

*Physicians' Desk Reference for Nonprescription Drugs and Dietary Supplements* is divided into two major sections. The first, entitled *Nonprescription Drug Information*, presents descriptions of conventional remedies marketed in compliance with the Code of Federal Regulations labeling requirements for over-the-counter drugs. The second section, entitled *Dietary Supplement Information*, contains information on herbal remedies and nutritional supplements marketed under the Dietary Supplement Health and Education Act of 1994. For your convenience, products in both sections are listed in the consolidated indices at the front of the book.

*Physicians' Desk Reference for Nonprescription Drugs and Dietary Supplements* is published annually by Thomson Medical Economics in cooperation with participating manufacturers. The function of the publisher is the compilation, organization, and distribution of product information obtained from manufacturers. Each product description has been prepared by the manufacturer, and edited and approved by the manufacturer's medical department, medical director, and/or medical consultant. During compilation of this information, the publisher has emphasized the necessity of describing products comprehensively, in order to provide all the facts necessary for sound and intelligent decision making. Descriptions seen here include all information made available by the manufacturer. Please note that descriptions of over-the-counter products marketed under the Dietary Supplement Health and Education Act of 1994 have not been evaluated by the Food and Drug Administration, and that such products are not intended to diagnose, treat, cure, or prevent any disease.

In organizing and presenting the material in *Physicians' Desk Reference For Nonprescription Drugs and Dietary Supplements*, the publisher does not warrant or guarantee any of the products described, or perform any independent analysis in connection with any of the product information contained herein. *Physicians' Desk Reference* does not assume, and expressly disclaims, any obligation to obtain and include any information other than that provided to it by the manufacturer. It should be understood that by making this material available the publisher is not advocating the use of any product described herein, nor is the publisher responsible for misuse of a product due to typographical error. Additional information on any product may be obtained from the manufacturer.

# CONTENTS

# MANUFACTURERS' INDEX

Listed in this index are all manufacturers that have supplied information in this edition. Each company's entry includes the address, phone, and fax number of its headquarters and regional offices, as well as contacts for inquiries, orders, and emergency information.

Products with entries in the Nonprescription Drug Information section are listed with their page numbers under the heading OTC Products Described. Products with entries in the Dietary Supplement Information section are listed with their page numbers under the

heading Dietary Supplements Described. Other OTC products and dietary supplements available from the manufacturer follow these two sections.

If an entry in the index lists multiple page numbers, the first one shown refers to the photograph of the product, the last one to its prescribing information.

- The ◆ symbol marks drugs shown in the Product Identification Guide.

- *Italic page numbers* signify partial information.

**A & Z PHARMACEUTICAL INC.**　503, 796

180 Oser Avenue, Suite 300
Hauppauge, NY 11788
**Direct Inquiries to:**
Customer Service
(631) 952-3800
FAX: (631) 952-3900

**Dietary Supplements Described:**
◆ D-Cal Chewable Caplets .........**503, 796**

**AK PHARMA INC.**　503, 796

P.O. Box 111
Pleasantville, NJ 08232-0111
**Direct Inquiries to:**
Elizabeth Klein
(609) 645-5100
FAX: (609) 645-0767
**For Medical Emergencies Contact:**
Alan E. Kligerman
(609) 645-5100

**Dietary Supplements Described:**
◆ Prelief Tablets and Granulate....**503, 796**

**ALPHARMA**　602

U.S. Pharmaceuticals Division
7205 Windsor Boulevard
Baltimore, MD 21244
**Direct Inquiries to:**
Customer Service
(800) 638-9096

**OTC Products Described:**
Permethrin Lotion......................**602**

**AMERICAN LONGEVITY**　797

2400 Boswell Road
Chula Vista, CA 91914
**Direct Inquiries to:**
Customer Service
(800) 982-3189
FAX: (619) 934-3205
www.americanlongevity.net

**Dietary Supplements Described:**
Plant Derived Minerals Liquid .........**797**
Ultimate Classic Liquid ...............**797**

**AWARENESS CORPORATION**　503, 798

1201 South Alma School Road
Suite 4750
Mesa, AZ 85210-1112
**Direct Inquiries to:**
(800) 69AWARE
www.awarenesshealth.com

**Dietary Supplements Described:**
◆ Awareness Clear Capsules ......**503, 798**
◆ Awareness Female Balance
　Capsules.....................**503, 798**
　Diabetic Balance Capsules............**798**
◆ Experience Capsules ...........**503, 798**

**BAYER CORPORATION CONSUMER CARE DIVISION**　503, 602

36 Columbia Road
P.O. Box 1910
Morristown, NJ 07962-1910

**Direct Inquiries to:**
Consumer Relations
(800) 331-4536
www.bayercare.com
**For Medical Emergencies Contact:**
Bayer Corporation
Consumer Care Division
(800) 331-4536

**OTC Products Described:**
◆ Aleve Tablets, Caplets and
　Gelcaps ......................**503, 602**
◆ Aleve Cold & Sinus Caplets......**503, 603**
◆ Aleve Sinus & Headache
　Caplets ......................**503, 604**
　Alka-Seltzer Original Antacid and
　Pain Reliever Effervescent
　Tablets.............................**604**
　Alka-Seltzer Cherry Antacid and
　Pain Reliever Effervescent
　Tablets.............................**604**
◆ Alka-Seltzer Lemon Lime
　Antacid and Pain Reliever
　Effervescent Tablets.........**503, 604**
　Alka-Seltzer Extra Strength
　Antacid and Pain Reliever
　Effervescent Tablets...............**604**
◆ Alka-Seltzer Morning Relief
　Tablets......................**503, 605**
◆ Alka-Seltzer Plus Cold
　Medicine Liqui-Gels .........**503, 608**
　Alka-Seltzer Plus Cold & Cough
　Medicine Effervescent Tablets ....**606**
　Alka-Seltzer Plus Cold & Sinus
　Medicine Effervescent Tablets ....**606**
◆ Alka-Seltzer Plus Night-Time
　Cold Medicine Liqui-Gels ....**503, 608**

## BEACH PHARMACEUTICALS     804

Division of Beach Products, Inc.
EXECUTIVE OFFICE:
5220 South Manhattan Avenue
Tampa, FL 33611
(813) 839-6565
**Direct Inquiries to:**
Richard Stephen Jenkins, Exec. V.P.:
(813) 839-6565
Clete Harmon, Dir. of Q.A.:
(864) 277-7282
**Manufacturing and Distribution:**
201 Delaware Street
Greenville, SC 29605
(800) 845-8210

## BEUTLICH LP PHARMACEUTICALS     623

1541 Shields Drive
Waukegan, IL 60085-8304

**Direct Inquiries to:**
(847) 473-1100
(800) 238-8542 in the U.S. and Canada
FAX: (847) 473-1122
www.beutlich.com
E-mail: beutlich@beutlich.com

## BODY WISE INTERNATIONAL INC.     804

2802 Dow Avenue
Tustin, CA 92780
**Direct Inquiries to:**
Wellness Research Center
(714) 505-6121
FAX: (714) 832-7247
E-mail: wellness@bodywise.com

## BOEHRINGER INGELHEIM CONSUMER HEALTHCARE PRODUCTS     505, 623

Division of Boehringer Ingelheim Pharmaceuticals, Inc.
900 Ridgebury Road
P.O. Box 368
Ridgefield, CT 06877
**Direct Inquiries to:**
(888) 285-9159

**OTC Products Described:**
- Dulcolax Bowel Prep Kit ......... **505, 623**
- Dulcolax Suppositories .......... **505, 624**
- Dulcolax Tablets ................. **505, 624**

## BOIRON, THE WORLD LEADER IN HOMEOPATHY   **625**

6 Campus Blvd.
Newtown Square, PA 19073
**Direct Inquiries to:**
Boiron Information Center
(800) 264-7661
FAX: (888) 264-7661
E-mail: info@boiron.com
**For Medical Emergencies Contact:**
Boiron Information Center
(800) 264-7661
E-mail: info@boiron.com

**OTC Products Described:**
Oscillococcinum Pellets ............... **625**

**Other Products Available:**
Acidil, for Heartburn
Arnica & Calendula Gel & Ointment
Camilia, for Baby Teething
Chestal Cough Syrup
Chestal For Children Cough Syrup
Cocyntal, for Baby Colic
Coldcalm, for Cold Symptoms
Cyclease, for Menstrual Cramps
Gasalia, for Gas
Ginsenique, for Fatigue
Homeodent Toothpaste
Natural Phases, for PMS
Optique 1 Eye Drops, for Eye Irritation
Quiétude, for Sleeplessness
Roxalia, for Sore Throat
Sabadil, for Allergies
Sedalia, for Nervousness Associated with Stress
Sinusalia, for Sinus Pain
Sportenine, for Cramps and Muscle Fatigue
Yeastaway, for Vaginal Yeast Infections

## BRISTOL-MYERS PRODUCTS   **505, 625**

A Bristol-Myers Squibb Company
345 Park Avenue
New York, NY 10154
**Direct Inquiries to:**
Bristol-Myers Products Division
Consumer Affairs Department
1350 Liberty Avenue
Hillside, NJ 07207
**Questions or Comments:**
(800) 468-7746

**OTC Products Described:**
- Multi-Sympton Comtrex Deep Chest Cold Softgels ......... **505, 627**
- Maximum Strength Comtrex Acute Head Cold Caplets .... **505, 626**
- Maximum Strength Comtrex Cold & Cough Day & Night Caplets (Daytime)............ **505, 626**
- Maximum Strength Comtrex Cold & Cough Day & Night Caplets (Nighttime) .......... **505, 626**

- Maximum Strength Comtrex Flu Therapy Day & Night Caplets (Daytime)............ **505, 627**
- Maximum Strength Comtrex Flu Therapy Day & Night Caplets (Nighttime) .......... **505, 627**
- Maximum Strength Comtrex Sinus & Nasal Decongestant Caplets ....... **505, 628**
- Aspirin Free Excedrin Caplets and Geltabs................. **506, 629**
- Excedrin Extra Strength Tablets, Caplets, and Geltabs ..................... **506, 629**
- Excedrin Migraine Tablets, Caplets, and Geltabs ........ **506, 630**
- Excedrin PM Tablets, Caplets, and Geltabs.................. **506, 630**

**Other Products Available:**
Alpha Keri Moisture Rich Cleansing Bar
Bufferin, Arthritis Strength Caplets
Bufferin, Extra Strength Tablets
4-Way Fast Acting Nasal Spray
4-Way Long Lasting Nasal Spray
4-Way Menthol Fast Acting Nasal Spray
4-Way Nasal Moisturizing Saline Mist
Maximum Strength Comtrex Nighttime Cold & Cough Caplets
Maximum Strength Comtrex Non-Drowsy Cold & Cough Caplets
Maximum Strength Comtrex Sore Throat Liquid
Therapeutic Mineral Ice Exercise Formula

## CELLTECH PHARMACEUTICALS, INC.   **631**

P.O. Box 31766
Rochester, NY 14603
**Direct Inquiries to:**
Customer Service Department
P.O. Box 31766
Rochester, NY 14603
(716) 274-5300
(888) 963-3382

**OTC Products Described:**
Delsym Extended-Release Suspension ........................ **631**

## CHATTEM, INC.   **631**

1715 West 38th Street
Chattanooga, TN 37409
**Direct Inquiries to:**
(423) 821-2037

**Dietary Supplements Described:**
Dexatrim Results Caplets ............. **631**
Dexatrim Results, Ephedrine Free Caplets ........................... **631**

## COVEX   **506, 806**

Sector Oficios 33, 1-3
28760 Tres Cantos
Madrid, Spain
**Direct Inquiries to:**
+34-91-804-4545
FAX: +34-91-804-3030
E-mail: vinpocetin@covex.es

**Dietary Supplements Described:**
- Intelectol Tablets ................ **506, 806**

## EFFCON LABORATORIES, INC.   **506, 632**

P.O. Box 7499
Marietta, GA 30065-1499
**Direct Inquiries to:**
J. Bradley Rivet
(800) 722-2428
FAX: (770) 428-6811
**For Medical Emergencies Contact:**
J. Bradley Rivet
(800) 722-2428
FAX: (770) 428-6811

**OTC Products Described:**
- Pin-X Pinworm Treatment ........ **506, 632**

## FLEMING & COMPANY   **632**

1600 Fenpark Dr.
Fenton, MO 63026
**Direct Inquiries to:**
Tom Fleming
(636) 343-8200
FAX: (636) 343-9865
www.flemingcompany.com
For product orders, call (800) 343-0164

**OTC Products Described:**
Chlor-3 Shaker......................... **632**
Nicotinex Elixir ......................... **807**
Ocean Nasal Mist..................... **633**
Purge Liquid .......................... **633**

**Dietary Supplements Described:**
Magonate Liquid....................... **807**
Magonate Natal Liquid .............. **807**
Magonate Tablets..................... **807**

## GLAXOSMITHKLINE CONSUMER HEALTHCARE, L.P.   **506, 633**

Post Office Box 1467
Pittsburgh, PA 15230
**Direct Inquiries to:**
Consumer Affairs
(800) 245-1040
**For Medical Emergencies Contact:**
Consumer Affairs
(800) 245-1040

**OTC Products Described:**
- Abreva Cream..................... **506, 633**
- Balmex Diaper Rash Ointment... **506, 633**
- Balmex Medicated Plus Baby Powder....................... **506, 633**
- BC Powder ......................... **634**
- BC Allergy Sinus Cold Powder ........ **634**
- Arthritis Strength BC Powder ......... **634**
- BC Sinus Cold Powder................. **634**
- Citrucel Caplets ...................... **635**
- Citrucel Orange Flavor Powder... **506, 635**
- Citrucel Sugar Free Orange Flavor Powder................ **506, 635**
- Contac Non-Drowsy 12 Hour Cold Caplets ....................... **636**
- Contac Non-Drowsy Timed Release 12 Hour Cold Caplets ...................... **506, 636**
- Contac Severe Cold and Flu Caplets Maximum Strength.................. **506, 637**
- Contac Severe Cold and Flu Caplets Non-Drowsy .............. **637**

**A. C. GRACE COMPANY          663**
1100 Quitman Rd.
P.O. Box 570
Big Sandy, TX 75755
**Direct Inquiries to:**
(903) 636-4368
**Orders Only:**
(800) 833-4368

**OTC Products Described:**

**HYLAND'S, INC.**
(See STANDARD HOMEOPATHIC
COMPANY)

**JOHNSON & JOHNSON •          509, 664
MERCK CONSUMER
PHARMACEUTICALS
CO.**
7050 Camp Hill Road
Fort Washington, PA 19034
**Direct Inquiries to:**
Consumer Affairs Department
(800) 469-5268
**For Medical Emergencies Contact:**
(800) 462-5268

**OTC Products Described:**

**KYOWA          509, 811
ENGINEERING-SUNDORY**
5-964 Nakamozu-Cho, Sakai-City
Osaka, Japan
**Direct Inquiries to:**
Consumer Relations
82-72-257-8568
Osaka
FAX: 81-722-57-8655
www.sundory.jp

**Dietary Supplements Described:**

**LEDERLE CONSUMER HEALTH          665**
A Division of Whitehall-Robins Healthcare
Five Giralda Farms
Madison, NJ 07940
**Direct Inquiries to:**
Lederle Consumer Product Information
(800) 282-8805

**OTC Products Described:**

**Dietary Supplements Described:**

**Other Products Available:**
   Centrum Focused Formulas Stress Tablets
   Centrum Kids Extra C Children's
   Chewables
   Centrum Kids Extra Calcium Children's
   Chewables
   Centrum Liquid

**LEGACY FOR LIFE          509, 816**
P.O. Box 410376
Melbourne, FL 32941-0376
**Direct Inquiries to:**
(800) 557-8477
www.legacyforlife.net

**Dietary Supplements Described:**

**Other Products Available:**
   BioChoice FLEX Capsules
   BioChoice SLIM Capsules

**MANNATECH, INC.          509, 816**
600 S. Royal Lane
Suite 200
Coppell, TX 75019
**Direct Inquiries to:**
Customer Service
(972) 471-8111
**For Medical Information Contact:**
Kia Gary, RN LNCC
(972) 471-8189
E-mail: Kgary@mannatech.com
www.mannatech.com
(for product information)
www.glycoscience.com
(for ingredient information)

**Dietary Supplements Described:**

**MILES INC. CONSUMER
HEALTHCARE PRODUCTS**
(See BAYER CORPORATION CONSUMER
CARE DIVISION)

**MISSION PHARMACAL        691
COMPANY**
10999 IH 10 West, Suite 1000
San Antonio, TX 78230-1355
**Direct Inquiries to:**
P.O. Box 786099
San Antonio, TX 78278-6099
(800) 292-7364
(210) 696-8400
FAX: (210) 696-6010
**For Medical Emergencies Contact:**
George Alexandrides
(830) 249-9822
FAX: (830) 816-2545

**OTC Products Described:**

**Dietary Supplements Described:**

**Other Products Available:**
Calcet Triple Calcium Supplement Tablets
Calcet Plus Multivitamin/Mineral Tablets
Citracal Prenatal Rx
Compete Multivitamin/Mineral Tablets
Fosfree Multivitamin/Mineral Tablets
Iromin-G Multivitamin/Mineral Tablets
Maxilube Personal Lubricant
Oncovite

**NOVARTIS CONSUMER      514, 691
HEALTH, INC.**
200 Kimball Drive
Parsippany, NJ 07054-0622

**Direct Inquiries to:**
Consumer and Professional Affairs
(800) 452-0051
FAX: (800) 635-2801
Or write to the above address

**OTC Products Described:**

**Dietary Supplements Described:**

**PARKE-DAVIS**
(See PFIZER CONSUMER HEALTHCARE,
PFIZER INC.)

**PFIZER CONSUMER       516, 707
GROUP, PFIZER INC.**
Consumer Health Products Group
201 Tabor Road
Morris Plains, NJ 07950
(See also Pfizer Consumer Healthcare,
Pfizer Inc.)

**Direct Inquiries to:**
(800) 223-0182

**For Consumer Product Information Call:**
(800) 524-2854 (Celestial Seasonings
Soothers only)
(800) 223-0182

**OTC Products Described:**

## PLOUGH, INC.
(See SCHERING-PLOUGH HEALTHCARE
PRODUCTS)

## PROCTER & GAMBLE          522, 744
P.O. Box 559
Cincinnati, OH 45201
**Direct Inquiries to:**
Consumer Relations
(800) 832-3064

**OTC Products Described:**

## PRODUCTS ON DEMAND          522, 755
1621 East Flamingo Road
Suite 15A
Las Vegas, NV 89119
**Direct Inquiries to:**
Shaina M. Toppo
(888) 806-0344
FAX: (888) 444-9844
www.vitara.com

**For Medical Emergencies Contact:**
(888) 806-0344
FAX: (888) 444-9844

**OTC Products Described:**

## THE PURDUE FREDERICK          523, 755
COMPANY
One Stamford Forum
Stamford, CT 06901-3431
**For Medical Information Contact:**
Medical Department
(888) 726-7535

**OTC Products Described:**

## REXALL SUNDOWN, INC.          523, 822
6111 Broken Sound Parkway NW
Boca Raton, FL 33487-2745
**Direct Inquiries to:**
(888) VITAHELP (848-2435)
www.osteobioflex.com

**Dietary Supplements Described:**

## RICHARDSON-VICKS, INC.
(See PROCTER & GAMBLE)

## SCHERING CORPORATION
(See SCHERING-PLOUGH HEALTHCARE
PRODUCTS)

## SCHERING-PLOUGH          523, 757
HEALTHCARE
PRODUCTS
3 Oak Way
Berkeley Heights, NJ 07922
**Direct Product Requests to:**
Schering-Plough HealthCare Products
Attn: Managed Care Department
3 Oak Way
Berkeley Heights, NJ 07922
(908) 679-1983
FAX: (908) 679-1776
**For Medical Emergencies Contact:**
Consumer Relations Department
(901) 320-2988 (Business Hours)
(901) 320-2364 (After Hours)

**SIGMA-TAU**                          **524, 823**
**HEALTHSCIENCE, INC.**

A division of Sigma-Tau HealthScience,
S.p.A.
800 South Frederick Avenue
Suite 102
Gaithersburg, MD 20877

---

**Direct Medical Inquiries to:**
(877) PROXEED (776-9333)
(301) 948-5450
FAX: (301) 948-5452
E-Mail: proxeedinfo@st-hs.com

**Direct Product Orders to:**
(877) PROXEED (776-9333)
www.proxeed.com

**STANDARD HOMEOPATHIC**          **767**
**COMPANY**

210 West 131st Street
Box 61067
Los Angeles, CA 90061

**Direct Inquiries to:**
Jay Borneman
(800) 624-9659, Ext. 20

**SUNPOWER NUTRACEUTICAL**         **825**
**INC.**

8850 Research Drive
Irvine, CA 92618

**Direct Inquiries to:**
(949) 833-8899

**UAS LABORATORIES**               **769**

5610 Rowland Road # 110
Minnetonka, MN 55343

**Direct Inquiries to:**
Dr. S.K. Dash
(952) 935-1707
FAX: (952) 935-1650

---

**For Medical Emergencies Contact:**
Dr. S.K. Dash
(952) 935-1707
FAX: (952) 935-1650

**UNITHER PHARMACEUTICALS**        **825**
**COMPANY**

1110 Spring Street
Silver Spring, MD 20910

**Direct Inquiries to:**
(321) 779-1441

**UPSHER-SMITH**                   **770**
**LABORATORIES, INC.**

14905 23rd Avenue N.
Plymouth, MN 55447

**Direct Inquiries to:**
Professional Services
(763) 475-3023
FAX: (763) 475-3410

**For Medical Emergencies Contact:**
Professional Services
(763) 475-3023
(800) 654-2299
FAX: (763) 475-3410

**Branch Offices:**
13700 1st Avenue N.
Plymouth, MN 55441
(763) 475-3023
FAX: (763) 475-3410

**WALLACE**                        **524, 770**
**PHARMACEUTICALS**

MedPointe Healthcare Inc.
Cranbury, NJ 08512

**Direct Inquiries to:**
Wallace Pharmaceuticals
MedPointe Healthcare Inc.
Cranbuy, NJ 08512
609-655-6000
**For Medical Information, Contact:**
**Generally:**
Professional Services
800-526-3840

**After Hours and Weekend Emergencies:**
609-655-6474

**WARNER-LAMBERT COMPANY**

(See PFIZER CONSUMER GROUP, PFIZER
INC.)

## WARNER-LAMBERT CONSUMER HEALTHCARE

(See PFIZER CONSUMER HEALTHCARE, PFIZER INC.)

## WELLNESS INTERNATIONAL NETWORK, LTD.     771

5800 Democracy Drive
Plano, TX 75024
**Direct Inquiries to:**
Product Coordinator
(972) 312-1100
FAX: (972) 943-5250

**OTC Products Described:**

**Dietary Supplements Described:**

## WHITEHALL LABORATORIES INC.

(See WHITEHALL-ROBINS HEALTHCARE)

## WHITEHALL-ROBINS HEALTHCARE     773

American Home Products Corporation
Five Giralda Farms
Madison, NJ 07940-0871

**Direct Inquiries to:**
Whitehall Consumer Product Information:
(800) 322-3129 (9-5 E.S.T.)
Robins Consumer Product Information:
(800) 762-4672 (9-5 E.S.T.)

**OTC Products Described:**

**Dietary Supplements Described:**

**Other Products Available:**

Anacin Caplets and Tablets
Aspirin Free Anacin Tablets
Maximum Strength Anacin Tablets
Regular Strength Anbesol Gel
Regular Strength Anbesol Liquid
Axid AR
Chapstick Flava-Craze
Chapstick Lip Balm
Chapstick Lip Moisturizer
Chapstick LipSations
Chapstick Medicated
Chapstick OverNight Lip Treatment
Chapstick Plus
Chapstick Sunblock 15 Lip Balm
Chapstick Ultra SPF 30
Denorex Advanced Formula
Denorex Extra Strength
Denorex Extra Strength with Conditioner
Denorex Mountain Fresh
Denorex Regular with Conditioner
Dimetapp Get Better Bear Sore Throat
  Pop
Dristan Cold Multi-Symptom Tablets
Dristan Cold Non-Drowsiness Formula
Dristan Maximum Strength Cold
  Non-Drowsiness Gel Caplets
Dristan Nasal Spray
Dristan Long-Lasting Nasal Spray
Dristan Sinus Caplets
Flexagen Caplets
Orudis KT Tablets
Riopan Plus Suspension
Riopan Plus Double Strength Suspension
Robitussin Cough & Congestion Liquid
Robitussin Maximum Strength Liquid
Robitussin Night Relief Liquid
Robitussin Pediatric Night Relief Drops
Robitussin Sugar-Free Cough Drops
Semicid Contraceptive Suppositories

## YOUNGEVITY, THE ANTI-AGING COMPANY     836

3227 Skylane Drive
Dallas, TX 75006
**Direct Inquiries to:**
(972) 239-6864, Ext. 108
FAX: (972) 404-3067
E-mail: asd@youngevity.com
www.youngevity.com

**Dietary Supplements Described:**

**ZILA PHARMACEUTICALS, INC.**                     792
5227 North 7th Street
Phoenix, AZ 85014-2800

**Direct Inquiries to:**
Diane Hammond
Associate Marketing Manager
(602) 266-6700
www.zila.com

**OTC Products Described:**

# SECTION 2

# PRODUCT NAME INDEX

This index includes all entries in the Product Information sections. Products are listed alphabetically by brand name.

If an entry in the index lists multiple page numbers, the first one shown refers to the photograph of the product, the last one to its prescribing information.

- **Bold page numbers** indicate full product information.

- *Italic page numbers* signify partial information.

*Italic Page Number* **Indicates Brief Listing**

*Italic Page Number* **Indicates Brief Listing**

# SECTION 3

# PRODUCT CATEGORY INDEX

This index cross-references each brand by pharmaceutical category. All fully-described products in the Product Information sections are included.

If an entry in the index lists multiple page numbers, the first one shown refers to the photograph of the product, the last one to its prescribing information.

The classification of each product is determined by the publisher in cooperation with the product's manufacturer or, when necessary, by the publisher alone.

**GENITAL WART PREPARATIONS**
(*see under:*
**SKIN & MUCOUS MEMBRANE AGENTS**
**WART PREPARATIONS**)

**GLAUCOMA PREPARATIONS**
(*see under:*
**OPHTHALMIC PREPARATIONS**
**SYMPATHOMIMETICS & COMBINATIONS**)

# H

**HAIR GROWTH STIMULANTS**
(*see under:*
**SKIN & MUCOUS MEMBRANE AGENTS**
**HAIR GROWTH STIMULANTS**)

**HEAD LICE RELIEF**
(*see under:*
**SKIN & MUCOUS MEMBRANE AGENTS**
**ANTI-INFECTIVES**
**SCABICIDES & PEDICULICIDES**)

**HEMATINICS**
(*see under:*
**DIETARY SUPPLEMENTS**
**BLOOD MODIFIERS**
**IRON & COMBINATIONS**)

**HEMORRHOIDAL PREPARATIONS**
(*see under:*
**SKIN & MUCOUS MEMBRANE AGENTS**
**ANORECTAL PREPARATIONS**)

## DECONGESTANTS, EXPECTORANTS & COMBINATIONS

## EXPECTORANTS & COMBINATIONS

## MISCELLANEOUS COLD & COUGH PRODUCTS

Preparation H Medicated Wipes
(Whitehall-Robins) ................... **782**
Tucks Pre-moistened Pads
(Pfizer Consumer
Healthcare) .................... **521, 736**

**MISCELLANEOUS VAGINAL PREPARATIONS**
Vitara Cream (Products on
Demand) ...................... **522, 755**

**VITAMINS**
(*see under:*
**DIETARY SUPPLEMENTS**
    **VITAMINS & COMBINATIONS)**

# W

**WART PREPARATIONS**
(*see under:*
**SKIN & MUCOUS MEMBRANE AGENTS**
    **WART PREPARATIONS)**

**WET DRESSINGS**
(*see under:*
**SKIN & MUCOUS MEMBRANE AGENTS**
    **WET DRESSINGS)**

**WOUND CARE**
(*see under:*
**SKIN & MUCOUS MEMBRANE AGENTS**
    **WOUND CARE PRODUCTS)**

# SECTION 4

# ACTIVE INGREDIENTS INDEX

This index cross-references each brand by its generic ingredients. All entries in the Product Information sections are included. Under each generic heading, all fully described products are listed first, followed by those with only partial descriptions.

If an entry in the index lists multiple page numbers, the first one shown refers to the photograph of the product, the last one to its prescribing information.

- **Bold page numbers** indicate full product information.

- *Italic page numbers* signify partial information.

Classification of products under these headings has been determined in cooperation with the products' manufacturers or, if necessary, by the publisher alone.

**LANOLIN**
A + D Original Ointment
(Schering-Plough) ............**523, 757**
Lubriderm Skin Therapy
Moisturizing Lotion (Pfizer
Consumer Healthcare)........**519, 726**

**LECITHIN**
Ambrotose with Lecithin Capsules
(Mannatech)..........................**816**
StePHan Bio-Nutritional Nightime
Moisture Creme (Wellness
International).........................**772**

**LEVMETAMFETAMINE**
Vicks Vapor Inhaler (Procter &
Gamble) ............................**754**

**LEVOCARNITINE FUMARATE**
Proceed Powder (Sigma-Tau)......**524, 823**

**LEVULOSE**
Emetrol Oral Solution (Lemon-Mint &
Cherry Flavors) (Pharmacia
Consumer) ..........................**741**

**LIDOCAINE**
Zilactin-L Liquid (Zila) ...................**792**

**LIDOCAINE HYDROCHLORIDE**
Bactine First Aid Liquid (Bayer
Consumer) ....................**503, 616**

**LIPOIC ACID**
Anti-Aging Daily Premium Pak
(Youngevity) ........................**837**

**LOPERAMIDE HYDROCHLORIDE**
Imodium A-D Liquid and
Caplets (McNeil Consumer) ..**510, 666**
Imodium Advanced Caplets
and Chewable Tablets
(McNeil Consumer) ...........**510, 666**

**M**

**MAGNESIUM CARBONATE**
Gaviscon Regular Strength
Liquid (GlaxoSmithKline)......**507, 641**
Gaviscon Extra Strength Liquid
(GlaxoSmithKline) .............**507, 641**
Gaviscon Extra Strength
Tablets (GlaxoSmithKline) ....**507, 641**

**MAGNESIUM CHLORIDE**
Chlor-3 Shaker (Fleming)................**632**

**MAGNESIUM GLUCONATE**
Magonate Liquid (Fleming)..............**807**
Magonate Natal Liquid (Fleming).......**807**
Magonate Tablets (Fleming) ............**807**

**MAGNESIUM HYDROXIDE**
Ex•Lax Milk of Magnesia
Liquid (Novartis Consumer) ..**514, 693**
Maalox Antacid/Anti-Gas Liquid
(Novartis Consumer)..........**515, 695**
Maalox Max Maximum
Strength Antacid/Anti-Gas
Liquid (Novartis Consumer) ..**515, 695**
Pepcid Complete Chewable
Tablets (J&J • Merck)........**509, 664**
Phillips' Chewable Tablets (Bayer
Consumer) ..........................**619**

Phillips' Milk of Magnesia
Liquid (Original, Cherry, &
Mint) (Bayer Consumer).......**505, 620**
Phillips' M-O Original Formula
Laxative (Bayer Consumer) ...**505, 620**
Phillips' M-O Refreshing Mint
Formula (Bayer Consumer) .........**620**
Rolaids Tablets (Pfizer
Consumer Healthcare)........**520, 728**
Extra Strength Rolaids Tablets
(Pfizer Consumer
Healthcare)....................**520, 728**

**MAGNESIUM OXIDE**
Beelith Tablets (Beach) ................**804**

**MAGNESIUM SALICYLATE**
Momentum Backache Relief Extra
Strength Caplets (Medtech) ........**690**

**MAGNESIUM TRISILICATE**
Gaviscon Regular Strength
Tablets (GlaxoSmithKline) ....**507, 641**

**MALT SOUP EXTRACT**
Maltsupex Powder, Liquid,
Tablets (Wallace)..............**524, 770**

**MECLIZINE HYDROCHLORIDE**
Bonine Chewable Tablets
(Pfizer Consumer
Healthcare)....................**518, 720**
Dramamine Less Drowsy Tablets
(Pharmacia Consumer) .............**740**

**MELATONIN**
VitaMist Intra-Oral Spray (Mayor).......**818**
Melatonin (Mayor).....................*818*

**MENTHOL**
BenGay External Analgesic
Products (Pfizer Consumer
Healthcare)....................**518, 719**
Celestial Seasonings Soothers
Throat Drops (Pfizer
Consumer Group) .............**516, 707**
Dermoplast Hospital Strength Spray
(Medtech) ..........................**689**
Halls Mentho-Lyptus Drops
(Pfizer Consumer Group)......**516, 707**
Halls Sugar Free
Mentho-Lyptus Drops
(Pfizer Consumer Group)......**516, 708**
Halls Sugar Free Squares
(Pfizer Consumer Group)......**516, 708**
Halls Plus Cough Drops (Pfizer
Consumer Group) .............**516, 708**
Listerine Mouthrinse (Pfizer
Consumer Healthcare)........**519, 724**
Cool Mint Listerine Mouthrinse
(Pfizer Consumer
Healthcare)....................**519, 724**
FreshBurst Listerine
Mouthrinse (Pfizer
Consumer Healthcare)........**519, 724**
Tartar Control Listerine
Mouthwash (Pfizer
Consumer Healthcare)........**519, 724**
Robitussin Cough Drops
(Whitehall-Robins).................**784**
Robitussin Honey Calmers Throat
Drops (Whitehall-Robins) ..........**788**
Robitussin Honey Cough Drops
(Whitehall-Robins).................**789**
Robitussin Sugar Free Throat Drops
(Whitehall-Robins).................**791**

Thera-Gesic Creme (Mission)...........**691**
Triaminic Vapor Patch-Cherry
Scent (Novartis Consumer)...**516, 707**
Triaminic Vapor Patch-Menthol
Scent (Novartis Consumer)...**516, 707**
Vicks Cough Drops, Menthol and
Cherry Flavors (Procter &
Gamble) .............................**750**
Vicks VapoRub Cream (Procter &
Gamble) .............................**754**
Vicks VapoRub Ointment (Procter &
Gamble) .............................**754**

**METHYL SALICYLATE**
BenGay External Analgesic
Products (Pfizer Consumer
Healthcare)....................**518, 719**
Listerine Mouthrinse (Pfizer
Consumer Healthcare)........**519, 724**
Cool Mint Listerine Mouthrinse
(Pfizer Consumer
Healthcare)....................**519, 724**
FreshBurst Listerine
Mouthrinse (Pfizer
Consumer Healthcare)........**519, 724**
Tartar Control Listerine
Mouthwash (Pfizer
Consumer Healthcare)........**519, 724**
Thera-Gesic Creme (Mission)...........**691**

**METHYLCELLULOSE**
Citrucel Caplets (GlaxoSmithKline).....**635**
Citrucel Orange Flavor Powder
(GlaxoSmithKline) .............**506, 635**
Citrucel Sugar Free Orange
Flavor Powder
(GlaxoSmithKline) .............**506, 635**

**MICONAZOLE NITRATE**
Desenex Liquid Spray (Novartis
Consumer) ..........................**691**
Desenex Shake Powder
(Novartis Consumer)..........**514, 691**
Desenex Spray Powder
(Novartis Consumer)..........**514, 691**
Desenex Jock Itch Spray Powder
(Novartis Consumer)...............**691**
Lotrimin AF Spray Powder,
Spray Liquid, Spray
Deodorant Powder, Shaker
Powder and Jock Itch Spray
Powder (Schering-Plough).....**524, 766**

**MILK OF MAGNESIA**
(*see under:* **MAGNESIUM HYDROXIDE**)

**MINERAL OIL**
Anusol Ointment (Pfizer
Consumer Healthcare)........**517, 710**
Lubriderm Skin Therapy
Moisturizing Lotion (Pfizer
Consumer Healthcare)........**519, 726**
Phillips' M-O Original Formula
Laxative (Bayer Consumer) ...**505, 620**
Phillips' M-O Refreshing Mint
Formula (Bayer Consumer) .........**620**
Preparation H Ointment
(Whitehall-Robins)..................**781**

**MINERALS, MULTIPLE**
Caltrate 600 PLUS Chewables
(Lederle Consumer) ................**813**
Caltrate 600 PLUS Tablets (Lederle
Consumer) ..........................**813**
Plant Derived Minerals Liquid
(American Longevity)...............**797**
Right Choice P.M. Multi Formula
Caplets (Body Wise) ...............**806**

# COMPANION DRUG INDEX

This index provides you with a quick-reference guide to over-the-counter products that may be used, in conjunction with prescription drug therapy, to reverse drug-induced side effects, relieve symptoms of the illness itself, or treat sequelae of the initial disease. All entries are derived from the FDA-approved prescribing information published by *PDR*.

The products listed are generally considered effective for temporary symptomatic relief. Please bear in mind, however, that they may not be appropriate for sustained therapy, and that certain common side effects may be harbingers of more serious reactions. Remember, too, that each case must be approached on an individual basis. When making a recommendation, be sure to adjust for the patient's age, concurrent

medical conditions, and complete drug regimen. Consider timing as well, since simultaneous ingestion may not be recommended in all instances.

Please note that only products fully described in *Physicians' Desk Reference* and its companion volumes are included in this index. The publisher therefore cannot guarantee that all entries are totally accurate or complete. Keep in mind, too, that although a given over-the-counter product is usually an appropriate companion for an entire class of prescription medications, certain drugs within the class may be exceptions. If you have any doubt about the suitability of a particular OTC product in a given situation, be sure to check the underlying *PDR* prescribing information and the relevant medical literature.

## ALCOHOLISM, VITAMINS AND MINERALS DEFICIENCY SECONDARY TO

Alcoholism may be treated with disulfiram or naltrexone hydrochloride. The following products may be recommended for relief of vitamins and minerals deficiency:

## ANCYLOSTOMIASIS, IRON-DEFICIENCY ANEMIA SECONDARY TO

Ancylostomiasis may be treated with mebendazole or thiabendazole. The following products may be recommended for relief of iron-deficiency anemia:

## ANEMIA, IRON-DEFICIENCY

May result from the use of chronic salicylate therapy or nonsteroidal anti-inflammatory drugs The following products may be recommended:

## ANGINA, UNSTABLE

May be treated with beta blockers, calcium channel blockers or nitrates. The following products may be recommended for relief of symptoms:

## ARTHRITIS

May be treated with corticosteroids or nonsteroidal anti-inflammatory drugs. The following products may be recommended for relief of symptoms:

## BRONCHITIS, CHRONIC, ACUTE EXACERBATION OF

May be treated with quinolones, sulfamethoxazole-trimethoprim, cefixime, cefpodoxime proxetil, cefprozil, ceftibuten dihydrate, cefuroxime axetil, cilastatin, clarithromycin, imipenem or loracarbef. The following products may be recommended for relief of symptoms:

## BURN INFECTIONS, SEVERE, NUTRIENTS DEFICIENCY SECONDARY TO

Severe burn infections may be treated with anti-infectives. The following products may be recommended for relief of nutrients deficiency:

## CANCER, NUTRIENTS DEFICIENCY SECONDARY TO

Cancer may be treated with chemotherapeutic agents. The following products may be recommended for relief of nutrients deficiency:

## CANDIDIASIS, VAGINAL

May be treated with antifungal agents. The following products may be recommended for relief of symptoms:

## CONGESTIVE HEART FAILURE, NUTRIENTS DEFICIENCY SECONDARY TO

Congestive heart failure may be treated with ace inhibitors, cardiac glycosides or diuretics. The following products may be recommended for relief of nutrients deficiency:

## CONSTIPATION

May result from the use of ace inhibitors, hmg-coa reductase inhibitors, anticholinergics, anticonvulsants, antidepressants, beta blockers, bile acid sequestrants, butyrophenones, calcium and aluminum-containing antacids, calcium channel blockers, ganglionic blockers, hematinics, monoamine oxidase inhibitors, narcotic analgesics, nonsteroidal anti-inflammatory drugs or phenothiazines. The following products may be recommended:

## CYSTIC FIBROSIS, NUTRIENTS DEFICIENCY SECONDARY TO

Cystic fibrosis may be treated with dornase alfa The following products may be recommended for relief of nutrients deficiency:

## DENTAL CARIES

May be treated with fluoride preparations or vitamin and fluoride supplements. The following products may be recommended for relief of symptoms:

## DIABETES MELLITUS, CONSTIPATION SECONDARY TO

Diabetes mellitus may be treated with insulins or oral hypoglycemic agents. The following products may be recommended for relief of constipation:

## DIABETES MELLITUS, POORLY CONTROLLED, CANDIDAL VULVOVAGINITIS SECONDARY TO

Diabetes mellitus may be treated with insulins or oral hypoglycemic agents. The following products may be recommended for relief of candidal vulvovaginitis:

## DIABETES MELLITUS, POORLY CONTROLLED, GINGIVITIS SECONDARY TO

Diabetes mellitus may be treated with insulins or oral hypoglycemic agents. The following products may be recommended for relief of gingivitis:

## DIABETES MELLITUS, POORLY CONTROLLED, VITAMINS AND MINERALS DEFICIENCY SECONDARY TO

Diabetes mellitus may be treated with insulins or oral hypoglycemic agents. The following products may be recommended for relief of vitamins and minerals deficiency:

## DIABETES MELLITUS, PRURITUS SECONDARY TO

Diabetes mellitus may be treated with insulins or oral hypoglycemic agents. The following products may be recommended for relief of pruritus:

## DIAPER DERMATITIS

May result from the use of cefpodoxime proxetil, cefprozil, cefuroxime axetil or varicella virus vaccine, live. The following products may be recommended:

## DIARRHEA

May result from the use of ace inhibitors, beta blockers, cardiac glycosides, chemotherapeutic agents, diuretics, magnesium-containing antacids, nonsteroidal anti-inflammatory drugs, potassium supplements, acarbose, alprazolam, colchicine, divalproex sodium, ethosuximide, fluoxetine hydrochloride, guanethidine monosulfate, hydralazine hydrochloride, levodopa, lithium carbonate, lithium citrate, mesna, metformin hydrochloride, misoprostol, olsalazine sodium, pancrelipase, procainamide hydrochloride, reserpine, succimer, ticlopidine hydrochloride or valproic acid. The following products may be recommended:

## DIARRHEA, INFECTIOUS

May be treated with sulfamethoxazole-trimethoprim, ciprofloxacin or furazolidone. The following products may be recommended for relief of symptoms:

## DYSPEPSIA

May result from the use of chronic systemic corticosteroid therapy, nonsteroidal anti-inflammatory drugs, ulcerogenic medications or mexiletine hydrochloride. The following products may be recommended:

## EMESIS, UNPLEASANT TASTE SECONDARY TO

Emesis may be treated with antiemetics. The following products may be recommended for relief of unpleasant taste:

## ENTEROBIASIS, PERIANAL PRURITUS SECONDARY TO

Enterobiasis may be treated with mebendazole. The following products may be recommended for relief of perianal pruritus:

## FEVER

May result from the use of immunization. The following products may be recommended:

## FLATULENCE

May result from the use of nonsteroidal anti-inflammatory drugs, potassium supplements, acarbose, cisapride, guanadrel sulfate, mesalamine, metformin hydrochloride, methyldopa, octreotide acetate or ursodiol. The following products may be recommended:

## FLU-LIKE SYNDROME

May result from the use of gemcitabine hydrochloride, interferon alfa-2b, recombinant, interferon alfa-n3 (human leukocyte derived), interferon beta-1b, interferon gamma-1b or succimer. The following products may be recommended:

**FLUSHING EPISODES**

May result from the use of lipid lowering doses of niacin. The following products may be recommended:

**GASTRITIS, IRON-DEFICIENCY SECONDARY TO**

Gastritis may be treated with histamine h2 receptor antagonists, proton pump inhibitors or sucralfate. The following products may be recommended for relief of iron deficiency:

**GASTROESOPHAGEAL REFLUX DISEASE**

May be treated with histamine h2 receptor antagonists, proton pump inhibitors or sucralfate. The following products may be recommended for relief of symptoms:

**GINGIVAL HYPERPLASIA**

May result from the use of calcium channel blockers, cyclosporine, fosphenytoin sodium or phenytoin. The following products may be recommended:

**HUMAN IMMUNODEFICIENCY VIRUS (HIV) INFECTIONS, NUTRIENTS DEFICIENCY SECONDARY TO**

HIV infections may be treated with non-nucleoside reverse transcriptase inhibitors, nucleoside reverse transcriptase inhibitors or protease inhibitors. The following products may be recommended for relief of nutrients deficiency:

**HUMAN IMMUNODEFICIENCY VIRUS (HIV) INFECTIONS, SEBORRHEIC DERMATITIS SECONDARY TO**

HIV infections may be treated with non-nucleoside reverse transcriptase inhibitors, nucleoside reverse transcriptase inhibitors or protease inhibitors. The following products may be recommended for relief of seborrheic dermatitis:

**HUMAN IMMUNODEFICIENCY VIRUS (HIV) INFECTIONS, XERODERMA SECONDARY TO**

HIV infections may be treated with non-nucleoside reverse transcriptase inhibitors, nucleoside reverse transcriptase inhibitors or protease inhibitors. The following products may be recommended for relief of xeroderma:

**HYPERTHYROIDISM, NUTRIENTS DEFICIENCY SECONDARY TO**

Hyperthyroidism may be treated with methimazole. The following products may be recommended for relief of nutrients deficiency:

**HYPOKALEMIA**

May result from the use of thiazides, thiazides, corticosteroids, diuretics, diuretics, aldesleukin, amphotericin b, carboplatin, etretinate, foscarnet sodium, mycophenolate mofetil, pamidronate disodium or tacrolimus. The following products may be recommended:

**HYPOMAGNESEMIA**

May result from the use of aldesleukin, aminoglycosides, amphotericin b, caroboplatin, cisplatin, cyclosporine, diuretics, foscarnet, pamidronate, sargramostim or tacrolimus. The following products may be recommended:

**HYPOPARATHYROIDISM**

May be treated with vitamin d sterols. The following products may be recommended for relief of symptoms:

**HYPOTHYROIDISM, CONSTIPATION SECONDARY TO**

Hypothyroidism may be treated with thyroid hormones. The following products may be recommended for relief of constipation:

**HYPOTHYROIDISM, XERODERMA SECONDARY TO**

Hypothyroidism may be treated with thyroid hormones. The following products may be recommended for relief of xeroderma:

**INFECTIONS, BACTERIAL, UPPER RESPIRATORY TRACT**

May be treated with amoxicillin-clavulanate, cephalosporins, doxycycline, erythromycin, macrolide antibiotics, penicillins or minocycline hydrochloride. The following products may be recommended for relief of symptoms:

## INFECTIONS, BACTERIAL, UPPER RESPIRATORY TRACT —cont.

## INFECTIONS, SKIN AND SKIN STRUCTURE

May be treated with aminoglycosides, amoxicillin, amoxicillin-clavulanate, cephalosporins, doxycycline, erythromycin, macrolide antibiotics, penicillins or quinolones. The following products may be recommended for relief of symptoms:

## IRRITABLE BOWEL SYNDROME

May be treated with anticholinergic combinations, dicyclomine hydrochloride or hyoscyamine sulfate. The following products may be recommended for relief of symptoms:

## ISCHEMIC HEART DISEASE

May be treated with beta blockers, calcium channel blockers, isosorbide dinitrate, isosorbide mononitrate or nitroglycerin. The following products may be recommended for relief of symptoms:

## KERATOCONJUNCTIVITIS, VERNAL

May be treated with ophthalmic mast cell stabilizers. The following products may be recommended for relief of symptoms:

## MYOCARDIAL INFARCTION, ACUTE

May be treated with ace inhibitors, anticoagulants, beta blockers, thrombolytic agents or nitroglycerin. The following products may be recommended for relief of symptoms:

## NASAL POLYPS, RHINORRHEA SECONDARY TO

Nasal polyps may be treated with nasal steroidal anti-inflammatory agents. The following products may be recommended for relief of rhinorrhea:

## NECATORIASIS, IRON-DEFICIENCY ANEMIA SECONDARY TO

Necatoriasis may be treated with mebendazole or thiabendazole The following products may be recommended for relief of iron-deficiency anemia:

## OSTEOPOROSIS

May be treated with biphosphonates, calcitonin or estrogens. The following products may be recommended for relief of symptoms:

## OSTEOPOROSIS, SECONDARY

May result from the use of chemotherapeutic agents, phenytoin, prolonged glucocorticoid therapy, thyroid hormones, carbamazepine or methotrexate sodium. The following products may be recommended:

## OTITIS MEDIA, ACUTE

May be treated with amoxicillin, amoxicillin-clavulanate, cephalosporins, erythromycin-sulfisoxazole, macrolide antibiotics or sulfamethoxazole-trimethoprim. The following products may be recommended for relief of symptoms:

**PANCREATIC INSUFFICIENCY, NUTRIENTS
DEFICIENCY SECONDARY TO**

Pancreatic insufficiency may be treated with
pancrelipase. The following products may be
recommended for relief of nutrients deficiency:

**PARKINSON'S DISEASE, CONSTIPATION
SECONDARY TO**

Parkinson's disease may be treated with cen-
trally active anticholinergic agents, dopaminer-
gic agents or selective inhibitor of mao type b.
The following products may be recommended
for relief of constipation:

**PARKINSON'S DISEASE, SEBORRHEIC
DERMATITIS SECONDARY TO**

Parkinson's disease may be treated with cen-
trally active anticholinergic agents, dopaminer-
gic agents or selective inhibitor of mao type b.
The following products may be recommended
for relief of seborrheic dermatitis:

**PEPTIC ULCER DISEASE**

May be treated with histamine h2 receptor
antagonists, proton pump inhibitors or sucralfate. The following products may be recommended for relief of symptoms:

**PEPTIC ULCER DISEASE, IRON DEFICIENCY SECONDARY TO**

Peptic ulcer disease may be treated with histamine h2 receptor antagonists, proton pump inhibitors or sucralfate. The following products may be recommended for relief of iron deficiency:

**PHARYNGITIS**

May be treated with cephalosporins, macrolide antibiotics or penicillins. The following products may be recommended for relief of symptoms:

**PHOTOSENSITIVITY REACTIONS**

May result from the use of thiazides, antidepressants, antihistamines, estrogens, nonsteroidal anti-inflammatory drugs, phenothiazines, quinolones, sulfonamides, sulfonylurea
hypoglycemic agents, tetracyclines, topical
retinoids, captopril, diltiazem hydrochloride,
enalapril maleate, fluorouracil, griseofulvin,
labetalol hydrochloride, lisinopril, methoxsalen,
methyldopa, minoxidil, nalidixic acid or nifedip-
ine. The following products may be recommended:

**PRURITUS, PERIANAL**

May result from the use of broad-spectrum
antibiotics. The following products may be recommended:

**PSORALEN WITH UV-A LIGHT (PUVA)
THERAPY**

May be treated with methoxsalen. The following
products may be recommended for relief of
symptoms:

**RENAL OSTEODYSTROPHY, HYPOCALCEMIA
SECONDARY TO**

Renal osteodystrophy may be treated with vitamin d sterols. The following products may be
recommended for relief of hypocalcemia:

**RESPIRATORY TRACT ILLNESS, INFLUENZA A
VIRUS-INDUCED**

May be treated with amantadine hydrochloride
or rimantadine hydrochloride. The following
products may be recommended for relief of
symptoms:

**RHINITIS, NONALLERGIC**

May be treated with nasal steroids or ipratropium bromide. The following products may be recommended for relief of symptoms:

**RHINITIS, NONALLERGIC VASOMOTOR**

May be treated with nasal steroids or ipratropium bromide. The following products may be recommended for relief of symptoms:

**SERUM-SICKNESSLIKE REACTIONS**

May result from the use of amoxicillin, amoxicillin-clavulanate, penicillins, sulfamethoxazole-trimethoprim, antivenin (crotalidae) polyvalent, antivenin (micrurus fulvius), metronidazole, ofloxacin, streptomycin sulfate, sulfadoxine, sulfamethoxazole or sulfasalazine. The following products may be recommended:

## SINUSITIS

May be treated with amoxicillin, amoxicillin-clavulanate, cefprozil, cefuroxime axetil, clarithromycin or loracarbef. The following products may be recommended for relief of symptoms:

## SINUSITIS —cont.

## SINUSITIS, HALITOSIS SECONDARY TO

Sinusitis may be treated with amoxicillin, amoxicillin-clavulanate, cefprozil, cefuroxime axetil, clarithromycin or loracarbef. The following products may be recommended for relief of halitosis:

## SKIN IRRITATION

May result from the use of transdermal drug delivery systems. The following products may be recommended:

## STOMATITIS, APHTHOUS

May result from the use of selective serotonin reuptake inhibitors, aldesleukin, clomipramine hydrochloride, didanosine, foscarnet sodium, indinavir sulfate, indomethacin, interferon alfa-2b, recombinant, methotrexate sodium, naproxen, naproxen sodium, nicotine polacrilex or stavudine. The following products may be recommended:

## TASTE DISTURBANCES

May result from the use of biguanides, acetazolamide, butorphanol tartrate, captopril, cefuroxime axetil, clarithromycin, etidronate disodium, felbamate, flunisolide, gemfibrozil, griseofulvin, interferon alfa-2b, recombinant, lithium carbonate, lithium citrate, mesna, metronidazole, nedocromil sodium, penicillamine, rifampin or succimer. The following products may be recommended:

## TONSILITIS, HALITOSIS SECONDARY TO

Tonsilitis may be treated with erythromycin, macrolide antibiotics, cefaclor, cefadroxil, cefixime, cefpodoxime proxetil, cefprozil, ceftibuten dihydrate or cefuroxime axetil. The following products may be recommended for relief of halitosis:

## TUBERCULOSIS, NUTRIENTS DEFICIENCY SECONDARY TO

Tuberculosis may be treated with capreomycin sulfate, ethambutol hydrochloride, ethionamide, isoniazid, pyrazinamide, rifampin or streptomycin sulfate. The following products may be recommended for relief of nutrients deficiency:

## VAGINOSIS, BACTERIAL

May be treated with sulfabenzamide/sulfacetamide/sulfathiozole or metronidazole. The following products may be recommended for relief of symptoms:

## VULVOVAGINITIS, CANDIDAL

May result from the use of estrogen-containing oral contraceptives, immunosuppressants or recent broad-spectrum antibiotic therapy. The following products may be recommended:

## XERODERMA

May result from the use of aldesleukin, protease inhibitors, retinoids, topical acne preparations, topical corticosteroids, topical retinoids, benzoyl peroxide, clofazimine, interferon alfa-2a, recombinant, interferon alfa-2b, recombinant or pentostatin.The following products may be recommended:

## XEROMYCTERIA

May result from the use of anticholinergics, antihistamines, retinoids, apraclonidine hydrochloride, clonidine, etretinate, ipratropium bromide, isotretinoin or lodoxamide tromethamine. The following products may be recommended:

## XEROSTOMIA

May result from the use of anticholinergics, antidepressants, diuretics, phenothiazines, alprazolam, bromocriptine mesylate, buspirone hydrochloride, butorphanol tartrate, clomipramine hydrochloride, clonidine, clozapine, dexfenfluramine hydrochloride, didanosine, disopyramide phosphate, etretinate, flumazenil, fluvoxamine maleate, guanfacine hydrochloride, isotretinoin, leuprolide acetate, pergolide mesylate, selegiline hydrochloride, tramadol hydrochloride or zolpidem tartrate. The following products may be recommended:

# PRODUCT IDENTIFICATION GUIDE

To aid in quick identification, this section provides full-color, actual-size photographs of tablets and capsules. A variety of other dosage forms and packages are shown at less than actual size. In all, the section contains some 700 photos.

Products in this section are arranged alphabetically by manufacturer. In some instances, not all dosage forms and sizes are pictured. For more information on any of the products in this section, please turn to the page indicated above the product's photo or check directly with the product's manufacturer.

While every effort has been made to guarantee faithful reproduction of the photos in this section, changes in size, color, and design are always a possibility. Be sure to confirm a product's identity with the manufacturer or your pharmacist.

# MANUFACTURER'S INDEX

## A & Z PHARMACEUTICAL INC.

A & Z Pharmaceutical Inc.
P. 796

Calcium Supplement with Fruit Flavor
Packages of 30 and 60 caplets

### D-Cal™

## AKPHARMA INC.

AkPharma Inc.
P. 796

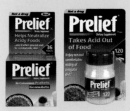

Dietary Supplement
Granulate and Tablets

### Prelief®

## AWARENESS CORPORATION

Awareness Corporation
P. 798

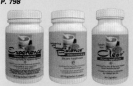

| Experience Weight Management & Natural Digestive Cleanse | Female Balance Natural Menopause & PMS Formula | Clear Helps with Candida, Fungus, Mold |

### Awareness Natural Dietary Supplements

## BAYER CORPORATION

Bayer Corporation
Consumer Care Division
P. 602

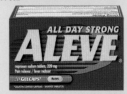

Tablets and Caplets available in
24, 50, 100 and 150 count.

Caplets also available in 200 count.

Gelcaps available in 20, 40
and 80 count.

### Aleve®

---

Bayer Corporation
Consumer Care Division
P. 603

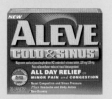

### Aleve® Cold & Sinus

Bayer Corporation
Consumer Care Division
P. 604

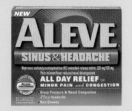

### Aleve® Sinus & Headache

Bayer Corporation
Consumer Care Division
P. 604

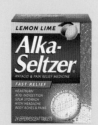

Lemon Lime Effervescent Antacid
and Pain Reliever

### Alka-Seltzer®

Bayer Corporation
Consumer Care Division
P. 605

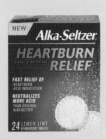

### Alka-Seltzer® Heartburn Relief

---

Bayer Corporation
Consumer Care Division
P. 605

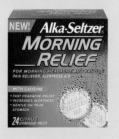

### Alka-Seltzer® Morning Relief™

Bayer Corporation
Consumer Care Division
P. 606

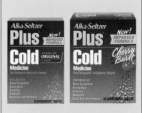

### Alka-Seltzer Plus® Cold Medicine

Bayer Corporation
Consumer Care Division
P. 608

Cold, Cold & Cough, Flu,
Cold & Sinus and Night-Time.

### Alka-Seltzer Plus® Cold Medicine Liqui-Gels®

---

Bayer Corporation
Consumer Care Division
P. 609

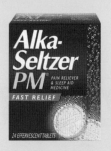

### Alka-Seltzer PM®

Bayer Corporation
Consumer Care Division
P. 616

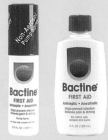

Antiseptic/Anesthetic
First Aid Spray and Liquid

### Bactine®

Bayer Corporation
Consumer Care Division
P. 611

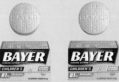

Low Strength, Chewable Aspirin
Orange and Cherry Flavors

### Aspirin Regimen BAYER® Children's

Bayer Corporation
Consumer Care Division
P. 615

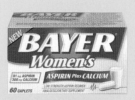

### BAYER® Women's Aspirin Plus Calcium

Bayer Corporation
Consumer Care Division
P. 610

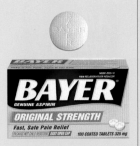

Ferrous Gluconate
Iron Supplement

**BAYER® Aspirin**

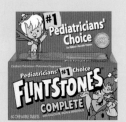

Genuine Bayer Tablets and Gelcaps,
Aspirin Regimen 81 mg,
Aspirin Regimen 325 mg

**BAYER® Aspirin**

---

Bayer Corporation
Consumer Care Division
P. 798

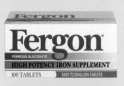

Ferrous Gluconate
Iron Supplement

**Fergon®**

Bayer Corporation
Consumer Care Division
P. 799

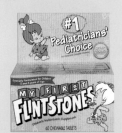

**Flintstones® Complete**

Bayer Corporation
Consumer Care Division
P. 799

Chewable Tablets

**My First Flintstones®**

Bayer Corporation
Consumer Care Division
P. 617

Maximum Strength
Caplets and Gelcaps

**Midol® Menstrual**

---

Bayer Corporation
Consumer Care Division
P. 618

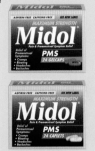

Maximum Strength
Gelcaps and Caplets

**Midol® PMS**

Bayer Corporation
Consumer Care Division
P. 617

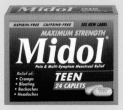

Maximum Strength Caplets

**Midol® Teen**

Bayer Corporation
Consumer Care Division
P. 618

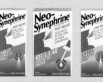

Nasal Decongestant
Spray and Drops
Available in Mild, Regular, Extra
Strength and Max 12-Hour Formula

**Neo-Synephrine®**

Bayer Corporation
Consumer Care Division
P. 619

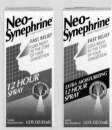

Nasal Spray in 12 hour and
12 hour Extra Moisturizing

**Neo Synephrine® 12 Hour**

---

Bayer Corporation
Consumer Care Division
P. 799

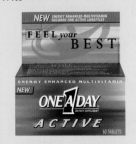

Energy Enhanced Multivitamin

**One-A-Day® Active**

Bayer Corporation
Consumer Care Division
P. 803

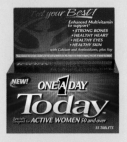

For Active Women 50 and over

**One-A-Day® Today™**

Bayer Corporation
Consumer Care Division
P. 800

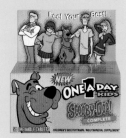

Kids Complete

**One-A-Day® Kids**

Bayer Corporation
Consumer Care Division
P. 800

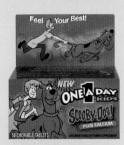

Kids Plus Calcium

**One-A-Day® Kids**

---

FACED WITH AN
Rx SIDE EFFECT?

Turn to the
Companion Drug Index
for products that provide
symptomatic relief.

Bayer Corporation
Consumer Care Division
*P. 620*

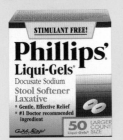

Stool Softener Laxative

## Phillips'® Liqui-Gels

Bayer Corporation
Consumer Care Division
*P. 620*

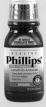

Original Flavor
Also available in
Mint and Cherry Flavors

## Phillips'®
## Milk of Magnesia

Bayer Corporation
Consumer Care Division
*P. 620*

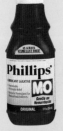

Lubricant Laxative in Original Formula.
Also available in Refreshing Mint Flavor.

## Phillips'® M-O

Bayer Corporation
Consumer Care Division
*P. 621*

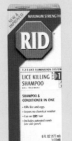

## Rid® Lice Killing
## Shampoo

---

Bayer Corporation
Consumer Care Division
*P. 621*

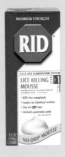

## Rid® Mousse

Bayer Corporation
Consumer Care Division
*P. 622*

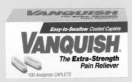

Extra-Strength Pain Formula

## Vanquish®

SEEKING AN
ALTERNATIVE?

Check the
Product Category Index,
where you'll find
alphabetical listings of
all the products in each
therapeutic class.

SEEKING AN
ALTERNATIVE?

Check the
Product Category Index,
where you'll find
alphabetical listings of
all the products in each
therapeutic class.

## BOEHRINGER INGELHEIM

Boehringer Ingelheim Consumer H.C.
*P. 623*

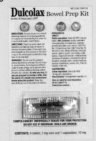

## Dulcolax® Bowel Prep Kit
brand of bisacodyl USP

---

Boehringer Ingelheim Consumer H.C.
*P. 624*

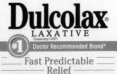

4 Comfort Shaped Suppositories

## Dulcolax® Laxative

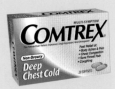

16 Comfort Shaped Suppositories

## Dulcolax® Laxative

Boehringer Ingelheim Consumer H.C.
*P. 624*

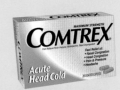

100 Comfort Coated Tablets

## Dulcolax® Laxative

LOOKING FOR
A PARTICULAR
COMPOUND?

In the
Active Ingredients Index
(Yellow Pages),
you'll find all the
brands that contain it.

LOOKING FOR
A PARTICULAR
COMPOUND?

In the
Active Ingredients Index
(Yellow Pages),
you'll find all the
brands that contain it.

---

## BRISTOL-MYERS PRODUCTS

Bristol-Myers Products
*P. 626*

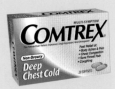

Comtrex® Deep
Chest Cold

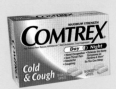

Comtrex®
Acute Head Cold

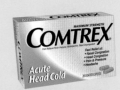

Comtrex® Cold & Cough
Day & Night
Also available in Non-Drowsy
and Nighttime formulas.

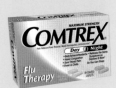

Comtrex® Flu
Therapy

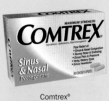

Comtrex®
Sinus & Nasal
Decongestant

## Comtrex®

Bristol-Myers Products
P. 629

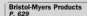
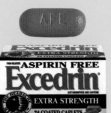
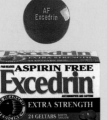

Bottles of 24, 50
and 100 caplets and geltabs

**Aspirin Free Excedrin®**

---

Bristol-Myers Products
P. 629

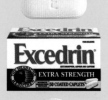

Bottles of 12, 24, 50, 100, 175
and 275, metal tins of 12 tablets
Bottles of 24, 50, 100, 175, 275
caplets and 24, 50 and 100 geltabs
(2 bottles of 50 each)

**Extra Strength Excedrin®**

---

Bristol-Myers Products
P. 630

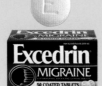

Bottles of 24, 50, 100, 175
and 275 tablets.
Bottles of 24, 50, 100 and 175 caplets.
Bottles of 24, 50 and 100 geltabs
(2 bottles of 50 each)

**Excedrin® Migraine**

---

Bristol-Myers Products
P. 630

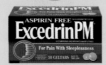

Tablets in bottles of 10
Tablets and Caplets in bottles of
24, 50 and 100
Geltabs in bottles of 24, 50 and 100

**Excedrin PM®**

---

Covex
P. 806

Powerful Memory Enhancer

**Intelectol™**

---

Effcon Laboratories
P. 632

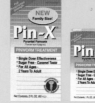

Oral Suspension available
in 60 mL and 30 mL.
For the treatment of
pinworm infections.

**Pin-X®**
(pyrantel pamoate)

---

GlaxoSmithKline Consumer Healthcare
P. 633

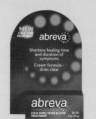

Cold Sore/Fever
Blister Treatment Cream

**Abreva™**

---

GlaxoSmithKline Consumer Healthcare
P. 633

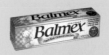

Available in 2 oz. and 4 oz. tubes
and 16 oz. jar

**Balmex®
Diaper Rash Ointment**

---

GlaxoSmithKline Consumer Healthcare
P. 633

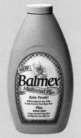

Available in 13 oz. bottle.

**Balmex® Medicated Plus
Baby Powder**

---

GlaxoSmithKline Consumer Healthcare
P. 635

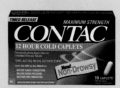

Fiber Therapy for Regularity
Sugar Free Orange available in:
8.6 oz., 16.9 oz., and 32 oz.
Regular Orange available in:
16 oz., 30 oz., and 50 oz. containers

**Citrucel®**

---

GlaxoSmithKline Consumer Healthcare
P. 636

Nasal Decongestant/Antihistamine
Packages of 10 and 20
Maximum Strength Caplets

**Contac® 12 Hour Cold**

---

GlaxoSmithKline Consumer Healthcare
P. 637

Multisymptom Cold & Flu Relief
Maximum Strength Formula:
Packages of 16 and 30 caplets
Non-Drowsy Formula:
Packages of 16 caplets

**Contac® Severe
Cold & Flu**

**GlaxoSmithKline Consumer Healthcare**
*P. 638*

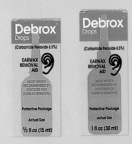

Drops
1/2 Fl. oz. 1 Fl. oz.

**Debrox®**

**GlaxoSmithKline Consumer Healthcare**
*P. 638*

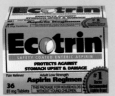

Adult Low Strength Tablets
in Bottles of 36

**Ecotrin®**

**GlaxoSmithKline Consumer Healthcare**
*P. 638*

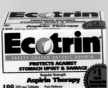

Regular Strength Tablets
in bottles of 100, 250

**Ecotrin®**

**GlaxoSmithKline Consumer Healthcare**
*P. 638*

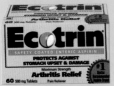

Maximum Strength Tablets
in bottles of 60, 150.

**Ecotrin®**

**GlaxoSmithKline Consumer Healthcare**
*P. 808*

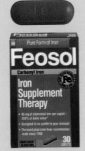

Packages of 30 caplets

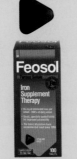

Packages of 100 tablets

**Feosol®**

**GlaxoSmithKline Consumer Healthcare**
*P. 641*

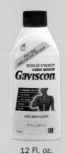

12 Fl. oz.

**Gaviscon® Regular
Strength Liquid Antacid**

**GlaxoSmithKline Consumer Healthcare**
*P. 641*

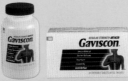

100-Tablet bottles
30-Tablet box (foil-wrapped 2s)

**Gaviscon® Regular
Strength Antacid**

**GlaxoSmithKline Consumer Healthcare**
*P. 641*

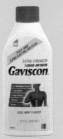

Extra Strength Formula
12 Fl. Oz.

**Gaviscon® Extra Strength
Liquid Antacid**

**GlaxoSmithKline Consumer Healthcare**
*P. 641*

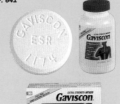

Extra Strength Formula
100-Tablet bottles
6 and 30-Tablet box
(foil-wrapped 2's)

**Gaviscon® Extra
Strength Antacid**

**GlaxoSmithKline Consumer Healthcare**
*P. 642*

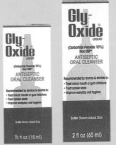

1/2 Fl. oz.        2 Fl. oz.

**Gly-Oxide® Liquid**

FACED WITH AN
Rx SIDE EFFECT?

Turn to the
Companion Drug Index
for products that provide
symptomatic relief.

**GlaxoSmithKline Consumer Healthcare**
*P. 644*

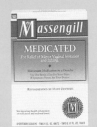

Medicated Disposable Douche
With Povidone-iodine
Available in single or twin packs

**Massengill®**

**GlaxoSmithKline Consumer Healthcare**
*P. 645*

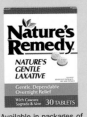

Available in packages of
15, 30 and 60 tablets.
A stimulant laxative with
natural active ingredients.

**Nature's Remedy®
Nature's Gentle Laxative**

**GlaxoSmithKline Consumer Healthcare**
*P. 645*

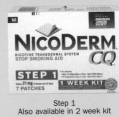

Step 1
Also available in 2 week kit

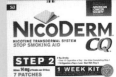

Step 2
Also available in 2 week kit

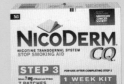

Step 3
Also available in 2 week kit

Includes User's Guide, Audio Tape and
Child Resistant Disposal Tray
Stop Smoking Aid
Nicotine Transdermal System

**NicoDerm® CQ™**

GlaxoSmithKline Consumer Healthcare
*P. 654*

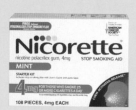

4 mg
For Smokers over 24
Cigarettes a day
Refill pack available
Stop Smoking Aid in Mint flavor
Nicotine Polacrilex Gum

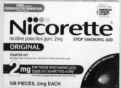

2 mg
For Smokers under 25
Cigarettes a day
Refill pack available in Mint Flavor
Stop Smoking Aid
Nicotine Polacrilex Gum

2 mg
For Smokers under 25
Cigarettes a day
Refill pack available
Stop Smoking Aid in Original flavor
Nicotine Polacrilex Gum

**Nicorette®**

GlaxoSmithKline Consumer Healthcare
*P. 658*

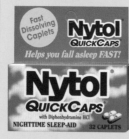

QuickCaps® and QuickGels™

**Nytol®**

GlaxoSmithKline Consumer Healthcare
*P. 809*

Calcium Supplement

**Os-Cal®**

GlaxoSmithKline Consumer Healthcare
*P. 658*

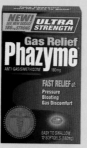

180 mg Softgels

**Gas Relief Phazyme®**

GlaxoSmithKline Consumer Healthcare
*P. 658*

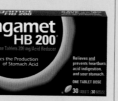

125 mg Chewable tablets

**Quick Dissolve
Phazyme®**

GlaxoSmithKline Consumer Healthcare
*P. 660*

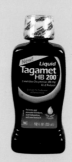

Acid Reducer
Packages of 6, 12, 18,
30, 50, 70 and 80

**Tagamet HB 200®**

GlaxoSmithKline Consumer Healthcare
*P. 660*

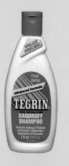

Liquid Tagamet HB 200®

GlaxoSmithKline Consumer Healthcare
*P. 661*

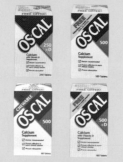

**Tegrin®
Dandruff Shampoo**

GlaxoSmithKline Consumer Healthcare
*P. 662*

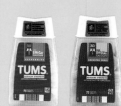

**Tegrin® Skin Cream
for Psoriasis**

GlaxoSmithKline Consumer Healthcare
*P. 662*

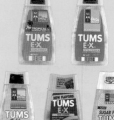

Peppermint and
Assorted Flavors

**Tums®**

GlaxoSmithKline Consumer Healthcare
*P. 662*

Tropical Fruit, Wintergreen,
Assorted Flavors, Assorted Berry
and SugarFree Orange Cream

**Tums E-X®**

GlaxoSmithKline Consumer Healthcare
*P. 662*

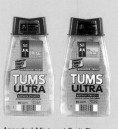

Assorted Mint and Fruit Flavors.
Also available in Tropical Fruit,
Assorted Berries and
Spearmint flavors

**Tums® Ultra™**

GlaxoSmithKline Consumer Healthcare
P. 663

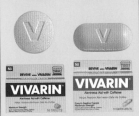

Alertness Aid with Caffeine
Available in tablets and caplets

**Vivarin®**

SEEKING AN
ALTERNATIVE?

Check the
Product Category Index,
where you'll find
alphabetical listings of
all the products in each
therapeutic class.

## J&J-MERCK CONSUMER

J&J-Merck Consumer
P. 664

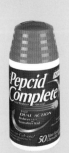

## Pepcid Complete®

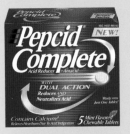

J&J-Merck Consumer
P. 664

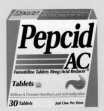

Tablets

Chewable Tablets

Gelcaps

**Pepcid AC®**

## KYOWA ENGINEERING-SUNDORY

Kyowa Engineering-Sundory
P. 811

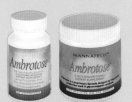

KYOWA's Agaricus Mushroom Extract
Dietary Supplement

**Sen-Sei-Ro Liquid Gold™**

Kyowa Engineering-Sundory
P. 811

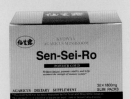

KYOWA's Agaricus Mushroom Powder
Dietary Supplement

**Sen-Sei-Ro Powder Gold™**

## LEGACY FOR LIFE

Legacy for Life™
P. 816

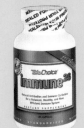

**BioChoice® immune²⁶**

## MANNATECH, INC.

Mannatech, Inc.
P. 816

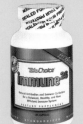

A Glyconutritional Dietary Supplement

**Ambrotose®**

Mannatech, Inc.
P. 817

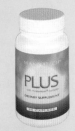

A Dietary Supplement of
Dried Fruits and Vegetables

**Phyt•Aloe®**

Mannatech, Inc.
P. 817

Dietary Supplement

**PLUS with
Ambrotose® complex**

## MATOL BOTANICAL
## INTERNATIONAL LTD.

Matol Botanical International Ltd.
P. 817

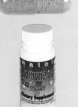

**Biomune OSF™
Plus**

LOOKING FOR
A PARTICULAR
COMPOUND?

In the
Active Ingredients Index
(Yellow Pages),
you'll find all the
brands that contain it.

## MCNEIL

**McNeil Consumer Healthcare**
*P. 818*

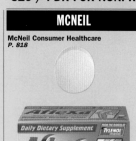

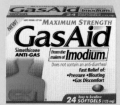

Tablets available in bottles of
50 and 110.

### Aflexa™ Tablets

**McNeil Consumer Healthcare**
*P. 666*

Softgels available in blister packs of
12, 24 and 48.

### Maximum Strength GasAid®

**McNeil Consumer Healthcare**
*P. 666*

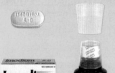

Available in 2 and 4 fl. oz. bottles
with a convenient dosage cup, and
caplets in 6's, 12's, 18's, 24's, 48's,
and 72's.

### Imodium® A-D

**McNeil Consumer Healthcare**
*P. 666*

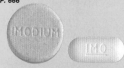

Vanilla mint chewable tablets
available in 6's, 12's, 18's,
30's and 42's. Caplets available
in 6's, 12's, 18's, and bottles of
30 and 42.

### Imodium® Advanced

---

**Lactaid Inc. Marketed By**
**McNeil Consumer Healthcare**
*P. 819*

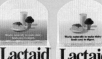

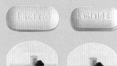

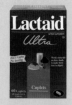

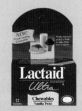

ORIGINAL STRENGTH available
in bottles of 120.
EXTRA STRENGTH available
in bottles of 50.
ULTRA CAPLETS available in
single serve packets of 12, 32
and 60 counts.
ULTRA CHEWABLE TABLETS available
in single serve packets of
12, 32, and 60 counts.

### Lactaid® Caplets and Chewable Tablets

**McNeil Consumer Healthcare**
*P. 668*

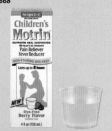

Available in Berry flavor in 4 fl. oz. with
child-resistant safety cap and
convenient dosage cup.

### Children's Motrin® Non-Staining Dye-Free Oral Suspension

---

**McNeil Consumer Healthcare**
*P. 668*

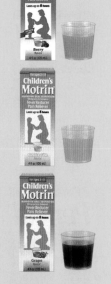

Available in Berry, Bubble Gum and
Grape flavors in 4 fl. oz. with
child-resistant safety cap
and convenient dosage cup.

### Children's Motrin® Oral Suspension

**McNeil Consumer Healthcare**
*P.*

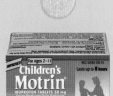

### Children's Motrin® Chewable Tablets

**McNeil Consumer Healthcare**
*P. 668*

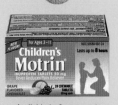

Available in Orange and
Grape-Flavored Chewable
Tablets of 50 mg.
Available in bottles of 24
with child-resistant safety cap.

### Children's Motrin® Chewable Tablets

---

**McNeil Consumer Healthcare**
*P. 670*

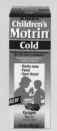
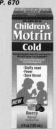

Available in Berry and Grape flavors in
4 fl. oz. with child-resistant safety cap
and convenient dosage cup.
Berry Flavor also available in
Non-Staining Dye-Free.

### Children's Motrin® Cold Oral Suspension

**McNeil Consumer Healthcare**
*P. 670*

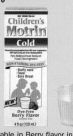

Available in Berry flavor in 4 fl. oz. with
child-resistant safety cap and
convenient dosage cup.

### Children's Motrin® Cold Non-Staining Dye-Free Oral Suspension

**McNeil Consumer Healthcare**
*P. 668*

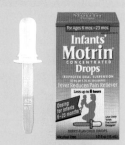

50 mg/1.25 mL
Available in 1/2 fl. oz. bottle.

### Infants' Motrin® Concentrated Drops

**McNeil Consumer Healthcare**
*P. 668*

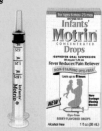

50 mg/1.25 mL
Available in 1 fl. oz. bottle.
New Syringe Dosing Device

### Infants' Motrin® Non-Staining Dye-Free Concentrated Drops

**McNeil Consumer Healthcare**
*P. 668*

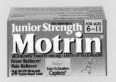

Available in bottles of 24 with child-resistant safety cap.

## Junior Strength Motrin® Caplets

**McNeil Consumer Healthcare**
*P. 668*

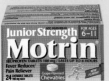

Available in Orange and Grape-flavored Chewable Tablets of 100 mg. Available in bottles of 24 with child-resistant safety cap.

## Junior Strength Motrin® Chewable Tablets

**McNeil Consumer Healthcare**
*P. 670*

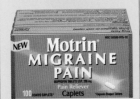

Caplets available in tamper-evident packaging of 24, 50 and 100.

## Motrin® Migraine Pain

---

**McNeil Consumer Healthcare**
*P. 667*

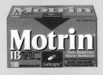

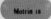

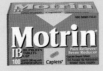

Gelcaps available in tamper evident packaging of 24, 50, and 100. Caplets available in tamper evident packaging of 24, 50, 60, 100, 165, 250, 300 and 500. Tablets available in tamper evident packaging of 24, 50, 100 and 165.

## Motrin® IB

**McNeil Consumer Healthcare**
*P. 668*

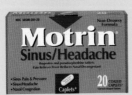

Caplets available in blister packs of 20's and 40's.

## Motrin® Sinus/Headache

**McNeil Consumer Healthcare**
*P. 672*

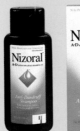

Available in 4 and 7 fl. oz. bottles.

## Nizoral® A-D

---

**McNeil Consumer Healthcare**
*P. 819*

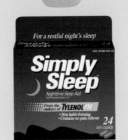

Chewable Tablets available in bottles of 60.

## Probiotica

**McNeil Consumer Healthcare**
*P. 672*

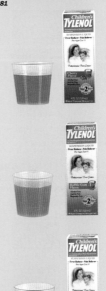

Mini-Caplets available in blister packs of 24, 48 and 72.

## Simply-Sleep™

**McNeil Consumer Healthcare**
*P. 681*

Available in Rich Cherry flavor in 2 and 4 fl. oz. bottles. Bubble Gum and Grape flavors in 4 fl. oz. with child-resistant safety cap and convenient dosage cup. Alcohol Free, 80 mg per 1/2 teaspoon.

## Children's TYLENOL® Suspension Liquid

---

**McNeil Consumer Healthcare**
*P. 681*

Fruit flavor: bottles of 30 with child-resistant safety cap and blister packs of 60 and 96.

Bubble Gum and Grape flavor bottles: of 30 with child-resistant safety cap.

## Children's TYLENOL® Soft Chews Chewable Tablets

**McNeil Consumer Healthcare**
*P. 682*

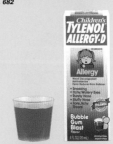

Available in Bubble Gum Blast flavor in child-resistant 4 fl. oz. bottles.

## Children's TYLENOL® Allergy-D Liquid

**McNeil Consumer Healthcare**
*P. 683*

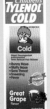

Available in 4 fl. oz. bottle with child-resistant safety cap and convenient dosage cup. Great Grape flavor.

## Children's TYLENOL® Cold Liquid

McNeil Consumer Healthcare
P. 683

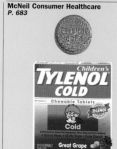

Available in blister pack of
24 chewable tablets.
Great Grape flavor.

**Children's TYLENOL® Cold
Chewable Tablets**

---

McNeil Consumer Healthcare
P. 687

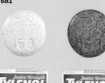

Available in Fruit Burst flavor in
child-resistant 4 fl. oz. bottles.

**Children's TYLENOL®
Sinus Liquid**

---

McNeil Consumer Healthcare
P. 681

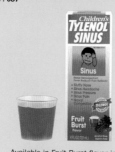

Available in blister pack of 24
chewable tablets. Fruit flavor and
Grape flavor.

**Junior Strength TYLENOL®
Soft Chews
Chewable Tablets**

---

McNeil Consumer Healthcare
P. 672

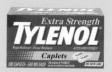

**Extra Strength TYLENOL®**

---

McNeil Consumer Healthcare
P. 683

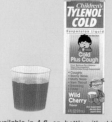

Available in 4 fl. oz. bottle with child-
resistant safety cap and convenient
dosage cup. Wild Cherry flavor.

**Children's TYLENOL®
Cold Plus Cough
Suspension Liquid**

---

McNeil Consumer Healthcare
P. 681

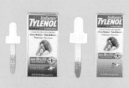

Available in Rich Cherry flavor and Rich
Grape flavor 1/2 oz. bottle with child-
resistant safety cap and calibrated
dropper. Rich Grape Flavor, Alcohol
Free, 80 mg per 0.8 mL. Cherry flavor
also available in 1 oz. bottle.

**Infants' TYLENOL®
Concentrated Drops**

---

McNeil Consumer Healthcare
P. 672

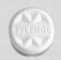

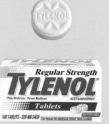

Tablets available in 100's.

**Regular Strength
TYLENOL®**

---

McNeil Consumer Healthcare
P. 672

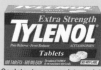

Caplets: tamper-resistant vials
of 10 and bottles of 24's, 50's,
100's, 150's and 250's.

Tablets: tamper-resistant vials
of 10 and bottles of 30's,
60's and 200's.

Liquid: tamper-evident
bottles of 8 fl. oz.

**Extra Strength TYLENOL®**

---

McNeil Consumer Healthcare
P. 683

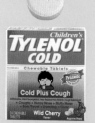

Available in blister pack of 24
chewable tablets. Wild Cherry flavor.

**Children's TYLENOL®
Cold Plus Cough
Chewable Tablets**

---

McNeil Consumer Healthcare
P. 683

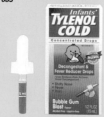

Available in 1/2 fl. oz. bottle with
child-resistant safety cap and
calibrated dropper. Bubble Gum flavor,
Alcohol-free.

**Infant's TYLENOL® Cold
Decongestant and Fever
Reducer Concentrated Drops**

---

McNeil Consumer Healthcare
P. 672

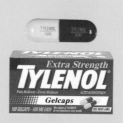

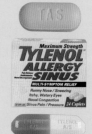

Gelcaps available in tamper-resistant
bottles of 24's, 50's, 100's, 150's
and 225's.

Geltabs available in tamper-resistant
bottles of 24's, 50's, 100's and 150's.

**Extra Strength TYLENOL®**

---

McNeil Consumer Healthcare
P. 674

Caplets in blister packs of 24 & 48.
Gelcaps in blister packs of 24 & 48.
Geltabs in blister packs of 24 & 48.

**Maximum Strength
TYLENOL® Allergy Sinus**

---

McNeil Consumer Healthcare
P. 687

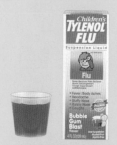

Available in Bubble Gum Blast flavor
in child-resistant 4 fl. oz. bottles.

**Children's TYLENOL®
Flu Suspension Liquid**

---

McNeil Consumer Healthcare
P. 683

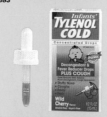

Available in 1/2 fl. oz. bottle with
child-resistant safety cap and
calibrated dropper. Wild Cherry flavor,
Alcohol-free.

**Infants' TYLENOL® Cold
Decongestant and Fever
Reducer Concentrated
Drops Plus Cough**

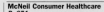

McNeil Consumer Healthcare
P. 674

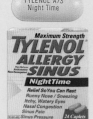

Caplets available in blister packs of 24's.

**Maximum Strength TYLENOL® Allergy Sinus NightTime**

McNeil Consumer Healthcare
P. 674

Caplets available in blister packs of 12's and 24's.

**TYLENOL® Severe Allergy**

McNeil Consumer Healthcare
P. 672

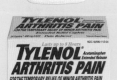

Caplets available in 24's, 50's, 100's, 150's, 250's and 290's.

**TYLENOL® Arthritis Pain Extended Relief**

McNeil Consumer Healthcare
P. 675

Caplets available in blister packs of 24.

**Multi-Symptom TYLENOL® Cold Complete Formula**

---

McNeil Consumer Healthcare
P. 675

Caplets available in blister packs of 24
Gelcaps available in blister packs of 24.

**Multi-Symptom TYLENOL® Cold Non-Drowsy**

McNeil Consumer Healthcare
P. 676

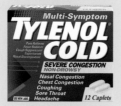

Available in blister packs of 24.

**TYLENOL® Cold Severe Congestion Non-Drowsy**

McNeil Consumer Healthcare
P. 677

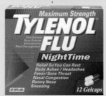

Gelcaps Available in blister packs of 12's and 24's.

**Maximum Strength TYLENOL® Flu NightTime**

McNeil Consumer Healthcare
P. 677

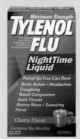

Available in 8 oz. bottles.

**Maximum Strength TYLENOL® Flu NightTime Liquid**

---

McNeil Consumer Healthcare
P. 677

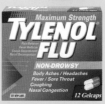

Gelcaps available in blister packs of 24.

**Maximum Strength TYLENOL® Flu Non-Drowsy**

McNeil Consumer Healthcare
P. 678

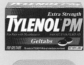

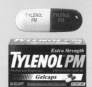

Geltabs available in tamper-resistant bottles of 24, 50 and 100.

Caplets available in tamper-resistant bottles of 24, 50, 100 and 150.

Gelcaps available in tamper-resistant bottles of 24 and 50.

Geltabs, Caplets and Gelcaps available in bottles of 50 for households without children.

**Extra Strength TYLENOL® PM**

McNeil Consumer Healthcare
P. 679

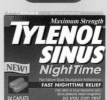

Available in blister packs of 24.

**Maximum Strength TYLENOL® Sinus NightTime Caplets**

---

McNeil Consumer Healthcare
P. 679

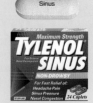

Caplets, Gelcaps and Geltabs in blister packs of 24 and 48.

**Maximum Strength TYLENOL® Sinus**

McNeil Consumer Healthcare
P. 680

Cherry and Honey Lemon flavors available in 8 fl. oz.

**Maximum Strength TYLENOL® Sore Throat**

McNeil Consumer Healthcare
P. 680

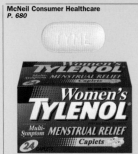

Caplets available in tamper-evident
bottles of 24 and 40.

**Women's TYLENOL®
Menstrual Relief**

Novartis Consumer Health, Inc.
P. 691

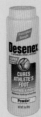

Powder          Spray Powder

**Desenex®**

FACED WITH AN
Rx SIDE EFFECT?

Turn to the
Companion Drug Index
for products that provide
symptomatic relief.

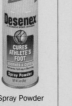

Antifungal Cream
Available in 12 g and 24 g

**Desenex®**

Novartis Consumer Health, Inc.
P. 820

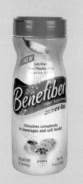

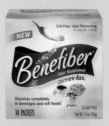

Available in 24 serving, 42 serving,
80 serving (club pack) bottles,
and 14 ct. packet carton.

**Benefiber®
Fiber Supplement**

Novartis Consumer Health, Inc.
P. 692

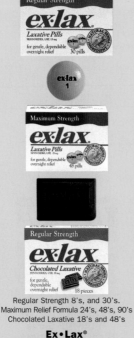

Regular Strength 8's, and 30's.
Maximum Relief Formula 24's, 48's, 90's
Chocolated Laxative 18's and 48's

**Ex·Lax®**

Novartis Consumer Health, Inc.
P. 693

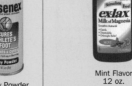

Mint Flavor
12 oz.

**Ex·Lax®
Milk of Magnesia**

Novartis Consumer Health, Inc.
P. 693

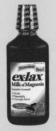

Chocolate Creme
12 oz.

**Ex·Lax®
Milk of Magnesia**

Novartis Consumer Health, Inc.
P. 693

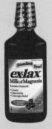

Raspberry Creme
12 oz.

**Ex·Lax®
Milk of Magnesia**

Novartis Consumer Health, Inc.
P. 693

Extra Strength Cherry 18's, 48's
Extra Strength Peppermint 18's, 48's
(125 mg simethicone)

**Gas-X®**

Novartis Consumer Health, Inc.
P. 693

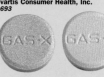

Cherry 12's, 36's
Peppermint 12's, 36's
(80 mg simethicone)

**Gas-X®**

Novartis Consumer Health, Inc.
P. 693

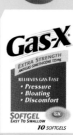

Extra Strength Softgels
in packs of 10's, 30's, 50's, 60's
(125 mg simethicone)

**Gas-X®**

Novartis Consumer Health, Inc.
P. 693

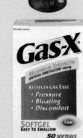

Maximum Strength Softgels
in packs of 50's
(166 mg simethicone)

**Gas-X®**

Novartis Consumer Health, Inc.
P. 693

Extra Strength Wild Berry 8's, 24's
Also available in Orange 8's, 24's

**Gas-X® with Maalox®**

Novartis Consumer Health, Inc.
P. 694

Athlete's Foot available in
12 g and 24 g
Jock Itch available in 12 g

## Lamisil AT® Cream

Novartis Consumer Health, Inc.
P. 694

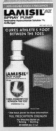

30 mL (1 oz)

## Lamisil AT®
## Athlete's Foot
## Solution Dropper

Novartis Consumer Health, Inc.
P. 694

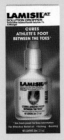

30 mL (1 oz)

## Lamisil AT®
## Athlete's Foot
## Spray Pump

Novartis Consumer Health, Inc.
P. 694

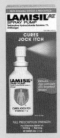

30 mL (1 oz)

## Lamisil AT®
## Jock Itch
## Spray Pump

---

Novartis Consumer Health, Inc.
P. 695

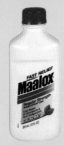

Cooling Mint Liquid
Also available in Smooth Cherry
Bottles of 5 (Mint Only), 12 & 26 oz.

## Maalox® Antacid

Novartis Consumer Health, Inc.
P. 695

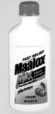

Cherry Liquid
Also available in Lemon,
Mint (12 & 26 oz.),
Vanilla Creme, Peaches N' Creme,
and Wild Berry (12 oz.)

## Maximum Strength
## Maalox® Antacid/Anti-Gas

Novartis Consumer Health, Inc.
P. 696

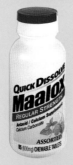

Assorted 85 and 145 ct
Wild Berry 45 ct
Lemon 45, 85 ct

## Maalox® Quick Dissolve
## Tablets Antacid/Calcium
## Supplement

---

Novartis Consumer Health, Inc.
P. 696

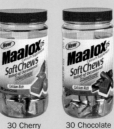

Assorted 35, 65, 90 ct
Wild Berry 35, 65 ct
Lemon 35, 65 ct

## Maximum Strength
## Maalox® Quick Dissolve
## Tablets Antacid/Anti-Gas

Novartis Consumer Health, Inc.
P. 821

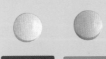

30 Cherry
Chews

30 Chocolate
Chews

## Maalox® DS Softchews

Novartis Consumer Health, Inc.
P. 821

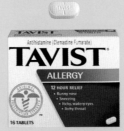

Slow Release Iron available
in 30, 60 and 90 ct.
Slow Release Iron & Folic Acid
available in 20 ct.

## SLOW FE®

Novartis Consumer Health, Inc.
P. 697

TAVIST

ALLERGY

## TAVIST® Allergy

8, 16 count

---

Novartis Consumer Health, Inc.
P. 697

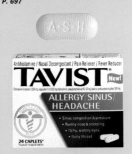

24, 48 count

## TAVIST® Allergy/Sinus/
## Headache

Novartis Consumer Health, Inc.
P. 698

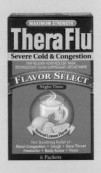

Flu & Congestion Non-Drowsy
Flu & Cough Night Time
Flu & Sore Throat Night Time
Severe Cold & Congestion Non-Drowsy
Formulas above available in 6 ct.
Severe Cold & Congestion Night Time
Available in 6 ct. and 12 ct.

Cold & Sore Throat Night Time
Available in 6 ct.
Cold & Cough Night Time
Available in 6 ct. and 12 ct.

Available in 12 ct. and 24 ct. caplets
Severe Cold & Congestion Night Time
Severe Cold & Congestion Non-Drowsy

## TheraFlu®

SEEKING AN
ALTERNATIVE?

Check the
Product Category Index,
where you'll find
alphabetical listings of
all the products in each
therapeutic class.

Novartis Consumer Health, Inc.
P. 705

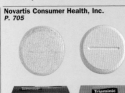

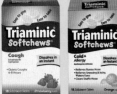

Cough

Cold & Allergy

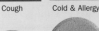

Cold & Cough

Cough &
Sore Throat

**Triaminic® Softchews®**

Novartis Consumer Health, Inc.
P. 704

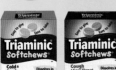

Allergy
Congestion

Allergy Runny
Nose & Congestion

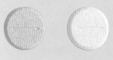

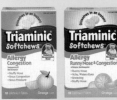

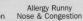
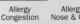

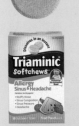

Allergy Sinus & Headache

**Triaminic® Softchews®
Allergy**

---

Novartis Consumer Health, Inc.
P. 701

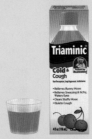

Cold & Cough

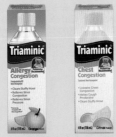

Allergy Congestion    Chest Congestion

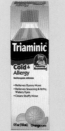

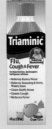

Cold & Allergy

Flu,
Cough & Fever

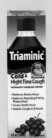

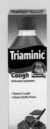

Cold & Night Time
Cough

Cough

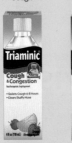

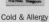

Cough & Congestion    Cough & Sore
Throat

**Triaminic®**

---

Novartis Consumer Health, Inc.
P. 707

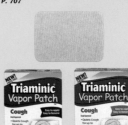

Menthol and
Mentholated Cherry Scents

**Triaminic® Vapor Patch**

Pfizer Consumer Group, Pfizer Inc.
P. 707

Herbal Throat Drops
Available in Honey-Lemon Chamomile,
Harvest Cherry and Sunshine Citrus

**Celestial Seasonings®
Soothers™**

Pfizer Consumer Group, Pfizer Inc.
P. 708

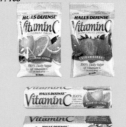

100% Daily Value
Vitamin C in each drop.
Available in Assorted Citrus
and Strawberry Flavors.

**Halls® Defense**

Pfizer Consumer Group, Pfizer Inc.
P. 708

Honey-Lemon, Mentho-Lyptus® & Cherry

**Halls® Plus
Cough Suppressant
Throat Drops
with Medicine Center**

---

Pfizer Consumer Group, Pfizer Inc.
P. 707

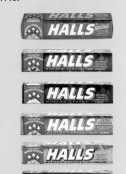

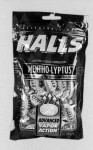

Cough Suppressant Drops
Spearmint, Mentho-Lyptus®,
Ice Blue, Honey-Lemon,
Cherry and Strawberry Flavors

**Halls® Mentho-Lyptus®**

Pfizer Consumer Group, Pfizer Inc.
P. 708

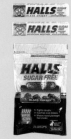

Cough Suppressant Drops
Black Cherry, Citrus Blend
and Mountain Menthol

**Halls® Sugar Free
Squares Mentho-Lyptus®**

Pfizer Consumer Group, Pfizer Inc.
P. 708

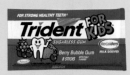

Sugarless Dental Gum available in
Berry Gum Flavor in a 8-stick pack.

**Trident for Kids™
with Recaldent™**

Pfizer Consumer Group, Pfizer Inc.
P. 709

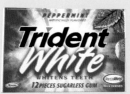

Available in Peppermint and
Wintergreen flavors in a 12-pellet
blister foil

**Trident White™
Sugarless Gum with
Recaldent™**

**PFIZER CONSUMER
HEALTHCARE, PFIZER INC.**

Pfizer Consumer Healthcare, Pfizer Inc.
P. 709

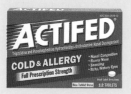

Available in boxes
of 12 and 24 tablets

**Actifed® Cold & Allergy**

Pfizer Consumer Healthcare, Pfizer Inc.
P. 709

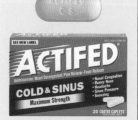

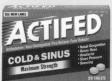

Available in boxes of
24 caplets and tablets

**Actifed® Cold & Sinus**

Pfizer Consumer Healthcare, Pfizer Inc.
P. 710

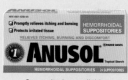

Ointment available in 1 oz. tubes

**Anusol®**

Pfizer Consumer Healthcare, Pfizer Inc.
P. 710

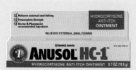

Suppositories available
in boxes of 12 and 24

**Anusol®**

Pfizer Consumer Healthcare, Pfizer Inc.
P. 711

Anti-Itch Hydrocortisone Ointment
Available in 0.7 oz. tube

**Anusol HC-1™**

Pfizer Consumer Healthcare, Pfizer Inc.
P. 711

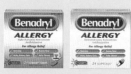

Tablets and Capsules
Available in boxes of 24 and 48
Tablets also available in
bottles of 100

**Benadryl® Allergy**

Pfizer Consumer Healthcare, Pfizer Inc.
P. 711

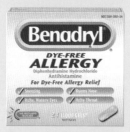

Available in boxes of 24 softgels

**Benadryl® Dye-Free
Allergy Liqui-Gels®
Softgels**

Pfizer Consumer Healthcare, Pfizer Inc.
P. 712

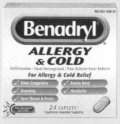

Available in boxes of 24 Tablets

**Benadryl®
Allergy & Cold**

Pfizer Consumer Healthcare, Pfizer Inc.
P. 712

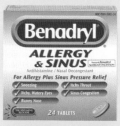

Available in boxes of 24 Tablets

**Benadryl® Allergy &
Sinus**

Pfizer Consumer Healthcare, Pfizer Inc.
P. 713

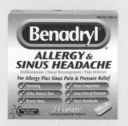

Available in boxes of 24 and 48
Caplets, and also available in
boxes of 72 Gelcaps

**Benadryl® Allergy &
Sinus Headache**

Pfizer Consumer Healthcare, Pfizer Inc.
P. 713

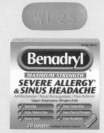

Available in boxes of 20 caplets

**Maximum Strength
Benadryl® Severe Allergy
& Sinus Headache**

Pfizer Consumer Healthcare, Pfizer Inc.
P. 714

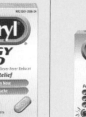

Available in boxes of
20 dissolving tablets

**Benadryl® Allergy &
Sinus FASTMELT™**

Pfizer Consumer Healthcare, Pfizer Inc.
P. 714

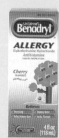

Available in 4 oz. and 8 oz. bottles

**Children's Benadryl®
Allergy Liquid Medication**

Pfizer Consumer Healthcare, Pfizer Inc.
P. 715

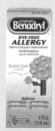

Available in 4 fl. oz. bottles

**Children's Benadryl®
Dye-Free Allergy Liquid
Medication**

Pfizer Consumer Healthcare, Pfizer Inc.
P. 715

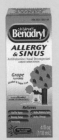

Available in 4 oz. bottles

### Children's Benadryl® Allergy & Sinus Liquid Medication

Pfizer Consumer Healthcare, Pfizer Inc.
P. 716

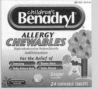

Available in boxes of 24 chewable Tablets

### Children's Benadryl® Allergy Chewables

Pfizer Consumer Healthcare, Pfizer Inc.
P. 716

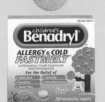

Available in boxes of 20 dissolving tablets

### Children's Benadryl® Allergy & Cold FASTMELT™

LOOKING FOR
A PARTICULAR
COMPOUND?

In the
Active Ingredients Index
(Yellow Pages),
you'll find all the
brands that contain it.

---

Pfizer Consumer Healthcare, Pfizer Inc.
P. 717

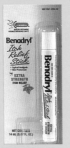

Extra Strength

### Benadryl® Itch Relief Stick

Pfizer Consumer Healthcare, Pfizer Inc.
P. 717

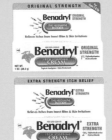

Original and Extra Strength

### Benadryl® Itch Stopping Cream

Pfizer Consumer Healthcare, Pfizer Inc.
P. 718

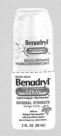 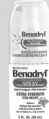

Original and Extra Strength

### Benadryl® Itch Stopping Spray

Pfizer Consumer Healthcare, Pfizer Inc.
P. 716

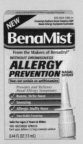

Available in in .44 and
.88 fl. oz., nasal sprays

### BenaMist™ Allergy Prevention Nasal Spray

---

Pfizer Consumer Healthcare, Pfizer Inc.
P. 719

Arthritis Formula, Greaseless,
Original Formula, Ultra Strength
and Vanishing Scent.

### BENGAY®

Pfizer Consumer Healthcare, Pfizer Inc.
P. 719

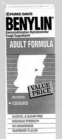

Available in 4 oz. bottles

### Benylin® Adult Cough Suppressant

Pfizer Consumer Healthcare, Pfizer Inc.
P. 719

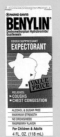

Available in 4 oz. bottles

### Benylin® Cough Suppressant Expectorant

---

Pfizer Consumer Healthcare, Pfizer Inc.
P. 720

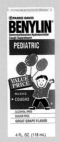

Available in 4 oz. bottles

### Benylin® Pediatric Cough Suppressant

Pfizer Consumer Healthcare, Pfizer Inc.
P. 720

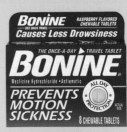

8 and 16 Chewable Tablets

### Bonine®

Pfizer Consumer Healthcare, Pfizer Inc.
P. 720

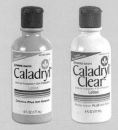

Itch Relief Plus Drying Action.
Available in Lotion, Clear Lotion

### Caladryl®

Pfizer Consumer Healthcare, Pfizer Inc.
P. 721

Kids available in 1 oz. Creme
Cortizone•5 available in 1 oz.
and 2 oz. Creme and 1 oz. Ointment

### Cortizone•5®

Pfizer Consumer Healthcare, Pfizer Inc.
P. 721

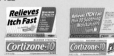

Cortizone•10 available in 1/2 oz., 1 oz., and 2 oz. Creme and 1 oz. and 2 oz. Ointment.
Cortizone•10 Plus available in 1 oz. and 2 oz. Creme.
Cortizone•10 Quick Shot Spray available in 1.5 oz.

**Cortizone•10®**

Pfizer Consumer Healthcare, Pfizer Inc.
P. 722

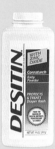

**DESITIN® Cornstarch Baby Powder**

Pfizer Consumer Healthcare, Pfizer Inc.
P. 722

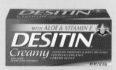
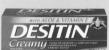

Diaper Rash Ointment

**DESITIN® Creamy**

Pfizer Consumer Healthcare, Pfizer Inc.
P. 722

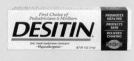
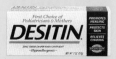

Diaper Rash Ointment

**DESITIN®**

Pfizer Consumer Healthcare, Pfizer Inc.
P. 723

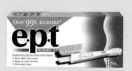

1 and 2 Pregnancy Test Kits Available One Step. Easy to read. Over 99% accurate in Laboratory Tests.

**e.p.t®**

Pfizer Consumer Healthcare, Pfizer Inc.
P. 724

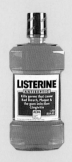

**Listerine® Antiseptic**

Pfizer Consumer Healthcare, Pfizer Inc.
P. 724

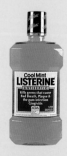

**Cool Mint Listerine® Antiseptic**

Pfizer Consumer Healthcare, Pfizer Inc.
P. 724

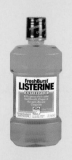

**FreshBurst Listerine® Antiseptic**

Pfizer Consumer Healthcare, Pfizer Inc.
P. 724

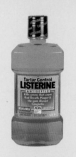

**Tartar Control Listerine® Antiseptic**

Pfizer Consumer Healthcare, Pfizer Inc.
P. 725

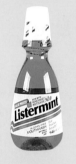

**Listermint® Alcohol-Free Mouthwash**

Pfizer Consumer Healthcare, Pfizer Inc.
P. 725

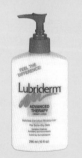

**Lubriderm® Advanced Therapy Creamy Lotion**

Pfizer Consumer Healthcare, Pfizer Inc.
P. 725

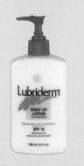

**Lubriderm® Daily UV Lotion with Sunscreen**

Pfizer Consumer Healthcare, Pfizer Inc.
P. 725

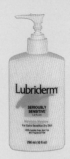

**Lubriderm® Seriously Sensitive® Lotion**

Pfizer Consumer Healthcare, Pfizer Inc.
P. 725

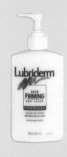

**Lubriderm® Skin Firming Body Lotion**

Pfizer Consumer Healthcare, Pfizer Inc.
P. 726

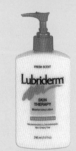

Available in Scented and Fragrance Free

**Lubriderm® Lotion**

Pfizer Consumer Healthcare, Pfizer Inc.
P. 726

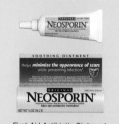

First Aid Antibiotic Ointment
Available in 1/2 oz. (14.2g) or 1 oz. (28.3g) tubes; 1/32 oz. (0.9 g) foil packets

**NEOSPORIN®**

Pfizer Consumer Healthcare, Pfizer Inc.
P. 726

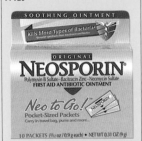

First Aid Antibiotic Ointment.
Available in Individual Foil Packets.
1/32 oz. (0.9 g) 10 packets per Box

**NEOSPORIN® Neo to Go!™**

---

Pfizer Consumer Healthcare, Pfizer Inc.
P. 727

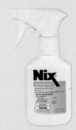

Lice Control Spray for
Bedding and Furniture
*NOT FOR HUMAN USE

**Nix®**

---

Pfizer Consumer Healthcare, Pfizer Inc.
P. 729

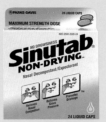

Available in Boxes of 24

**Sinutab® Non-Drying
Liquid Caps**

---

Pfizer Consumer Healthcare, Pfizer Inc.
P. 731

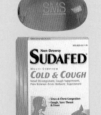

Available in 10's or 20's Liquid Caps

**Sudafed® Cold & Cough**

---

Pfizer Consumer Healthcare, Pfizer Inc.
P. 726

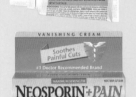

First Aid Antibiotic
Pain Relieving Cream
Available in 1/2 oz. (14.2g) tubes

**NEOSPORIN®+ Pain Relief**

---

Pfizer Consumer Healthcare, Pfizer Inc.
P. 728

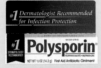

First Aid Antibiotic Powder & Ointment
Powder, 0.35 oz. (10g) Ointment,
1/2 oz. (14.2g) and 1 oz. (28.3g)
tubes and 1/32 oz (0.9g) foil packets

**Polysporin®**

---

Pfizer Consumer Healthcare, Pfizer Inc.
P. 730

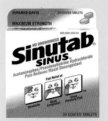

Maximum Strength
Without Drowsiness Formula
Available in 24 Caplets or Tablets

**Sinutab® Sinus**

---

Pfizer Consumer Healthcare, Pfizer Inc.
P. 733

Available in boxes of
10 and 20 liquid caps

**Sudafed®
Sinus and Cold**

---

Pfizer Consumer Healthcare, Pfizer Inc.
P. 726

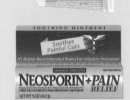

First Aid Antibiotic/
Pain Relieving Ointment
Available in 1/2 oz. (14.2g)
and 1 oz. (28.3g) tubes

**NEOSPORIN®+ Pain Relief**

---

Pfizer Consumer Healthcare, Pfizer Inc.
P. 728

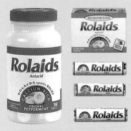

Fast, Effective Relief from
Heartburn, Acid Indigestion or
Sour Stomach
Original Peppermint,
Spearmint, and Cherry Flavors

**Rolaids®**

---

Pfizer Consumer Healthcare, Pfizer Inc.
P. 729

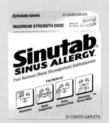

Maximum Strength Formula
Available in 24 Caplets or Tablets

**Sinutab® Sinus Allergy**

---

Pfizer Consumer Healthcare, Pfizer Inc.
P. 731

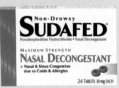

30 mg Tablets
Available in 24, 48 and 96

**Sudafed®
Nasal Decongestant**

---

Pfizer Consumer Healthcare, Pfizer Inc.
P. 726

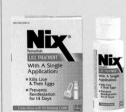

Lice Treatment Creme Rinse
2 fl. oz. (59 mL)
Also available in:
2-bottle family pack

**Nix®**

---

Pfizer Consumer Healthcare, Pfizer Inc.
P. 728

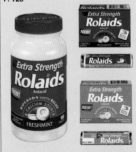

Freshmint and fruit

**Extra Strength Rolaids®**

---

Pfizer Consumer Healthcare, Pfizer Inc.
P. 732

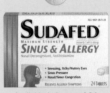

Available in boxes of 24

**Sudafed® Sinus
and Allergy**

---

Pfizer Consumer Healthcare, Pfizer Inc.
P. 732

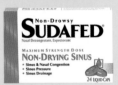

Available in 24 Liquid Caps

**Sudafed® Non-Drying
Sinus Liquid Caps**

Pfizer Consumer Healthcare, Pfizer Inc.
P. 732

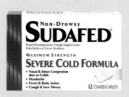

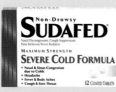

Available in 12's or 24's
caplets, 12's in tablets

**Sudafed®
Severe Cold Formula**

Pfizer Consumer Healthcare, Pfizer Inc.
P. 730

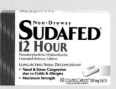

12 Hour Caplets
Available in 10 and 20 caplets

**Sudafed® 12 Hour**

Pfizer Consumer Healthcare, Pfizer Inc.
P. 730

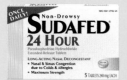

Available in boxes of 5 and 10 tablets.

**Sudafed® 24 Hour**

---

Pfizer Consumer Healthcare, Pfizer Inc.
P. 733

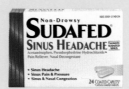

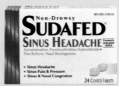

Available in 24's or 48's caplets;
24's tablets

**Sudafed® Sinus
Headache**

Pfizer Consumer Healthcare, Pfizer Inc.
P. 734

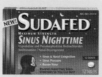

Maximum Strength
Available in 12 tablets

**Sudafed® Sinus
Nighttime**

Pfizer Consumer Healthcare, Pfizer Inc.
P. 734

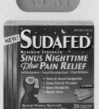

Maximum Strength
Available in 20 caplets

**Sudafed® Sinus
Nighttime Plus Pain
Relief**

---

Pfizer Consumer Healthcare, Pfizer Inc.
P. 734

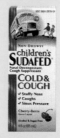

Available in 4 fl. oz. bottles

**Children's Sudafed®
Cold & Cough
Liquid Medication**

Pfizer Consumer Healthcare, Pfizer Inc.
P. 735

Available in boxes of
24 chewable tablets

**Children's Sudafed®
Nasal Decongestant**

Pfizer Consumer Healthcare, Pfizer Inc.
P. 735

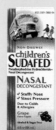

Available in 4 fl. oz. bottles

**Children's Sudafed®
Nasal Decongestant
Liquid Medication**

Pfizer Consumer Healthcare, Pfizer Inc.
P. 736

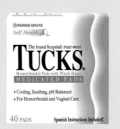

Pre-Moistened Pads
Available in 40 and 100 pad packages
Tucks® Take Alongs available in 12
individually packed towelettes.

**Tucks®**

---

Pfizer Consumer Healthcare, Pfizer Inc.
P. 736

Nighttime Sleep Aid
SleepGels available in
8, 16 and 32 softgels
SleepTabs available in
8, 16, 32 and 48 tablets

**Unisom®**

Pfizer Consumer Healthcare, Pfizer Inc.
P. 737

Advanced Relief, Original,
L.R. Long Lasting and
A.C. Seasonal Relief.

**Visine®**

Pfizer Consumer Healthcare, Pfizer Inc.
P. 737

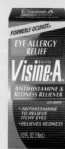

Eye Allergy Relief

**Visine®-A™**

Pfizer Consumer Healthcare, Pfizer Inc.
P. 738

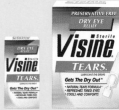

Dry Eye Relief

**Visine® Tears™**

Pfizer Consumer Healthcare, Pfizer Inc.
P. 739

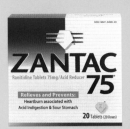

Available in boxes of
4, 10, 20, 30, 60, 80 and 110 tablets

**Zantac® 75**

FACED WITH AN
Rx SIDE EFFECT?

Turn to the
Companion Drug Index
for products that provide
symptomatic relief.

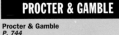

## PROCTER & GAMBLE

Procter & Gamble
P. 744

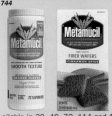

Available in 30, 48, 72, 114 and 180
dose canisters and cartons of 30
one-dose packets.
Also available in sugar free.
Cinnamon Spice and Apple Crisp
Wafers available in 12-dose cartons.

**Metamucil®**

Procter & Gamble
P. 745

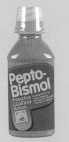

Also available in Maximum Strength
Liquid, Chewable Tablets and
Swallowable Caplets

**Pepto-Bismol®**

Procter & Gamble
P. 747

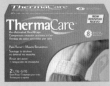

Back Wrap for Pain Relief
and Muscle Relaxation

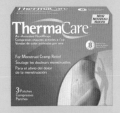

Patches For Menstrual Cramp Relief

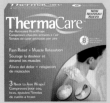

Neck to Arm Wrap for Pain Relief
and Muscle Relaxation
Air-Activated Heat Wraps

**ThermaCare™**

Procter & Gamble
P. 748

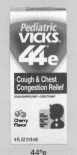

44®e
Cough & Chest Congestion Relief

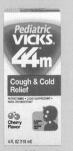

44®m
Cough & Cold Relief

**Pediatric VICKS®**

Procter & Gamble
P. 747

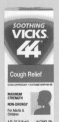

VICKS® 44®
Cough Relief

VICKS® 44®D
Cough & Head Congestion Relief

VICKS® E
Cough & Chest Congestion Relief

VICKS44® M
Cough, Cold & Flu Relief

**VICKS®**

Procter & Gamble
P. 750

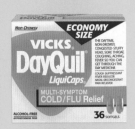

Multi-Symptom
Cold/Flu Relief

**VICKS® DayQuil®
LiquiCaps®**

Procter & Gamble
P. 749

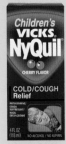

Cherry Flavor
Cold/Cough Relief

**Children's VICKS® NyQuil®**

Procter & Gamble
P. 751

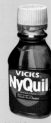

Multi-Symptom
Cold/Flu Relief

**VICKS® NyQuil®
Liquid**

Procter & Gamble
P. 751

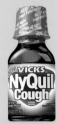

Cough Relief

**VICKS® NyQuil®
Cough**

## PRODUCTS ON DEMAND

Products On Demand
P. 755

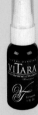

1 oz

**Vitara™
Feminine Cream**

## PURDUE FREDERICK

**The Purdue Frederick Company**
P. 756

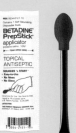

Topical Antiseptic

### Betadine® PrepStick®

**The Purdue Frederick Company**
P. 756

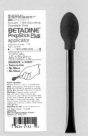

Topical Antiseptic

### Betadine® PrepStick® Plus™

**The Purdue Frederick Company**
P. 755

Maximum Strength Ointment

Antibiotics + Moisturizer

Antibiotics + Pain Reliever

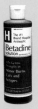

Solution

### Betadine®

---

**The Purdue Frederick Company**
P. 757

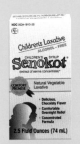

Natural Vegetable Laxative
Children's Syrup

### Senokot®

**The Purdue Frederick Company**
P. 757

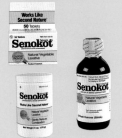

Natural Vegetable Laxative
Available in Tablets, Granules,
and Syrup.

### Senokot®

**The Purdue Frederick Company**
P. 757

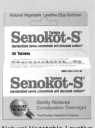

Natural Vegetable Laxative
Plus Softener Tablets

### Senokot-S®

## REXALL SUNDOWN

**Rexall Sundown**
P. 823

Double Strength

Triple Strength

### Osteo Bi-Flex®

---

## SCHERING-PLOUGH

**Schering-Plough HealthCare Products**
P. 757

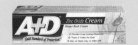

Original Ointment and
Cream with Zinc Oxide

### A and D® Ointment

**Schering-Plough HealthCare Products**
P. 757

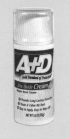

### A and D®
### Zinc Oxide Cream

**Schering-Plough HealthCare Products**
P. 758

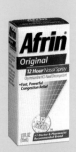

### Afrin® Original 12 Hour
### Nasal Spray

**Schering-Plough HealthCare Products**
P. 758

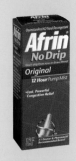

### Afrin® No Drip
### 12 Hour Nasal Spray

---

**Schering-Plough HealthCare Products**
P. 759

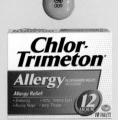

12 Hour Allergy Tablets

### Chlor-Trimeton®

**Schering-Plough HealthCare Products**
P. 757

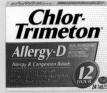

12 Hour Allergy Decongestant Tablets

### Chlor-Trimeton®

**Schering-Plough HealthCare Products**
P. 760

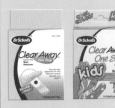

### Clear Away® One Step
### Wart Removers

**Schering-Plough HealthCare Products**
P. 761

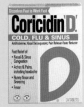

For Relief Of Cold,
Flu & Sinus Symptoms

### Coricidin´D´®

Schering-Plough HealthCare Products
P. 761

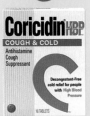

Cough and Cold Relief for people with
High Blood Pressure

**Coricidin HBP®**

Schering-Plough HealthCare Products
P. 761

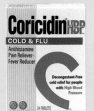

Cold and Flu Relief for people with
High Blood Pressure

**Coricidin HBP®**

Schering-Plough HealthCare Products
P. 761

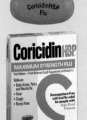

Maximum Strength Flu Relief
for people with High Blood Pressure

**Coricidin HBP®**

Schering-Plough HealthCare Products
P. 762

Available in
Laxative Tablets and Caplets,
Combination Vegetable Laxative
Plus Stool Softener and
Stool Softener Gelcaps.

**Correctol®**

Schering-Plough HealthCare Products
P. 763

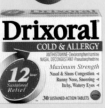

12 Hour Sustained-Action Tablets

**Drixoral®
Cold & Allergy**

Schering-Plough HealthCare Products
P. 764

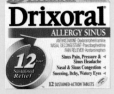

12 Hour Sustained-Action Tablets

**Drixoral®
Allergy Sinus**

Schering-Plough HealthCare Products
P. 764

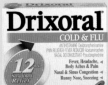

12 Hour Sustained-Action Tablets

**Drixoral®
Cold & Flu**

Schering-Plough HealthCare Products
P. 763

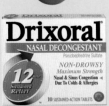

12 Hour Sustained-Action Tablets

**Drixoral®
Nasal Decongestant**

Schering-Plough HealthCare Products
P. 765

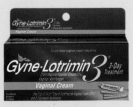

3-Day Treatment
Vaginal Cream

**Gyne-Lotrimin 3®**

Schering-Plough HealthCare Products
P. 765

Also available in 10 mL solution for
Athlete's Foot and 20 mL lotion for
Jock Itch.

**Lotrimin® AF**

Schering-Plough HealthCare Products
P. 766

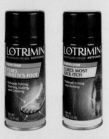

Also available for Athlete's Foot:
Powder Spray, Deodorant Powder
Spray, Shaker Powder

**Lotrimin® AF**

Schering-Plough HealthCare Products
P. 766

**Lotrimin® Ultra™**

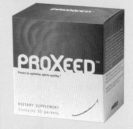
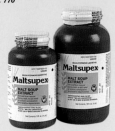
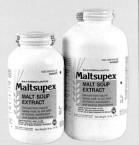

# SECTION 7

# NONPRESCRIPTION DRUG INFORMATION

This section presents information on nonprescription drugs, self-testing kits, and other medical products marketed for home use by consumers. It is made possible through the courtesy of the manufacturers whose products appear on the following pages. The information concerning each product has been prepared, edited, and approved by professional staff of the manufacturer.

Pharmaceutical product descriptions in this section must be in compliance with the Code of Federal Regulations labeling requirements for over-the-counter drugs. The descriptions are designed to provide all information necessary for informed use, including, when applicable, active ingredients, inactive ingredients, indications, actions, warnings, cautions, drug interactions, symptoms and treatment of oral overdosage, dosage and directions for use, professional labeling, and how supplied. In some cases, additional information has been supplied to complement the standard labeling.

In compiling this section, the publisher has emphasized the necessity of describing products comprehensively. The descriptions seen here include all information made available by the manufacturer. The publisher does not warrant or guarantee any product described here, and does not perform any independent analysis of the information provided. Inclusion of a product in this book does not represent an endorsement, and the publisher does not necessarily advocate the use of any product listed.

# Alpharma
## U.S. Pharmaceuticals Division

**7205 WINDSOR BOULEVARD
BALTIMORE, MD 21244**

**For General Inquiries Contact:**
Customer Service
(800) 638-9096

---

**PERMETHRIN LOTION 1%**
Lice Treatment

**Description:**
**EACH FLUID OUNCE CONTAINS:** Active Ingredient: Permethrin 280 mg (1%). Inactive Ingredients: Balsam fir canada, cetyl alcohol, citric acid, FD&C Yellow No. 6, fragrance, hydrolyzed animal protein, hydroxyethyl cellulose, polyoxyethylene 10 cetyl ether, propylene glycol, stearalkonium chloride, water, isopropyl alcohol 5.6 g (20%), methylparaben 56 mg (0.2%), and propylparaben 22 mg (0.08%).
Permethrin Lotion 1% kills lice and their unhatched eggs with usually only one application. Permethrin Lotion 1% protects against head lice reinfestation for 14 days. The creme rinse formula leaves hair manageable and easy to comb.

**Indications:** For the treatment of head lice. For prophylactic use during head lice epidemics.

**Warnings:** For external use only. Keep out of eyes when rinsing hair. Adults and children: Close eyes and do not open eyes until product is rinsed out. If product gets into the eyes, immediately flush with water. Do not use near the eyes or permit contact with mucous membranes, such as inside the nose, mouth, or vagina, as irritation may occur. Children: Also protect children's eyes with a washcloth, towel or other suitable material or method. This product should not be used on pediatric patients less than 2 months of age. Itching, redness, or swelling of the scalp may occur. If skin irritation persists or infection is present or develops, discontinue use and consult a doctor. Consult a doctor if infestation of eyebrows or eyelashes occurs. This product may cause breathing difficulty or an asthmatic episode in susceptible persons. As with any drug, if you are pregnant or nursing a baby, seek the advice of a health professional before using this product. Keep this and all drugs out of the reach of children. In case of accidental ingestion, seek professional assistance or contact a Poison Control Center immediately.

**Dosage and Administration:**
**Treatment:** Permethrin Lotion 1% should be used after hair has been washed with patient's regular shampoo, rinsed with water and towel dried. A sufficient amount should be applied to satu-rate hair and scalp (especially behind the ears and on the nape of the neck). Leave on hair for 10 minutes but not longer. Rinse with water. A single application is usually sufficient. If live lice are observed seven days or more after the first application of this product, a second treatment should be given. For proper head lice management, remove nits with the nit comb provided.
Head lice live on the scalp and lay small white eggs (nits) on the hair shaft close to the scalp. The nits are most easily found on the nape of the neck or behind the ears. All personal headgear, scarfs, coats, and bed linen should be disinfected by machine washing in hot water and drying, using the hot cycle of a dryer for at least 20 minutes. Personal articles of clothing or bedding that cannot be washed may be dry-cleaned, sealed in a plastic bag for a period of about 2 weeks, or sprayed with a product specifically designed for this purpose. Personal combs and brushes may be disinfected by soaking in hot water (above 130°F) for 5 to 10 minutes. Thorough vacuuming of rooms inhabited by infected patients is recommended.
**Prophylaxis:** Prophylactic use of Permethrin Lotion 1% is only recommended for individuals exposed to head lice epidemics in which at least 20% of the population at an institution are infested and for immediate household members of infested individuals. Casual use is strongly discouraged.
The method of application of Permethrin Lotion 1% for prophylaxis is identical to that described above for treatment of a lice infestation except nit removal is not required.

**Directions For Use:** One application of Permethrin Lotion 1% has been shown to protect greater than 95% of patients against reinfestation for at least two weeks. In epidemic settings, a second prophylactic application is recommended two weeks after the first because the life cycle of a head louse is approximately four weeks.

**How Supplied:** Bottles of 2 fl. oz. (59 mL) with nit removal comb and Family Pack of 2 bottles, 2 fl. oz. (59 mL) each, with 2 nit removal combs.
Store at 15° to 25°C (59° to 77°F).
Manufactured by
**Alpharma USPD Inc.**
Baltimore, MD 21244
FORM NO. 5242          Rev. 9/99
                        VC1587

---

**IF YOU SUSPECT
AN INTERACTION. . .**
The 1,800-page
*PDR Companion Guide*™ can help.
Use the order form
in the front of this book.

---

# Bayer Corporation
## Consumer Care Division

**36 COLUMBIA ROAD
P.O. BOX 1910
MORRISTOWN, NJ 07962-1910**

**Direct Inquiries to:**
Consumer Relations
(800) 331-4536
www.bayercare.com

**For Medical Emergency Contact:**
Bayer Corporation
Consumer Care Division
(800) 331-4536

---

**ALEVE®**
**All Day Strong**
**naproxen sodium tablets, 220 mg**
**Pain reliever/fever reducer**

**ALEVE®** Caplets*, Gelcaps**, or Tablets
Naproxen Sodium Tablets, USP

**Active Ingredient:**          **Purpose:**
**(in each tablet/caplet/gelcap)**
Naproxen sodium 220 mg (naproxen 200 mg) ...... Pain reliever/Fever reducer

**Uses:** Temporarily relieves minor aches and pains due to:
• common cold
• headache
• toothache
• muscular aches
• backache
• menstrual cramps
• minor pain of arthritis
temporarily reduces fever

**Warnings: Allergy Alert:** Naproxen sodium may cause a severe allergic reaction which may include:
• hives
• facial swelling
• asthma (wheezing)
• shock

**Alcohol warning:** If you consume 3 or more alcoholic drinks every day, ask your doctor whether you should take naproxen sodium or other pain relievers/fever reducers. Naproxen sodium may cause stomach bleeding.

**Do not use** if you have ever had an allergic reaction to any other pain reliever/fever reducer

**Ask a doctor before use if you have** had serious side effects from any pain reliever/fever reducer

**Ask a doctor or pharmacist before use if you are**
• taking any other product that contains naproxen sodium or any other pain reliever/fever reducer
• taking other drugs on a regular basis
• under a doctor's care for any continuing condition

**Stop use and ask a doctor if:**
• an allergic reaction occurs. Seek medical help right away.
• any new or unexpected symptoms occur
• symptoms continue or worsen

| Over age 65 | 1 caplet every 12 hours. Do not exceed 1 caplet in 12 hours, unless directed by a doctor. |
|---|---|
| 12–65 years | take 1 caplet every 8 to 12 hours. For the first dose you may take 2 caplets within the first hour. Do not take more than 2 caplets in any 8 to 12 hours, or 3 caplets in a 24 hour period. The smallest effective dose should be used. |
| under 12 years | • ask a doctor |

| Over age 65 | 1 gelcap every 12 hours. Do not exceed 1 gelcap in 12 hours, unless directed by a doctor. |
|---|---|
| 12–65 years | take 1 gelcap every 8 to 12 hours. For the first dose you may take 2 gelcaps within the first hour. Do not take more than 2 gelcaps in any 8 to 12 hours, or 3 gelcaps in a 24 hour period. The smallest effective dose should be used. |
| under 12 years | • ask a doctor |

| Over age 65 | 1 tablet every 12 hours. Do not exceed 1 tablet in 12 hours, unless directed by a doctor. |
|---|---|
| 12–65 years | take 1 tablet every 8 to 12 hours. For the first dose you may take 2 tablets within the first hour. Do not take more than 2 tablets in any 8 to 12 hours, or 3 tablets in a 24 hour period. The smallest effective dose should be used. |
| under 12 years | • ask a doctor |

• you have difficulty swallowing or it feels like the pill is stuck in your throat
• you develop heartburn
• stomach pain occurs with use of this product or if even mild symptoms persist
• pain worsens or lasts for more than 10 days
• fever lasts for more than 3 days
• painful area is red or swollen

**If pregnant or breast-feeding,** ask a health professional before use. It is especially important not to use naproxen sodium during the last 3 months of pregnancy unless definitely directed to do so by a doctor because it may cause problems in the unborn child or complications during delivery.

**Keep out of reach of children.** In case of overdose, get medical help or contact a Poison Control Center right away.

**Directions:**
• do not take more than directed
• **drink a full glass of water with each dose**

**ALEVE® Caplets**
[See first table above]

**ALEVE® Gelcaps**
[See second table above]

**ALEVE® Tablets**
[See third table above]

**Other Information:**
• store at 20–25°C (68–77°F)
• avoid high humidity and excessive heat 40°C (104°F)

**ALEVE® Caplets**
• **each caplet contains:** sodium 20 mg

**ALEVE® Gelcaps**
• **each gelcap contains:** sodium 20 mg

**ALEVE® Tablets**
• **each tablet contains:** sodium 20 mg

**Inactive Ingredients:**
**ALEVE® Caplets:** Magnesium stearate, microcrystalline cellulose, opadry YS-1-4215, povidone, talc.
**ALEVE® Gelcaps:** D&C yellow #10 lake, disodium EDTA, edible ink, FD&C blue #1, FD&C yellow #6 lake, gelatin, glycerin, hydroxypropyl methylcellulose, magnesium stearate, microcrystalline cellulose, polyethylene glycol, povidone, stearic acid, talc, titanium dioxide, triacetin.
**ALEVE® Tablets** Magnesium stearate, microcrystalline cellulose, opadry YS-1-4215, povidone, talc.

---

\* capsule-shaped tablet(s)
\*\* gelatin coated capsule-shaped tablet(s)

**How Supplied:**
**ALEVE® Caplets** in boxes of 8, 24, 50, 100, 150, 200.
**ALEVE® Gelcaps** in boxes of 20, 40, 80.
**ALEVE® Tablets** in boxes of 24, 50, 100, 150.

***Questions or comments?*** call **1-800-395-0689** or www.aleve.com

Do not use if carton is open or if foil seal imprinted with "Safety *SQUEASE®*" on bottle opening is missing or broken.

Distributed by
Bayer Corporation
PO Box 1910
Morristown, NJ 07962-1910 USA
B-R LLC
*Read Consumer*
*Leaflet Before Use*

*Shown in Product Identification Guide, page 503*

## ALEVE® COLD & SINUS
**Pain reliever/fever reducer/nasal decongestant**

**Active ingredients:**
**(in each caplet)**                    **Purpose:**
Naproxen sodium 220 mg
(naproxen 200 mg) ... Pain reliever/fever reducer
Pseudoephedrine HCl 120 mg, extended-release ..... Nasal decongestant

**Uses:** temporarily relieves these cold, sinus and flu symptoms:
• sinus pressure
• minor body aches and pains
• headache
• nasal and sinus congestion (promotes sinus drainage and restores freer breathing through the nose)
• fever

**Warnings:**
**Allergy alert:** Naproxen sodium may cause a severe allergic reaction which may include:
• hives
• facial swelling
• asthma (wheezing)
• shock

**Alcohol warning:** If you consume 3 or more alcoholic drinks every day, ask your doctor whether you should take naproxen sodium or other pain relievers/fever reducers. Naproxen sodium may cause stomach bleeding.

**Do not use if you**
• have ever had an allergic reaction to any other pain reliever/fever reducer
• are now taking a prescription monoamine oxidase inhibitor (MAOI) (certain drugs for depression, psychiatric or emotional conditions, or Parkinson's disease), or for 2 weeks after stopping the MAOI drug. If you do not know if your prescription drug contains an MAOI, ask a doctor or pharmacist before taking this product.

**Ask a doctor before use if you have**
• heart disease
• high blood pressure
• thyroid disease
• diabetes
• trouble urinating due to an enlarged prostate gland
• had serious side effects from any pain reliever/fever reducer

**Ask a doctor or pharmacist before use if you are**
• using any other product containing naproxen or pseudoephedrine
• taking any other pain reliever/fever reducer or nasal decongestant
• under a doctor's care for any continuing medical condition
• taking other drugs on a regular basis

**When using this product**
• **do not use more than directed**

**Stop use and ask a doctor if**
• an allergic reaction occurs. Seek medical help right away.
• you get nervous, dizzy, or sleepless
• you develop heartburn
• nasal congestion lasts more than 7 days
• symptoms continue or get worse
• you have trouble swallowing or the caplet feels stuck in your thoat
• new or unexpected symptoms occur

***Continued on next page***

## Aleve Cold & Sinus—Cont.

- stomach pain occurs with use of this product or if even mild symptoms persist
- fever lasts for more than 3 days

**If pregnant or breast-feeding,** ask a health professional before use.

It is especially important not to use naproxen sodium during the last 3 months of pregnancy unless definitely directed to do so by a doctor because it may cause problems in the unborn child or complications during delivery.

**Keep out of reach of children.** In case of overdose, get medical help or contact a Poison Control Center right away.

**Directions:**
- **swallow whole;** do not crush or chew
- **drink a full glass of water with each dose**
- adults and children 12 years and older: **1 caplet every 12 hours;** do not take more than 2 caplets in 24 hours
- children under 12 years: ask a doctor

**Other information:**
- **each caplet contains:** sodium 20 mg
- store at 20 to 25° C (68–77°F)
- store in a dry place

**Inactive Ingredients:** colloidal silicon dioxide, FD&C blue #1 lake, hydroxypropyl methylcellulose, lactose, magnesium stearate, microcrystalline cellulose, pharmaceutical glaze, polyethylene glycol, povidone, propylene glycol, talc, titanium dioxide

**Questions or Comments?** call **1-800-395-0689**

**How Supplied:** Boxes of 10 or 20 caplets (capsule-shaped tablets)
Distributed by: Bayer Corporation
Consumer Care Division
Morristown, NJ 07960 USA     B-R LLC
*Shown in Product Identification Guide, page 503*

---

## ALEVE® SINUS & HEADACHE
**Pain reliever/fever reducer/nasal decongestant**

**Active ingredients**
**(in each caplet)**          **Purpose:**
Naproxen sodium 220 mg
(naproxen 200 mg) ... Pain reliever/fever reducer
Pseudoephedrine HCl 120 mg,
extended-release ..... Nasal decongestant

**Uses:** temporarily relieves these cold, sinus and flu symptoms:
- sinus pressure
- minor body aches and pains
- headache
- nasal and sinus congestion (promotes sinus drainage and restores freer breathing through the nose)
- fever

**Warnings:  Allergy alert:** Naproxen sodium may cause a severe allergic reaction which may include:
- hives
- facial swelling
- asthma (wheezing)
- shock

**Alcohol warning:** If you consume 3 or more alcoholic drinks every day, ask your doctor whether you should take naproxen sodium or other pain relievers/fever reducers. Naproxen sodium may cause stomach bleeding.

**Do not use if you**
- have ever had an allergic reaction to any other pain reliever/fever reducer
- are now taking a prescription monoamine oxidase inhibitor (MAOI) (certain drugs for depression, psychiatric or emotional conditions, or Parkinson's disease), or for 2 weeks after stopping the MAOI drug. If you do not know if your prescription drug contains an MAOI, ask a doctor or pharmacist before taking this product.

**Ask a doctor before use if you have**
- heart disease
- high blood pressure
- thyroid disease
- diabetes
- trouble urinating due to an enlarged prostate gland
- had serious side effects from any pain reliever/fever reducer

**Ask a doctor or pharmacist before use if you are**
- using any other product containing naproxen or pseudoephedrine
- taking any other pain reliever/fever reducer or nasal decongestant
- under a doctor's care for any continuing medical condition
- taking other drugs on a regular basis

**When using this product • do not use more than directed**

**Stop use and ask a doctor if:**
- an allergic reaction occurs. Seek medical help right away.
- you get nervous, dizzy, or sleepless
- you develop heartburn
- nasal congestion lasts more than 7 days
- symptoms continue or get worse
- you have trouble swallowing or the caplet feels stuck in your throat
- new or unexpected symptoms occur
- stomach pain occurs with use of this product or if even mild symptoms persist
- fever lasts for more than 3 days

**If pregnant or breast-feeding,** ask a health professional before use. If is especially important not to use naproxen sodium during the last 3 months of pregnancy unless definitely directed to do so by a doctor because it may cause problems in the unborn child or complications during delivery.

**Keep out of reach of children.** If case of overdose, get medical help or contact a Poison Control Center right away.

**Directions:**
- **swallow whole;** do not crush or chew
- **drink a full glass of water with each dose**
- adults and children 12 years and older: **1 caplet every 12 hours;** do not take more than 2 caplets in 24 hours
- children under 12 years: ask a doctor

**Other Information: • each caplet contains:** sodium 20 mg
- store at 20 to 25°C (68–77°F)
- store in a dry place

**Inactive Ingredients:** Colloidal silicon dioxide, D&C yellow #10 lake, FD&C blue #1 lake, hydroxypropyl methylcellulose, lactose, magnesium stearate, microcrystalline cellulose, pharmaceutical glaze, polyethylene glycol, povidone, propylene glycol, talc, titanium dioxide

**Question or comments?** call **1-800-395-0689**

**How Supplied:** Box of 10 Caplets (Capsule-Shaped Tablets).
Visit our website at www.aleve.com
Distributed by:
Bayer Corporation
Consumer Care Division
PO Box 1910
Morristown, NJ 07962-1910 USA
B-R LLC
154043
*Shown in Product Identification Guide, page 503*

---

## ALKA-SELTZER® Original
## ALKA-SELTZER® Cherry
## ALKA-SELTZER® Extra Strength
## ALKA-SELTZER® Lemon Lime
**Effervescent Antacid Pain Reliever**

**Active Ingredients:**
**ALKA-SELTZER® Original, Cherry, and Lemon Lime:** Aspirin 325 mg, Citric acid 1000 mg, Sodium bicarbonate (heat-treated) 1916 mg.
**ALKA-SELTZER® Extra Strength:** Aspirin 500 mg, Citric acid 1000 mg, Sodium bicarbonate (heat-treated) 1985 mg.

**Inactive Ingredients:**
**ALKA-SELTZER® Original:** none.
**ALKA-SELTZER® Cherry:** artificial flavor, asparatame, dimethicone, docusate sodium, flavor, povidone, sodium benzoate, tableting aids.
**ALKA-SELTZER® Extra Strength:** flavors.
**ALKA-SELTZER® Lemon Lime:** aspartame, dimethicone, dimethyl polysiloxane, docusate sodium, flavor, povidone, sodium benzoate
**ALKA-SELTZER® Original:** 567 mg.
**ALKA-SELTZER® Cherry and Lemon Lime:** 503 mg.
**ALKA-SELTZER® Extra Strength:** 588 mg.

**Uses:** For fast relief of heartburn, acid indigestion, and sour stomach when accompanied with headache or body aches and pains, upset stomach with headache from over-indulgence in food and drink, pain alone (headache or body and muscular aches and pains).

**Warnings:  Reye's syndrome:** Children and teenagers should not use this medicine for chicken pox or flu symptoms before a doctor is consulted about Reye's syndrome, a rare but serious illness reported to be associated with aspirin.
**Alcohol warning:** If you consume 3 or more alcoholic drinks every day, ask your doctor whether you should take aspirin or other pain relievers/fever reducers. Aspirin may cause stomach bleeding.
**Do not use** if you have ever had an allergic reaction to aspirin or any other pain reliever/fever reducer.

**Ask a doctor before use if you have:**
- asthma
- ulcers
- bleeding problems
- stomach problems that last or come back frequently, such as heartburn, upset stomach, or pain

**Ask a doctor or pharmacist before use if you are**
- presently taking a prescription drug. Antacids may interact with certain prescription drugs
- taking a prescription drug for anticoagulation (thinning the blood)
- diabetes
- gout
- arthritis
- on a sodium restricted diet.

**Stop use and ask a doctor if:**
- an allergic reaction occurs. Seek medical help right away.
- symptoms get worse or last for more than 10 days.
- new symptoms occur.
- ringing in the ears or loss of hearing occurs.
- redness or swelling is present.

**If pregnant or breast-feeding,** ask a health professional before use. **It is especially important not to use aspirin during the last three months of pregnancy unless definitely directed to do so by a doctor because it may cause problems in the unborn child or complications during delivery.**

**Keep out of reach of children.** In case of accidental overdose, get medical help or contact a Poison Control Center right away.

**Other Information:**
**ALKA SELTZER® Original**
- **each tablet contains:** sodium 567 mg
- protect from excessive heat
- Alka-Seltzer in water contains principally the antacid sodium citrate and the analgesic sodium acetylsalicylate

**ALKA SELTZER® Cherry**
- **each tablet contains:** sodium 503 mg
- **phenylketonurics:** contains phenylalanine 12.3 mg per tablet
- protect from excessive heat
- Alka-Seltzer Cherry in water contains principally the antacid sodium citrate and the analgesic sodium acetylsalicylate

**ALKA SELTZER® Lemon-Lime**
- **each tablet contains:** sodium 503 mg
- **phenylketonurics:** contains phenylalanine 9 mg per tablet
- protect from excessive heat
- Alka-Seltzer Lemon-Lime in water contains principally the antacid sodium citrate and the analgesic sodium acetylsalicylate

**ALKA SELTZER® Extra Strength**
- **each tablet contains:** sodium 588 mg
- protect from excessive heat
- Alka-Seltzer Extra Strength in water contains principally the antacid sodium citrate and the analgesic sodium acetylsalicylate.

**Directions:**
**ALKA SELTZER® Original**
**ALKA SELTZER® Cherry**
**ALKA SELTZER® Lemon Lime**
Do not exceed recommended dosage. Fully dissolve tablets in 4 ounces of water before taking.
Adults and Children 12 years and over: 2 tablets every 4 hours, or as directed by a doctor not to exceed 8 tablets in 24 hours. (60 years or older, 2 tablets

| adults and children 12 years and older | 2 tablets every 4 hours as needed, or as directed by a doctor. | do not exceed 8 tablets in 24 hours or as directed by a doctor. |
|---|---|---|
| adult 60 years of age and older | 2 tablets every 4 hours as needed, or as directed by a doctor. | do not exceed 4 tablets in 24 hours or as directed by a doctor. |
| children under 12 years | Ask a doctor. | |

every 4 hours, or as directed by a doctor not to exceed 4 tablets in 24 hours).

**ALKA SELTZER® Extra Strength**
**Do not exceed recommended dosage.** Fully dissolve tablets in 4 ounces of water before taking.
Adults and Children 12 years and over: 2 tablets every 6 hours, or as directed by a doctor not to exceed 7 tablets in 24 hours. (60 years or older, 2 tablets every 6 hours, or as directed by a doctor not to exceed 4 tablets in 24 hours).

Place two (2) tablets in 4 oz of water. Dissolve tablets completely. You do not have to drink any of the residue that may be on the bottom of the glass. The medicines of Alka-Seltzer are in the water.

Take Alka-Seltzer any time—morning, noon, or night—when you need relief from heartburn, acid indigestion, sour stomach with headache, or body aches and pains.

**How Supplied:** 24 Foil Packs of Effervecent Tablets.
For more information visit our web site at www.alka-seltzer.com
**Questions or comments?**
Please call **1-800-800-4793**.
Made in U.S.A.
Bayer Corporation, Consumer Care Division
P.O. Box 1910
Morristown, NJ 07962-1910 USA
*Shown in Product Identification Guide, page 503*

---

## ALKA-SELTZER® HEARTBURN RELIEF
**Antacid Medicine**

**Active Ingredients:**      **Purpose:**
**(In each tablet)**
Citric acid 1000 mg ..................... antacid
Sodium bicarbonate (heat-treated) 1940 mg ........................................ antacid

**Inactive Ingredients:** acesulfame potassium, aspartame, flavor enhancer, flavors, magnesium stearate, mannitol

**Uses:**
Provides relief of:
- heartburn
- acid indigestion
- upset stomach associated with the above conditions

**Warnings:**
**Do not use** this product if you are on a sodium-restricted diet unless directed by a doctor.

**Ask a doctor or pharmacist before use if you are** presently taking a prescription drug. Antacids may interact with certain prescription drugs.
**When using this product do not exceed recommended dosage.**
**Stop use and ask a doctor if** symptoms last for more than 2 weeks.
**If pregnant or breast-feeding,** ask a health professional before use.
**Keep out of reach of children.**

**Directions:** Fully dissolve tablets in 4 ounces of water before taking.
[See table above]

**Other Information:**
- **each tablet contains:** sodium 578 mg.
- **phenylketonurics:** contains phenylalanine 5.6 mg per tablet
- Alka-Seltzer Heartburn Relief in water contains the antacid sodium citrate as the principal active ingredient.

**How Supplied:** Alka-Seltzer Heartburn Relief is available in 24 or 36 count packages in lemon lime flavor.
***Questions or comments:*** 1-800-800-4793 or www.alka-seltzer.com
Bayer Corporation
Consumer Care Division
Morristown, NJ 07960
USA
*Shown in Product Identification Guide, page 503*

---

## ALKA-SELTZER® MORNING RELIEF
**Pain Reliever, Alertness Aid**
**For Morning Headache and Fatigue with Caffeine**
- Fast Headache Relief
- Increases Alertness
- Gentle on your stomach

**Active Ingredients:**      **Purpose:**
**(in each tablet)**
Aspirin 500 mg .......................... analgesic
Caffeine 65 mg ........... alertness aid/pain reliever aid

**Inactive Ingredients:** acesulfame potassium, aspartame, citric acid, dimethicone, docusate sodium, flavor, mannitol, povidone, sodium benzoate, sodium bicarbonate

**Uses:**
- for the temporary relief of minor aches and pains with fatigue or drowsiness associated with a hangover
- also effective for headaches, body aches and pains alone

**Warnings:**
**Reye's syndrome:** Children and teenagers should not use this medicine for chicken pox or flu symptoms before a doctor is consulted about Reye's syndrome, a rare but serious illness reported to be associated with aspirin.

*Continued on next page*

| adults and children 12 years and over | 2 tablets every 6 hours, as needed, or as directed by a doctor | do not exceed 8 tablets in 24 hours or as directed by a doctor |
|---|---|---|
| adults 60 years and over | 2 tablets every 6 hours, as needed, or as directed by a doctor | do not exceed 4 tablets in 24 hours or as directed by a doctor |
| children under 12 years | do not use | |

## Alka-Seltzer Morning—Cont.

**Alcohol warning:** If you consume 3 or more alcoholic drinks every day, ask your doctor whether you should take aspirin or other pain relievers/fever reducers. Aspirin may cause stomach bleeding.

**Do not use:**
- if you have ever had an allergic reaction to any pain reliever/fever reducer
- this product if you are on a sodium restricted diet unless directed by a doctor
- in children under 12 years of age

**Ask a doctor before use if you have:**
- asthma
- ulcers
- bleeding problems
- stomach problems that last or come back, such as heartburn, upset stomach, or pain

**Ask a doctor or pharmacist before use if you are** taking a prescription drug for
- anticoagulation (blood thinning)
- gout
- diabetes
- arthritis

**When using this product**
- limit the use of caffeine-containing medications, foods, beverages because too much caffeine may cause nervousness, irritability, sleeplessness, and occasionally, rapid heart beat. The recommended dose of this product contains about as much caffeine as a cup of coffee.
- if fatigue or drowsiness persists or continues to recur, consult a doctor. For occasional use only. Not intended for use as a substitute for sleep.

**Stop use and ask a doctor if:**
- allergic reaction occurs. Seek medical attention right away
- pain gets worse or lasts more than 10 days
- new symptoms occur
- ringing in the ears or loss of hearing occurs
- redness or swelling is present

**If pregnant or breast-feeding,** ask a health professional before use. **It is especially important not to use aspirin during the last 3 months of pregnancy unless definitely directed to do so by a doctor because it may cause problems in the unborn child or complications during delivery.**

**Keep out of reach of children.** In case of overdose, get medical help or contact a Poison Control Center right away.

**Directions:**
- do not exceed recommended dosage
- do not use for more than 2 days for hangover
- fully dissolve Alka-Seltzer Morning Relief tablets in 4 ounces of water before taking
[See table above]

**Other Information:**
- **each tablet contains:** sodium 415 mg
- **phenylketonurics:** contains phenylalanine 9 mg per tablet

**How Supplied:** Packet of 24 Citrus Effervescent Tablets
*Questions or comments?*
**1-800-800-4793** or www.alka-seltzer.com
For more information visit our website at www.alka-seltzer.com
Questions? Comments?
Please call 1-800-800-4793.
Bayer Corporation
Consumer Care Division
P.O. Box 1910
Morristown, NJ 07962-1910 USA
*Shown in Product Identification Guide, page 503*

---

## ALKA-SELTZER PLUS® COLD MEDICINE
**Analgesic, Antihistamine, Nasal Decongestant**

## ALKA-SELTZER PLUS® COLD MEDICINE
Also in **Cherry Burst and Orange Zest Flavors**
**Analgesic, Antihistamine, Nasal Decongestant**

## ALKA-SELTZER PLUS® COLD & SINUS MEDICINE
**Non-Drowsy Medicine**
**Analgesic, Nasal Decongestant**

## ALKA-SELTZER PLUS® COLD & COUGH MEDICINE
**Antihistamine, Cough Suppressant, Nasal Decongestant**

## ALKA-SELTZER PLUS® NIGHT-TIME COLD MEDICINE
**Cough Suppressant, Antihistamine, Nasal Decongestant**

## ALKA-SELTZER PLUS® FLU MEDICINE
**Analgesic, Cough Suppressant, Nasal Decongestant**

[See table below]
[See first table at top of next page]

**Uses:**
[See second table at top of next page]

**Directions:**
[See table at top of page 608]

**WARNINGS:**
(Specific to Flu formula:)
**Reye's syndrome:** Children and teenagers should not use this medicine for chicken pox or flu symptoms before a doctor is consulted about Reye's syndrome, a rare but serious illness reported to be associated with aspirin.

**Alcohol Warning:** If you consume 3 or more alcoholic drinks every day, ask your doctor whether you should take aspirin or other pain relievers/fever reducers. Aspirin may cause stomach bleeding.

(Specific to Cold, Cold & Sinus formula:)
**Alcohol Warning:** If you consume 3 or more alcoholic drinks every day, ask your doctor whether you should take acetaminophen or other pain relievers/fever reducers. Acetaminophen may cause liver damage.

**Active Ingredients:**

| per tablet | Cold | Cherry Burst | Orange Zest | Cold & Sinus | Cold & Cough | Night-Time | Flu |
|---|---|---|---|---|---|---|---|
| Aspirin 500 mg | | | | | | | √ |
| Acetaminophen 250 mg | √ | √ | √ | √ | | | |
| Chlorpheniramine maleate 2 mg | √ | √ | √ | | | | √ |
| Dextromethorphan HBr 10 mg | | | | | √ | √ | |
| Dextromethorphan HBr 15 mg | | | | | | | √ |
| Doxylamine succinate 6.25 mg | | | | | | √ | |
| Phenylephrine HCl 5 mg | √ | √ | √ | √ | √ | √ | |

## Inactive Ingredients:

| per softgel | Cold | Cherry Burst | Orange Zest | Cold Sinus | Cold & Cough | Night-Time | Flu |
|---|---|---|---|---|---|---|---|
| FD&C Red #40 | | √ | √ | | | | √ |
| FD&C Yellow #6 | | | √ | | | | √ |
| acesulfame potassium | √ | √ | √ | √ | | √ | |
| aspartame | √ | √ | √ | √ | | √ | √ |
| citric acid | √ | √ | √ | √ | √ | √ | √ |
| dimethicone | | | | | | | √ |
| docusate sodium | | | | | | | √ |
| flavors | √ | √ | √ | √ | √ | √ | √ |
| fumaric acid | √ | √ | √ | √ | √ | √ | √ |
| glyceryl behenate | √ | √ | √ | √ | √ | √ | |
| maltodextrin | √ | √ | √ | √ | √ | √ | |
| mannitol | | | | | | | √ |
| povidone | | | | | | | √ |
| poyethylene glycol behenate | √ | √ | √ | √ | √ | √ | |
| sodium benzoate | | | | | | | √ |
| sodium bicarbonate | √ | √ | √ | √ | √ | √ | |
| sodium saccharin | | | | | | | √ |
| sorbitol | √ | √ | √ | √ | √ | √ | |

| per tablet | Cold | Cherry Burst | Orange Zest | Cold & Sinus | Cold & Cough | Night-Time | Flu |
|---|---|---|---|---|---|---|---|
| body aches & pains | √ | √ | √ | | | | √ |
| headache | √ | √ | √ | √ | | | √ |
| coughing | | | | | √ | √ | √ |
| fever | √ | √ | √ | | | | √ |
| runny nose | √ | √ | √ | | √ | √ | √ |
| sinus pain & pressure | | | | √ | | | |
| sneezing | √ | √ | √ | | | | √ |
| nasal & sinus congestion | √ | √ | √ | √ | √ | √ | |
| sore throat | √ | √ | √ | | | | √ |

**(Specific to Cold, Flu formula:)**
**Sore throat warning:** If sore throat is severe, persists for more than 2 days, is accompanied or followed by fever, headache, rash, nausea, or vomiting, consult a doctor promptly.
**Do not use:**
• if you are now taking a prescription monoamine oxidase inhibitor (MAOI) (certain drugs for depression, psychiatric or emotional conditions, or Parkinson's disease), or for 2 weeks after stopping the MAOI drug. If you are uncertain whether your prescription drug contains an MAOI, ask a doctor or pharmacist before taking this product.

**(Specific to Flu formula:)**
• if you are allergic to aspirin or any other pain reliever/fever reducer.
**(Specific to Cold, Cold & Sinus:)**
• with any other products containing acetaminophen
**Ask a doctor before use if you have**
• difficulty in urination due to enlargement of the prostate gland
• a breathing problem such as emphysema or chronic bronchitis
**(Specific to Cold & Cough, Night-Time, Flu formula:)**
• persistent or chronic cough such as occurs with smoking, asthma, or emphysema
• cough with excessive phlegm (mucus)

**(Specific to Flu formula:)**
• a breathing problem such as emphysema or chronic bronchitis, or asthma
• stomach problems that persist or recur
**(Specific to Cold, Cold & Sinus, Cold & Cough, Night-Time formula:)**
• heart disease, high blood pressure, diabetes, thyroid disease
**(Specific to Cold, Cold & Cough, Night-Time, Flu formula:)**
• glaucoma
**Ask a doctor or pharmacist before use if you are:**
**(Specific to Cold, Cold & Cough, Night-Time, Flu formula:)**
• taking sedatives or tranquilizers
**(Specific to Cold & Cough, Night-Time, Flu formula:)**
• on a sodium restricted diet
**(Specific to Flu formula:)**
• taking a prescription drug for anticoagulation (blood thinning), diabetes, gout, arthritis
**When using this product:**
• **do not exceed recommended dosage (Specific to Cold, Cold & Cough, Flu formula:)**
• you may get drowsy
**(Specific to Night-Time formula:)**
• you may get markedly drowsy
**(Specific to Cold, Cold & Cough, Night-Time, Flu formula:)**
• avoid alcoholic drinks
• excitability may occur, especially in children
• alcohol, sedatives, and tranquilizers may increase drowsiness
• be careful when driving a motor vehicle or operating machinery
**Stop use and ask a doctor if:**
• nervousness, dizziness, or sleeplessness occurs
• symptoms do not improve within 7 days or are accompanied by a fever
• fever gets worse or lasts for more than 3 days
• redness or swelling is present
• new symptoms occur
**(Specific to Cold & Cough, Night-Time, Flu formula:)**
• cough persists for more than 7 days, tends to recur, or is accompanied by a fever, rash, or persistent headache. These may be signs of a serious condition.
**(Specific to Flu formula:)**
• ringing in the ears or loss of hearing occurs
**If pregnant or breast-feeding,** ask a health professional before use.
**(Specific to Flu formula:)**
**Keep out of reach of children.** In case of overdose, get medical help or contact a Poison Control Center right away. Prompt medical attention is critical for adults as well as children even if you do not notice any signs or symptoms.
**Other Information:**
• this product does not contain phenylpropanolamine (PPA)
• protect from excessive heat
**How Supplied:**
**Specific to Cold Medicine:** Contains 12, 20, and 36 Effervescent Tablets.
**Specific to Cold & Sinus Medicine, Cold & Cough Medicine, Night-Time Cold Medicine, Flu Medicine:** Contains 20 Effervescent Tablets.
*Questions or comments?*
1-800-800-4793 or
www.alka-seltzerplus.com

*Continued on next page*

**ALKA-SELTZER PLUS® COLD MEDICINE (Cherry Burst and Orange Zest)**
**ALKA-SELTZER PLUS® COLD & SINUS MEDICINE**
**ALKA-SELTZER PLUS® COLD & COUGH MEDICINE**

| adults and children 12 years and over | take 2 tablets fully dissolved in 4 oz. of water every 4 hours | do not exceed 8 tablets in 24 hours or as directed by a doctor |
|---|---|---|
| children under 12 years | consult a doctor | |

**ALKA-SELTZER PLUS® NIGHT-TIME COLD MEDICINE**

| adults and children 12 years and over | take 2 tablets fully dissolved in 4 oz. of water at bedtime (may be taken every 4 hours) | do not exceed 8 tablets in 24 hours or as directed by a doctor |
|---|---|---|
| children under 12 years | consult a doctor | |

**ALKA-SELTZER PLUS® FLU MEDICINE**

| adults and children 12 years and over | take 2 tablets fully dissolved in 4 oz. of water every 6 hours | do not exceed 8 tablets in 24 hours or as directed by a doctor |
|---|---|---|
| children under 12 years | consult a doctor | |

**Alka-Seltzer Plus Cold—Cont.**

Bayer Corporation
Consumer Care Division
Morristown, NJ 07960 USA
*Shown in Product Identification
Guide, page 503*

---

**ALKA-SELTZER PLUS®
COLD MEDICINE
LIQUI-GELS®**
Analgesic, Antihistamine, Nasal
Decongestant

**ALKA-SELTZER PLUS®
COLD& SINUS MEDICINE
LIQUI-GELS®**
Analgesic, Nasal Decongestant

**ALKA-SELTZER PLUS®
COLD& COUGH MEDICINE
LIQUI-GELS®**
Analgesic, Antihistamine, Cough
Suppressant, Nasal Decongestant

**ALKA-SELTZER PLUS®
NIGHT-TIME COLD MEDICINE
LIQUI-GELS®**
Analgesic, Cough Suppressant,
Antihistamine, Nasal Decongestant

**ALKA-SELTZER PLUS®
FLU MEDICINE
LIQUI-GELS®**
Analgesic, Cough Suppressant, Nasal
Decongestant

[See first table to the right]
[See second table to the right]
[See first table at top of next page]
[See second table at top of next page]

**Warnings:**
**Alcohol warning:** If you consume 3 or more alcoholic drinks every day, ask your doctor whether you should take acetaminophen or other pain relievers/fever reducers.
Acetaminophen may cause liver damage.
**Specific to Cold, Cold & Cough, Night-Time, Flu formulas:**

**Sore throat warning:** If sore throat is severe, persists for more than 2 days, is accompanied or followed by fever, headache, rash, nausea, or vomiting, consult a doctor promptly.

**Do not use:**
• with any other products containing acetaminophen
• if you are now taking a prescription monoamine oxidase inhibitor (MAOI) (certain drugs for depression, psychiatric or emotional conditions, or Parkinson's disease), or for 2 weeks after stopping the MAOI drug. If you are uncertain whether your prescription drug contains an MAOI, ask a doctor or pharmacist before taking this product.

**Ask a doctor before use if you have:**
• heart disease, high blood pressure, diabetes, thyroid disease
• difficulty in urination due to enlargement of the prostate gland

**Specific to Cold, Cold & Cough, Night-Time formulas:**
• breathing problems such as emphysema or chronic bronchitis
• glaucoma

**Specific to Cold & Cough, Night-Time, Flu formulas:**
• persistent or chronic cough such as occurs with smoking, asthma, or emphysema

**Active Ingredients:**

| Per softgel | Cold | Cold & Sinus | Cold & Cough | Night-Time | Flu |
|---|---|---|---|---|---|
| Acetaminophen 325 mg | √ | √ | √ | √ | √ |
| Chlorpheniramine maleate 2 mg | √ | | √ | | |
| Dextromethorphan hydrobromide 10 mg | | | √ | √ | √ |
| Doxylamine succinate 6.25 mg | | | | √ | |
| Pseudophedrine HCl 30 mg | √ | √ | √ | √ | √ |

**Inactive Ingredients:**

| per softgel | Cold | Cold & Sinus | Cold & Cough | Night-Time | Flu |
|---|---|---|---|---|---|
| FD&C blue #1 | √ | | √ | √ | |
| FD&C red #40 | √ | √ | | | √ |
| D&C red #33 | | √ | | | |
| D&C yellow #10 | | | | √ | |
| gelatin | √ | √ | √ | √ | √ |
| glycerin | √ | √ | √ | √ | √ |
| polyethylene glycol | √ | √ | √ | √ | √ |
| polyvinyl acetate phthalate | √ | √ | √ | √ | √ |
| potassium acetate | √ | √ | √ | √ | √ |
| povidone | √ | √ | √ | √ | √ |
| propylene glycol | √ | √ | √ | √ | √ |
| sorbitol | √ | √ | √ | √ | √ |
| titanium dioxide | √ | √ | √ | √ | √ |
| Water | √ | √ | √ | √ | √ |

## Uses:

| | Cold | Cold & Sinus | Cold & Cough | Night-Time | Flu |
|---|:---:|:---:|:---:|:---:|:---:|
| body aches & pains | √ | | √ | √ | √ |
| headache | √ | √ | √ | √ | √ |
| coughing | | | √ | √ | √ |
| fever | √ | | √ | √ | √ |
| runny nose | √ | | √ | √ | |
| sinus pain & pressure | | √ | | | |
| sneezing | √ | | √ | √ | |
| nasal & sinus congestion | √ | √ | √ | √ | √ |
| sore throat | √ | | √ | √ | √ |

## Directions:

### ALKA-SELTZER PLUS® COLD MEDICINE LIQUI-GELS®

| adults and children 12 years and over | swallow 2 softgels with water every 4 hours | do not exceed 8 softgels in 24 hours or as directed by a doctor |
|---|---|---|
| children under 12 years | consult a doctor | |

### ALKA-SELTZER PLUS® NIGHT-TIME COLD MEDICINE LIQUI-GELS®

| adults and children 12 years and over | swallow 2 softgels with water at bedtime (may be taken every 6 hours) | do not exceed 8 softgels in 24 hours or as directed by a doctor |
|---|---|---|
| children under 12 years | consult a doctor | |

### ALKA-SELTZER PLUS® COLD & SINUS MEDICINE LIQUI-GELS®
### ALKA-SELTZER PLUS® COLD & COUGH MEDICINE LIQUI-GELS®
### ALKA-SELTZER PLUS® FLU MEDICINE LIQUI-GELS®

| adults and children 12 years and over | swallow 2 softgels with water every 4 hours | do not exceed 8 softgels in 24 hours or as directed by a doctor |
|---|---|---|
| children 6 to under 12 years | take 1 softgel with water every 4 hours | do not exceed 4 softgels in 24 hours or as directed by a doctor |
| children under 6 years | consult a doctor | |

• cough with excessive phlegm (mucus)

**Specific to Cold, Cold & Cough, Night-Time formulas:**

**Ask a doctor or pharmacist before use if you are** taking sedatives or tranquilizers.

**When using this product:**
• **do not exceed recommended dosage**

**Specific to Cold & Cough, Night-Time formulas:**
• you may get markedly drowsy

**Specific to Cold, Cold & Sinus formula:**
• you may get drowsy

**Specific to Cold, Cold & Cough, Night-Time formulas:**
• avoid alcoholic drinks
• excitability may occur, especially in children
• alcohol, sedatives, and tranquilizers may increase drowsiness
• be careful when driving motor vehicle or operating machinery

**Stop use and ask a doctor if:**
• nervousness, dizziness, or sleeplessness occurs
• symptoms do not improve within 7 days or are accompanied by a fever
• fever gets worse or lasts for more than 3 days
• redness or swelling is present
• new symptoms occur

**Specific to Cold & Cough, Night-Time, Flu formulas:**
• cough persists for more than 7 days, tends to recur, or is accompanied by a fever, rash, or persistent headache. These may be signs of a serious condition.

**If pregnant or breast-feeding,** ask a health professional before use.

**Keep out of reach of children.** In case of overdose, get medical help or contact a Poison Control Center right away. Prompt medical attention is critical for adults as well as children even if you do not notice any signs or symptoms.

## Other Information:
• this product does not contain phenylpropanolamine (PPA)
• store at room temperature and avoid excessive heat

**How Supplied:** ALKA-SELTZER PLUS® Cold Medicine, ALKA-SELTZER PLUS® Cold & Cough Medicine, ALKA-SELTZER PLUS® Night-Time Cold Medicine: Carton of 20 softgels. ALKA-SELTZER PLUS® Cold & Sinus Medicine, ALKA-SELTZER PLUS® Flu Non-Drowsy Medicine: Carton of 12 softgels.

*Questions or comments?* 1-800-800-4793 or www.alka-seltzerplus.com
Distributed by:
Bayer Corporation
PO Box 1910
Morristown, NJ 07962-1910 USA
Liqui-Gels is a registered trademark of R.P. Scherer Corporation.

*Shown in Product Identification Guide, page 503*

---

## ALKA-SELTZER PM™
[əl-ka sēl-sur]
## PAIN RELIEVER &
## SLEEP AID MEDICINE

| **Active ingredients:** (in each tablet) | **Purpose:** |
|---|---|
| Aspirin 325 mg | Pain reliever |
| Diphenhydramine citrate 38 mg | Sleep aid |

**Inactive Ingredients:** acesulfame potassium, aspartame, citric acid, dimethicone, docusate sodium, flavors, povidone, sodium benzoate, sodium bicarbonate

**Uses:** For the temporary relief of occasional headache and minor aches and pains with accompanying sleeplessness.

**Warnings: Reye's syndrome:** Children and teenagers should not use this medicine for chicken pox or flu symptoms before a doctor is consulted about Reye's syndrome, a rare but serious illness reported to be associated with aspirin.

**Alcohol warning:** If you consume 3 or more drinks every day, ask your doctor whether you should take aspirin or other pain relievers/fever reducers. Aspirin may cause stomach bleeding.

**Do not use** if you are allergic to aspirin. Avoid alcoholic beverages while taking this product.

• this product if you are on a sodium restricted diet
• in children under 12 years of age

**Ask a doctor before use if you have:**
• bleeding problems
• breathing problems such as emphysema, chronic bronchitis
• asthma
• ulcers
• glaucoma
• stomach problems (such as heartburn, upset stomach, or stomach pain) that persist or recur
• difficulty in urination due to enlargement of the prostate gland

*Continued on next page*

## Alka-Seltzer PM—Cont.

**Ask a doctor or pharmacist before use if you are:**
- taking sedatives or tranquilizers
- taking a prescription drug for
  - anticoagulation (blood thinning)
  - diabetes
  - gout
  - arthritis

**When using this product avoid alcoholic drinks.**

**Stop use and ask a doctor if:**
- an allergic reaction occurs. Seek medical help right away.
- pain gets worse or lasts for more than 10 days.
- new symptoms.
- ringing in the ears or loss of hearing occurs.
- redness or swelling is present.
- sleeplessness (insomnia) persists for more than 2 weeks

These could be signs of a serious condition.

**If pregnant or breast-feeding,** ask a health professional before use. **It is especially important not to use aspirin during the last 3 months of pregnancy unless definitely directed to do so by a doctor because it may cause problems in the unborn child or complications during delivery.**

**Keep out of reach of children.** In case of overdose, get medical help or contact a Poison Control Center right away.

**Directions:**
- do not exceed recommended dosage.
- fully dissolve tablets in 4 ounces of water before taking.

| adults and children 12 years and over | take 2 tablets with water at bedtime, if needed, or as directed by a doctor. |
|---|---|
| children under 12 years | do not use. |

**Other Information:**
- **each tablet contains:** sodium 503 mg
- **phenylketonurics:** contains phenylalanine 4.0 mg per tablet.
- Store at room temperature.

Place two (2) tablets in 4 oz of water. Dissolve tablets completely.

Drink Alka-Seltzer. You do not have to drink any of the residue that may be on the bottom of the glass. The medicines of Alka-Seltzer are in the water.

**How Supplied** Foil Packs of 24 Effervescent Tablets.
*FOIL SEALED FOR YOUR SAFETY. DO NOT USE IF FOIL PACKS ARE TORN OR BROKEN.*
***Questions or comments?***
1-800-800-4793 or www.alka-seltzer.com
For more information, visit our website at www.alka-seltzer.com

Questions or comments?
Please call 1-800-800-4793.
Made in the U.S.A.
Bayer Corporation
Consumer Care Division
P.O. Box 1910
Morristown, NJ 07962-1910 USA
*Shown in Product Identification Guide, page 503*

---

## Genuine BAYER® Aspirin
## Caplets, Gelcaps, and Tablets

**Active Ingredient:**    **Purposes:**
(in each caplet, gelcap, tablet)
Aspirin
325 mg ..... pain reliever/fever reducer

**Uses:** Temporarily relieves:
- headache
- muscle pain
- toothache
- menstrual pain
- pain and fever of colds
- minor pain of arthritis

**Warnings: Reye's syndrome:** Children and teenagers should not use this medicine for chicken pox or flu symptoms before a doctor is consulted about Reye's syndrome, a rare but serious illness reported to be associated with aspirin.

**Alcohol warning:** If you consume 3 or more alcoholic drinks every day, ask your doctor whether you should take aspirin or other pain relievers/fever reducers. Aspirin may cause stomach bleeding.

**Do not use** if you are allergic to aspirin or any other pain reliever/fever reducer.

**Ask a doctor before use if you have:**
- stomach problems (such as heartburn, upset stomach, or stomach pain) that continue or come back
- bleeding problems
- ulcers
- asthma

**Ask a doctor or pharmacist before use if you are** taking a prescription drug for
- anticoagulation (blood thinning)
- gout
- diabetes
- arthritis

**Stop use and ask a doctor if:**
- an allergic reaction occurs. Seek medical help right away.
- pain gets worse or lasts for more than 10 days
- fever lasts for more than 3 days
- new symptoms occur
- ringing in the ears or loss of hearing occurs
- redness or swelling is present

**If pregnant or breast-feeding,** ask a health professional before use. **It is especially important not to use aspirin during the last 3 months of pregnancy unless definitely directed to do so by a doctor because it may cause problems in the unborn child or complications during delivery.**

**Keep out of reach of children.** In case of overdose, get medical help or contact a Poison Control Center right away.

**Directions:**
- drink a full glass of water with each dose
- adults and children 12 years and over: take 1 or 2 caplets every 4 hours not to exceed 12 caplets in 24 hours

- children under 12 years: consult a doctor

**Other Information:**
- save carton for full directions and warnings
- store at room temperature

**Inactive Ingredients:**
**BAYER® Genuine Aspirin Caplets:** Cellulose, hydroxypropyl methylcellulose, starch, triacetin
**BAYER® Genuine Aspirin Gelcaps:** Butylparaben, D&C Yellow #10 Aluminum Lake, FD&C Blue #1 Aluminum Lake, Gelatin, Glycerin, Hydroxypropyl Methylcellulose, Methylparaben, Polyvinylpyrrolidone, Propylene Glycol, Propylparaben, Shellac, Sodium Lauryl Sulfate, Sorbitan Trioleate, Starch, Titanium Dioxide, Triacetin
**BAYER® Genuine Aspirin Tablets:** Cellulose, Hydroxypropyl Methylcellulose, Starch, Triacetin

**How Supplied:** BAYER® Genuine Aspirin Original Strength 325 mg is available in bottles of 100 coated caplets, in bottles of 80 Gelcaps, and in bottles of 100 coated tablets.
**Questions or comments?**
1-800-331-4536 or
www.bayeraspirin.com
Bayer Corporation
PO Box 1910
Morristown, NJ 07962-1910 USA
*Shown in Product Identification Guide, page 504*

---

## ASPIRIN REGIMEN BAYER® 81 mg
## ASPIRIN REGIMEN BAYER® 325 mg
**Delayed Release Enteric Aspirin Adult Low Strength 81 mg Tablets and Regular Strength 325 mg Caplets**

**Active Ingredient:**
(in each tablet)    **Purpose:**
Aspirin 81 mg ..................... Pain reliever
Aspirin 325 mg ................. Pain reliever

**Uses:** For the temporary relief of minor aches and pains or as recommended by your doctor. **Because of its delayed action, this product will not provide fast relief of headaches or other symptoms needing immediate relief.**

**Warnings: Reye's syndrome:** Children and teenagers should not use this medicine for chicken pox or flu symptoms before a doctor is consulted about Reye's syndrome, a rare but serious illness reported to be associated with aspirin.

**Alcohol warning:** If you consume 3 or more alcoholic drinks every day, ask your doctor whether you should take aspirin or other pain relievers/fever reducers. Aspirin may cause stomach bleeding.

**Do not use** if you are allergic to aspirin or any other pain reliever/fever reducer.

**Ask a doctor before use if you have:**
- stomach problems (such as heartburn, upset stomach, or stomach pain) that continue or come back
- bleeding problems
- ulcers
- asthma

**Ask a doctor or pharmacist before use if you are** taking a prescription drug for
- anticoagulation (blood thinning)
- gout
- diabetes
- arthritis

**Stop use and ask a doctor if**
- an allergic reaction occurs. Seek medical help right away.
- pain gets worse or lasts for more than 10 days
- new symptoms occur
- ringing in the ears or loss of hearing occurs
- redness or swelling is present

**If pregnant or breast-feeding,** ask a health professional before use. **It is especially important not to use aspirin during the last 3 months of pregnancy unless definitely directed to do so by a doctor because it may cause problems in the unborn child or complications during delivery.**

**Keep out of reach of children.** In case of overdose, get medical help or contact a Poison Control Center right away.

**Directions:**

**ASPIRIN REGIMEN BAYER® 81 mg:**
- drink a full glass of water with each dose
- adults and children 12 years and over: take 4 to 8 tablets every 4 hours not to exceed 48 tablets in 24 hours unless directed by a doctor
- children under 12 years: consult a doctor

**ASPIRIN REGIMEN BAYER® 325 mg:**
- drink a full glass of water with each dose
- adults and children 12 years and over: take 1 or 2 caplets every 4 hours not to exceed 12 caplets in 24 hours unless directed by a doctor
- children under 12 years: consult a doctor

**Other Information:**
- save carton for full directions and warnings
- store at room temperature

**Inactive Ingredients:**

**ASPIRIN REGIMEN BAYER® 81 mg:** Carnauba wax, cellulose, croscarmellose sodium, D&C yellow #10 aluminum lake, FD&C yellow #6 aluminum lake, hydroxypropyl methylcellulose, iron oxides, lactose, methacrylic acid copolymer, microcrystalline cellulose, polysorbate 80, propylene glycol, shellac, sodium lauryl sulfate, starch, titanium dioxide, triacetin

**ASPIRIN REGIMEN BAYER® 325 mg:** Carnauba wax, cellulose, D&C yellow #10 aluminum lake, FD&C yellow #6 aluminum lake, hydroxypropyl methylcellulose, iron oxides, methacrylic acid copolymer, polysorbate 80, propylene gylcol, shellac, sodium lauryl sulfate, starch, titanium dioxide, triacetin

| Weight (lb) | Age (years) | Dosage | Maximum Dosage |
|---|---|---|---|
| under 32 | children under 3 | consult a doctor | |
| 32 to 35 | 3 to under 4 | 2 tablets | repeat every 4 hours while symptoms persist up to a maximum of 5 doses in 24 hours or as directed by a doctor |
| 36 to 45 | 4 to under 6 | 3 tablets | |
| 46 to 65 | 6 to under 9 | 4 tablets | |
| 66 to 76 | 9 to under 11 | 4 to 5 tablets | |
| 77 to 83 | 11 to under 12 | 4 to 6 tablets | |
| | adults and children 12 years and over | 5 to 8 tablets | |

**How Supplied:**

**ASPIRIN REGIMEN BAYER® 81 mg:** Bottle of 120 tablets delayed release enteric safety coated aspirin.

**ASPIRIN REGIMEN BAYER® 325 mg:** Bottle of 100 caplets delayed release enteric safety coated aspirin.

***Questions or comments?***
1-800-331-4536 or
www.bayeraspirin.com
***USE ONLY IF SEAL UNDER BOTTLE CAP WITH BLUE "Bayer Corporation" PRINT IS INTACT.***
Bayer Corporation
PO Box 1910
Morristown, NJ 07962-1910 USA
*Shown in Product Identification Guide, page 504*

---

**BAYER® Children's Chewable Tablets**
**Genuine Aspirin**
**Cherry & Orange Flavored**

**Active Ingredient:**
**(in each tablet)**     **Purposes:**
Aspirin
81 mg ......... Pain reliever/fever reducer

**Uses:** For the temporary relief of:
- minor aches, pains, and headaches
- to reduce fever associated with colds, sore throats, and teething

**Warnings: Reye's syndrome:** Children and teenagers should not use this medicine for chicken pox or flu symptoms before a doctor is consulted about Reye's syndrome, a rare but serious illness reported to be associated with aspirin.
**Alcohol warning:** If you consume 3 or more alcoholic drinks every day, ask your doctor whether you should take aspirin or other pain relievers/fever reducers. Aspirin may cause stomach bleeding.
**Sore throat warning:** If sore throat is severe, persists for more than 2 days, is accompanied or followed by fever, headache, rash, nausea, or vomiting, consult a doctor promptly.
**Do not use:**
- if you are allergic to aspirin or any other pain reliever/fever reducer
- for at least 7 days after tonsillectomy or oral surgery
**Ask a doctor before use if you have:**
- stomach problems (such as heartburn, upset stomach, or stomach pain) that continue or come back

- bleeding problems
- ulcers
- asthma
- a child experiencing arthritis pain

**Ask a doctor or pharmacist before use if you are** taking a prescription drug for
- anticoagulation (blood thinning)
- gout
- diabetes
- arthritis

**Stop use and ask a doctor if:**
- an allergic reaction occurs. Seek medical help right away.
- pain gets worse or lasts more than 10 days (for adults) or 5 days (for children)
- fever gets worse or lasts more than 3 days
- new symptoms occur
- ringing in the ears or loss of hearing occurs
- redness or swelling is present

**If pregnant or breast-feeding,** ask a health professional before use. **It is especially important not to use aspirin during the last 3 months of pregnancy unless definitely directed to do so by a doctor because it may cause problems in the unborn child or complications during delivery.**

**Keep out of reach of children.** In case of overdose, get medical help or contact a Poison Control Center right away.

**Directions:**
- drink a full glass of water with each dose
- to be administered only under adult supervision
- if possible use weight to dose. Otherwise use age.
[See table above]

**Other Information:**
- save carton for full directions and warnings
- store at room temperature.

**Inactive Ingredients:**
**BAYER® Children's Chewable: Cherry Flavored:** D&C Red #27 Aluminum Lake, Dextrose, FD&C Red #40 Aluminum Lake, Flavor, Saccharin Sodium, Starch

**BAYER Children's Chewable: Orange Flavored:** Dextrose, FD&C Yellow #6 Aluminum Lake, Flavor, Sodium Saccharin, starch

**How Supplied:** Bottle of 36 chewable tablets.

*Continued on next page*

## Bayer Children's—Cont.

**USE ONLY IF SEAL UNDER BOTTLE CAP WITH WHITE "Bayer Corporation" PRINT IS INTACT.**
Questions or comments?
1-800-331-4536 or
www.bayeraspirin.com
Bayer Corporation
PO Box 1910
Morristown, NJ 07962-1910 USA
*Shown in Product Identification Guide, page 503*

---

## PROFESSIONAL LABELING

**Genuine Bayer Aspirin
Aspirin Regimen Bayer 325 mg
Aspirin Regimen Bayer 81 mg
Bayer Women's Aspirin with Calcium
Aspirin Regimen Bayer Childrens
Chewable 81 mg**

**Professional Labeling:**

**Indications And Usage:** Vascular Indications (Ischemic Stroke, TIA, Acute MI, Prevention of Recurrent MI, Unstable Angina Pectoris, and Chronic Stable Angina Pectoris): Aspirin is indicated to: (1) Reduce the combined risk of death and nonfatal stroke in patients who have had ischemic stroke or transient ischemia of the brain due to fibrin platelet emboli, (2) reduce the risk of vascular mortality in patients with a suspected acute MI, (3) reduce the combined risk of death and nonfatal MI in patients with a previous MI or unstable angina pectoris, and (4) reduce the combined risk of MI and sudden death in patients with chronic stable angina pectoris.
Revascularization Procedures (Coronary Artery Bypass Graft (CABG), Percutaneous Transluminal Coronary Angioplasty (PTCA), and Carotid Endarterectomy): Aspirin is indicated in patients who have undergone revascularization procedures (i.e., CABG, PTCA, or carotid endarterectomy) when there is a preexisting condition for which aspirin is already indicated.
Rheumatologic Disease Indications (Rheumatoid Arthritis, Juvenile Rheumatoid Arthritis, Spondyloarthropathies, Osteoarthritis, and the Arthritis and Pleurisy of Systemic Lupus Erythematosus (SLE)): Aspirin is indicated for the relief of the signs and symptoms of rheumatoid arthritis, juvenile rheumatoid arthritis, osteoarthritis, spondyloarthropathies, and arthritis and pleurisy associated with SLE.

**Contraindications:** Allergy: Aspirin is contraindicated in patients with known allergy to nonsteroidal anti-inflammatory drug products and in patients with the syndrome of asthma, rhinitis, and nasal polyps. Aspirin may cause severe urticaria, angioedema, or bronchospasm (asthma).
Reye's syndrome: Aspirin should not be used in children or teenagers for viral infections, with or without fever, because of the risk of Reye's syndrome with concomitant use of aspirin in certain viral illnesses.

**Warnings:** Alcohol Warning: Patients who consume three or more alcoholic drinks every day should be counseled about the bleeding risks involved with chronic, heavy alcohol use while taking aspirin.
Coagulation Abnormalities: Even low doses of aspirin can inhibit platelet function leading to an increase in bleeding time. This can adversely affect patients with inherited (hemophilia) or acquired (liver disease or vitamin K deficiency) bleeding disorders.
GI Side Effects: GI side effects include stomach pain, heartburn, nausea, vomiting, and gross GI bleeding. Although minor upper GI symptoms, such as dyspepsia, are common and can occur anytime during therapy, physicians should remain alert for signs of ulceration and bleeding, even in the absence of previous GI symptoms. Physicians should inform patients about the signs and symptoms of GI side effects and what steps to take if they occur.
Peptic Ulcer Disease: Patients with a history of active peptic ulcer disease should avoid using aspirin, which can cause gastric mucosal irritation and bleeding.

**Precautions:**

**General:** Renal Failure: Avoid aspirin in patients with severe renal failure (glomerular filtration rate less than 10 mL/minute).
Hepatic Insufficiency: Avoid aspirin in patients with severe hepatic insufficiency.
Sodium Restricted Diets: Patients with sodium-retaining states, such as congestive heart failure or renal failure, should avoid sodium-containing buffered aspirin preparations because of their high sodium content.
Laboratory Tests: Aspirin has been associated with elevated hepatic enzymes, blood urea nitrogen and serum creatinine, hyperkalemia, proteinuria, and prolonged bleeding time.
**Drug Interactions:** Angiotensin Converting Enzyme (ACE) Inhibitors: The hyponatremic and hypotensive effects of ACE inhibitors may be diminished by the concomitant administration of aspirin due to its indirect effect on the renin-angiotensin conversion pathway.
Acetazolamide: Concurrent use of aspirin and acetazolamide can lead to high serum concentrations of acetazolamide (and toxicity) due to competition at the renal tubule for secretion.
Anticoagulant Therapy (Heparin and Warfarin): Patients on anticoagulation therapy are at increased risk for bleeding because of drug-drug interactions and the effect on platelets. Aspirin can displace warfarin from protein binding sites, leading to prolongation of both the prothrombin time and the bleeding time.

Aspirin can increase the anticoagulant activity of heparin, increasing bleeding risk.
Anticonvulsants: Salicylate can displace protein-bound phenytoin and valproic acid, leading to a decrease in the total concentration of phenytoin and an increase in serum valproic acid levels.
Beta Blockers: The hypotensive effects of beta blockers may be diminished by the concomitant administration of aspirin due to inhibition of renal prostaglandins, leading to decreased renal blood flow, and salt and fluid retention.
Diuretics: The effectiveness of diuretics in patients with underlying renal or cardiovascular disease may be diminished by the concomitant administration of aspirin due to inhibition of renal prostaglandins, leading to decreased renal blood flow and salt and fluid retention.
Methotrexate: Salicylate can inhibit renal clearance of methotrexate, leading to bone marrow toxicity, especially in the elderly or renal impaired.
Nonsteroidal Anti-inflammatory Drugs (NSAID's): The concurrent use of aspirin with other NSAID's should be avoided because this may increase bleeding or lead to decreased renal function.
Oral Hypoglycemics: Moderate doses of aspirin may increase the effectiveness of oral hypoglycemic drugs, leading to hypoglycemia.
Uricosuric Agents (Probenecid and Sulfinpyrazone): Salicylates antagonize the uricosuric action of uricosuric agents.
Carcinogenesis, Mutagenesis, Impairment of Fertility: Administration of aspirin for 68 weeks at 0.5 percent in the feed of rats was not carcinogenic. In the Ames Salmonella assay, aspirin was not mutagenic; however, aspirin did induce chromosome aberrations in cultured human fibroblasts. Aspirin inhibits ovulation in rats. (See Pregnancy.)
Pregnancy: Pregnant women should only take aspirin if clearly needed. Because of the known effects of NSAID's on the fetal cardiovascular system (closure of the ductus arteriosus), use during the third trimester of pregnancy should be avoided. Salicylate products have also been associated with alterations in maternal and neonatal hemostasis mechanisms, decreased birth weight, and with perinatal mortality.
Labor and Delivery: Aspirin should be avoided 1 week prior to and during labor and delivery because it can result in excessive blood loss at delivery. Prolonged gestation and prolonged labor due to prostaglandin inhibition have been reported.
Nursing Mothers: Nursing mothers should avoid using aspirin because salicylate is excreted in breast milk. Use of high doses may lead to rashes, platelet abnormalities, and bleeding in nursing infants.
Pediatric Use: Pediatric dosing recommendations for juvenile rheumatoid arthritis are based on well-controlled clinical studies. An initial dose of 90–130 mg/kg/day in divided doses, with an increase as needed for anti-inflamma-

tory efficacy (target plasma salicylate levels of 150–300 mcg/mL) are effective. At high doses (i.e., plasma levels of greater than 200 mcg/mL), the incidence of toxicity increases.

**Adverse Reactions:** Many adverse reactions due to aspirin ingestion are dose-related. The following is a list of adverse reactions that have been reported in the literature. (See **Warnings**.)

Body as a Whole: Fever, hypothermia, thirst.

Cardiovascular: Dysrhythmias, hypotension, tachycardia.

Central Nervous System: Agitation, cerebral edema, coma, confusion, dizziness, headache, subdural or intracranial hemorrhage, lethargy, seizures.

Fluid and Electrolyte: Dehydration, hyperkalemia, metabolic acidosis, respiratory alkalosis.

Gastrointestinal: Dyspepsia, GI bleeding, ulceration and perforation, nausea, vomiting, transient elevations of hepatic enzymes, hepatitis, Reye's Syndrome, pancreatitis.

Hematologic: Prolongation of the prothrombin time, disseminated intravascular coagulation, coagulopathy, thrombocytopenia.

Hypersensitivity: Acute anaphylaxis, angioedema, asthma, bronchospasm, laryngeal edema, urticaria.

Musculoskeletal: Rhabdomyolysis.

Metabolism: Hypoglycemia (in children), hyperglycemia.

Reproductive: Prolonged pregnancy and labor, stillbirths, lower birth weight infants, antepartum and postpartum bleeding.

Respiratory: Hyperpnea, pulmonary edema, tachypnea.

Special Senses: Hearing loss, tinnitus. Patients with high frequency hearing loss may have difficulty perceiving tinnitus. In these patients, tinnitus cannot be used as a clinical indicator of salicylism.

Urogenital: Interstitial nephritis, papillary necrosis, proteinuria, renal insufficiency and failure.

**Drug Abuse And Dependence:** Aspirin is nonnarcotic. There is no known potential for addiction associated with the use of aspirin.

**Overdosage:** Salicylate toxicity may result from acute ingestion (overdose) or chronic intoxication. The early signs of salicylic overdose (salicylism), including tinnitus (ringing in the ears), occur at plasma concentrations approaching 200 mcg/mL. Plasma concentrations of aspirin above 300 mcg/mL are clearly toxic. Severe toxic effects are associated with levels above 400 mcg/mL. (See **Clinical Pharmacology**.) A single lethal dose of aspirin in adults is not known with certainty but death may be expected at 30 g. For real or suspected overdose, a Poison Control Center should be contacted immediately. Careful medical management is essential.

Signs and Symptoms: In acute overdose, severe acid-base and electrolyte disturbances may occur and are complicated by hyperthermia and dehydration. Respiratory alkalosis occurs early while hyperventilation is present, but is quickly followed by metabolic acidosis.

Treatment: Treatment consists primarily of supporting vital functions, increasing salicylate elimination, and correcting the acid-base disturbance. Gastric emptying and/or lavage is recommended as soon as possible after ingestion, even if the patient has vomited spontaneously. After lavage and/or emesis, administration of activated charcoal, as a slurry, is beneficial, if less than 3 hours have passed since ingestion. Charcoal adsorption should not be employed prior to emesis and lavage.

Severity of aspirin intoxication is determined by measuring the blood salicylate level. Acid-base status should be closely followed with serial blood gas and serum pH measurements. Fluid and electrolyte balance should aslo be maintained.

In severe cases, hyperthermia and hypovolemia are the major immediate threats to life. Children should be sponged with tepid water. Replacement fluid should be administered intravenously and augmented with correction of acidosis. Plasma electrolytes and pH should be monitored to promote alkaline diuresis of salicylate if renal function is normal. Infusion of glucose may be required to control hypoglycemia.

Hemodialysis and peritoneal dialysis can be performed to reduce the body drug content. In patients with renal insufficiency or in cases of life-threatening intoxication, dialysis is usually required. Exchange transfusion may be indicated in infants and young children.

**Dosage and Administration:** Each dose of aspirin should be taken with a full glass of water unless patient is fluid restricted. Anti-inflammatory and analgesic dosages should be individualized. When aspirin is used in high doses, the development of tinnitus may be used as a clinical sign of elevated plasma salicylate levels except in patients with high frequency hearing loss.

Ischemic Stroke and TIA: 50–325 mg once a day. Continue therapy indefinitely.

Suspected Acute MI: The initial dose of 160–162.5 mg is administered as soon as an MI is suspected. The maintenance dose of 160–162.5 mg a day is continued for 30 days post-infarction. After 30 days, consider further therapy based on dosage and administration for prevention of recurrent MI.

Prevention of Recurrent MI: 75–325 mg once a day. Continue therapy indefinitely.

Unstable Angina Pectoris: 75–325 mg once a day. Continue therapy indefinitely.

Chronic Stable Angina Pectoris: 75–325 mg once a day. Continue therapy indefinitely.

CABG: 325 mg daily starting 6 hours post-procedure. Continue therapy for 1 year post-procedure.

PTCA: The initial dose of 325 mg should be given 2 hours presurgery. Maintenance dose is 160–325 mg daily. Continue therapy indefinitely.

Carotid Endarterectomy: Doses of 80 mg once daily to 650 mg twice daily, started presurgery, are recommended. Continue therapy indefinitely.

Rheumatoid Arthritis: The initial dose is 3 g a day in divided doses. Increase as needed for anti-inflammatory efficacy with target plasma salicylate levels of 150–300 mcg/mL. At high doses (i.e., plasma levels of greater than 200 mcg/mL), the incidence of toxicity increases.

Juvenile Rheumatoid Arthritis: Initial dose is 90–130 mg/kg/day in divided doses. Increase as needed for anti-inflammatory efficacy with target plasma salicylate levels of 150–300 mcg/mL. At high doses (i.e., plasma levels of greater than 200 mcg/mL), the incidence of toxicity increases.

Spondyloarthropathies: Up to 4 g per day in divided doses.

Osteoarthritis: Up to 3 g per day in divided doses.

Arthritis and Pleurisy of SLE: The initial dose is 3 g a day in divided doses. Increase as needed for anti-inflammatory efficacy with target plasma salicylate levels of 150–300 mcg/mL. At high doses (i.e., plasma levels of greater than 200 mcg/mL), the incidence of toxicity increases.

---

## Extra Strength BAYER® Aspirin Arthritis Pain
## Caplets

**Active Ingredient:**      **Purpose:**
**(in each caplet)**
Aspirin 500 mg .................. Pain reliever

**Uses:** For the temporary relief of minor aches and pains of arthritis or as recommended by your doctor.
**Because of its delayed action, this product will not provide fast relief of headaches, or other symptoms needing immediate relief.**

**Warnings: Reye's syndrome:** Children and teenagers should not use this medicine for chicken pox or flu symptoms before a doctor is consulted about Reye's syndrome, a rare but serious illness reported to be associated with aspirin.

**Alcohol warning:** If you consume 3 or more alcoholic drinks every day, ask your doctor whether you should take aspirin or other pain relievers/fever reducers. Aspirin may cause stomach bleeding.

**Do not use** if you are allergic to aspirin or any other pain reliever/fever reducer.

**Ask a doctor before use if you have:**
- stomach problems (such as heartburn, upset stomach, or stomach pain) that continue or come back
- bleeding problems
- ulcers
- asthma

*Continued on next page*

## Bayer Arthritis Pain E.S.—Cont.

**Ask a doctor or pharmacist before use if you are** taking a prescription drug for
- anticoagulation (blood thinning)
- gout
- diabetes
- arthritis

**Stop use and ask a doctor if:**
- an allergic reaction occurs. Seek medical help right away.
- pain gets worse or lasts for more than 10 days
- new symptoms occur
- ringing in the ears or loss of hearing occurs
- redness or swelling is present

**If pregnant or breast-feeding,** ask a health professional before use. **It is especially important not to use aspirin during the last 3 months of pregnancy unless definitely directed to do so by a doctor because it may cause problems in the unborn child or complications during delivery.**

**Keep out of reach of children.** In case of overdose, get medical help or contact a Poison Control Center right away.

**Directions:**
- drink a full glass of water with each dose
- adults and children 12 years and over: take 2 caplets every 6 hours not to exceed 8 caplets in 24 hours unless directed by a doctor
- children under 12 years: consult a doctor

**Other Information:**
- save carton for full directions and warnings.
- store at room temperature.

**Inactive Ingredients:** Carnauba wax, cellulose, D&C yellow #10 aluminum lake, FD&C yellow #6 aluminum lake, hydroxypropyl methylcellulose, iron oxides, methacrylic acid copolymer, polysorbate 80, propylene glycol, shellac, sodium lauryl sulfate, starch, titanium dioxide, triacetin.

**How Supplied:** Bottle of 50 caplets delayed release aspirin (enteric safety coated

**USE ONLY IF SEAL UNDER BOTTLE CAP WITH BLUE "Bayer Corporation" PRINT IS INTACT.**
Questions or comments?
1-800-331-4536 or
www.bayeraspirin.com
Bayer Corporation
PO Box 1910
Morristown, NJ 07962-1910 USA

---

## Extra Strength BAYER® Aspirin Caplets, and Gelcaps

| **Active Ingredient:** (in each caplet) | **Purposes:** |
|---|---|

Aspirin
500 mg ...... Pain reliever/fever reducer

**Uses:** For the temporary relief of
- headache
- pain and fever of colds
- muscle pain
- menstrual pain
- toothache
- minor pain of arthritis

**Warnings: Reye's syndrome:** Children and teenagers should not use this medicine for chicken pox or flu symptoms before a doctor is consulted about Reye's syndrome, a rare but serious illness reported to be associated with aspirin.

**Alcohol warning:** If you consume 3 or more alcoholic drinks every day, ask your doctor whether you should take aspirin or other pain relievers/fever reducers. Aspirin may cause stomach bleeding.

**Do not use** if you are allergic to aspirin or any other pain reliever/fever reducer.

**Ask a doctor before use if you have:**
- stomach problems (such as heartburn, upset stomach, or stomach pain) that last or come back
- bleeding problems
- ulcers
- asthma

**Ask a doctor or pharmacist before use if you are** taking a prescription drug for
- anticoagulation (blood thinning)
- gout
- diabetes
- arthritis

**Stop use and ask a doctor if:**
- an allergic reaction occurs. Seek medical help right away.
- pain gets worse or lasts for more than 10 days
- fever lasts for more than 3 days
- new symptoms occur
- ringing in the ears or loss of hearing occurs
- redness or swelling is present

**If pregnant or breast-feeding,** ask a health professional before use. **It is especially important not to use aspirin during the last 3 months of pregnancy unless definitely directed to do so by a doctor because it may cause problems in the unborn child or complications during delivery.**

**Keep out of reach of children.** In case of overdose, get medical help or contact a Poison Control Center right away.

**Directions:**
- drink a full glass of water with each dose
- adults and children 12 years and over: take 1 or 2 caplets every 4 to 6 hours not to exceed 8 caplets in 24 hours
- children under 12 years: consult a doctor

**Other Information:**
- save carton for full directions and warnings
- store at room temperature

**Inactive Ingredients: Extra Strength BAYER® Aspirin Caplets:** Carnauba Wax, Cellulose, D&C Red #7 Calcium Lake, FD&C Blue #2 Aluminum Lake, FD&C Red #40 Aluminum Lake, Hydroxypropyl Methylcellulose, Propylene Glycol, Shellac, Starch, Titanium Dioxide, Triacetin

**Extra Strength BAYER® Aspirin Gelcaps:** Butylparaben, D&C Yellow #10 Aluminum Lake, FD&C Blue #1 Aluminum Lake, FD&C Red #40, Gelatin, Glycerin, Hydroxypropyl Methylcellulose, Methylparaben, Polyvinylpyrrolidone, Propylene Glycol, Propylparaben,

Shellac, Sodium Lauryl Sulfate, Sorbitan Trioleate, Starch, Titanium Dioxide, Triacetin

**How Supplied:**
**Extra Strength BAYER® Aspirin Caplets:** Bottle of 50 coated caplets (500 mg).
**Extra Strength BAYER® Aspirin Gelcaps:** Bottle of 80 gelcaps (500 mg).
**Questions or comments?**
**1-800-331-4536 or www.bayeraspirin-.com**
**USE ONLY IF SEAL UNDER BOTTLE CAP WITH BLUE "Bayer Corporation" PRINT IS INTACT.**
Bayer Corporation
PO Box 1910
Morristown, NJ 07962-1910 USA

---

## Extra Strength BAYER® PLUS Buffered Aspirin Caplets

| **Active Ingredient:** (in each caplet) | **Purposes:** |
|---|---|

Aspirin
500 mg ....... Pain reliever/fever reducer

**Uses:** For the temporary relief of
- headache
- pain and fever of colds
- muscle pain
- menstrual pain
- toothache
- minor pain of arthritis

**Warnings: Reye's syndrome:** Children and teenagers should not use this medicine for chicken pox or flu symptoms before a doctor is consulted about Reye's syndrome, a rare but serious illness reported to be associated with aspirin.

**Alcohol warning:** If you consume 3 or more alcoholic drinks every day, ask your doctor whether you should take aspirin or other pain relievers/fever reducers. Aspirin may cause stomach bleeding.

**Do not use** if you are allergic to aspirin or any other pain reliever/fever reducer.

**Ask a doctor before use if you have:**
- stomach problems (such as heartburn, upset stomach, or stomach pain) that continue or come back
- bleeding problems
- ulcers
- asthma

**Ask a doctor or pharmacist before use if you are** taking a prescription drug for
- anticoagulation (blood thinning)
- gout
- diabetes
- arthritis

**Stop use and ask a doctor if:**
- an allergic reaction occurs. Seek medical help right away.
- pain gets worse or lasts for more than 10 days
- fever lasts for more than 3 days
- new symptoms occur
- ringing in the ears or loss of hearing occurs
- redness or swelling is present

**If pregnant or breast-feeding,** ask a health professional before use. **It is especially important not to use aspirin during the last 3 months of pregnancy unless definitely directed to do so by a**

doctor because it may cause problems in the unborn child or complications during delivery.

**Keep out of reach of children.** In case of overdose, get medical help or contact a Poison Control Center right away.

## Directions:
- drink a full glass of water with each dose
- adults and children 12 years and over: take 1 or 2 caplets every 4 to 6 hours as needed, not to exceed 8 caplets in 24 hours
- children under 12 years: consult a doctor

## Other Information:
- contains calcium carbonate (350 mg = 140 mg elemental calcium)
- save carton for full directions and warnings
- store at room temperature

**Inactive Ingredients:** Calcium carbonate, carnauba wax, colloidal silicon dioxide, D&C red #7 calcium lake, FD&C blue #2 aluminum lake, FD&C red #40 aluminum lake, hydroxypropyl methylcellulose, microcrystalline cellulose, propylene glycol, shellac, sodium starch glycolate, starch, titanium dioxide, zinc stearate

**How Supplied:** Bottle of 50 buffered caplets (500 mg).

**Questions or comments?**
1-800-331-4536 or
www.bayeraspirin.com
**USE ONLY IF SEAL UNDER BOTTLE CAP WITH GREEN "Bayer Corporation" PRINT IS INTACT.**
Bayer Corporation
PO Box 1910
Morristown, NJ 07962-1910 USA

---

**Extra Strength BAYER® PM For Pain with Sleeplessness Caplets**

**Active Ingredients:**
(in each caplet)                    Purpose:
Aspirin 500 mg .................. Pain reliever
Diphenhydramine citrate
  38.3 mg ...................... Sleep aid

**Uses:** For the temporary relief of occasional headache and minor aches and pains with accompanying sleeplessness

**Warnings: Reye's syndrome:** Children and teenagers should not use this medicine for chicken pox or flu symptoms before a doctor is consulted about Reye's syndrome, a rare but serious illness reported to be associated with aspirin.

**Alcohol warning:** If you consume 3 or more alcoholic drinks every day, ask your doctor whether you should take aspirin or other pain relievers/fever reducers. Aspirin may cause stomach bleeding.

**Do not use** if you are allergic to aspirin or any other pain reliever/fever reducer.

**Ask a doctor before use if you have:**
- stomach problems (such as heartburn, upset stomach, or stomach pain) that continue or come back
- bleeding problems
- ulcers

- a breathing problem such as emphysema, chronic bronchitis, or asthma
- glaucoma
- difficulty in urination due to enlargement of the prostate gland

**Ask a doctor or pharmacist before use if you are:**
- taking sedatives or tranquilizers
- taking a prescription drug for
  - anticoagulation (blood thinning)
  - gout
  - diabetes
  - arthritis

**When using this product** avoid alcoholic drinks.

**Stop use and ask a doctor if:**
- an allergic reaction occurs. Seek medical help right away.
- pain gets worse or lasts for more than 10 days
- new symptoms occur
- ringing in the ears or loss of hearing occurs
- redness or swelling is present
- sleeplessness lasts for more than 2 weeks. Insomnia may be a symptom of a serious condition.

**If pregnant or breast-feeding,** ask a health professional before use. **It is especially important not to use aspirin during the last 3 months of pregnancy unless definitely directed to do so by a doctor because it may cause problems in the unborn child or complications during delivery.**

**Keep out of reach of children.** In case of overdose, get medical help or contact a Poison Control Center right away.

## Directions:
- do not exceed recommended dosage
- drink a full glass of water with each dose
- adults and children 12 years and over: take 2 caplets at bedtime, if needed, or as directed by a doctor.
- children under 12 years: consult a doctor

## Other Information:
- save carton for full directions and warnings
- store at room temperature

**Inactive Ingredients:** Carnauba wax, citric acid, colloidal silicon dioxide, FD&C blue #1 aluminum lake, FD&C blue #2 aluminum lake, hydroxypropyl methylcellulose, microcrystalline cellulose, propylene glycol, shellac, starch, titanium dioxide, zinc stearate

**How Supplied:** Bottle of 40 caplets.
**Questions or comments?**
1-800-331-4536 or
www.bayeraspirin.com
**USE ONLY IF SEAL UNDER BOTTLE CAP WITH BLUE "Bayer Corporation" PRINT IS INTACT.**
Bayer Corporation
PO Box 1910
Morristown, NJ 07962-1910 USA

---

**BAYER® WOMEN'S ASPIRIN PLUS CALCIUM**
**Low Strength Aspirin Regimen**
**Analgesic/Dietary Supplement**
**81 mg Aspirin-300 mg Calcium**

**Directions:** For calcium, take up to 4 caplets per day.

Serving Size: One Caplet

|  | Amount Per Serving | % Daily Value |
|---|---|---|
| Calcium (elemental) | 300 mg | 30% |

**Ingredients:** Calcium Carbonate, Microcrystalline Cellulose, Aspirin, Lactose, Cellulose, Maltodextrin, Starch, Carnauba Wax, Hydroxypropyl Methylcellulose, Polydextrose, Titanium Dioxide, Triacetin, Sodium Starch Glycolate, Colloidal Silicon Dioxide, Zinc Stearate, Mineral Oil, Crospovidone, Magnesium Stearate, Stearic Acid.

**What you should know about Osteoporosis**
Menopausal women and women with a family history of the disease are groups at risk for developing osteoporosis. Adequate calcium intake throughout life, along with a healthy diet and regular exercise, builds and maintains good bone health and may reduce the risk of osteoporosis. While adequate calcium intake is important, daily intakes above 2,000 mg may not provide additional benefits.

**Active Ingredient:**
(in each caplet)                    Purpose:
Aspirin 81 mg ..................... Pain reliever

**Uses:** For the temporary relief of minor aches and pains or as recommended by your doctor

**Warnings: Reye's syndrome:** Children and teenagers should not use this medicine for chicken pox or flu symptoms before a doctor is consulted about Reye's syndrome, a rare but serious illness reported to be associated with aspirin.

**Alcohol warning:** If you consume 3 or more alcoholic drinks every day, ask your doctor whether you should take aspirin or other pain relievers/fever reducers. Aspirin may cause stomach bleeding.

**Do not use** if you are allergic to aspirin or any other pain reliever/fever reducer.

**Ask a doctor before use if you have:**
- stomach problems (such as heartburn, upset stomach, or stomach pain) that continue or come back
- bleeding problems
- ulcers
- asthma

**Ask a doctor or pharmacist before use if you are** taking a prescription drug for
- anticoagulation (blood thinning)
- gout
- diabetes
- arthritis

**Stop use and ask a doctor if:**
- an allergic reaction occurs. Seek medical help right away.
- pain gets worse or lasts for more than 10 days
- new symptoms occur
- ringing in the ears or loss of hearing occurs
- redness or swelling is present

**If pregnant or breast-feeding,** ask a health professional before use. **It is espe-**

*Continued on next page*

## Bayer Women's—Cont.

cially important not to use aspirin during the last 3 months of pregnancy unless definitely directed to do so by a doctor because it may cause problems in the unborn child or complications during delivery.

**Keep out of reach of children.** In case of overdose, get medical help or contact a Poison Control Center right away.

**Directions:**
• talk to your doctor about regimen use of aspirin
• drink a full glass of water with each dose
• for pain, adults and children 12 years and over: take 4 caplets not to exceed 4 caplets in 24 hours
• children under 12 years: consult a doctor

**Other Information:**
• save carton for full directions and warnings
• store at room temperature

**Inactive Ingredients:** Calcium carbonate, carnauba wax, cellulose, colloidal silicon dioxide, crospovidone, hydroxypropyl methylcellulose, lactose, magnesium stearate, maltodextrin, microcrystalline cellulose, mineral oil, polydextrose, sodium starch glycolate, starch, stearic acid, titanium dioxide, triacetin, zinc stearate.

**How Supplied:** Bottle of 90 Caplets
Aspirin is not appropriate for everyone, so be sure to talk to your doctor before you begin an aspirin regimen.
*Ideal for women on an aspirin regimen, as directed by a doctor, who need a head start on their daily calcium requirements to help fight Osteoporosis.*
*For more information on how to fight heart disease and stroke, visit the American Heart Association Web Site at www.americanheart.org.*
**USE ONLY IF SEAL UNDER BOTTLE CAP WITH GREEN "Bayer Corporation" PRINT IS INTACT.**
*Questions or comments?*
**1-800-331-4536** or
www.bayeraspirin.com
Bayer Corporation
Consumer Care Division
PO Box 1910
Morristown, NJ 07962-1910 USA
*Shown in Product Identification Guide, page 503*

---

**BACTINE® Antiseptic-Anesthetic First Aid Liquid**

## Product Information

**Active Ingredients:** Benzalkonium chloride 0.13% w/w, and lidocaine Hydrochloride 2.5% w/w.

**Inactive Ingredients:** Disodium EDTA, fragrances, octoxynol 9, propylene glycol, water.

**Indications:** First aid to help prevent bacterial contamination or skin infection

and for the temporary relief of pain and itching in minor cuts, scrapes, and burns.

**Directions:** Adults and children 2 years of age and older: Clean the affected area. Apply a small amount of this product on the area 1 to 3 times daily. May be covered with a sterile bandage. If bandaged, let dry first. Children under 2 years of age: ask a doctor.

**Warnings:**
**For external use only**
**Ask a doctor before use if you have**
• deep or puncture wounds
• animal bites
• serious burns
**When using this product:**
• do not use in or near the eyes
• do not apply over large areas of the body or in large quantities
• do not apply over raw surfaces or blistered areas
**Stop use and ask a doctor if:**
• condition worsens
• symptoms persist for more than 7 days, or clear up and occur again within a few days
**Keep out of reach of children.** If swallowed, get medical help or contact a Poison Control Center right away
Protect from excessive heat.

**How Supplied:** Bactine Antiseptic-Anesthetic First Aid Liquid is available as 2 oz, 4 oz, and 16 oz. liquid with child resistant closures and 5.0 oz. pump spray.
*Shown in Product Identification Guide, page 503*

---

**DOMEBORO® Astringent SOLUTION (Powder Packets)**
**DOMEBORO® Astringent SOLUTION (Effervescent Tablets)**

**Active Ingredients:**
**DOMEBORO® Astringent Solution Powder Packets**

| Active Ingredient: | Purpose: |
|---|---|
| Aluminum Acetate ............... | Astringent |

(Each powder packet, when dissolved in water and ready for use, provides the active ingredient Aluminum Acetate resulting from the reaction of Calcium Acetate 938 mg, and Aluminum Sulfate 1191 mg. The resulting astringent solution is buffered to an acid pH.)
**DOMEBORO® Astringent Solution Effervescent Tablets**

| Active Ingredient: | Purpose: |
|---|---|
| (in each tablet)* | |
| Aluminum Acetate 525 mg .. | Astringent |

**Uses:** Temporarily relieves minor skin irritations due to:
• poison ivy
• poison oak
• poison sumac
• insect bites
• athlete's foot
• rashes caused by soaps, detergents, cosmetics, or jewelry
**Warnings: For external use only. Avoid contact with the eyes.**
**When using this product,** do not cover compress or wet dressing with plastic to prevent evaporation.

**Stop use and ask a doctor if** condition worsens or symptoms persist for more than 7 days. These could be signs of a serious condition.

**Keep out of reach of children.** If swallowed, get medical help or contact a Poison Control Center right away.

**Directions:**
**DOMEBORO® Astringent Solution Powder Packets**
• Dissolve one, two, or three packets of Domeboro® powder in 16 ounces of water to obtain the following modified Burow's Solution:

| Number of Packets | Dilution | % Aluminum acetate |
|---|---|---|
| one packet | 1:40 dilution | 0.16% |
| two packets | 1:20 dilution | 0.32% |
| three packets | 1:13 dilution | 0.48% |

• Do not strain or filter the solution.
• Can be used as a compress, wet dressing, or as a soak.

AS A COMPRESS OR WET DRESSING:
• Saturate a clean, soft, white cloth (such as a diaper or torn sheet) in the solution.
• Gently squeeze and apply loosely to the affected area.
• Saturate the cloth in the solution every 15 to 30 minutes and apply to the affected area.
• Discard the solution after each use.
• Repeat as often as necessary.
AS A SOAK:
• Soak affected area in the solution for 15 to 30 minutes.
• Discard solution after each use.
• Repeat 3 times a day.
**DOMEBORO® Astringent Solution Effervescent Tablets**
• Dissolve one, two, or three tablets in 12 ounces of water and stir the solution until fully dissolved to obtain the following modified Burow's Solution.

| Number of Tablets | Dilution | % Aluminum Acetate |
|---|---|---|
| one tablet | 1:40 dilution | 0.16% |
| two tablets | 1:20 dilution | 0.32% |
| three tablets | 1:13 dilution | 0.48% |

• Do not strain or filter the solution.
• Can be used as a compress, wet dressing, or as a soak.

AS A COMPRESS OR WET DRESSING:
• Saturate a clean, soft, white cloth (such as a diaper or torn sheet) in the solution.
• Gently squeeze and apply loosely to the affected area.
• Saturate the cloth in the solution every 15 minutes and apply to the affected area.
• Discard the solution after each use.
• Repeat as often as necessary.

**AS A SOAK:**
- Soak affected area in the solution for 15 to 30 minutes.
- Discard solution after each use.
- Repeat 3 times a day.

**Other information:**
**DOMEBORO® Astringent Solution Effervescent Tablets:**
Each tablet, when dissolved in water and ready for use, provides the active ingredient Aluminum Acetate, resulting from the reaction of Calcium Acetate 606 mg and Aluminum Sulfate 879 mg. The resulting astringent solution is buffered to an acid pH.

**Inactive Ingredients:**
**DOMEBORO® Astringent Solution Powder Packets:** Dextrin.
**DOMEBORO® Astringent Solution Effervescent Tablets:** Dextrin, Polyethylene Glycol, Sodium Bicarbonate

**How Supplied:**
**DOMEBORO® Astringent Solution Powder Packets:** 12 Powder Packets.
**DOMEBORO® Astringent Solution Effervescent Tablets:** 12 Effervescent Tablets.

*Questions or comments?* 1-800-800-4793 weekdays 8:30-5:00 (Eastern Standard Time)
www.bayercare.com
DOMEBORO provides soothing, effective relief of minor skin irritations. For over 50 years doctors have been recommending DOMEBORO ASTRINGENT SOLUTION to help relieve minor skin irritations.
Bayer Corporation
Consumer Care Division
Morristown, NJ 07960 USA   MADE IN USA

---

**Maximum Strength**
**MIDOL® Teen**
**Pain & Multi-Symptom Menstrual Relief**
**Aspirin Free/Caffeine Free**
**Caplet**

Midol. Because your period's more than a pain.™

**Active Ingredients:**
| (in each caplet) | Purpose: |
|---|---|
| Acetaminophen 500 mg | Pain reliever |
| Pamabrom 25 mg | Diuretic |

**Uses:** For the temporary relief of these symptoms associated with menstrual periods:
- cramps
- bloating
- water-weight gain
- headache
- backache
- muscle aches

**Warnings: Alcohol warning:** If you consume 3 or more alcoholic drinks every day, ask your doctor whether you should take acetaminophen or other pain relievers/fever reducers. Acetaminophen may cause liver damage.

**Do not use** with any other product containing acetaminophen.
**Stop use and ask a doctor if:**
- new symptoms occur
- redness or swelling is present
- pain gets worse or lasts for more than 10 days

**If pregnant or breast-feeding,** ask a health professional before use.
**Keep out of reach of children.** In case of overdose, get medical help or contact a Poison Control Center right away. Prompt medical help is critical for adults as well as children even if you do not notice any signs or symptoms.

**Directions:**
- adults and children 12 years and older
- take 2 caplets with water
- repeat every 6 hours, as needed
- do not exceed 8 caplets per day
- children under 12 years, consult a doctor

**Other Information:** Store at room temperature

**Inactive Ingredients:** Carnauba Wax, Croscarmellose sodium, D&C Red #7 calcium Lake, FD&C Blue #2 Aluminum Lake, Hydroxypropyl methylcellulose, Magnesium Stearate, Microcrystalline cellulose, Propylene glycol, Shellac, Starch, Titanium Dioxide, Triacetin

**How Supplied:** Caplets-White capsule-shaped caplets available in packages of 24 caplets containing 3 blisters of 8 caplets each.
**Questions? Comments?**
**Please call 1-800-331-4536.**
**Visit our website at**
**www.bayercare.com**
**ASPIRIN-FREE   CAFFEINE-FREE**
Distributed by:
Bayer Corporation
Consumer Care Division
Morristown, NJ 07960 USA
*Shown in Product Identification Guide, page 504*

---

**Maximum Strength**
**MIDOL® Menstrual**
**Pain & Multi-Symptom Menstrual Relief**
**Aspirin Free**
**Caplets and Gelcaps**

**Active Ingredients:**
| (in each caplet and gelcap) | Purpose: |
|---|---|
| Acetaminophen 500 mg | Pain reliever |
| Caffeine 60 mg | Stimulant |
| Pyrilamine maleate 15 mg | Diuretic |

**Uses:** For the temporary relief of these symptoms associated with menstrual periods:
- cramps
- bloating
- water-weight gain
- breast tenderness
- headache
- backache
- muscle aches
- fatigue

**Warnings: Alcohol warning:** If you consume 3 or more alcoholic drinks every day, ask your doctor whether you should take acetaminophen or other pain relievers/fever reducers. Acetaminophen may cause liver damage.
**Do not use** with any other product containing acetaminophen.
**Ask a doctor before use if you have:**
- glaucoma
- difficulty in urination due to enlargement of the prostate gland
- a breathing problem such as emphysema or chronic bronchitis

**Ask a doctor or pharmacist before use if you are** taking sedatives or tranquilizers.
**When using this product:**
- you may get drowsy
- avoid alcoholic drinks
- excitability may occur, especially in children
- alcohol, sedatives, and tranquilizers may increase drowsiness
- be careful when driving a motor vehicle or operating machinery
- limit the use of caffeine-containing medications, foods, or beverages. Too much caffeine may cause nervousness, irritability, sleeplessness, and occasionally, rapid heartbeat.

**Stop use and ask a doctor if:**
- new symptoms occur
- redness or swelling is present
- pain gets worse or lasts for more than 10 days

**If pregnant or breast-feeding,** ask a health professional before use.
**Keep out of reach of children.** In case of overdose, get medical help or contact a Poison Control Center right away. Prompt medical help is critical for adults as well as children even if you do not notice any signs or symptoms.

**Directions:**
**MIDOL® Extra Strength Caplets:**
- adults and children 12 years and older
  - take 2 caplets with water
  - repeat every 4 hours, as needed
  - do not exceed 8 caplets per day
- children under 12 years, consult a doctor

**MIDOL® Extra Strength Gelcaps:**
- adults and children 12 years and older
  - take 2 gelcaps with water
  - repeat every 6 hours, as needed
  - do not exceed 8 gelcaps per day
- children under 12 years, consult a doctor

**Other Information:**
- store at room temperature
- avoid excessive heat 104°F (40°C)
- the recommended dose of this product contains about as much caffeine as a cup of coffee

**Inactive Ingredients:**

**MIDOL® Extra Strength Caplets:** Croscarmellose Sodium, FD&C Blue #2, Hydroxypropyl Methylcellulose, Magnesium Stearate, Microcrystalline Cellulose, Pregelatinized Starch, Triacetin.

**MIDOL® Extra Strength Gelcaps:** Carnauba Wax, Croscarmellose Sodium, D&C Red #33 Lake, Disodium EDTA, FD&C Blue #1 Lake, Gelatin, Glycerin, Hydroxypropyl Methylcellulose, Iron Oxide, Lecithin, Magnesium Stearate, Microcrystalline Cellulose, Pharmaceutical

*Continued on next page*

## Midol—Cont.

Glaze, Simethicone, Starch, Stearic Acid, Titanium Dioxide, Triacetin

**How Supplied:**
**MIDOL® Extra Strength Caplets:**
Capsule-shaped caplets available in packages of 24 caplets containing 3 blisters of 8 capsules each.
**MIDOL® Extra Strength Gelcaps:**
Capsule-shaped gelcaps available in packages of 24 gelcaps containing 3 blisters of 8 gelcaps each.
Use only if blister unit is unbroken.
Store at room temperature; avoid excessive heat 40°C (104°F).
**Questions? Comments?**
**Please call 1-800-331-4536.**
**Visit our website at www.bayercare.com**
ASPIRIN-FREE
B-R LLC
Distributed by:
Bayer Corporation
Consumer Care Division
Morristown, NJ 07960 USA
*Shown in Product Identification Guide, page 504*

---

Maximum Strength
**MIDOL® PMS**
Pain & Premenstrual Symptom Relief
Aspirin Free/Caffeine Free
Caplets and Gelcaps

**Active Ingredients:**
**(in each caplet
and in each gelcap)          Purpose:**
Acetaminophen 500 mg .... Pain reliever
Pamabrom 25 mg ........................ Diuretic
Pyrilamine maleate 15 mg ....... Diuretic

**Uses:** For the temporary relief of these symptoms associated with menstrual periods:
• bloating
• water-weight gain
• cramps
• breast tenderness
• headache
• backache

**Warnings: Alcohol warning:** If you consume 3 or more alcoholic drinks every day, ask your doctor whether you should take acetaminophen or other pain relievers/fever reducers. Acetaminophen may cause liver damage.
**Do not use** with any other product containing acetaminophen.
**Ask a doctor before use if you have:**
• glaucoma
• difficulty in urination due to enlargement of the prostate gland
• a breathing problem such as emphysema or chronic bronchitis
**Ask a doctor or pharmacist before use if you are** taking sedatives or tranquilizers.
**When using this product:**
• you may get drowsy
• excitability may occur, especially in children
• alcohol, sedatives, and tranquilizers may increase drowsiness

• avoid alcoholic drinks
• be careful when driving a motor vehicle or operating machinery
**Stop use and ask a doctor if:**
• new symptoms occur
• redness or swelling is present
• pain gets worse or lasts for more than 10 days
**If pregnant or breast-feeding,** ask a health professional before use.
**Keep out of reach of children.** In case of overdose, get medical help or contact a Poison Control Center right away. Prompt medical help is critical for adults as well as for chilren even if you do not notice any signs or symptoms.

**Directions:**
**MIDOL® Maximum Strength PMS Caplets:**
• adults and children 12 years and older
  • take 2 caplets with water
  • repeat every 6 hours, as needed
  • do not exceed 8 caplets per day
• children under 12 years, consult a doctor
**MIDOL® Maximum Strength PMS Gelcaps:**
• adults and children 12 years and older
  • take 2 gelcaps with water
  • repeat every 6 hours, as needed
  • do not exceed 8 gelcaps per day
• children under 12 years, consult a doctor
**Other Information:** Store at room temperature

**Inactive Ingredients:**
**MIDOL® Maximum Strength PMS:** Carnauba Wax, Croscarmellose Sodium, D&C Red #30 Aluminum Lake, D&C Yellow #10 Aluminum Lake, Hydroxypropyl Methylcellulose, Magnesium Stearate, Microcrystalline Cellulose, Propylene Glycol, Shellac, Starch, Titanium Dioxide, Triacetin
**MIDOL® Maximum Strength PMS Gelcaps:** Croscarmellose Sodium, D&C Red #27 Lake, EDTA Disodium, FD&C Blue #1, FD&C Red #40 Lake, Gelatin, Glycerin, Hydroxypropyl Methylcellulose, Iron Oxide, Magnesium Stearate, Microcrystalline Cellulose, Starch, Stearic Acid, Titanium Dioxide, Triacetin.

**How Supplied:**
**MIDOL® Maximum Strength PMS Caplets:** Capsule-shaped caplets available in packages of 24 caplets containing 3 blisters of 8 caplets each.
**MIDOL® Maximum Strength PMS Gelcaps:** Capsule-shaped gelcaps available in packages of 24 gelcaps containing 3 blisters of 8 gelcaps each.
Use only if blister unit is unbroken.
Store at room temperature; avoid excessive heat 40°C (104°F).
**Questions? Comments?**
**Please call 1-800-331-4536.**
**Visit our website at www.bayercare.com**
ASPIRIN-FREE CAFFEINE-FREE
B-R LLC
Distributed by:
Bayer Corporation
Consumer Care Division
Morristown, NJ 07960 USA
*Shown in Product Identification Guide, page 504*

**NEO-SYNEPHRINE®**
Mild Formula, Regular Strength, Extra Strength

**Active Ingredients:**
**Neo-Synephrine® Extra Strength Drops**
**Neo-Synephrine® Extra Strength Spray**
**Active Ingredient:          Purpose:**
Phenylephrine
Hydrochloride 1.0% ........................ Nasal decongestant
**Neo-Synephrine® Regular Strength Drops**
**Neo-Synephrine® Regular Strength Spray**
**Active Ingredient:          Purpose:**
Phenylephrine
Hydrochloride 0.5% ........................ Nasal decongestant
**Neo-Synephrine® Mild Formula Spray**
**Active Ingredient:          Purpose:**
Phenylephrine
Hydrochloride 0.25% ........................ Nasal decongestant

**Uses:** • Temporarily relieves nasal congestion:
  — due to common cold
  — due to hay fever or other respiratory allergies (allergic rhinitis)
  — associated with sinusitis
• Temporarily relieves stuffy nose.
• Helps clear nasal passages; shrinks swollen membranes.
• Temporarily restores freer breathing through the nose.
• Helps decongest sinus openings and passages;
• temporarily relieves sinus congestion and pressure.

**Warnings: Do not exceed recommended dosage.**
**Ask a doctor before use if you have**
• heart disease
• high blood pressure
• thyroid disease
• diabetes
• difficulty in urination due to enlargement of the prostate gland
**When using this product** temporary discomfort may occur such as:
• burning
• stinging
• sneezing
• increase in nasal discharge
• use by more than one person may spread infection.
**Stop use and ask a doctor if** symptoms persist. Do not use for more than 3 days. Use only as directed. Frequent or prolonged use may cause nasal congestion to recur or worsen.
**If pregnant or breast-feeding,** ask a health professional before use.
**Keep out of reach of children.** If swallowed, get medical help or contact a Poison Control Center right away.

**Directions:**
**Neo-Synephrine® Extra Strength Drops**
**Neo-Synephrine® Regular Strength Drops**

| Adults and children 12 years of age and over | 2 or 3 drops in each nostril not more often than every 4 hours. |
|---|---|
| Children under 12 years | Ask a doctor. |

**Neo-Synephrine® Extra Strength Spray**
**Neo-Synephrine® Regular Strength Spray**
To spray, squeeze bottle quickly and firmly.

| Adults and children 12 years of age and over | 2 or 3 sprays in each nostril not more often than every 4 hours. |
|---|---|
| Children under 12 years | Ask a doctor. |

**Neo-Synephrine® Mild Formula Spray**
To spray, squeeze bottle quickly and firmly.

| Adults and children 6 to under 12 years of age ( with adult supervision) | 2 or 3 sprays in each nostril not more often than every 4 hours. |
|---|---|
| Children under 6 years | Ask a doctor. |

**Other Information:**
- Store at room temperature.
- Protect from light.

**Inactive Ingredients:** Benzalkonium Chloride, Citric Acid, Sodium Chloride, Sodium Citrate, Thimerosal, Water

**How Supplied:**
**Neo-Synephrine® Regular Strength Drops;**
**Neo-Synephrine® Extra Strength Drops:** 15 mL (0.5%).
DO NOT USE IF IMPRINTED BOTTLE OVERWRAP IS BROKEN OR MISSING.
**Neo-Synephrine® Regular Strength Spray;**
**Neo-Synephrine® Extra Strength Spray:** 15 mL (1.0%).
USE ONLY IF NECKBAND PRINTED WITH "Bayer" IS INTACT.
**Neo-Synephrine® Mild Formula Spray:** 15 mL (0.25%).
USE ONLY IF NECKBAND PRINTED WITH "Bayer" IS INTACT.
*Shown in Product Identification Guide, page 504*

---

**NEO-SYNEPHRINE®**
**12 Hour**
**(nasal spray)**
**12 Hour Extra Moisturizing**
**(nasal spray)**

**Active Ingredients:**            **Purpose:**
Oxymetazoline
  hydrochloride 0.05% ................... Nasal
                                        decongestant

**Uses:** Temporarily relieves nasal congestion:
— due to common cold
— due to hay fever or other respiratory allergies
— associated with sinusitis
- temporarily relieves stuffy nose.
- helps clear nasal passages; shrinks swollen membranes.
- temporarily restores freer breathing through the nose.
- helps decongest sinus openings and passages; temporarily relieves sinus congestion and pressure.

**Warnings:  Do not exceed recommended dosage.**
**Ask a doctor before use if you have**
- heart disease
- high blood pressure
- thyroid disease
- diabetes
- difficulty in urination due to enlargement of the prostate gland
**When using this product**
- temporary discomfort such as burning, stinging, sneezing, and increase in nasal discharge may occur
- use by more than one person may spread infection
**Stop use and ask a doctor if** symptoms persist for more than 3 days. Frequent or prolonged use may cause nasal congestion to recur or worsen.
**If pregnant or breast-feeding,** ask a health professional before use.
**Keep out of reach of children.** If swallowed, get medical help or contact a Poison Control Center right away.
**Directions:**
- use only as directed
- to spray, squeeze bottle quickly and firmly

| adults and children 6 to under 12 years (with adult supervision) | 2 to 3 sprays in each nostril not more often than every 10 to 12 hours. Do not exceed 2 doses in 24 hours. |
|---|---|
| children under 6 years | ask a doctor. |

**Other Information:**
- store at room temperature.
- protect from light.
**Inactive Ingredients:**
**NEO-SYNEPHRINE® 12 Hour Spray:** Benzalkonium chloride, disodium phosphate, EDTA disodium, sodium chloride, sodium phosphate, water
**NEO-SYNEPHRINE® 12 Hour Extra Moisturizing Spray:** Benzalkonium chloride, disodium phosphate, EDTA disodium, glycerin, sodium chloride, sodium phosphate, water

**How Supplied:** Plastic squeeze bottle of 15 ml (½ Fl oz).
USE ONLY IF NECKBAND PRINTED WITH "Bayer" IS INTACT.
*Shown in Product Identification Guide, page 504*

---

**PHILLIPS'® CHEWABLE TABLETS ANTACID-LAXATIVE STIMULANT FREE**

**Indications:**
**As A Laxative:** To relieve occasional constipation (irregularity). This product generally produces bowel movement in 1/2 to 6 hours.
**As An Antacid:** To relieve acid indigestion, sour stomach, and heartburn.

**Active Ingredient per tablet:** Magnesium Hydroxide 311 mg.

**Inactive Ingredients:** Colloidal Silicon Dioxide, Dextrates, Magnesium Stearate, Maltodextrin, Natural Flavor, Starch, Sucrose.

Sodium Content: 0.92 mg per tablet.

**Directions:**
**As A Laxative:** Take preferably before bedtime, followed with a full glass (8 oz.) of liquid. **Adults and Children 12 years and older,** Chew 6–8 tablets. **Children 6–11 years,** Chew 3–4 tablets. **2–5 years,** Chew 1–2 tablets. **Under 2,** Consult a doctor.

**As An Antacid:** Take up to 4 times a day or as directed by a doctor. **Adults,** Chew 2–4 tablets. **Children 7–14 years,** Chew 1 tablet.

**Warnings:**

**As A Laxative:** Do not take any laxative if abdominal pain, nausea, vomiting or kidney disease are present unless directed by a doctor. If you have noticed a sudden change in bowel habits persisting for over 2 weeks, consult a doctor before using a laxative. Laxative products should not be used for a period longer than 1 week, unless directed by a doctor. Rectal bleeding or failure to have a bowel movement after use of a laxative may indicate a serious condition. Discontinue use and consult your doctor.

**As An Antacid:** Do not take more than the maximum recommended daily dosage in a 24-hour period, or use the maximum dosage of this product for more than 2 weeks, or use this product if you have kidney disease, except under the advice and supervision of a doctor. May have a laxative effect.

**Drug Interaction Precaution:** May interact with certain prescription drugs. If you are presently taking a prescription drug, do not take this product without checking with your doctor or other healthcare professional.

Keep this and all drugs out of the reach of children. In case of accidental overdose, seek professional assistance or contact a Poison Control Center immediately. As with any drug, if you are pregnant or nursing a baby, seek the advice of a healthcare professional before using this product.

**How Supplied:** Bottles of 100 Tablets and 200 Tablets

**Questions? Comments?**
**Please call 1-800-331-4536.**
**Visit our website at**
**www.bayercare.com**

*Continued on next page*

## PHILLIP'S® LIQUI-GELS®

**Uses:**
- For the relief of occasional constipation (irregularity).
- This product generally produces a bowel movement in 12–72 hours.

**Active ingredient**
(in each softgel):        **Purpose:**
Docusate sodium
  100 mg .............. Stool softener laxative

**Inactive ingredients:** FD&C blue #2 lake, gelatin, glycerin, methylparaben, polyethylene glycol, propylene glycol, propylparaben, shellac, sorbitol, titanium dioxide

Phillips' Liqui-Gels are a very low sodium product. Each softgel contains 5 mg of sodium.

**Directions:**
Take softgels with a full glass (8 oz) of water.

| adults and children 12 years and over | Take 1 to 3 softgels daily or as directed by a doctor. This dose may be taken as a single daily dose or in divided doses. |
|---|---|
| children 6 to under 12 years | Take 1 softgel daily or as directed by a doctor. |
| children under 6 years of age | consult a doctor. |

**Warnings:** **Do not use** laxative products for a period longer than 1 week unless directed by a doctor. **Ask a doctor before use if you have** abdominal pain, nausea, vomiting or if you have noticed a sudden change in bowel habits that persists over a period of 2 weeks. **Ask a doctor or pharmacist before use if you are** presently taking mineral oil. **Stop use and ask a doctor if** you have rectal bleeding or failure to have a bowel movement after use. These could be signs of a serious condition. **If pregnant or breast-feeding,** ask a health professional before use. **Keep out of reach of children.** In case of overdosage, get medical help or contact a Poison Control Center right away.

**Storage:** Store at room temperature. Avoid excessive heat 104°F (40°C).

**Questions?** 1-800-331-4536 or www.bayercare.com

**How Supplied:** Blister packs of 10, 30 & 50 Liqui-Gels.

Liqui-Gels is a registered trademark of R.P. Scherer Corp.

*Shown in Product Identification Guide, page 505*

## PHILLIPS'® MILK OF MAGNESIA
**Original Formula**
**Cherry Formula**
**Mint Formula**

**Active Ingredients:**
*Original Formula:* Magnesium Hydroxide 400 mg per teaspoon (5 ml).
*Cherry Formula:* Magnesium Hydroxide 400 mg per teaspoon (5 ml).
*Mint Formula:* Magnesium Hydroxide 400 mg per teaspoon (5 ml).

**Inactive Ingredients:**
*Original Formula:* Purified Water.
*Cherry Formula:* Carboxymethylcellulose Sodium, Citric Acid, D&C Red #28, Flavor, Glycerin, Microcrystalline Cellulose, Purified Water, Sodium Citrate, Sodium Hypochlorite, Sucrose, Xanthan Gum.
*Mint Formula:* Artifical and Natural Flavors, Mineral Oil, Purified Water, Sodium Saccarin.

**Indications: AS A LAXATIVE**—To relieve occasional constipation (irregularity). This product generally produces bowel movement in $^1/_2$ to 6 hours.

**AS AN ANTACID**—To relieve acid indigestion, sour stomach and heartburn.

**Directions: For Laxative Use** - SHAKE WELL BEFORE USING. Adults and Children 12 years & older: 2–4 tablespoonful at bedtime or upon arising, followed by a full glass (8 oz.) of liquid.
**Children: DO NOT USE DOSAGE CUP.** Children 6–11 years: 1–2 tablespoonful, followed by a full glass (8 oz.) of liquid. Children 2–5 years: 1–3 teaspoonful, followed by a full glass (8 oz.) of liquid. Children under 2 years: Consult a doctor.

**Directions: For Antacid Use** - SHAKE WELL BEFORE USING. **DO NOT USE DOSAGE CUP.** Adults and Children 12 years & older: 1–3 teaspoonful with a little water, up to four times a day or as directed by a doctor.

**Drug Interaction Precaution:** Antacids may interact with certain prescription drugs. If you are presently taking a prescription drug, do not take this product without checking with your doctor or other health professional.

**Laxative Warnings:** Do not take any laxative if abdominal pain, nausea, vomiting or kidney disease are present unless directed by a doctor. If you have noticed a sudden change in bowel habits persisting for over 2 weeks, consult a doctor before using a laxative. Laxative products should not be used for a period longer than 1 week, unless directed by a doctor. Rectal bleeding or failure to have a bowel movement after use of a laxative may indicate a serious condition. Discontinue use and consult your doctor.

Phillips' Milk of Magnesia is a saline laxative.

**Antacid Warnings:** Do not take more than the maximum recommended daily dosage in a 24 hour period (See Directions), or use the maximum dosage of this product for more than two weeks, or use this product if you have kidney disease, except under the advice and supervision of a doctor. May have laxative effect.

If pregnant or breast-feeding, ask a health professional before use. Keep this and all drugs out of the reach of children. In case of accidental overdose, seek professional assistance or contact a Poison Control Center immediately.

**Storage:** Keep tightly closed and avoid freezing.

**How Supplied:** Phillips' Milk of Magnesia is available in Original, Mint, and Cherry formulas and comes in 4 oz., 12 oz., and 26 oz. bottles. Also available in chewable tablets and concentrated liquid formulas.

*Shown in Product Identification Guide, page 505*

---

## PHILLIPS'® M-O
**Lubricant Laxative**
**Original Formula**
**Refreshing Mint Formula**

**Active Ingredients:**
*Original Formula:* Magnesium Hydroxide 301 mg, Mineral Oil 1.25 ml per 5 ml teaspoonful
*Refreshing Mint Formula:* Magnesium Hydroxide 300 mg, Mineral Oil 1.25 ml per 5 ml teaspoonful.

**Inactive Ingredients:**
*Original Formula:* Purified Water, Sodium Citrate.
*Refreshing Mint Formula:* Flavor, Glycerin, Microcrystalline Cellulose, Sodium Carboxymethylcellulose, Sodium Citrate, Sodium Hypochlorite, Sodium Saccharin, Water.

**Indications:**
For the relief of occasional constipation or irregularity accompanied by hemorrhoids. This product generally produces bowel movement in 6 to 8 hours.

**Directions for Use:**
Shake well before using. Store at room temperature. Keep from freezing. Laxative Dosage Cup, for adults† only, should be washed before and after use. Do not take with meals.
**FOR CONSTIPATION RELIEF**
†**ADULTS** and **CHILDREN 12 years and over:** 2–4 tablespoonsful at bedtime or upon arising, followed by a full glass (8 oz.) of liquid.**

**CHILDREN 6 to 11 years: DO NOT USE DOSAGE CUP:** 1 teaspoonful to 1 tablespoonful at bedtime or upon arising, followed by a full glass (8 oz.) of liquid.**
Children under 6 years: Consult a doctor.

*Lubricant Saline Laxative. **As bowel function improves, reduce dose gradually.

**Warnings:** Do not use laxative products when abdominal pain, nausea, vomiting or kidney disease are present unless directed by a doctor. If you have noticed a sudden change in bowel habits persisting for over 2 weeks, consult a doctor before using a laxative. Laxative products should not be used for a period longer than 1 week, unless directed by a doctor. Rectal bleeding or failure to have a bowel movement after use may indicate a serious condition. Discontinue use and consult a doctor. Do not administer to children under 6 years of age, to pregnant women, to bedridden patients or to persons with difficulty in swallowing. Do not take with meals. Keep this and all drugs out of the reach of children. In case of accidental overdose, seek professional assistance or contact a Poison Control Center immediately. **If pregnant or breast-feeding,** ask a health professional before use. **DRUG INTERACTION PRECAUTION:** Do not take this product if you are presently taking a stool softener laxative unless directed by a doctor.

**How Supplied:** **Original:** Bottle of 12 fl oz (354 ml). **Refreshing Mint:** Bottles of 12 fl oz (354 ml) and 26 fl oz (769 ml).

Questions? Comments?
Please call **1-800-331-4536.**
Visit our website at
www.bayercare.com

Bayer Corporation
Consumer Care Division
Morristown, NJ 07960 USA
*Shown in Product Identification
Guide, page 505*

---

**1-2-3 LICE ELIMINATION SYSTEM**
**LICE KILLING SHAMPOO**
**LICE TREATMENT**
**SHAMPOO & CONDITIONER IN ONE**

- Kills lice and eggs
- Leaves no chemical residue
- Use on **DRY** hair
- Includes patented comb

**Active Ingredients:**     **Purpose:**
Piperonyl butoxide
(4%) ................. Lice Treatment
Pyrethrum extract (equivalent to
0.33% pyrethrins) ........ Lice Treatment

**Uses:** Treats head, pubic (crab), and body lice

**Warnings:**
- **For external use only**
**Do not use** near the eyes or permit contact with the inside of the nose, mouth, or vagina. Irritation may occur.
**Ask a doctor before use if you have** an allergy to ragweed.
**When using this product:**
- keep out of eyes and do not open eyes until product is rinsed out of hair.
- protect eyes with washcloth, towel, or other suitable method

---

- if product gets into the eyes, immediately flush with water
**Stop use and ask a doctor if:**
- skin irritation or infection is present or develops
- infestation of eyebrows or eyelashes occurs
**Keep out of reach of children.** If swallowed, get medical help or contact a Poison Control Center right away.

**Directions:**
- **Important: Read warnings and complete directions in the Consumer Information Insert before using.**
- Apply to **DRY HAIR** only. Massage until hair and scalp are thoroughly wet with product (see insert)
- After completing application, allow product to remain on hair for 10 minutes but no longer.
- Add sufficient warm water to form a lather and shampoo as usual. Rinse thoroughly.
- A fine-toothed comb or a special lice/nit removing comb (included) must be used to help remove dead lice, eggs, and nits from hair.
- **A second treatment must be done in 10 days to kill any newly hatched lice.**
**Other Information:**
- It is important to wash in hot water (130°F) all clothing, bedding, towels, and hair products (combs, brushes) used by infested persons.
- Dry clean non-washable fabrics.
- To eliminate infestation of furniture and bedding that cannot be washed or dry cleaned, a multi-use lice spray may be used.
- Store at room temperature: 59°–86°F (15°–30°C).

**Inactive Ingredients** Water, SD Alcohol, PEG-25 Hydrogenated Castor Oil, Ammonium Laureth Sulfate, Polyquaternium-10, Fragrance

RID Lice Killing Shampoo will kill lice completely without leaving a chemical residue. To help prevent reinfestation, use it twice (Day 1 and Day 10). Amount of shampoo needed will vary by hair length. See below for guidelines:

| Hair Length | Approximate Dosage for 1 Adult/Child: |
|---|---|
| Short (ear length or shorter) | Day 1: 1 oz - 2 oz<br>Day 10: 1 oz - 2 oz<br>**Total: 2 oz - 4 oz** |
| Medium (shoulder length) | Day 1: 2 oz - 3 oz<br>Day 10: 2 oz - 3 oz<br>**Total: 4 oz - 6 oz** |
| Long (past shoulder length) | Day 1: 3 oz - 4 oz<br>Day 10: 3 oz - 4 oz<br>**Total: 6 oz - 8 oz** |

The patented RID® comb is proven 100% effective as demonstrated in laboratory studies performed by trained testers. Individual results may vary.

RID 1-2-3 LICE Elimination System Completely eliminate lice from your family and home.
Step 1—Kill Lice
- Apply RID Lice Killing Shampoo according to label directions.
- Repeat this step 10 days later to help prevent reinfestation.

---

Step 2—Comb-Out Eggs & Nits
- After Step 1, apply RID® Egg & Nit Comb-Out Gel on damp hair to make removal faster and easier.
*(Purchase separately)*
- Comb out the eggs and nits in the hair with a fine-toothed comb or with the RID® patented comb (included).
Step 3—Clean Home
- Use RID® **Home Lice Control Spray** to kill lice and their eggs on mattresses, furniture, car interiors, and other non-washable items.
*(Purchase separately)*
- Wash bed linens, clothing, and other items in hot water and dry in high heat.

**How Supplied:** 6 FL OZ (177 ml), 1 Comb.

**Questions or comments?**
1-800-RID-LICE (1-800-743-5423)
www.ridlice.com

Distributed by: Bayer Corporation
P.O. Box 1910
Morristown, NJ 07962-1910 USA
*Shown in Product Identification
Guide, page 505*

---

**1-2-3 LICE ELIMINATION SYSTEM**
**LICE KILLING NO-DRIP MOUSSE**
**pyrethrum extract*/piperonyl butoxide**
**aerosolized foam Lice Treatment**

- Kills lice completely
- Leaves no chemical residue
- Use on **DRY** hair
- Includes patented comb

**Active Ingredients:**     **Purpose:**
**(calculated without propellant)**
Piperonyl butoxide
(4%) ................. Lice Treatment
Pyrethrum extract* (equivalent to
0.33% pyrethrins) ........ Lice Treatment

**Uses:** Treats head, pubic (crab), and body lice

**Warnings:**
- **For external use only**
- **Flammable:** Keep away from fire or flame
**Do not use** near the eyes or permit contact with the inside of the nose, mouth, or vagina. Irritation may occur.
**Ask a doctor before use if you have** an allergy to ragweed
**When using this product:**
- keep out of eyes when rinsing hair
- close eyes tightly and do not open eyes until product is rinsed out of hair
- protect eyes with washcloth, towel, or other suitable method
- if product gets into the eyes, immediately flush with water
- do not inhale; use in a well ventilated area
- do not puncture or incinerate. Contents under pressure.
**Stop use and ask a doctor if:**
- skin irritation or infection is present or develops
- infestation of eyebrows or eyelashes occurs
**Keep out of reach of children.** If swallowed, get medical help or contact a Poison Control Center right away.

*Continued on next page*

## 1-2-3 Lice Elimination—Cont.

**Directions:**
- **Important: Read warnings and complete directions in the Consumer Information Insert before using.**
- Shake well before using.
- Holding the can upside down, apply RID® No-Drip Mousse to **DRY hair** or other affected area. Massage until hair and scalp are thoroughly wet with product.
- After completing application, allow product to remain on the hair for 10 minutes but no longer.
- Rinse thoroughly with warm water and wash hair with soap or regular shampoo.
- A fine-toothed comb or a special lice/nit removing comb (included) must be used to help remove dead lice or their eggs (nits) from hair.
- A second treatment must be done in 7 to 10 days to kill any newly hatched lice.

**Other Information:**
- It is important to wash in hot water (130°F) all clothing, bedding, towels, and hair products (combs, brushes) used by infested persons.
- Dry clean non-washable fabrics.
- To eliminate infestation of furniture and bedding that cannot be washed or dry cleaned, a multi use lice spray may be used.
- Store at 20°–25°C (68°–77°F).
- Do not store at temperature above 43°C (110°F).
- Keep in a cool place out of the sun.

**Inactive Ingredients:** cetearyl alcohol, isobutane, PEG-20 stearate, propane, propylene glycol, purified water, quaternium-52, SD Alcohol 3-C (26.5% w/w)

**Questions? call 1-800-RID-LICE** (1-800-743-5423)
www.ridlice.com

RID Lice Killing No-Drip Mousse will kill lice completely without leaving a chemical residue. To help prevent reinfestation, use it **twice** (Day 1 and Day 10)†. Amount of Mousse needed will vary by hair length. See below for guidelines:

| Hair Length | Approximate Dosage for 1 Adult/Child: |
|---|---|
| Short (ear length or shorter) | Day 1: 1 oz – 2 oz<br>Day 10: 1 oz – 2 oz<br>**Total: 2 oz – 4 oz** |
| Medium (shoulder length) | Day 1: 2 oz – 3 oz<br>Day 10: 2 oz – 3 oz<br>**Total: 4 oz – 6 oz** |
| Long (past shoulder length) | Day 1: 3 oz – 4 oz<br>Day 10: 3 oz – 4 oz<br>**Total: 6 oz – 8 oz** |

†While you must apply the 2nd application within 7–10 days of the 1st treatment, it is strongly recommended to wait until Day 10 for maximum effectiveness. Use RID Egg & Nit Comb-Out Gel after each treatment application to remove eggs & nits and help prevent reinfestation.

The patented RID® comb is proven 100% effective as demonstrated in laboratory studies performed by trained testers. Individual results may vary.

## RID 1-2-3 LICE ELIMINATION SYSTEM

Completely eliminate lice from your family and home.

Step 1– Kill Lice
- Apply RID **Lice Killing Mousse** according to label directions.
- Repeat this step 7 to 10 days later to help prevent reinfestation.

Step 2– Comb-Out Eggs & Nits
- After Step 1, apply RID® Egg & Nit Comb-Out Gel on damp hair to make removal faster and easier. *(Purchase separately)*
- Comb out the eggs and nits in the hair with a fine-toothed comb or with the RID® patented comb (included).

Step 3– Clean Home
- Use RID® **Home Lice Control Spray** to kill lice and their eggs on mattresses, furniture, car interiors, and other non-washable items. *(Purchase separately)*
- Wash bed linens, clothing, and other items in hot water and dry in high heat.

**How Supplied:** 5.5 oz (156 g), 1 Comb.

*50% extract (not USP)
Distributed by:
Bayer Corporation
P.O. Box 1910
Morristown, NJ 07962-1910 USA
*Shown in Product Identification Guide, page 505*

## VANQUISH®
**Extra Strength Pain Reliever Analgesic Caplets**

**Active Ingredient:**     **Purpose:**
**(in each caplet)**
Aspirin 227 mg .................... Pain reliever
Acetaminophen 194 mg .... Pain reliever
Caffeine 33 mg ............. Pain reliever aid

**Uses:** Temporarily relieves minor aches and pains due to
- headache
- backache
- menstrual cramps
- arthritis
- colds and flu
- muscle aches and pains

**Warnings: Reye's syndrome:** Children and teenagers should not use this medicine for chicken pox or flu symptoms before a doctor is consulted about Reye's syndrome, a rare but serious illness reported to be associated with aspirin.

**Alcohol warning:** If you consume 3 or more alcoholic drinks every day, ask your doctor whether you should take acetaminophen and aspirin or other pain relievers/fever reducers. Acetaminophen and aspirin may cause liver damage and stomach bleeding.

**Do not use:**
- if you have had an allergic reaction to any other pain reliever/fever reducer
- with any other product containing acetaminophen.

**Ask a doctor before use if you have:**
- asthma
- ulcers
- bleeding problems
- stomach problems that last or come back such as heartburn, upset stomach or stomach pain

**Ask a doctor or pharmacist before use if you are taking a prescription drug for:**
- diabetes
- gout
- arthritis
- anticoagulation (blood thinning)

**Stop use and ask doctor if:**
- an allergic reaction occurs. Seek medical help right away.
- pain gets worse or lasts more than 10 days
- new symptoms occur
- ringing in the ears or loss of hearing occurs
- redness or swelling is present

**If pregnant or breast-feeding,** ask a health professional before use. **It is especially important not to use aspirin during the last 3 months of pregnancy unless definitely directed to do so by a doctor because it may cause problems in the unborn child or complications during delivery.**

**Keep out of reach of children.** In case of overdose, get medical help or contact a Poison Control Center right away. Prompt medical attention is critical for adults as well as children even if you do not notice any signs or symptoms.

**Directions:**
- adults and children 12 years and over: take 2 caplets with water every 6 hours, not to exceed 8 caplets in 24 hours unless directed by a doctor
- children under 12 years: consult a doctor

**Other Information:**
- save carton for full directions and warnings
- store at room temperature 20°–25°C (68°–77°F)
- buffered with aluminum hydroxide and magnesium hydroxide

**Inactive Ingredients:** Aluminum hydroxide, colloidal silicon dioxide, hydroxypropyl methylcellulose, magnesium hydroxide, microcrystalline cellulose, propylene glycol, starch, titanium dioxide, zinc stearate

**How Supplied:** Bottle of 100 analgesic caplets.
USE ONLY IF SEAL UNDER BOTTLE CAP WITH GREEN "Bayer Corporation" PRINT IS INTACT.
**Questions or comments?**
1-800-331-4536 or www.bayercare.com
Distributed by:
Bayer Corporation
PO Box 1910
Morristown, NJ 07962-1910
*Shown in Product Identification Guide, page 505*

## Beutlich LP Pharmaceuticals

**1541 SHIELDS DRIVE
WAUKEGAN, IL 60085-8304**

**Direct Inquiries to:**
847-473-1100
800-238-8542 in US & Canada
FAX 847–473-1122
www.beutlich.com
e-mail beutlich@beutlich.com

### CEO–TWO® Evacuant
Laxative Adult Rectal Suppository

NDC #0283-0763-09

**Composition:** Each suppository contains sodium bicarbonate and potassium bitartrate in a special blend of water-soluble polyethylene glycols.

**Indications:** For relief of occasional constipation, irregularity or for bowel training programs. CEO-TWO generally produces a bowel movement in 5–30 minutes. The lubrication provided by the emollient base combined with the gentle pressure of the released carbon dioxide slowly distends the rectal ampulla stimulating peristalsis. CEO-TWO does not interfere with normal digestion, is not habit forming, won't cause cramping or irritation or alter the normal peristaltic reflex, and it leaves no residue.

**Administration and Dosage:** Adults and children over 12 years of age. Rectal dosage is one suppository containing 0.6 gram of sodium bicarbonate and 0.9 gram potassium bitartrate in a single daily dose. For children under 12 years of age: consult a doctor. For most effective results and ease of insertion, moisten a CEO-TWO suppository by placing it under a warm water tap for 30 seconds or in a cup of water for 10 seconds before insertion. Insert rectally past the largest diameter of the suppository. Patient should retain in the rectum as long as possible (usually about 5–30 minutes).

**Warnings:** For rectal use only. Do not use this product if you are on a low salt diet unless directed by a doctor. (172 milligrams of sodium per suppository) Do not lubricate with mineral oil or petrolatum prior to use. Do not use when abdominal pain, nausea or vomiting are present unless directed by a doctor. Laxative products should not be used for longer than one week unless directed by a doctor. If you have noticed a sudden change of bowel habits that persists over a period of 2 weeks, consult a doctor before using a laxative. Rectal bleeding or failure to have a bowel movement after use of a laxative may indicate a serious problem. Discontinue use and consult your doctor.

**How Supplied:** In box of 10 individually foil wrapped white opaque suppositories. Keep in cool dry place. **DO NOT REFRIGERATE**

### HURRICAINE® TOPICAL ANESTHETIC

**Composition:** HURRICAINE contains 20% benzocaine in a flavored, water soluble polyethylene glycol base.

**Action and Indications:** HURRICAINE is a topical anesthetic that provides rapid anesthesia on all accessible mucous membrane in 15 to 30 seconds, short duration of 15 minutes, has virtually no systemic absorption, and tastes good. Hurricaine is used as a lubricant and topical anesthetic to facilitate passage of fiberoptic gastroscopes, laryngoscopes, proctoscopes and sigmoidoscopes. In addition, Hurricaine is effective in suppressing the pharyngeal and tracheal gag reflex during the placement of nasogastric tubes. Hurricaine is used to control pain and discomfort during certain gynecological procedures such as IUD insertion, vaginal speculum placement, and as a preinjection anesthesia prior to LEEP procedures and paracervical blocks. Hurricaine is also effective for the temporary relief of pain due to sore throat, stomatitis and mucositis. It is also effective in controlling various types of pain associated with dental procedures and the temporary relief of minor mouth irritations, canker sores and irritation to the mouth and gums caused by dentures or orthodontic appliances.

**Contraindications:** Patients with a known hypersensitivity to benzocaine should not use HURRICAINE. True allergic reactions are rare.

**Adverse Reactions:** Methemoglobinemia has been reported following the use of benzocaine on extremely rare occasions. Intravenous methylene blue is the specific therapy for this condition.

**Cautions: DO NOT USE IN THE EYES.
NOT FOR INJECTION.
KEEP THIS AND ALL DRUGS OUT OF THE REACH OF CHILDREN.**

**Packaging Available**
**GEL**
1 oz. Jar Fresh Mint NDC #0283-0998-31
1 oz. Jar Wild Cherry NDC #0283-0871-31
1 oz. Jar Pina Colada NDC #0283-0886-31
1 oz. Jar Watermelon NDC #0283-0293-31
1/6 oz. Tube Wild Cherry NDC #0283-0871-75
1/6 oz. Tube Watermelon NDC #0283-0293-75
**LIQUID**
1 fl. oz. Jar Wild Cherry NDC #0283-0569-31
1 fl. oz. Jar Pina Colada NDC #0283-1886-31
1/6 oz. Tube Wild Cherry NDC #0283-0569-75
.25 ml Dry Handle Swab Wild Cherry 100 Each Per Box NDC #0283-0693-01

.25 ml Dry Handle Swab Wild Cherry 6 Each Per Travel Pack NDC #0283-0693-36
**SPRAY**
2 oz. Aerosol Wild Cherry NDC #0283-0679-02
**SPRAY KIT**
2 oz. Aerosol Wild Cherry NDC #0283-0183-02 with 200 Disposable Extension Tubes

### PERIDIN-C®

**Composition:** Each orange colored tablet contains 2 popular antioxidants; Vitamin C and Natural Bioflavonoids.
Ascorbic Acid 200 mg.
Hesperidin Complex 150 mg.
Hesperidin Methyl Chalcone 50 mg.
F.D. & C. #6. Sugar Free.

**Dosage:** 1 tablet daily or as directed.

**How Supplied:** In bottles of:
100 tablets NDC #0283-0597-01
500 tablets NDC #0283-0597-05

## Boehringer Ingelheim Consumer Healthcare Products Division of Boehringer Ingelheim Pharmceuticals Inc.

**900 RIDGEBURY ROAD
P.O. BOX 368
RIDGEFIELD, CT 06877**

**For direct inquiries contact:**
1-888-285-9159

### DULCOLAX® Bowel Prep Kit
**brand of bisacodyl USP**

**Indications:** For use as part of a bowel cleansing regimen in preparing patients for surgery or for preparing the colon for x-ray or endoscopic examination.

**Directions:** Read the entire label and directions on back at least 24 hours in advance of examination. Follow each step and complete all instructions or the entire x-ray or the endoscopic examination may have to be repeated.

**Warnings:** Do not use this product unless directed by a doctor. Do not chew or crush tablets. Do not give to children under 6 years of age, or to persons who cannot swallow without chewing unless directed by a doctor. **As with any drug, if you are pregnant or nursing a baby, seek the advice of a health care pro-**

*Continued on next page*

## Dulcolax Bowel Prep—Cont.

fessional before using this product.
Keep this and all drugs out of the reach
of children.

### Ingredients
**TABLET**

**Active Ingredient:** bisacodyl USP
5 mg per tablet. **Also Contains:** acacia,
acetylated monoglyceride, carnauba wax,
cellulose acetate phthalate, corn starch,
D&C Red No. 30 aluminum lake, D&C
Yellow No. 10 aluminum lake, dibutyl
phthalate, docusate sodium, gelatin,
glycerin, iron oxides, kaolin, lactose,
magnesium stearate, methylparaben,
pharmaceutical glaze, polyethylene glycol, povidone, propylparaben, sodium
benzoate, sorbitan monooleate, sucrose,
talc, titanium dioxide, white wax.

**SUPPOSITORY**

**Active Ingredient:** bisacodyl USP
10 mg per suppository.
**Also Contains:** hydrogenated vegetable
oil.
**Store at controlled room temperature
20–25°C (68–77°F).**
**Protect from moisture.**
**TAMPER EVIDENT. INDIVIDUALLY
SEALED FOR YOUR PROTECTION. DO
NOT USE IF INDIVIDUAL SEALS ARE
BROKEN.**
**Preparation Instructions for surgery or
x-ray of colon or endoscopic examination.**
**For your examination to be performed
properly, you must prepare yourself as
outlined in the directions. Preparation
begins at 12 noon the day before your
x-ray appointment.**
**Follow these directions exactly. Take
the medication, food and water in the
amounts shown and at the times
shown.**

### Directions
**12 Noon**
**Lunch**—Eat only the following:
1 cup bouillon soup and crackers
1 chicken or turkey white meat sand-
wich
(no butter, mayonnaise, lettuce, etc.)
1/2 glass clear apple juice or clear grape
juice
1 serving plain gelatin (no cream, fruit,
etc.)
1 glass skimmed milk or nonfat dry milk
**1 P.M.**
Drink one full glass or more of water
**3 P.M.**
Drink one full glass or more of water
**5 P.M.**
**Supper**—Eat only the following:
1 cup bouillon soup and crackers
1 glass clear apple juice or clear grape
juice
1 serving plain gelatin (no cream, fruit,
etc.)
**7 P.M.**
Drink one full glass or more of water
**8 P.M.**

Drink the entire amount of the liquid
laxative your doctor has prescribed to go
along with this kit.
**10 P.M.**
Take either three or four **Dulcolax®** Tablets (per your doctor's instructions) with
one full glass or more of water. **Do not
crush or chew tablets. Swallow them
whole. Do not take tablets within one
hour of consuming antacids or milk.**
**12 Midnight**
Drink one full glass or more of water
**If your physician has requested an ex-
amination of your urinary tract (an IVP)
in addition to your barium enema, the
7 A.M. procedures that follow should
not be carried out until after the IVP has
been completed.**
**7 A.M.**
If you are scheduled for a *barium enema
only,* do the following:
Drink one and one-half glasses of water
Use one **Dulcolax®** rectal suppository as
follows:
1. Unwrap suppository
2. Lie on left side with right thigh raised
3. Insert suppository into rectum,
pointed end first, as high as possible.
Make sure that some part of the suppository touches the wall of the rectum.
4. Close thighs to aid in retaining suppository.
5. Retain suppository at least 15–20
minutes, if possible. A bowel evacuation
usually occurs in 15 minutes to one hour.

**How Supplied:** 4 tablets, 5 mg each
and 1 suppository, 10 mg
**Questions about Dulcolax**
Call toll-free 1-888-285-9159
Distributed by:
Boehringer Ingelheim Consumer
Healthcare Products
Division of Boehringer Ingelheim
Pharmaceuticals, Inc. Ridgefield, CT
06877
©Boehringer Ingelheim Pharmaceuti-
cals, Inc.
*Shown in Product Identification
Guide, page 505*

---

## DULCOLAX®
[*dul 'cō-Lax*]
**brand of bisacodyl USP**
**Tablets of 5 mg**
**Laxative**

**Indications:** For relief of occasional
constipation and irregularity.

**Active ingredient:** bisacodyl USP
5 mg per tablet.

**Inactive ingredients:** acacia, acetylated monoglyceride, carnauba wax, cellulose acetate phthalate, corn starch, dibutyl phthalate, docusate sodium, gelatin, glycerin, iron oxides, kaolin, lactose,
magnesium stearate, methylparaben,
pharmaceutical glaze, polyethylene glycol, povidone, propylparaben, Red No. 30
lake, sodium benzoate, sorbitan monooleate, sucrose, talc, titanium dioxide,
white wax, Yellow No. 10 lake. Sodium
content: less than 0.2 mg/tablet.

**Directions:** Adults and children 12
years of age and over: Take 1 to 3 tablets
(usually 2) in a single dose once daily.
Children 6 to 12 years of age: Take 1 tablet once daily. Children under 6 years of
age: Consult a physician. Expect results
in 8–12 hours if taken at bedtime or
within 6 hours if taken before breakfast.

**Warnings:** Do not chew or crush. Do
not give to children under 6 years of age,
or to persons who cannot swallow without chewing, unless directed by a physician. Do not take this product within 1
hour after taking an antacid or milk. Do
not use laxative products when abdominal pain, nausea, or vomiting are present
unless directed by a physician. If you
have noticed a sudden change in bowel
habits that persists over a period of 2
weeks, consult a physician before using a
laxative. Restoration of normal bowel
function by using this product may cause
abdominal discomfort including cramps.
Laxative products should not be used for
a period longer than 1 week unless directed by a physician. Rectal bleeding or
failure to have a bowel movement after
use of a laxative may indicate a serious
condition. Discontinue use and consult
your physician. As with any drug, if you
are pregnant or nursing a baby, seek the
advice of a health care professional before using this product. KEEP THIS
AND ALL DRUGS OUT OF REACH OF
CHILDREN. In case of accidental overdose, seek professional assistance or contact a poison control center immediately.

**How Supplied:** Blister Pack of 10, 25,
50 or 100 Comfort Coated Tablets–5 mg
each–Enteric coated
**Questions about Dulcolax**
Call toll-free 1-888-285-9159

Boehringer Ingelheim Consumer
Healthcare Products
Division of Boehringer Ingelheim
Pharmaceuticals Inc., Ridgefield, CT
06877 MADE IN MEXICO
© Boehringer Ingelheim Pharmaceuti-
cals, Inc.
*Shown in Product Identification
Guide, page 505*

---

## DULCOLAX®
[*dul' co-lax*]
**brand of bisacodyl USP**
**Suppositories of 10 mg**
**Laxative**

**Drug Facts:**

**Active Ingredient:**          **Purpose:**
**(in each suppository)**
Bisacodyl USP, 10 mg ............. Laxative

**Uses:**
• Relieves occasional constipation and
  irregularity.
• This product usually causes bowel
  movement in 15 minutes to 1 hour.

**Warnings:**
**For rectal use only**
**Do not use**
- When abdominal pain, nausea, or vomiting are present.

**Ask a doctor before use if you have:**
- Stomach pain, nausea, or vomiting.
- A sudden change in bowel habits that lasts more than 2 weeks.

**When using this product:**
You may have abdominal discomfort, faintness, rectal burning and mild cramps.

**Stop use and ask a doctor if:**
- Rectal bleeding occurs, or you fail to have a bowel movement after using a laxative. This may indicate a serious condition.
- You need to use a laxative for more than 1 week.

**If pregnant or breast-feeding,** ask a doctor before use. **Keep out of reach of children.**
If swallowed, get medical help or contact a Poison Control Center right away.

**Directions:**

| Adults and children 12 years and over | 1 suppository once daily. Remove foil. Insert suppository well into rectum, pointed end first. Retain about 15 to 20 minutes. |
|---|---|
| Children 6 to under 12 years | 1/2 suppository once daily. |
| Children under 6 years | Ask a doctor |

**Other Information**
- Store at controlled room temperature 20–25°C (68–77°F)

**Inactive Ingredients:** Hydrogenated vegetable oil.

**How Supplied:** Comfort shaped suppositories of 10 mg each in boxes of 4, 8, 16 or 50.

**Questions about Dulcolax?**
Call toll-free 1-888-285-9159

Boehringer Ingelheim Consumer Healthcare Products.
Division of Boehringer Ingelheim Pharmaceuticals, Inc., Ridgefield, CT 06877    Made in Italy.

©Boehringer Ingelheim Pharmaceuticals, Inc.
*Shown in Product Identification Guide, page 505*

---

# BOIRON

**6 CAMPUS BLVD.**
**NEWTOWN SQUARE, PA 19073**

**Direct Inquiries and Medical Emergencies:**
Boiron Information Center
info@boiron.com
(800)264-7661

## OSCILLOCOCCINUM®

*[oh-sill'o-cox-see'num']*

**Active Ingredients:** Anas barbariae hepatis et cordis extractum 200CK. *Made according to the Homeopathic Pharmacopeia of the United States.*

**Inactive Ingredients:** sucrose, lactose.

**Use:** For temporary relief of symptoms of flu such as fever, chills, body aches and pains.

**Directions:** (Adults and children 2 years of age and older):
Take 1 dose at the onset of symptoms (dissolve entire contents of one tube in the mouth).
Repeat for 2 more doses at 6 hour intervals.

**Warnings: Do not use** if the label sealing the cap is broken.
**Ask a doctor before** use in children under 2 years of age.
**Stop using this product** and consult a doctor if symptoms persist for more than 3 days or worsen.
As with any drug, if pregnant or nursing a baby, ask a health professional before use.
Keep this and all medication out of reach of children.
**Diabetics:** this product contains sugar.

**How Supplied:** White pellets in unit dose containers of 0.04 oz. (1 gram) each. Supplied in boxes of 3 unit doses or 6 unit doses.
NDC #0220-9280-32 (3 doses) and NDC #0220-9280-33 (6 doses)
Made in France

---

---

# Bristol-Myers Products

(A Bristol-Myers Squibb Company)
**345 PARK AVENUE**
**NEW YORK, NY 10154**

**Direct Inquiries to:**
Bristol-Myers Products Division
Consumer Affairs Department
1350 Liberty Avenue
Hillside, NJ 07207

**Questions or Comments?**
1-(800) 468-7746

## OVERDOSE PROFESSIONAL INFORMATION FOR COMTREX® & EXCEDRIN® PRODUCTS

All of the following listed Comtrex and Excedrin drug products contain acetaminophen. In case of overdose, please read the following Acetylcysteine information:

**Overdose Information:**
**Acetylcysteine As An Antidote For Acetaminophen Overdose**
Acetaminophen is rapidly absorbed from the upper gastrointestinal tract with peak plasma levels occurring between 30 and 60 minutes after therapeutic doses and usually within 4 hours following an overdose. The parent compound, which is nontoxic, is extensively metabolized in the liver to form principally the sulfate and glucuronide conjugates which are also nontoxic and are rapidly excreted in the urine. A small fraction of an ingested dose is metabolized in the liver by the cytochrome P-450 mixed function oxidase enzyme system to form a reactive, potentially toxic, intermediate metabolite which preferentially conjugates with hepatic glutathione to form the nontoxic cysteine and mercapturic acid derivatives which are then excreted by the kidney. Therapeutic doses of acetaminophen do not saturate the glucuronide and sulfate conjugation pathways and do not result in the formation of sufficient reactive metabolite to deplete glutathione stores. However, following ingestion of a large overdose (150 mg/kg or greater) the glucuronide and sulfate conjugation pathways are saturated resulting in a larger fraction of the drug being metabolized via the P-450 pathway. The increased formation of reactive metabolite may deplete the hepatic stores of glutathione with subsequent binding of the metabolite to protein molecules within the hepatocyte resulting in cellular necrosis. Acetylcysteine has been shown to reduce the extent of liver injury following acetaminophen overdose.
Early symptoms following a potentially hepatotoxic overdose may include: nausea, vomiting, diaphoresis and general malaise. Clinical and laboratory evidence of hepatic toxicity may not be ap-

*Continued on next page*

## Comtrex Prof. Info.—Cont.

parent until 48 to 72 hours postingestion. In most adults and adolescents, regardless of the quantity of acetaminophen reported to have been ingested, administer acetylcysteine immediately. Acetylcysteine therapy should be initiated and continued for a full course of therapy. Its effectiveness depends on early administration, with benefit seen principally in patients treated within 16 hours of the overdose.

If acetaminophen plasma assay capability is not available, and the estimated acetaminophen ingestion exceeds 150 mg/kg, acetylcysteine therapy should be initiated and continued for a full course of therapy.

For full prescribing information, refer to the acetylcysteine package insert. Do not await the results of assays for acetaminophen level before initiating treatment with acetylcysteine. The following additional procedures are recommended: the stomach should be emptied promptly by lavage or by induction of emesis with syrup of ipecac.

A serum acetaminophen assay should be obtained as early as possible, but no sooner than four hours following ingestion. Liver function studies should be obtained initially and repeated at 24-hour intervals.

For additional emergency information call your regional poison center or toll-free (1-800-525-6115) to the Rocky Mountain Poison Center for assistance in diagnosis and for directions in the use of acetylcysteine as an antidote.

---

**Maximum Strength
COMTREX® COLD & COUGH
DAY & NIGHT**

**Active Ingredients:** Each daytime caplet contains: Acetaminophen 500 mg, Pseudoephedrine HCl 30 mg and Dextromethorphan HBr 15 mg.
Each nighttime caplet contains: Acetaminophen 500 mg, Chlorpheniramine maleate 2 mg, Dextromethorphan HBr 15 mg, and Pseudoephedrine HCl 30 mg.

**Uses:**
- **daytime** (orange caplets) – for temporary relief of the following symptoms associated with a cold:
  - headache
  - sore throat pain
  - cough
  - minor aches and pains
  - nasal congestion
  - reduction of fever
- **nighttime** (blue caplets) – provides the same relief as the daytime caplets plus temporarily relieves:
  - runny nose
  - sneezing

**Warnings: Alcohol warning:** If you consume 3 or more alcoholic drinks every day, ask your doctor whether you should take acetaminophen or other pain relievers/fever reducers. Acetaminophen may cause liver damage.

**Sore throat warning:** Severe or persistent sore throat or sore throat accompanied by high fever, headache, nausea, and vomiting may be serious. Ask a doctor right away. Do not use for more than 2 days or give to children under 3 years of age unless directed by a doctor.

**Do not use:**
- for more than 7 days
- if you are now taking a prescription monoamine oxidase inhibitor (MAOI) (certain drugs for depression, psychiatric or emotional conditions, or Parkinson's disease), or for 2 weeks after stopping the MAOI drug. If you do not know if your prescription drug contains an MAOI, ask a doctor or pharmacist before taking this product.
- with any other products containing acetaminophen. Taking more than directed may cause liver damage.

**Ask a doctor before use if you have:**
- heart disease
- high blood pressure
- diabetes
- glaucoma
- thyroid disease
- trouble urinating due to an enlarged prostate gland
- cough that occurs with too much phlegm (mucus)
- chronic cough that lasts or as occurs with smoking or asthma
- a breathing problem such as emphysema or chronic bronchitis

**Ask a doctor or pharmacist before use if you are** taking sedatives or tranquilizers.

**When using this product:**
- **do not use more than directed**
- when using nighttime product:
  - excitability may occur, especially in children
  - marked drowsiness may occur
  - alcohol, sedatives and tranquilizers may increase drowsiness
  - avoid alcoholic drinks
  - be careful when driving a motor vehicle or operating machinery

**Stop use and ask a doctor if:**
- new symptoms occur
- you get nervous, dizzy, or sleepless
- symptoms do not get better or worsen
- redness or swelling is present
- you need to use for more than 7 days
- fever gets worse or lasts more than 3 days
- cough lasts for more than 7 days, comes back, or occurs with rash, headache, or fever that lasts more than 3 days. These could be signs of a serious condition.

**If pregnant or breast-feeding,** ask a health professional before use.

**Keep out of reach of children.** In case of overdose, get medical help or contact a Poison Control Center right away. Quick medical attention is critical for adults as well as children even if you do not notice any signs or symptoms.

**Directions:**
- children under 12 years of age: ask a doctor
- adults and children 12 years of age and over:
  - **daytime** – take 2 orange caplets every 6 hours while symptoms persist, not to exceed 4 daytime caplets in 24 hours, or as directed by your doctor.
  - **nighttime** – take 2 blue caplets, if needed, to be taken no sooner than 6

hours after the last daytime caplets, not to exceed 2 nighttime caplets in 24 hours, or as directed by your doctor

**Other Information:**
- store at room temperature

**Inactive Ingredients:**
- **daytime caplet** – benzoic acid, carnauba wax, corn starch, D&C yellow no. 10*, D&C yellow no.10 lake, FD&C red no. 40*, FD&C red no. 40 lake, hydroxypropyl methylcellulose, magnesium stearate, methylparaben, mineral oil, polysorbate 20, povidone, propylene glycol, propylparaben, simethicone emulsion, sorbitan monolaurate, stearic acid, titanium dioxide, *may contain these ingredients
- **nighttime caplet** – benzoic acid, carnauba wax, corn starch, D&C yellow no. 10 lake, FD&C blue no. 1 lake, hydroxypropyl methylcellulose, magnesium stearate, methylparaben, mineral oil, polysorbate 20, povidone, propylene glycol, propylparaben, simethicone emulsion, sodium citrate, sorbitan monolaurate, stearic acid, titanium dioxide.

**Overdose: Acetylcysteine as an antidote for acetaminophen overdose.** See OVERDOSE PROFESSIONAL INFORMATION FOR COMTREX & EXCEDRIN PRODUCTS section at the beginning of Bristol-Myers Products listing.

**How Supplied:** 10 Daytime orange caplets debossed with "CxD" on one side and 10 Nighttime blue caplets debossed with "Cx" on one side

**Other COMTREX products available:** Nighttime Cold & Cough, Cold & Cough non-Drowsy, Sinus & Nasal Decongestant, Acute Head Cold, Deep Chest Cold, Sore Throat, Flu Therapy Day/Night

*Shown in Product Identification Guide, page 505*

---

**Maximum Strength
COMTREX®
ACUTE HEAD COLD**

**Active Ingredients:** Each caplet contains: Acetaminophen 500 mg, Brompheniramine maleate 2 mg and Pseudoephedrine HCl 30 mg.

**Uses:**
for temporary relief of the following symptoms associated with a cold:
- headache
- nasal congestion
- sinus pressure
- runny nose
- sneezing
- sore throat pain

**Warnings: Alcohol warning:** If you consume 3 or more alcoholic drinks every day, ask your doctor whether you should take acetaminophen or other pain relievers/fever reducers. Acetaminophen may cause liver damage.

**Sore throat warning:** Severe or persistent sore throat or sore throat accompanied by high fever, headache, nausea, and vomiting may be serious. Ask a doctor right away. Do not use for more than 2 days or give to children under 3 years of age unless directed by a doctor.

**Do not use:**
- for more than 7 days
- if you are now taking a prescription monoamine oxidase inhibitor (MAOI) (certain drugs for depression, psychiatric or emotional conditions, or Parkinson's disease), or for 2 weeks after stopping the MAOI drug. If you do not know if your prescription drug contains an MAOI, ask a doctor or pharmacist before taking this product.
- with any other products containing acetaminophen. Taking more than directed may cause liver damage.

**Ask a doctor before use if you have:**
- a breathing problem such as emphysema or chronic bronchitis
- heart disease
- high blood pressure
- thyroid disease
- diabetes
- glaucoma
- trouble urinating due to an enlarged prostate gland

**Ask a doctor or pharmacist before use if you are** taking sedatives or tranquilizers.

**When using this product:**
- **do not use more than directed**
- drowsiness may occur
- avoid alcoholic drinks
- excitability may occur, especially in children
- alcohol, sedatives and tranquilizers may increase drowsiness
- be careful when driving a motor vehicle or operating machinery

**Stop use and ask a doctor if:**
- symptoms do not get better or worsen
- you get nervous, dizzy, or sleepless
- new symptoms occur
- redness or swelling is present
- you need to use for more than 7 days
- fever occurs and lasts more than 3 days

**If pregnant or breast-feeding,** ask a health professional before use.

**Keep out of reach of children.** In case of overdose, get medical help or contact a Poison Control Center right away. Quick medical attention is critical for adults as well as children even if you do not notice any signs or symptoms.

**Directions**
- children under 12 years of age: ask a doctor
- adults and children 12 years of age and over: take 2 caplets every 6 hours, while symptoms persist, not more than 8 caplets in 24 hours, or as directed by your doctor.

**Other Information:**
- store at room temperature

**Inactive Ingredients:** Benzoic acid, carnauba wax, corn starch, croscarmellose sodium, FD&C red no. 40 lake, hydroxypropyl methylcellulose, magnesium stearate, methylparaben, microcrystalline cellulose, polyethylene glycol, polysorbate 80, povidone, propylparaben, stearic acid, titanium dioxide

**Overdose: Acetylcysteine as an antidote for acetaminophen overdose.** See OVERDOSE PROFESSIONAL INFORMATION FOR COMTREX & EX-

CEDRIN PRODUCTS section at the beginning of Bristol-Myers Products listing.

**How Supplied:** COMTREX® Acute Head Cold is supplied as coated red caplets debossed with "Cx H", in blister packages of 20's

**Other COMTREX products available:** Nighttime Cold & Cough, Cold & Cough non-Drowsy, Deep Chest Cold, Sinus & Nasal Decongestant, Sore Throat, Cold & Cough Day/Night, and Flu Therapy Day/Night

*Shown in Product Identification Guide, page 505*

---

**Multi-Symptom
COMTREX®
Deep Chest Cold**

**Active Ingredients:** Each softgel contains: Acetaminophen 250 mg, Dextromethorphan HBr 10 mg, Guaifenesin 100 mg and Pseudoephedrine HCl 30 mg.

**Uses:** • for temporary relief of the following symptoms associated with a cold:
- minor aches
- pain
- headache
- muscular aches
- sore throat pain
- nasal congestion
- cough
- helps loosen phlegm (mucus) and thin bronchial secretions to drain bronchial tubes to make coughs more productive

**Warnings: Alcohol warning:** If you consume 3 or more alcoholic drinks every day, ask your doctor whether you should take acetaminophen or other pain relievers/fever reducers. Acetaminophen may cause liver damage.

**Sore throat warning:** Severe or persistent sore throat or sore throat accompanied by high fever, headache, nausea, and vomiting may be serious. Ask a doctor right away. Do not use for more than 2 days or give to children under 3 years of age unless directed by a doctor.

**Do not use:**
- for more than 7 days
- if you are now taking a prescription monoamine oxidase inhibitor (MAOI) (certain drugs for depression, psychiatric or emotional conditions, or Parkinson's disease), or for 2 weeks after stopping the MAOI drug. If you do not know if your prescription drug contains an MAOI, ask a doctor or pharmacist before taking this product.
- with any other products containing acetaminophen. Taking more than directed may cause liver damage.

**Ask a doctor before use if you have:**
- heart disease
- high blood pressure
- thyroid disease
- diabetes
- trouble urinating due to an enlarged prostate gland
- cough that occurs with too much phlegm (mucus)
- chronic cough that lasts or as occurs with smoking, asthma, chronic bronchitis or emphysema

**When using this product:**
- **do not use more than directed**

**Stop use and ask a doctor if:**
- symptoms do not get better or worsen
- you need to use more than 7 days
- new symptoms occur
- redness or swelling is present
- you get nervous, dizzy, or sleepless
- fever gets worse or lasts more than 3 days
- cough lasts more than 7 days, comes back, or occurs with fever, rash or headache that lasts. These could be signs of a serious condition.

**If pregnant or breast-feeding,** ask a health professional before use.

**Keep out of reach of children.** In case of overdose, get medical help or contact a Poison Control Center right away. Quick medical attention is critical for adults as well as children even if you do not notice any signs or symptoms.

**Directions:**
- children under 12 years of age: ask a doctor
- adults and children 12 years of age and over: take 2 softgels every 4 hours, while symptoms persist, not more than 12 softgels in 24 hours, or as directed by your doctor

**Other Information:**
- store at controlled room temperature 20° – 25° C (68° – 77° F)

**Inactive Ingredients:** FD&C yellow no. 6, gelatin, glycerin, polyethylene glycol, povidone, propylene glycol, sorbitol, water.

**Overdose: Acetylcysteine as an antidote for acetaminophen overdose.** See OVERDOSE PROFESSIONAL INFORMATION FOR COMTEX & EXCEDRIN PRODUCTS section at the beginning of Bristol-Myers Products listing.

**How Supplied:** COMTREX® Deep Chest Cold is supplied as orange oval shaped softgel imprinted in white with "COMTREX CC", in blister packages of 20's

**Other COMTREX products available:** Nighttime Cold & Cough, Cold & Cough non-Drowsy, Acute Head Cold, Sinus & Nasal Decongestant, Sore Throat, Cold & Cough Day/Night, and Flu Therapy Day/Night

*Shown in Product Identification Guide, page 505*

---

**Maximum Strength
COMTREX® FLU THERAPY
DAY & NIGHT**

**Active Ingredients:** Each daytime caplet contains: Acetaminophen 500 mg, and Pseudoephedrine HCl 30 mg. Each nighttime caplet contains: Acetaminophen 500 mg, Chlorpheniramine maleate 2 mg, and Pseudoephedrine HCl 30 mg.

**Uses:**
- **daytime** (orange caplets)—for temporary relief of the following symptoms associated with the flu:

*Continued on next page*

## Comtrex Flu—Cont.

- muscular aches and pains
- sore throat pain
- headache
- nasal congestion
- temporarily reduces fever
- **nighttime** (green caplets)—provides the same relief as the daytime caplets plus temporarily relieves:
  - runny nose
  - sneezing

**Warnings:**

**Alcohol warning:** If you consume 3 or more alcoholic drinks every day, ask your doctor whether you should take acetaminophen or other pain relievers/fever reducers. Acetaminophen may cause liver damage.

**Sore throat warning:** Severe or persistent sore throat or sore throat accompanied by high fever, headache, nausea, and vomiting may be serious. Ask a doctor right away. Do not use for more than 2 days or give to children under 3 years of age unless directed by a doctor.

**Do not use:**

- for more than 7 days
- if you are now taking a prescription monoamine oxidase inhibitor (MAOI) (certain drugs for depression, psychiatric or emotional conditions, or Parkinson's disease), or for 2 weeks after stopping the MAOI drug. If you do not know if your prescription drug contains an MAOI, ask a doctor or pharmacist before taking this product.
- with any other products containing acetaminophen. Taking more than directed may cause liver damage.

**Ask a doctor before use if you have:**

- heart disease
- high blood pressure
- thyroid disease
- diabetes
- glaucoma
- trouble urinating due to an enlarged prostate gland
- a breathing problem such as emphysema or chronic bronchitis

**Ask a doctor or pharmacist before use if you are** taking sedatives or tranquilizers.

**When using this product**

- **do not use more than directed**
- when using nighttime product:
  - excitability may occur, especially in children
  - drowsiness may occur
  - alcohol, sedatives and tranquilizers may increase drowsiness
  - avoid alcoholic drinks
  - be careful when driving a motor vehicle or operating machinery

**Stop use and ask a doctor if:**

- new symptoms occur
- you get nervous, dizzy, or sleepless
- symptoms do not get better or worsen
- redness or swelling is present
- you need to use for more than 7 days
- fever gets worse or lasts more than 3 days

**If pregnant or breast-feeding,** ask a health professional before use.

**Keep out of reach of children.** In case of overdose, get medical help or contact a Poison Control Center right away. Quick medical attention is critical for adults as well as children even if you do not notice any signs or symptoms.

**Directions:**

- children under 12 years of age: ask a doctor
- adults and children 12 years of age and over:
  - **daytime** – take 2 orange caplets every 6 hours while symptoms persist, not to exceed 4 daytime caplets in 24 hours, or as directed by your doctor.
  - **nighttime** – take 2 green caplets, if needed, to be taken no sooner than 6 hours after the last daytime caplets, not to exceed 2 nighttime caplets in 24 hours, or as directed by your doctor.

**Other Information:**

- store at room temperature

**Inactive Ingredients:**

- **daytime caplet**–benzoic acid, carnauba wax, corn starch, D&C yellow no. 10, D&C yellow no. 10 lake, FD&C red no. 40, FD&C red no. 40 lake, hydroxypropyl methylcellulose, mineral oil, polysorbate 20, povidone, propylene glycol, simethicone emulsion, sorbitan monolaurate, stearic acid, titanium dioxide.
- **nighttime caplet**–benzoic acid, carnauba wax, corn starch, D&C yellow no. 10 lake, FD&C blue no. 1 lake, FD&C red no. 40 lake, hydroxypropyl methylcellulose, magnesium stearate, methylparaben, mineral oil, polysorbate 20, povidone, propylene glycol, propylparaben, simethicone emulsion, sodium citrate, sorbitan monolaurate, stearic acid, titanium dioxide.

**Overdose: Acetylcysteine as an antidote for acetaminophen overdose.** See OVERDOSE PROFESSIONAL INFORMATION FOR COMTREX & EXCEDRIN PRODUCTS section at the beginning of Bristol-Myers Products listing.

**How Supplied:** 10 Daytime orange caplets debossed with "CxF" on one side and 10 Nighttime green caplets debossed with "CxR" on one side

**Other COMTREX products available:** Nighttime Cold & Cough, Cold & Cough non-Drowsy, Sinus & Nasal Decongestant, Acute Head Cold, Deep Chest Cold, Sore Throat, and Cold & Cough Day/Night

*Shown in Product Identification Guide, page 505*

---

Maximum Strength
**COMTREX®**
Sinus & Nasal Decongestant

**Active Ingredients:** Each caplet contains: Acetaminophen 500 mg, Chlorpheniramine maleate 2 mg, and Pseudoephedrine HCl 30 mg.

**Uses:**

- temporarily relieves these symptoms associated with a cold or upper respiratory allergies:
  - runny nose
  - sneezing
  - itching of the nose or throat
  - itchy, watery eyes
  - nasal congestion
  - sinus pressure
  - headache pain

**Warnings: Alcohol warning:** If you consume 3 or more alcoholic drinks every day, ask your doctor whether you should take acetaminophen or other pain relievers/fever reducers. Acetaminophen may cause liver damage.

**Do not use:**

- for more than 7 days
- if you are now taking a prescription monoamine oxidase inhibitor (MAOI) (certain drugs for depression, psychiatric or emotional conditions, or Parkinson's disease), or for 2 weeks after stopping the MAOI drug. If you do not know if your prescription drug contains an MAOI, ask a doctor or pharmacist before taking this product.
- with any other products containing acetaminophen. Taking more than directed may cause liver damage.

**Ask a doctor before use if you have:**

- heart disease
- high blood pressure
- thyroid disease
- diabetes
- glaucoma
- trouble urinating due to an enlarged prostate gland
- a breathing problem such as emphysema or chronic bronchitis

**Ask a doctor or pharmacist before use if you are** taking sedatives or tranquilizers.

**When using this product:**

- **do not use more than directed**
- drowsiness may occur
- alcohol, sedatives and tranquilizers may increase drowsiness
- avoid alcoholic drinks
- be careful when driving a motor vehicle or operating machinery
- excitability may occur, especially in children

**Stop use and ask a doctor if:**

- symptoms do not get better or worsen
- you get nervous, dizzy, or sleepless
- new symptoms occur
- redness or swelling is present
- you need to use more than 7 days
- fever gets worse or lasts more than 3 days

**If pregnant or breast-feeding,** ask a health professional before use.

**Keep out of reach of children.** In case of overdose, get medical help or contact a Poison Control Center right away. Quick medical attention is critical for adults as well as children even if you do not notice any signs or symptoms.

**Directions:**

- children under 12 years of age: ask a doctor
- adults and children 12 years of age and over: take 2 caplets every 6 hours, while symptoms persist, not more than 8 caplets in 24 hours, or as directed by your doctor

**Other Information:**

- store at room temperature

**Inactive Ingredients:** Benzoic acid, carnauba wax, corn starch, D&C yellow no. 10 lake, FD&C blue no. 1 lake, FD&C red no. 40 lake, hydroxypropyl methylcellulose, magnesium stearate, methylparaben, mineral oil, polysorbate 20, povidone, propylene glycol, propylparaben, simethicone emulsion, sodium citrate, sorbitan monolaurate, stearic acid, titanium dioxide.

**Overdose: Acetylcysteine as an antidote for acetaminophen overdose.** See OVERDOSE PROFESSIONAL INFORMATION FOR COMTREX & EXCEDRIN PRODUCTS section at the beginning of Bristol-Myers Products listing.

**How Supplied:** COMTREX® Sinus & Nasal Decongestant is supplied as coated green caplets debossed with "CxR" on one side, in blister packages of 20's

**Other COMTREX products available:** Nighttime Cold & Cough, Cold & Cough non-Drowsy, Acute Head Cold, Deep Chest Cold, Sore Throat, Cold & Cough Day/Night, and Flu Therapy Day/Night

*Shown in Product Identification Guide, page 505*

---

## Aspirin Free EXCEDRIN®
[ĕx "cĕd 'rin]
**Pain Reliever**

**Active Ingredients:** Each caplet and geltab contains Acetaminophen 500 mg and Caffeine 65 mg.

**Inactive Ingredients:** (caplet) benzoic acid, carnauba wax, corn starch, croscarmellose sodium, D&C Red # 27 Lake, D&C Yellow # 10 Lake, FD&C Blue # 1 Lake, FD&C Red # 40, hydroxypropyl methylcellulose, magnesium stearate, methylparaben, microcrystalline cellulose, mineral oil, polysorbate 20, povidone, propylene glycol, propylparaben, simethicone emulsion, sorbitan monolaurate, stearic acid, titanium dioxide.

**Inactive Ingredients:** (geltab) benzoic acid, corn starch, croscarmellose sodium, FD&C Blue # 1, FD&C Red # 40, FD&C Yellow # 6, gelatin, glycerin, hydroxypropyl methylcellulose, magnesium stearate, methylparaben, microcrystalline cellulose, mineral oil, polysorbate 20, povidone, propylene glycol, propylparaben, simethicone emulsion, sorbitan monolaurate, stearic acid, titanium dioxide.

**Indications:** For the temporary relief of minor aches and pains associated with headache, sinusitis, a cold, muscular aches, premenstrual and menstrual cramps, toothache, and for the minor pain from arthritis.

**Alcohol Warning:** If you consume 3 or more alcoholic drinks every day, ask your doctor whether you should take acetaminophen or other pain relievers/fever reducers. Acetaminophen may cause liver damage.

**Warnings: Keep out of reach of children.** In case of overdose, get medical help or contact a Poison Control Center right away. Do not take with any other products containing acetaminophen. Taking more than directed may cause liver damage. Prompt medical attention is critical for adults as well as for children even if you do not notice any signs or symptoms. As with any drug, if you are pregnant or nursing a baby, seek the advice of a health professional before using this product. Do not take this product for pain for more than 10 days or for fever for more than 3 days unless directed by a doctor. If pain or fever persists or gets worse, if new symptoms occur, of if redness or swelling is present, consult a doctor because these could be signs of a serious condition. Consult a dentist promptly for toothache.

**Directions:** Adults: 2 caplets or geltabs every 6 hours while symptoms persist, not to exceed 8 caplets or geltabs in 24 hours, or as directed by a doctor. Children under 12 years of age: consult a doctor.

**Overdose: Acetylcysteine as an antidote for acetaminophen overdose.** See OVERDOSE PROFESSIONAL INFORMATION FOR COMTREX AND EXCEDRIN PRODUCTS section at the beginning of the Bristol-Myers Products listing.

**How Supplied:** Aspirin Free EXCEDRIN® is supplied as: Coated red caplets with "AF Excedrin" printed in white on one side in bottles of 24's, 50's and 100's. Easy to swallow red geltabs with "AF Excedrin" printed in white on one side supplied in bottles of 24's, 50's, 100's.

Store at room temperature.

*Shown in Product Identification Guide, page 506*

---

## EXCEDRIN® Extra-Strength
**Pain Reliever**
[ĕx "cĕd 'rin ]

**Active Ingredients:** Each tablet, caplet, or geltab contains Acetaminophen 250 mg, Aspirin 250 mg, and Caffeine 65 mg.

**Inactive Ingredients:** (tablet, caplet) benzoic acid, carnauba wax, hydroxypropylcellulose, hydroxypropyl methylcellulose, microcrystalline cellulose, mineral oil, polysorbate 20, povidone, propylene glycol, simethicone emulsion, sorbitan monolaurate, stearic acid.
May also contain: FD&C blue # 1, titanium dioxide.

**Inactive Ingredients:** (geltab) benzoic acid, D&C yellow #10 lake, disodium EDTA, FD&C blue #1 lake, FD&C red # 40 lake, ferric oxide, gelatin, glycerin, hydroxypropylcellulose, hydroxypropyl methylcellulose, maltitol solution, microcrystalline cellulose, mineral oil, pepsin, polysorbate 20, povidone, propylene glycol, propyl gallate, simethicone emulsion, sorbitan monolaurate, stearic acid, titanium dioxide.

**Uses:** For the temporary relief of minor aches and pains associated with headache, sinusitis, a cold, muscular aches, premenstrual and menstrual cramps, toothache, and for the minor pain from arthritis.

**Warnings:**

**Warning:** Children and teenagers should not use this medicine for chicken pox or flu symptoms before a doctor is consulted about Reye's syndrome, a rare but serious illness reported to be associated with aspirin.

**Alcohol Warning:** If you consume 3 or more alcoholic drinks every day, ask your doctor whether you should take acetaminophen and aspirin or other pain relievers/fever reducers. Acetaminophen and aspirin may cause liver damage and stomach bleeding.

**Keep out of reach of children.** In case of overdose, get medical help or contact a Poison Control Center right away. Do not take with any other products containing acetaminophen. Taking more than directed may cause liver damage. Prompt medical attention is critical for adults as well as for children even if you do not notice any signs or symptoms. As with any drug, if you are pregnant or nursing a baby, seek the advice of a health professional before using this product. **IT IS ESPECIALLY IMPORTANT NOT TO USE ASPIRIN DURING THE LAST 3 MONTHS OF PREGNANCY UNLESS SPECIFICALLY DIRECTED TO DO SO BY A DOCTOR BECAUSE IT MAY CAUSE PROBLEMS IN THE UNBORN CHILD OR COMPLICATIONS DURING DELIVERY.** Do not take this product for pain for more than 10 days or for fever for more than 3 days unless directed by a doctor. If pain or fever persists or gets worse, if new symptoms occur, or if redness or swelling is present, consult a doctor because these could be signs of a serious condition. Consult a dentist promptly for toothache. Do not take this product if you are allergic to aspirin, have asthma, have stomach problems (such as heartburn, upset stomach or stomach pain) that persist or recur, or if you have ulcers or bleeding problems, unless directed by a doctor. If ringing in the ears or loss of hearing occurs, consult a doctor before taking any more of this product.

**Drug Interaction Precaution:** Do not take this product if you are taking a prescription drug for anticoagulation (thinning the blood), diabetes, gout or arthritis unless directed by a doctor.

**Directions:** Adults: 2 tablets, caplets or geltabs with water every 6 hours while symptoms persist, not to exceed 8 tablets, caplets or geltabs in 24 hours, or as directed by a doctor. Children under 12 years of age: consult a doctor.

**Overdose: Acetylcysteine as an antidote for acetaminophen overdose.** See OVERDOSE PROFESSIONAL INFORMATION FOR COMTREX AND

*Continued on next page*

## Excedrin Extra-Strength—Cont.

EXCEDRIN PRODUCTS section at the beginning of the Bristol-Myers Products listing.

**How Supplied:** Extra Strength EXCEDRIN® is supplied as:
Coated white circular tablet with letter "E" debossed on one side. Supplied in bottles of 12's, 24's, 50's, 100's, 175's, 275's.
Coated white caplets with "E" debossed on one side. Supplied in bottles of 24's, 50's, 100's, 175's, 275's.
Gel-coated round geltabs–green on one side, white on the other, printed with black "E" on one side. Supplied in bottles of 24's, 50's and 100's (2 bottles of 50 each).
Store at room temperature.

*Shown in Product Identification
Guide, page 506*

---

## EXCEDRIN® MIGRAINE
[*ĕx" cĕd' rin*]
**Pain Reliever/Pain Reliever Aid**

**Active Ingredients:** Each tablet, caplet or geltab contains Acetaminophen 250 mg, Aspirin 250 mg and Caffeine 65 mg.

**Inactive Ingredients:** (tablet and caplet) benzoic acid, carnauba wax, hydroxypropylcellulose, hydroxypropyl methylcellulose, microcrystalline cellulose, mineral oil, polysorbate 20, povidone, propylene glycol, simethicone emulsion, sorbitan monolaurate, stearic acid, may also contain: FD&C blue no. 1, titanium dioxide.

**Inactive Ingredients:** (geltab) benzoic acid, D&C yellow #10 lake, disodium EDTA, FD&C blue #1 lake, FD&C red #40 lake, ferric oxide, gelatin, glycerin, hydroxypropylcellulose, hydroxypropyl methylcellulose, maltitol solution, microcrystalline cellulose, mineral oil, pepsin, polysorbate 20, povidone, propylene glycol, propyl gallate, simethicone emulsion, sorbitan monolaurate, stearic acid, titanium dioxide.

**Use:** Treats migraine.

**Warnings:**
**Reye's Syndrome:** Children and teenagers should not use this drug for chicken pox, or flu symptoms before a doctor is consulted about Reye's syndrome, a rare but serious illness reported to be associated with aspirin.
**Allergy alert:** aspirin may cause a severe allergic reaction which may include: • hives • facial swelling • asthma (wheezing) • shock
**Alcohol warning:** If you consume 3 or more alcoholic drinks every day, ask your doctor whether you should take acetaminophen and aspirin or other pain relievers/fever reducers. Acetaminophen and aspirin may cause liver damage and stomach bleeding.
**Caffeine warning:** The recommended dose of this product contains about as much caffeine as a cup of coffee. Limit

the use of caffeine-containing medications, foods, or beverages while taking this product because too much caffeine may cause nervousness, irritability, sleeplessness, and, occasionally, rapid heart beat.
**Do not use** • if you have ever had an allergic reaction to any other pain reliever/fever reducer
**Ask a doctor before use if you have**
• never had migraines diagnosed by a health professional
• a headache that is different from your usual migraines
• the worst headache of your life
• fever and stiff neck
• headaches beginning after or caused by head injury, exertion, coughing or bending
• experienced your first headache after the age of 50
• daily headaches
• asthma
• bleeding problems
• ulcers
• stomach problems such as heartburn, upset stomach, or stomach pain that do not go away or recur
• a migraine so severe as to require bed rest
• problems or serious side effects from taking pain relievers or fever reducers
**Ask a doctor or pharmacist before use if you are** taking a prescription drug for:
• anticoagulation (thinning of the blood)
• diabetes
• gout
• arthritis
**Stop use and ask a doctor if**
• an allergic reaction occurs. Seek medical help right away.
• your migraine is not relieved or worsens after first dose
• new or unexpected symptoms occur
• ringing in the ears or loss of hearing occurs
**If pregnant or breast-feeding,** ask a health professional before use. It is especially important not to use aspirin during the last 3 months of pregnancy unless definitely directed to do so by a doctor because it may cause problems in the unborn child or complications during delivery.
**Keep out of reach of children.** In case of overdose, get medical help or contact a Poison Control Center right away. Quick medical attention is critical for adults as well as for children even if you do not notice any signs or symptoms.

**Directions:**
• adults: take 2 (tablets, caplets or geltabs) with a glass of water
• if symptoms persist or worsen, ask your doctor
• do not take more than 2 (tablets, caplets, or geltabs) in 24 hours, unless directed by a doctor
• under 18 years of age: ask a doctor

**Overdose: Acetylcysteine as an antidote for acetaminophen overdose.** See OVERDOSE PROFESSIONAL INFORMATION FOR COMTREX AND EXCEDRIN PRODUCTS section at the beginning of the Bristol-Myers Products listing.

**How Supplied:** EXCEDRIN® MIGRAINE is supplied as:
Coated white circular tablets or coated white caplets with letter "E" debossed on

one side. Supplied in bottles of 24's, 50's, 100's, and 175's. 275's (tablets) are available in club store packages. Coated round geltabs–green on one side, white on the other, printed with black "E" on one side. Supplied in bottles of 24's, 50's and 100's (2 bottles of 50 each).
Store at 20–25°C (68–77°F).

*Shown in Product Identification
Guide, page 506*

---

## EXCEDRIN® PM
[*ĕx "cĕd 'rĭn* ]
**Pain Reliever/Nighttime Sleep-Aid**

**Active Ingredients:** Each tablet, caplet or geltab contains: Acetaminophen 500 mg and Diphenhydramine citrate 38 mg.

**Inactive Ingredients:** (Tablet and Caplet) benzoic acid, corn starch, D&C yellow #10 lake, FD&C blue #1 lake, hydroxypropyl methylcellulose, magnesium stearate, mineral oil, polysorbate 20, povidone, propylene glycol, simethicone emulsion, sodium citrate, sorbitan monolaurate, stearic acid, titanium dioxide, may also contain: carnauba wax, croscarmellose sodium, methylparaben, microcrystalline cellulose, propylparaben, sodium starch glycolate.
(Geltab) benzoic acid, corn starch, D&C red #33 lake, edetate disodium, FD&C blue #1, FD&C blue #1 lake, gelatin, glycerin, hydroxypropyl methylcellulose, magnesium stearate, mineral oil, polysorbate 20, povidone, propylene glycol, simethicone emulsion, sorbitan monolaurate, stearic acid, titanium dioxide, may also contain: croscarmellose sodium, methylparaben, microcrystalline cellulose, propylparaben, sodium starch glycolate.

**Uses:** For temporary relief of occasional headaches and minor aches and pains with accompanying sleeplessness.

**Warnings**
**Alcohol Warning:** If you consume 3 or more alcoholic drinks every day, ask your doctor whether you should take acetaminophen or other pain relievers/fever reducers. Acetaminophen may cause liver damage.
**Do not use**
• in children under 12 years of age
• with other diphenhydramine products, including one applied topically
**Ask a doctor before use if you have**
• glaucoma
• a breathing problem such as emphysema or chronic bronchitis
• trouble urinating due to an enlarged prostate gland
**Ask a doctor or pharmacist before use if you are** taking sedatives or tranquilizers
**When using this product**
• avoid alcoholic drinks
**Stop use and ask a doctor if**
• new symptoms occur
• sleeplessness lasts continuously for more than 2 weeks. Insomnia may be a symptom of serious underlying medical illness.

- pain gets worse or lasts for more than 10 days
- redness or swelling is present
- fever gets worse or lasts for more than 3 days

**If pregnant or breast-feeding,** ask a health professional before use.

**Keep out of reach of children.** In case of overdose, get medical help or contact a Poison Control Center right away. Do not take with any other products containing acetaminophen. Taking more than directed may cause liver damage. Quick medical attention is critical for adults as well as for children even if you do not notice any signs or symptoms.

**Directions**
- children under 12 years of age: consult a doctor
- adults and children 12 years and over: take 2 tablets, caplets or geltabs at bedtime, if needed, or as directed by a doctor.

**Overdose: Acetylcysteine as an antidote for acetaminophen overdose.** See OVERDOSE PROFESSIONAL INFORMATION FOR COMTREX AND EXCEDRIN PRODUCTS section at the beginning of the Bristol-Myers Products listing.

**How Supplied:** EXCEDRIN PM® is supplied as:
Light blue circular coated tablets with "PM" debossed on one side. Supplied in bottles of 10's, 24's, 50's, 100's.
Light blue coated caplet with "PM" debossed on one side. Supplied in bottles of 24's, 50's, 100's.
Gel coated-light blue and white geltabs with "PM" printed in black on one side. Supplied in bottles of 24's, 50's, 100's.
Store at room temperature.

*Shown in Product Identification Guide, page 506*

---

# Celltech Pharmaceuticals, Inc.
**PO BOX 31710 ROCHESTER, NY 14603**

**Direct Inquiries to:**
Customer Service Department
P.O. Box 31766
Rochester, NY 14603
(716) 274-5300
(888) 963-3382

**DELSYM® Cough Formula**
*[del 'sĭm ]*
**(dextromethorphan polistirex)**
**Extended-Release Suspension**
**12-Hour Cough Relief**

**Active Ingredient:** Each teaspoonful (5 mL) contains dextromethorphan polistirex equivalent to 30 mg dextromethorphan hydrobromide.

**Inactive Ingredients:** Alcohol 0.26%, citric acid, ethylcellulose, FD&C Yellow No. 6, flavor, high fructose corn syrup, methylparaben, polyethylene glycol 3350, polysorbate 80, propylene glycol, propylparaben, purified water, sucrose, tragacanth, vegetable oil, xanthan gum.

**Indications:** Temporarily relieves cough due to minor throat and bronchial irritation as may occur with the common cold or inhaled irritants.

**Warnings:** Do not take this product for persistent or chronic cough such as occurs with smoking, asthma, or emphysema, or if cough is accompanied by excessive phlegm (mucus) unless directed by a physician. A persistent cough may be a sign of a serious condition. If cough persists for more than 1 week, tends to recur, or is accompanied by fever, rash, or persistent headache, consult a physician. As with any drug, if you are pregnant or nursing a baby, seek the advice of a health professional before using this product. **Keep this and all drugs out of the reach of children.** In case of accidental overdose, seek professional assistance or contact a Poison Control Center immediately.

**Drug Interaction Precaution:** Do not use this product if you are now taking a prescription monoamine oxidase inhibitor (MAOI) (certain drugs for depression, psychiatric or emotional conditions, or Parkinson's disease), or for 2 weeks after stopping the MAOI drug. If you are uncertain whether your prescription drug contains an MAOI, consult a health professional before taking this product.

**Directions: Shake Bottle Well Before Using.** Dose as follows or as directed by a physician.
**Adults and Children 12 years of age and over:** 2 teaspoonfuls every 12 hours, not to exceed 4 teaspoonfuls in 24 hours.
**Children 6 to under 12 years of age:** 1 teaspoonful every 12 hours, not to exceed 2 teaspoonfuls in 24 hours.
**Children 2 to under 6 years of age:** $1/2$ teaspoonful every 12 hours, not to exceed 1 teaspoonful in 24 hours.

**Children under 2 years of age:** Consult a physician.

**How Supplied:** 89 mL (3 fl oz) bottles NDC 53014-842-61
**Store at 15°–30°C (59°–86°F).**
®Celltech Manufacturing, Inc.
Celltech Pharmaceuticals, Inc.
Rochester, NY 14623 USA

---

# Chattem, Inc.
**1715 WEST 38th STREET CHATTANOOGA, TN 37409**

**Direct Inquiries to:**
(423) 821-2037

**DEXATRIM RESULTS**
**DEXATRIM RESULTS, Ephedrine Free Formula**

DEXATRIM RESULTS: Supplement Facts:
[See table below]
DEXATRIM RESULTS, Ephedrine Free Formula: Supplement Facts:
[See table at bottom of next page]
**Other Ingredients:** Gelatin, microcrystalline cellulose, croscarmellose sodium, stearic acid, silicon dioxide, pharmaceutical glaze, carnauba wax.

**Warnings:** FOR ADULT USE ONLY. NOT FOR USE BY INDIVIDUALS UNDER 18 YEARS OF AGE. DO NOT TAKE MORE THAN THREE CAPLETS PER DAY (24 HOURS). Do not exceed recommended serving size. Exceeding the recommended dose has not been shown to result in greater effectiveness. Do not use if pregnant or nursing. Consult a physician or licensed qualified health care professional before using this product if you have, or have a family history of heart disease, thyroid disease, diabetes, high blood pressure, recurrent headaches, depression or other psychiatric condition, glaucoma, difficulty in uri-

*Continued on next page*

---

|  | Amount Per Caplet | % Daily Value |
|---|---|---|
| Vitamin C | 10 mg | 17 |
| Vitamin E | 5 IU | 17 |
| Vitamin B6 | 2 mg | 100 |
| Pantothenic acid | 5 mg | 50 |
| Calcium | 97 mg | 9.7 |
| Iron | 0.54 mg | 3 |
| Phosphorous | 70 mg | 7 |
| Magnesium | 6.7 mg | 2 |
| Zinc | 2.5 mg | 17 |
| Manganese (as amino acid chelate) | 0.67 mg | 34 |
| Chromium (as amino acid chelate) | 40 mcg | 33 |
| Proprietary herbal blend #1: Ephedra stem, Yohimbe bark, Siberian ginseng root, licorice root, rutin, kelp, fenugreek seed, hesperidin complex | 185 mg | † |
| Proprietary herbal blend #2: CocoGen™, caffeine, green tea leaf extract. | 130 mg | † |

## Dexatrim—Cont.

nation, prostate enlargement, or seizure disorder, if you are using a monoamine oxidase inhibitor (MAOI) or any other dietary supplement, prescription drug or over-the-counter drug containing ephedrine, pseudoephedrine, or phenylpropanolamine (ingredients found in certain allergy, asthma, cough/cold and weight control products).

Discontinue use and call a physician or licensed qualified health care professional immediately if you experience rapid heartbeat, dizziness, severe headache, shortness of breath, or other similar symptoms. INDIVIDUALS WHO CONSUME CAFFEINE WITH THIS PRODUCT MAY EXPERIENCE SERIOUS ADVERSE HEALTH EFFECTS. EXCEEDING RECOMMENDED SERVING MAY CAUSE SERIOUS ADVERSE HEALTH EFFECTS INCLUDING HEART ATTACK AND STROKE. **KEEP OUT OF REACH OF CHILDREN.**

DEXATRIM RESULTS: This product contains 12 mg of naturally-occurring concentrated ephedrine group alkaloids per serving in the form of herbal extracts, 0.3 mg of Yohimbine and 40 mg of naturally-occurring caffeine per serving (equivalent to one-half cup of coffee). DEXATRIM RESULTS, Ephedrine Free Formula: This product contains 40 mg of naturally-occurring caffeine per serving (equivalent to one-half cup of coffee). Improper use of these products may be hazardous to a person's health.

**Suggested Use:** Take one caplet 3 times per day.

**How Supplied:** Tamper-resistant bottles of 60 caplets.

**Product Identification:** DEXATRIM RESULTS: natural light tannish-gray speckled caplet-shaped tablet with pharmaceutical glaze. DEXATRIM RESULTS, Ephedrine Free Formula; natural brown caplet-shaped tablet with pharmaceutical glaze.

| | Amount Per Caplet | % Daily Value |
|---|---|---|
| Vitamin C | 10 mg | 17 |
| Vitamin E | 5 IU | 17 |
| Vitamin B6 | 2 mg | 100 |
| Pantothenic acid | 5 mg | 50 |
| Calcium | 90 mg | 9 |
| Phosphorous | 70 mg | 7 |
| Magnesium | 6.7 mg | 2 |
| Zinc | 2.5 mg | 17 |
| Manganese (as amino acid chelate) | 0.67 mg | 34 |
| Chromium (as amino acid chelate) | 40 mcg | 33 |
| Proprietary herbal blend #1: Bitter orange peel extract, Yohimbe bark, Siberian ginseng root, licorice root, rutin, kelp, fenugreek seed, hesperidin complex | 202 mg | † |
| Proprietary herbal blend #2: CocoGen™, caffeine, green tea leaf extract. | 130 mg | † |

† Daily value not established.

---

To report adverse events call FDA's MEDWATCH at 1-800-332-1088

## Effcon™ Laboratories, Inc.

**P.O. BOX 7499**
**MARIETTA, GA 30065-1499**

**Address inquiries to:**
Brad Rivet
(800-722-2428)
Fax: (770-428-6811)

**For Medical Emergency Contact:**
Brad Rivet
(800-722-2428)
Fax: (770-428-6811)

## PIN-X®
### Pinworm Treatment

**Description:** Each 1 mL of liquid for oral administration contains:
Pyrantel base ...................... 50 mg
    (as Pyrantel Pamoate)

**Indication:** For the treatment of pinworms.

**Warnings:** Keep this and all drugs out of the reach of children. In case of accidental overdose, seek professional assistance or contact a poison control center immediately.
If you are pregnant or have liver disease, do not take this product unless directed by a doctor.

**Directions for Use:** Adults and children 2 years to under 12 years of age: oral dosage is a single dose of 5 milligrams of pyrantel base per pound, or 11 milligrams per kilogram, of body weight not to exceed 1 gram. Dosage information is summarized on the following dosing schedule:

| Weight | | Dosage |
|---|---|---|
| | | (taken as a single dose) |
| 25 to 37 lbs. | = | $1/2$ tsp. |
| 38 to 62 lbs. | = | 1 tsp. |
| 63 to 87 lbs. | = | $1^1/2$ tsp. |
| 88 to 112 lbs. | = | 2 tsp. |
| 113 to 137 lbs. | = | $2^1/2$ tsp. |
| 138 to 162 lbs. | = | 3 tsp. (1 tbsp.) |
| 163 to 187 lbs. | = | $3^1/2$ tsp. |
| 188 lbs. & over | = | 4 tsp. |

SHAKE WELL BEFORE USING

**How Supplied:** Pin-X is supplied as a tan to yellowish, caramel-flavored suspension which contains 50 mg of pyrantel base (as pyrantel pamoate) per mL, in bottles of 30 mL (1 fl oz). NDC 55806-024-10 and in bottles of 60 mL (2 fl oz) NDC 55806-024-11

Store at controlled room temperature 15°–30°C (59°–86°F).

Manufactured for:
**Effcon™ Laboratories Inc.**
Marietta, GA 30065-1499
Rev. 1/89
Code 587A00
*Shown in Product Identification Guide, page 506*

---

Patient Education Brochures—Pin-X® Pinworm Treatment

Effcon Laboratories provides complimentary Patient Education Brochures for patient counseling regarding the treatment and prevention of pinworm infestation. Brochures are available for all healthcare professionals and may be requested by phone (800-722-2428); fax (770-428-6811); or through Effcon's web page (www.effcon.com).

---

## Fleming & Company
**1600 FENPARK DR.**
**FENTON, MO 63026**

**Direct Inquiries to:**
Tom Fleming
636 343-8200
FAX (636) 343-9865
e-mail: info@flemingcompany.com

## CHLOR–3
### Medicinal Condiment

### DESCRIPTION
Medical condiment containing sodium chloride 50%; potassium chloride 30%; magnesium chloride 20%.

**Active Ingredients:** A mixture of sodium chloride (50% 24.3 mEq/half tsp. iodized); potassium chloride (30% 11.5 mEq/half tsp.); magnesium chloride (20% 5.7 mEq/half tsp.).

**Indications:** The first medicinal condiment to restore needed K+& Mg++ lost during diuresis, at the expense of Na+. To restore electrolytes lost by overcooking foods, or to add to diets that lack green vegetables, bananas, etc. And to replace conventional salting of foods in culinary and gourmet arts.

**Symptoms and Treatment of Oral Overdosage:** Hyperkalemia and hypermagnesemia are not end-stage results of usage.

**How Supplied:** In 8-oz plastic shaker, tamper-evident bottles.

---

### OCEAN® Nasal Mist
**(buffered isotonic saline)**

**Description:** A 0.65% special saline made isotonic by the addition of a dual preservative system and buffering excipients prevent nasal irritation.

**Ingredients:** 0.65% Sodium Chloride and Phenylcarbinol and Benzalkonium Chloride as preservatives.

**Action and Uses:** For dry nasal membranes including rhinitis medicamentosa, rhinitis sicca and atrophic rhinitis. For patients 'hooked on nose drops' and glaucoma patients on diuretics having dry nasal capillaries. OCEAN® may also be used as a mist or drop. Upright delivers a spray; horizontally a stream; upside down a drop.

**Administration and Dosage:** For dry nasal membranes, two squeezes in each nostril P.R.N.

**Supplied:** Plastic 45cc spray bottles and pints.

---

### PURGE
**(Flavored Castor Oil Stimulant Laxative)**

**Composition:** Contains 95% castor oil (USP) in a sweetened lemon flavored base that completely masks the odor and taste of the oil.

**Indications:** Preparation of the bowel for x-ray, surgery and proctological procedures, IVPs, and constipation.

**Dosage:** Adults and children 12 years of age and over: 15–60 mL (1–4 tbsp) in a single dose. Children 2 to under 12 years of age: 5–15 mL (1–3 tsp) in a single dose. Children under 2 years: consult a physician.

**Precaution:** Not indicated when nausea, vomiting, abdominal pain or symptoms of appendicitis occur. Pregnancy, use only on advice of physician.

**Supplied:** Plastic 1 oz. & 2 oz. bottles.

---

**GlaxoSmithKline Consumer Healthcare, L.P.**

P.O. BOX 1467
PITTSBURGH, PA 15230

**Direct Inquiries to:**
Consumer Affairs
1-800-245-1040

**For Medical Emergencies Contact:**
Consumer Affairs
1-800-245-1040

---

### ABREVA™
**Cold Sore/Fever Blister Treatment Cream**
**Docosanol 10% Cream**

**Uses:**
- Treats cold sore/fever blisters on the face or lips
- Shortens healing time and duration of symptoms: tingling, pain, burning, and/or itching

**Active Ingredient:**          **Purpose:**
Docosanol 10% ... Cold sore/fever blister treatment

**Inactive Ingredients:** Benzyl alcohol, light mineral oil, propylene glycol, purified water, sucrose distearate, sucrose stearate.

**Directions:**
- **adults and children 12 years or over:**
  - wash hands before and after applying cream
  - apply to affected area on face or lips at the first sign of cold sore/fever blister (tingle). Early treatment ensures the best results.
  - rub in gently but completely
  - use 5 times a day until healed
- **children under 12 years:** ask a doctor

**Warnings:**
**For external use only.**
**Do not use**
- if you are allergic to any ingredient in this product
**When using this product**
- apply only to affected areas
- do not use in or near the eyes
- avoid applying directly inside your mouth
- do not share this product with anyone. This may spread infection.
**Stop use and ask a doctor if**
- your cold sore gets worse or the cold sore is not healed within 10 days
- **Keep out of reach of children.** If swallowed, get medical help or contact a poison control center right away.
**Other Information:**
- store at 20°–25°C (68°–77°F)
- do not freeze

**How Supplied:** Abreva Cream is supplied in 2.0 g [.07 oz] tubes.
**Question?** Call 1-877-709-3539 weekdays

*Shown in Product Identification Guide, page 506*

---

### BALMEX®
**Medicated Plus™ Baby Powder**

**Description:** Balmex® Medicated Plus™ Baby Powder helps prevent and treat diaper rash with cornstarch (86.9%) and zinc oxide (10%), plus it contains WATER LOCK®, a patented, safe, super absorbing ingredient that helps keep your baby dry.

**Indications and Uses:** Balmex Medicated Plus Baby Powder helps treat and prevent diaper rash, protects chafed skin associated with diaper rash and helps protect from wetness. The cornstarch and zinc oxide based formulation provides a protective barrier on the skin against the natural causes of irritation, a super absorbing starch copolymer which allows our formula to absorb 2 times more moisture than cornstarch alone.

**Directions:** Change wet and soiled diapers promptly, cleanse the diaper area, and allow to dry. Apply powder liberally as often as necessary, with each diaper change, especially at bedtime or anytime when exposure to wet diapers may be prolonged. Apply powder close to the body away from the child's face. Carefully shake the powder into the diaper or into the hand and apply to diaper area.

**Warnings:** Avoid contact with eyes. Keep powder away from child's face to avoid inhalation, which can cause breathing problems. For external use only. Do not use on broken skin. If condition worsens or does not improve within 7 days, contact a physician. Keep out of reach of children. If swallowed, get medical help or contact a Poison Control Center right away.

**Active Ingredients:** Topical starch (cornstarch) 86.9%. zinc oxide 10%.

**Inactive Ingredients:** Fragrance, Starch Copolymer (WATER LOCK®), Tribasic Calcium Phosphate

**How Supplied:** 13 oz. (368g.) Bottle WATER LOCK® is a registered trademark of Grain Processing Corporation
*Shown in Product Identification Guide, page 506*

---

### BALMEX®
**Diaper Rash Ointment (Zinc Oxide) With Aloe & Vitamin E**

**Description:** Balmex® Diaper Rash Ointment with Aloe & Vitamin E contains Zinc Oxide (11.3%) in a unique formulation including Peruvian Balsam suitable for topical application for the treatment and prevention of diaper rash.

**Indications and Uses:** Balmex helps treat and prevent diaper rash while it moisturizes and nourishes the skin. The zinc oxide based formulation provides a protective barrier on the skin against the

*Continued on next page*

## Balmex—Cont.

natural causes of irritation. Balmex spreads on smooth and wipes off the baby easily, without causing irritation to the affected area. Balmex tactile properties promote compliance amongst mothers.

**Directions:** Change wet and soiled diapers promptly, cleanse the diaper area, and allow to dry. Apply ointment liberally as often as necessary, with each diaper change, especially at bedtime or anytime when exposure to wet diapers may be prolonged.

**Warnings:** Avoid contact with the eyes. For external use only. If condition worsens or does not improve within 7 days, contact a physician. Keep out of reach of children. If swallowed, get medical help or contact a Poison Control Center right away.

**Active Ingredient:** Zinc Oxide (11.3%).

**Inactive Ingredients:** Aloe Vera Gel, Balsan (Specially Purified Balsam Peru), Beeswax, Benzoic Acid, Dimethicone, Methylparaben, Mineral Oil, Propylparaben, Purified Water, Sodium Borate, Tocopheryl (Vitamin E Acetate).

**How Supplied:** 2 oz. (57g.) and 4 oz. (113g.) tubes and 16 oz. (454g.) jar.

*Shown in Product Identification Guide, page 506*

---

## BC® POWDER
## ARTHRITIS STRENGTH BC® POWDER
## BC® COLD POWDER LINE

**Description:** BC® POWDER: Active Ingredients: Each powder contains Aspirin 650 mg, Salicylamide 195 mg and Caffeine 33.3 mg. Inactive Ingredients: Dioctylsodium Sulfosuccinate, Fumaric Acid, Lactose and Potassium Chloride. ARTHRITIS STRENGTH BC® POWDER: Active Ingredients: Each powder contains Aspirin 742 mg, Salicylamide 222 mg and Caffeine 38 mg. Inactive Ingredients: Dioctylsodium Sulfosuccinate, Fumaric Acid, Lactose and Potassium Chloride.
BC® ALLERGY SINUS COLD POWDER

**Active Ingredients:** Aspirin 650 mg, Pseudoephedrine Hydrochloride 60 mg and Chlorpheniramine Maleate 4 mg per powder. Inactive Ingredients: Fumaric Acid, Glycine, Lactose, Potassium Chloride, Silica, Sodium Lauryl Sulfate. BC® SINUS COLD POWDER. **Active Ingredients:** Aspirin 650 mg and Pseudoephedrine Hydrochloride 60 mg. per powder. **Inactive Ingredients:** Fumaric Acid, Glycine, Lactose, Potassium Chloride, Silica, Sodium Lauryl Sulfate.

**Indications:** BC Powder is for relief of simple headache; for temporary relief of minor arthritic pain, neuralgia, neuritis and sciatica; for relief of muscular aches, discomfort and fever of colds; and for relief of normal menstrual pain and pain of tooth extraction.

Arthritis Strength BC Powder is specially formulated to fight occasional minor pain and inflammation of arthritis. Like Original Formula BC, Arthritis Strength BC provides fast temporary relief of minor arthritis pain and inflammation, neuralgia, neuritis and sciatica; relief of muscular aches, discomfort and fever of colds; and pain of tooth extraction.

BC Allergy Sinus Cold Powder is for relief of multiple symptoms such as body aches, fever, nasal congestion, sneezing, running nose, and watery itchy eyes associated with allergy and sinus attacks and the onset of colds. BC Sinus Cold Powder is for relief of such symptoms as body aches, fever, and nasal congestion.

BC Powder®, Arthritis
Strength BC® Powder:

**Warnings: Children and teenagers should not use this medicine for chicken pox or flu symptoms before a doctor is consulted about Reye's Syndrome, a rare but serious illness reported to be associated with aspirin. Keep this and all medicines out of children's reach. In case of accidental overdose, contact a physician or poison control center immediately.**

As with any drug, if you are pregnant or nursing a baby seek the advice of a health professional before using this product.

**IT IS ESPECIALLY IMPORTANT NOT TO USE ASPIRIN DURING THE LAST 3 MONTHS OF PREGNANCY UNLESS SPECIFICALLY DIRECTED TO DO SO BY A DOCTOR BECAUSE IT MAY CAUSE PROBLEMS IN THE UNBORN CHILD OR COMPLICATIONS DURING DELIVERY.**

**Alcohol Warning:** If you consume 3 or more alcoholic drinks every day, ask your doctor whether you should take aspirin or other pain relievers/fever reducers. Aspirin may cause stomach bleeding.

This product contains aspirin and should not be taken by individuals who are sensitive to aspirin. If pain persists for more than 10 days, or redness is present, consult a physician immediately.

**BC Cold Powder Line:**

**Warnings: Children and teenagers should not use BC for chicken pox or flu symptoms before a doctor is consulted about Reye's Syndrome, a rare but serious illness reported to be associated with aspirin. Keep BC and all medicines out of children's reach. In case of accidental overdose, contact a physician or poison control center immediately.**

As with any drug, if you are pregnant or nursing a baby seek the advice of a health professional before using BC.

**Alcohol Warning:** If you consume 3 or more alcoholic drinks every day, ask your doctor whether you should take aspirin or other pain relievers/fever reducers. Aspirin may cause stomach bleeding.

**IT IS ESPECIALLY IMPORTANT NOT TO USE ASPIRIN DURING THE LAST 3 MONTHS OF PREGNANCY UNLESS SPECIFICALLY DIRECTED TO DO SO BY A DOCTOR BECAUSE IT MAY CAUSE PROBLEMS IN THE UNBORN CHILD OR COMPLICATIONS DURING DELIVERY.**

**Do not exceed recommended dosage.** If nervousness, dizziness, or sleeplessness occur, discontinue use and consult a doctor. If symptoms do not improve within 7 days, or are accompanied by fever that lasts more than 3 days, or if new symptoms occur, consult a physician before continuing use. Do not take BC if you are sensitive to aspirin, or have heart disease, high blood pressure, thyroid disease, diabetes, asthma, glaucoma, emphysema, chronic pulmonary disease, shortness of breath, difficulty in breathing or difficulty in urination due to enlargement of the prostate gland, or if you are presently taking a prescription antihypertensive or antidepressant drug unless directed by a doctor. *"Drug interaction precaution.* Do not use this product if you are now taking a prescription monoamine oxidase inhibitor (MAOI) (certain drugs for depression, psychiatric or emotional conditions, or Parkinson's disease), or for 2 weeks after stopping the MAOI drug. If you are uncertain whether your prescription drug contains an MAOI, consult a health professional before taking this product." BC Allergy Sinus Cold Powder with antihistamine may cause drowsiness. Avoid alcoholic beverages when taking this product because it may increase drowsiness. Use caution when driving a motor vehicle or operating machinery. May cause excitability, especially in children.

**Overdosage:** In case of accidental overdosage, contact a physician or poison control center immediately.

**Dosage and Administration:** BC® Powder, Arthritis Strength BC® Powder, BC® Cold Powder Line:

Place one powder on tongue and follow with liquid. If you prefer, stir powder into glass of water or other liquid. May be used every three to four hours, (every 4–6 hours for BC® Cold Powder Line, (up to 3 powders each 24 hours.) For BC® Powder and Arthritis Strength BC® up to 4 powders each 24 hours. For children under 12, consult a physician.

**How Supplied:** BC Powder: Available in tamper evident overwrapped envelopes of 2 or 6 powders, as well as tamper evident boxes of 24 and 50 powders.

Arthritis Strength BC Powder: Available in tamper evident over wrapped envelopes of 6 powders, and tamper evident overwrapped boxes of 24 and 50 powders.

BC Cold Powder Line:
Available in tamper-evident over-wrapped envelopes of 6 powders, as well as tamper-evident boxes of 12 powders.

---

## Orange Flavor
### CITRUCEL®
[sĭt ′rə-sĕl ]
**(Methylcellulose)**
**Bulk-forming Fiber Laxative**

**Description:** Each 19 g adult dose (approximately one heaping measuring tablespoonful) contains Methylcellulose 2 g. Each 9.5 g child's dose (one-half the adult dose) contains Methylcellulose 1 g. Methylcellulose is a nonallergenic fiber. Also contains: Citric Acid, FD&C Yellow No. 6 Lake, Orange Flavors (natural and artificial), Potassium Citrate, Riboflavin, Sucrose, and other ingredients. Each adult dose contains approximately 3 mg of sodium and contributes 60 calories from Sucrose.

**Actions:** Promotes elimination by providing additional fiber (bulk) to the diet. This product generally produces bowel movement in 12 to 72 hours.

**Indications:** For relief of constipation (irregularity). May also be used for relief of constipation associated with other bowel disorders such as irritable bowel syndrome, diverticular disease, and hemorrhoids as well as for bowel management during postpartum, postsurgical, and convalescent periods when recommended by a physician.

**Contraindications:** Intestinal obstruction, fecal impaction, known hypersensitivity to formula ingredients.

**Warnings:** Patients should be instructed to consult their physician before using any laxative if they have noticed a sudden change in bowel habits which persists for two weeks. Unless directed by a physician, patients should be advised not to use laxative products when abdominal pain, nausea, or vomiting is present. Patients should also be advised to discontinue use and consult a physician if rectal bleeding or failure to have a bowel movement occurs after use of any laxative product. Unless recommended by a physician, patients should not exceed the recommended maximum daily dose. Patients should not use laxative products for a period longer than one week unless directed by a physician. TAKING THIS PRODUCT WITHOUT ADEQUATE FLUID MAY CAUSE IT TO SWELL AND BLOCK YOUR THROAT OR ESOPHAGUS AND MAY CAUSE CHOKING. DO NOT TAKE THIS PRODUCT IF YOU HAVE DIFFICULTY IN SWALLOWING. IF YOU EXPERIENCE CHEST PAIN, VOMITING, OR DIFFICULTY IN SWALLOWING OR BREATHING AFTER TAKING THIS PRODUCT, SEEK IMMEDIATE MEDICAL ATTENTION. KEEP THIS AND ALL DRUGS OUT OF THE REACH OF CHILDREN.

**Dosage and Administration:** Adult Dose: dissolve one leveled scoop (one heaping tablespoon – 19g) in 8 ounces of cold water up to three times daily at the first sign of constipation. Children age 6 to 12 years of age: *one-half the adult dose* stirred briskly in 8 ounces of cold water, once daily at the first sign of constipation. The mixture should be administered promptly and drinking another glass of water is highly recommended (see warnings). Children under 6 years of age: *Use only as directed by a physician.* Continued use for 12 to 72 hours may be necessary for full benefit.
TAKE THIS PRODUCT (CHILD OR ADULT DOSE) WITH AT LEAST 8 OZ. (A FULL GLASS) OF WATER OR OTHER FLUID. TAKING THIS PRODUCT WITHOUT ENOUGH LIQUID MAY CAUSE CHOKING. SEE WARNINGS.

**How Supplied:** 16 oz., 30 oz., and 50 oz. containers.
Boxes of 20-single-dose packets.
Store below 86°F (30°C). Protect contents from humidity; keep tightly closed.
*Shown in Product Identification Guide, page 506*

---

## Sugar Free Orange Flavor
### CITRUCEL®
[sĭt ′rə-sĕl ]
**(Methylcellulose)**
**Bulk-forming Fiber Laxative**

**Description:** Each 10.2 g adult dose (approximately one rounded measuring tablespoonful) contains Methylcellulose 2 g. Each 5.1 g child's dose (one-half the adult dose) contains Methylcellulose 1 g. Methylcellulose is a nonallergenic fiber. Also contains: Aspartame, Dibasic Calcium Phosphate, FD&C Yellow No. 6 Lake, Malic Acid, Maltodextrin, Orange Flavors (natural and artificial), Potassium Citrate, and Riboflavin. Each 10.2 g dose contains approximately 3 mg of sodium and contributes 24 calories from Maltodextrin.

**Actions:** Promotes elimination by providing additional fiber (bulk) to the diet. This product generally produces bowel movement in 12 to 72 hours.

**Indications:** For relief of constipation (irregularity). May also be used for relief of constipation associated with other bowel disorders such as irritable bowel syndrome, diverticular disease, and hemorrhoids as well as for bowel management during postpartum, postsurgical, and convalescent periods when recommended by a physician.

**Contraindications and Warnings:** See entry for "Orange Flavor Citrucel".

**Phenylketonurics:** CONTAINS PHENYLALANINE 52 mg per adult dose. Individuals with phenylketonuria and other individuals who must restrict their intake of phenylalanine should be warned that each 10.2 g adult dose contains aspartame which provides 52 mg of phenylalanine.

**Dosage and Administration:** Adult Dose: dissolve one leveled scoop (one rounded measuring tablespoon – 10.2 g) in 8 ounces of cold water up to three times daily at the first sign of constipation. Children age 6 to 12 years of age: *one-half the adult dose* stirred briskly into at least 8 ounces of cold water, once daily at the first sign of constipation. The mixture should be administered promptly and drinking another glass of water is highly recommended (see warnings). Children under 6 years of age: *Use only as directed by a physician.* Continued use for 12 to 72 hours may be necessary for full benefit.
TAKE THIS PRODUCT (CHILD OR ADULT DOSE) WITH AT LEAST 8 OZ. (A FULL GLASS) OF WATER OR OTHER FLUID. TAKING THIS PRODUCT WITHOUT ENOUGH LIQUID MAY CAUSE CHOKING. SEE WARNINGS.

**How Supplied:**
8.6 oz, 16.9 oz, and 32 oz containers.
Boxes of 20 single-dose packets.
Store below 86°F (30°C). Protect contents from humidity; keep tightly closed.
*Shown in Product Identification Guide, page 506*

---

### CITRUCEL®
**(methylcellulose)**
**Soluble Fiber Caplet**
**Bulk-Forming Fiber Laxative**

**Uses:** Helps restore and maintain regularity. Helps relieve constipation. Also useful in treatment of constipation (irregularity) associated with other bowel disorders when recommended by a physician. This product generally produces a bowel movement in 12 to 72 hours.

**Active Ingredient:** Each caplet contains 500mg Methylcellulose.

**Inactive Ingredients:** Crospovidone, Dibasic Calcium Phosphate, FD&C Yellow No. 6 Aluminum Lake, Magnesium Stearate, Maltodextrin, Povidone, Sodium Lauryl Sulfate.

**Directions:** Adult dose: Take two caplets as needed with 8 ounces of liquid, up to six times daily. Children (6–12 years): Take one caplet with 8 ounces of liquid, up to six times per day. The dosage requirement may vary according to the severity of constipation. Children under 6 years: consult a physician. TAKE THIS PRODUCT (CHILD OR ADULT DOSE) WITH AT LEAST 8 OUNCES (A FULL GLASS) OF WATER OR OTHER FLUID. TAKING THIS PRODUCT WITHOUT ENOUGH LIQUID MAY CAUSE CHOKING. SEE WARNINGS.

**Directions for Use:** Take each dose with 8oz. of liquid.

*Continued on next page*

## Citrucel Caplets—Cont.

| Age | Dose | Daily Maximum |
|---|---|---|
| Adults & Children over 12 years | 2 Caplets | Up to 6 times daily* |
| Children (6 to 12 years) | 1 Caplet | Up to 6 times daily* |
| Children under 6 years | Consult a physician | |

*Refer to directions below.

**Warnings:** Consult a physician before using any laxative product if you have noticed a sudden change in bowel habits which persists for two weeks. Unless directed by a physician, do not use laxative products when abdominal pain, nausea, or vomiting are present. Discontinue use and consult a physician if rectal bleeding or failure to produce a bowel movement occurs after use of any laxative product. Unless recommended by a physician, do not exceed recommended maximum daily dose. Laxative products should not be used for a period longer than a weak unless directed by a physician. If sensitive to any of the ingredients, do not use. **TAKING THIS PRODUCT WITHOUT ADEQUATE FLUID MAY CAUSE IT TO SWELL AND BLOCK YOUR THROAT OR ESOPHAGUS AND MAY CAUSE CHOKING. DO NOT TAKE THIS PRODUCT IF YOU HAVE DIFFI-CULTY IN SWALLOWING. IF YOU EXPERIENCE CHEST PAIN, VOMIT-ING, OR DIFFICULTY IN SWALLOW-ING OR BREATHING AFTER TAKING THIS PRODUCT, SEEK IMMEDIATE MEDICAL ATTENTION. KEEP THIS AND ALL DRUGS OUT OF THE REACH OF CHILDREN.**

Store at room temperature 15–30°C (59–86°F). Protect contents from moisture.

Tamper evident feature: Bottle sealed with printed foil under cap. Do not use if foil is torn or broken.

**How Supplied:** Bottles of 100 caplets

**Questions or comments?**

Call toll-free 1-800-897-6081 weekdays.

Patents Pending

The various Citrucel Logos and design elements of the packaging are Registered Trademarks of GlaxoSmith-Kline.

©2001 GlaxoSmithKline

Distributed by:

*GlaxoSmithKline Consumer Healthcare*

GlaxoSmithKline Consumer Healthcare, L.P.

Pittsburgh, PA 15230, Made in Canada.

## CONTAC® Non-Drowsy Decongestant 12 Hour Cold Caplets

**Product Information:** Each Maximum Strength Contac 12 Hour Cold Caplet provides up to 12 hours of relief. Part of the caplet goes to work right away for fast relief; the rest is released gradually to provide up to 12 hours of prolonged relief. With just one caplet in the morning and one at bedtime, you feel better all day, sleep better at night, breathing freely without congestion or sinus pressure.

**Indications:** Temporarily relieves nasal congestion due to the common cold, hay fever or other upper respiratory allergies and associated with sinusitis. Helps decongest sinus openings and passages; temporarily relieves sinus congestion and pressure.

**Directions:** Adults and children over 12 years of age: One caplet every 12 hours, not to exceed 2 caplets in 24 hours, or as directed by a doctor. Children under 12 years of age: consult a doctor.

**TAMPER-EVIDENT PACKAGING FEATURES FOR YOUR PROTEC-TION:** Each caplet is encased in a plastic cell with a foil back; do not use if cell or foil is broken.

**Warnings:** Do not exceed the recommended dosage. If nervousness, dizziness, or sleeplessness occur, discontinue use and consult a doctor. If symptoms do not improve within 7 days or are accompanied by high fever, consult a doctor. Do not take this product, unless directed by a doctor, if you have heart disease, high blood pressure, thyroid disease, diabetes, glaucoma or difficulty in urination due to enlargement of the prostate gland. KEEP THIS AND ALL DRUGS OUT OF REACH OF CHILDREN. IN CASE OF ACCIDENTAL OVERDOSE, SEEK PROFESSIONAL ASSISTANCE OR CONTACT A POISON CONTROL CENTER IMMEDIATELY. As with any drug, if you are pregnant or nursing a baby, seek the advice of a health professional before using this product.

**Drug Interaction Precaution:** Do not use this product if you are now taking a prescription monoamine oxidase inhibitor (MAOI) (certain drugs for depression, psychiatric or emotional conditions, or Parkinson's disease), or for 2 weeks after stopping the MAOI drug. If you are uncertain whether your prescription drug contains an MAOI, consult a health professional before taking this product.

**Active Ingredient:** Pseudoephedrine Hydrochloride 120 mg.

Store at 15° to 25°C (59° to 77°F) in a dry place and protest from light.

**Each Caplet Also Contains:** Carnauba Wax, Colloidal Silicon Dioxide, Dibasic Calcium Phosphate, Hydroxypropyl Methylcellulose, Magnesium Stearate, Microcrystalline Cellulose, Polyethylene Glycol, Polysorbate 80, Titanium Dioxide.

**How Supplied:** Consumer packages of 10 and 20 caplets.

**Note: There are other CONTAC products. Make sure this is the one you are interested in. See the table below for all of the products in the CONTAC line.**

*Shown in Product Identification Guide, page 506*

## CONTAC® Non-Drowsy Timed Release-Maximum Strength 12 Hour Cold Caplets

**Indications:** For the temporary relief of nasal congestion due to the common cold, hay fever or other upper respiratory allergies, and nasal congestion associated with sinusitis. Promotes nasal and/or sinus drainage; temporarily relieves sinus congestion and pressure. Temporarily restores freer breathing through the nose.

Each Maximum Strength Contac 12-Hour Cold caplet provides up to 12 hours of relief. Part of the caplet goes to work right away for fast relief; the rest is released gradually to provide up to 12 hours of prolonged relief. With just one caplet in the morning and one at bedtime, you feel better all day, sleep better at night, breathing freely without congestion or sinus pressure.

**Active Ingredient:** Each coated extended-release caplet contains Pseudoephedrine Hydrochloride 120 mg.

**Inactive Ingredients:** carnauba wax, collodial silicon dioxide, dibasic calcium phosphate, hydroxypropyl methylcellulose, magnesium stearate, microcrystalline cellulose, polyethylene glycol, polysorbate 80, titanium dioxide.

**Directions:** Adults and children 12 years of age and over – One caplet every 12 hours, not to exceed two caplets in 24 hours. This product is not recommended for children under 12 years of age.

**Warnings: Do not exceed recommended dosage.** If nervousness, dizziness, or sleeplessness occur, discontinue use and consult a doctor. If symptoms do not improve within 7 days or are accompanied by fever, consult a doctor. Do not take this product if you have heart disease, high blood pressure, thyroid disease, diabetes, or difficulty in urination due to enlargement of the prostate gland unless directed by a doctor. As with any drug, if you are pregnant or nursing a baby, seek the advice of a health professional before using this product.

**Drug Interaction Precaution:** Do not use this product if you are now taking a prescription monoamine oxidase inhibitor (MAOI) (certain drugs for depression, psychiatric or emotional conditions, or Parkinson's disease), or for 2 weeks after stopping the MAOI drug. If you are uncertain whether your prescription contains an MAOI, consult a health professional before taking this product.

**KEEP THIS AND ALL DRUGS OUT OF THE REACH OF CHILDREN.** In case of ac-

**PDR For Nonprescription Drugs**

| | CONTAC Non-Drowsy 12 Hour Cold Caplets | CONTAC 12 Hour Cold Capsules | CONTAC Severe Cold and Flu Caplets Maximum Strength (each 2 caplet dose) | CONTAC Severe Cold and Flu Non-Drowsy Caplets (each 2 caplet dose) | CONTAC Day & Night Cold & Flu Day Caplets | CONTAC Day & Night Cold & Flu Night Caplets |
|---|---|---|---|---|---|---|
| Phenylpropanolamine HCl | — | 75.0 mg | — | — | — | — |
| Chlorpheniramine Maleate | — | 8.0 mg | 4.0 mg | — | — | — |
| Pseudoephedrine HCl | 120 mg | — | 60 mg | 60.0 mg | 60.0 mg | 60.0 mg |
| Acetaminophen | — | — | 1000.0 mg | 650.0 mg | 650.0 mg | 650.0 mg |
| Dextromethorphan Hydrobromide | — | — | 30.0 mg | 30.0 mg | 30.0 mg | 30.0 mg |
| Diphenhydramine HCl | — | — | — | — | — | 50.0 mg |

cidental overdose, seek professional assistance or contact a Poison Control Center immediately.
Store at 15° to 25°C (59° to 77°F) in a dry place and protect from light.

**How Supplied:** Packets of 10 and 20 Caplets
U.S. Patent No. 5,895,663
*Comments or questions?*
Call toll-free 1-800-245-1040 weekdays.

---

**CONTAC®**
**Severe Cold and Flu**
**Caplets Maximum Strength**
**Analgesic• Decongestant**
**Antihistamine• Cough Suppressant**
**CONTAC®**
**Severe Cold and Flu**
**Caplets Non-Drowsy**
**Nasal Decongestant • Analgesic•**
**Cough Suppressant**

**Active Ingredients:** Each *Non-Drowsy Caplet* contains Acetaminophen 325 mg, Psudoephedrine HCl 30 mg and Dextromethorphan Hydrobromide 15 mg.
Each *Maximum Strength Caplet* contains Acetaminophen 500 mg, Dextromethorphan Hydrobromide 15 mg, Pseudoephedrine HCl 30 mg and chlorpheniromine Maleate 2 mg.

**Product Information:** Two caplets every 6 hours to help relieve the discomforts of severe colds with flu-like symptoms.

**Indications:** *Non-Drowsy & Maximum Strength Caplets:* Temporarily relieves nasal congestion & coughing due to the common cold. Provides temporary relief of fever, sore throat, headache & minor aches associated with the common cold or the flu.
*Maximum Strength Caplets:* Temporarily relieves runny nose, sneezing, itchy and watery eyes due to the common cold.

**Directions:** Adults (12 years and older): Two caplets every 6 hours, not to exceed 8 caplets in any 24-hour period, or as directed by a doctor. Children under 12 years of age: consult a doctor.

**TAMPER-EVIDENT PACKAGING FEATURES FOR YOUR PROTECTION:**
Caplets are encased in a plastic cell with a foil back; do not use if cell or foil is broken. The letters ND SCF for non-drowsy and SCF for maximum strength appear on each caplet; do not use this product if these letters are missing.

**Warnings: For *Non-Drowsy and Maximum Strength Caplets:* Do not exceed recommended dosage.** If nervousness, dizziness, or sleeplessness occur, discontinue use and consult a doctor. If symptoms do not improve or are accompanied by fever that lasts for more than 3 days, or if new symptoms occur, consult a doctor. If sore throat is severe, persists for more than 2 days, is accompanied or followed by fever, headache, rash, nausea, or vomiting, consult a doctor promptly. A persistent cough may be a sign of a serious condition. If cough persists for more than 7 days, tends to recur, or is accompanied by rash, persistent headache, fever that lasts for more than 3 days, or if new symptoms occur, consult a doctor. Do not take this product for persistent or chronic cough such as occurs with smoking, asthma, emphysema, or if cough is accompanied by excessive phlegm (mucus) unless directed by a doctor. Do not take this product if you have heart disease, high blood pressure, thyroid disease, diabetes, glaucoma or difficulty in urination due to enlargement of the prostate gland unless directed by a doctor. **Alcohol Warning:** If you consume 3 or more alcoholic drinks every day, ask your doctor whether you should take acetaminophen or other pain relievers/fever reducers. Acetaminophen may cause liver damage. **KEEP THIS AND ALL DRUGS OUT OF THE REACH OF CHILDREN.** Prompt medical attention is critical for adults as well as for children even if you do not notice any signs or symptoms. In case of accidental overdose, seek professional assistance or contact a Poison Control Center immediately. As with any drug, if you are pregnant or nursing a baby, seek the advice of a health professional before using this product.

**Additional Warnings for *Maximum Strength Caplets:*** May cause excitability especially in children. Do not take this product, unless directed by a doctor, if you have a breathing problem such as emphysema or chronic bronchitis. May cause marked drowsiness: alcohol, sedatives, and tranquilizers may increase the drowsiness effect. Avoid taking alcoholic beverages while taking this product. Do not take this product if you are taking sedatives or tranquilizers, without first consulting your doctor. Use caution when driving a motor vehicle or operating machinery.

**Drug Interaction Precaution:** Do not use this product if you are now taking a prescription monoamine oxidase inhibitor (MAOI) (certain drugs for depression, psychiatric or emotional conditions, or Parkinson's disease), or for 2 weeks after stopping the MAOI drug. If you are uncertain whether your prescription drug contains an MAOI, consult a health professional before taking this product.

**Inactive Ingredients:** Each *Non-Drowsy and Maximum Strength Caplet* contains: Carnauba Wax, Colloidal Silicon Dioxide, Hydroxypropyl Methylcellulose, Magnesium stearate, Microcrystalline Cellulose, Polyethylene Glycol, Polysorbate 80, Starch, Stearic Acid, Titanium Dioxide.
Each *Maximum Strength Caplet* also contains: FD&C Blue #1 Al Lake.

Avoid storing at high temperature (greater than 100°F).

**How Supplied:** *Non-Drowsy:* Consumer packages of 16.
*Maximum Strength:* Consumer packages of 16 & 30.
*Shown in Product Identification Guide, page 506*

**Product Change:** Maximum Strength Caplets now with new decongestant (pseudoephedrine HCl).

**Note: There are other CONTAC products. Make sure this is the one you are interested in.** See the table below for all of the products in the CONTAC line.
[See table above]

*Continued on next page*

## DEBROX® Drops
## Ear Wax Removal Aid

**Description:** Carbamide peroxide 6.5%. Also contains citric acid, glycerin, propylene glycol, sodium stannate, water, and other ingredients.

**Actions:** DEBROX®, used as directed, cleanses the ear with sustained microfoam. DEBROX Drops foam on contact with earwax due to the release of oxygen (there may be an associated crackling sound). DEBROX Drops provide a safe, nonirritating method of softening and removing ear wax.

**Indications:** For occasional use as an aid to soften, loosen, and remove excessive earwax.

**Directions:** FOR USE IN THE EAR ONLY. Adults and children over 12 years of age: tilt head sideways and place 5 to 10 drops into ear. Tip of applicator should not enter ear canal. Keep drops in ear for several minutes by keeping head tilted or placing cotton in the ear. Use twice daily for up to four days if needed, or as directed by a doctor. Any wax remaining after treatment may be removed by gently flushing the ear with warm water, using a soft rubber bulb ear syringe. Children under 12 years of age: consult a doctor.

**Warnings:** Do not use if you have ear drainage or discharge, ear pain, irritation or rash in the ear, or are dizzy; consult a doctor. Do not use if you have an injury or perforation (hole) of the eardrum or after ear surgery unless directed by a doctor. Do not use for more than four days. If excessive earwax remains after use of this product, consult a doctor. Avoid contact with the eyes.

**Cautions:** Avoid exposing bottle to excessive heat and direct sunlight. Keep tip on bottle when not in use. Keep this and all drugs out of the reach of children. In case of accidental ingestion, seek professional assistance or contact a poison control center immediately.

**How Supplied:** DEBROX Drops are available in $^1/_2$- or 1-fl-oz (15 or 30 ml) plastic squeeze bottles with applicator spouts.

*Shown in Product Identification Guide, page 507*

---

## ECOTRIN
### Enteric-Coated Aspirin
Antiarthritic, Antiplatelet
COMPREHENSIVE PRESCRIBING INFORMATION

**Description:** Ecotrin enteric coated aspirin (acetylsalicylic acid) tablets available in 81mg, 325mg and 500 mg tablets for oral administration. The 325 mg and 500 mg tablets contain the following inactive ingredients: Carnuba Wax, Colloidal Silicon Dioxide, FD&C Yellow No. 6, Hydroxypropyl Methylcellulose, Methacrylic Acid Copolymer, Microcrystalline Cellulose, Pregelatinized Starch, Propylene Glycol, Simethicone, Sodium Starch Glycolate, Stearic Acid, Talc, Titanium Dioxide, and Triethyl Citrate. The 81 mg tablets contain Carnuba Wax, Corn Starch, D&C Yellow No. 10, FD&C Yellow No. 6, Hydroxypropyl Methylcellulose, Methacrylic Acid Copolymer, Microcrystalline Cellulose, Propylene Glycol, Simethicone, Stearic Acid, Talc and Triethyl Citrate.

Aspirin is an odorless white, needle-like crystalline or powdery substance. When exposed to moisture, aspirin hydrolyzes into salicylic and acetic acids, and gives off a vinegary-odor. It is highly lipid soluble and slightly soluble in water.

**Clinical Pharmacology:** Mechanism of Action: Aspirin is a more potent inhibitor of both prostaglandin synthesis and platelet aggregation than other salicylic acid derivatives. The differences in activity between aspirin and salicylic acid are thought to be due to the acetyl group on the aspirin molecule. This acetyl group is responsible for the inactivation of cyclooxygenase via acetylation.

### PHARMACOKINETICS
Absorption: In general, immediate release aspirin is well and completely absorbed from the gastrointestinal (GI) tract. Following absorption, aspirin is hydrolyzed to salicylic acid with peak plasma levels of salicylic acid occurring within 1–2 hours of dosing (see Pharmacokinetics—Metabolism). The rate of absorption from the GI tract is dependent upon the dosage form, the presence or absence of food, gastric pH (the presence or absence of GI antacids or buffering agents), and other physiologic factors. Enteric coated aspirin products are erratically absorbed from the GI tract.

Distribution: Salicylic acid is widely distributed to all tissues and fluids in the body including the central nervous system (CNS), breast milk, and fetal tissues. The highest concentrations are found in the plasma, liver, renal cortex, heart, and lungs.

The protein binding of salicylate is concentration-dependent, i.e., non-linear. At low concentrations ($< 100$ mcg/mL) approximately 90 percent of plasma salicylate is bound to albumin while at higher concentrations ($> 400$ mcg/mL), only about 75 percent is bound. The early signs of salicylic overdose (salicylism), including tinnitus (ringing in the ears), occur at plasma concentrations approximating 200 mcg/mL. Severe toxic effects are associated with levels $> 400$ mcg/mL (See Adverse Reactions and Overdosage.)

Metabolism: Aspirin is rapidly hydrolyzed in the plasma to salicylic acid such that plasma levels of aspirin are essentially undetectable 1–2 hours after dosing. Salicylic acid is primarily conjugated in the liver to form salicyluric acid, a phenolic glucuronide, an acyl glucuronide, and a number of minor metabolites. Salicylic acid has a plasma half-life of approximately 6 hours. Salicylate metabolism is saturable and total body clearance decreases at higher serum concentrations due to the limited ability of the liver to form both salicyluric acid and phenolic glucuronide. Following toxic doses (10–20 grams (g)), the plasma half-life may be increased to over 20 hours.

Elimination: The elimination of salicylic acid follows zero order pharmacokinetics; (i.e., the rate of drug elimination is constant in relation to plasma concentration). Renal excretion of unchanged drug depends upon urine pH. As urinary pH rises above 6.5, the renal clearance of free salicylate increases from $< 5$ percent to $> 80$ percent. Alkalinization of the urine is a key concept in the management of salicylate overdose. (See Overdosage.) Following therapeutic doses, approximately 10 percent is found excreted in the urine as salicylic acid, 75 percent as salicyluric acid, as the phenolic and acyl glucuronides, respectively.

Pharmacodynamics: Aspirin affects platelet aggregation by irreversibly inhibiting prostaglandin cyclo-oxygenase. This effect lasts for the life of the platelet and prevents the formation of the platelet aggregating factor thromboxane A2. Non-acetylated salicylates do not inhibit this enzyme and have no effect on platelet aggregation. At somewhat higher doses, aspirin reversibly inhibits the formation of prostaglandin $1_2$ (prostacyclin), which is an arterial vasodilator and inhibits platelet aggregation.

At higher doses aspirin is an effective anti-inflammatory agent, partially due to inhibition of inflammatory mediators via cyclooxygenase inhibition in peripheral tissues. In vitro studies suggest that other mediators of inflammation may also be suppressed by aspirin administration, although the precise mechanism of action has not been elucidated. It is this non-specific suppression of cyclooxygenase activity in peripheral tissues following large doses that leads to its primary side effect of gastric irritation. (See Adverse Reactions.)

**Clinical Studies:** Ischemic Stroke and Transient Ischemic Attack (TIA): In clinical trials of subjects with TIA's due to fibrin platelet emboli or ischemic stroke, aspirin has been shown to significantly reduce the risk of the combined endpoint of stroke or death and the combined endpoint of TIA, stroke, or death by about 13–18 percent.

Suspect Acute Myocardial Infarction (MI): In a large, multi-center study of aspirin, streptokinase, and the combination of aspirin and streptokinase in 17,187 patients with suspected acute MI, aspirin treatment produced a 23-percent reduction in the risk of vascular mortality. Aspirin was also shown to have an additional benefit in patients given a thrombolytic agent.

Prevention of Recurrent MI and Unstable Angina Pectoris: These indications are supported by the results of six large, randomized, multi-center, placebo-controlled trials of predominantly male post-MI subjects and one randomized placebo-controlled study of men with unstable angina pectoris. Aspirin therapy in MI subjects was associated with a significant reduction (about 20 percent) in the risk of the combination endpoint of subsequent death and/or nonfatal reinfarction in these patients. In aspirin-treated unstable angina patients the event rate was reduced to 5 percent from the 10 percent rate in the placebo group.

Chronic Stable Angina Pectoris: In a randomized, multi-center, double-blind trial designed to assess the role of aspirin for prevention of MI in patients with chronic stable angina pectoris, aspirin significantly reduced the primary combined endpoint of nonfatal MI, fatal MI, and sudden death by 34 percent. The secondary endpoint for vascular events (first occurrence of MI, stroke, or vascular death) was also significantly reduced (32 percent).

Revascularization Procedures: Most patients who undergo coronary artery revascularization procedures have already had symptomatic coronary artery disease for which aspirin is indicated. Similarly, patients with lesions of the carotid bifurcation sufficient to require carotid endarterectomy are likely to have had a precedent event. Aspirin is recommended for patients who undergo revascularization procedures if there is a pre-existing condition for which aspirin is already indicated.

Rheumatologic Diseases: In clinical studies in patients with rheumatoid arthritis, juvenile rheumatoid arthritis, ankylosing spondylitis and osteoarthritis, aspirin has been shown to be effective in controlling various indices of clinical disease activity.

**Animal Toxicology:** The acute oral 50 percent lethal dose in rats is about 1.5 g/kg and in mice 1.1 g/kg. Renal papillary necrosis and decreased urinary concentrating ability occur in rodents chronically administered high doses. Dose-dependent gastric mucosal injury occurs in rats and humans. Mammals may develop aspirin toxicosis associated with GI symptoms, circulatory effects, and central nervous system depression. (See Overdosage.)

**Indications and Usage:** Vascular Indications (Ischemic Stroke, TIA, Acute MI, Prevention of Recurrent MI, Unstable Angina Pectoris, and Chronic Stable Angina Pectoris): Aspirin is indicated to: (1) Reduce the combined risk of death and nonfatal stroke in patients who have had ischemic stroke or transient ischemia of the brain due to fibrin platelet emboli, (2) reduce the risk of vascular mortality in patients with a suspected acute MI, (3) reduce the combined risk of death and nonfatal MI in patients with a previous MI or unstable angina pectoris,

and (4) reduce the combined risk of MI and sudden death in patients with chronic stable angina pectoris.

Revascularization Procedures (Coronary Artery Bypass Graft (CABG), Percutaneous Transluminal Coronary Angioplasty (PTCA), and Carotid Endarterectomy): Aspirin is indicated in patients who have undergone revascularization procedures (i.e., CABG, PTCA, or carotid endarterectomy) when there is a preexisting condition for which aspirin is already indicated.

Rheumatologic Disease Indications (Rheumatoid Arthritis, Juvenile Rheumatoid Arthritis, Spondyloarthropathies, Osteoarthritis, and the Arthritis and Pleurisy of Systemic Lupus Erythematosus (SLE)): Aspirin is indicated for the relief of the signs and symptoms of rheumatoid arthritis, juvenile rheumatoid arthritis, osteoarthritis, spondyloarthropathies, and arthritis and pleurisy associated with SLE.

**Contraindications:** Allergy: Aspirin is contraindicated in patients with known allergy to nonsteroidal anti-inflammatory drug products and in patients with the syndrome of asthma, rhinitis, and nasal polyps. Aspirin may cause severe urticaria, angioedema, or bronchospasm (asthma).

Reye's Syndrome: Aspirin should not be used in children or teenagers for viral infections, with or without fever, because of the risk of Reye's syndrome with concomitant use of aspirin in certain viral illnesses.

**Warnings:** Alcohol Warning: Patients who consume three or more alcoholic drinks every day should be counseled about the bleeding risks involved with chronic, heavy alcohol use while taking aspirin.

Coagulation Abnormalities: Even low doses of aspirin can inhibit platelet function leading to an increase in bleeding time. This can adversely affect patients with inherited (hemophilia) or acquired (liver disease or vitamin K deficiency) bleeding disorders.

GI Side Effects: GI side effects include stomach pain, heartburn, nausea, vomiting, and gross GI bleeding. Although minor upper GI symptoms, such as dyspepsia, are common and can occur anytime during therapy, physicians should remain alert for signs of ulceration and bleedings, even in the absence of previous GI symptoms. Physicians should inform patients about the signs and symptoms of GI side effects and what steps to take if they occur.

Peptic Ulcer Disease: Patients with a history of active peptic ulcer disease should avoid using aspirin, which can cause gastric mucosal irritation and bleeding.

**Precautions**
**General**
Renal Failure: Avoid aspirin in patients with severe renal failure (glomerular filtration rate less than 10 mL/minute).

Hepatic Insufficiency: Avoid aspirin in patients with severe hepatic insufficiency.

Sodium Restricted Diets: Patients with sodium-retaining states, such as congestive heart failure or renal failure, should avoid sodium-containing buffered aspirin preparations because of their high sodium content.

Laboratory Tests: Aspirin has been associated with elevated hepatic enzymes, blood urea nitrogen and serum creatinine, hyperkalemia, proteinuria, and prolonged bleeding time.

**Drug Interactions**
Angiotensin Converting Enzyme (ACE) Inhibitors: The hyponatremic and hypotensive effects of ACE inhibitors may be diminished by the concomitant administration of aspirin due to its direct effect on the renin-angiotensin conversion pathway.

Acetazolamide: Concurrent use of aspirin and acetazolamide can lead to high serum concentrations of acetazolamide (and toxicity) due to competition at the renal tubule for secretion.

Anticoagulant Therapy (Heparin and Warfarin): Patients on anticoagulation therapy are at increased risk for bleeding because of drug-drug interactions and the effect on platelets. Aspirin can displace warfarin from protein binding sites, leading to prolongation of both the prothrombin time and the bleeding time. Aspirin can increase the anticoagulant activity of heparin, increasing bleeding risk.

Anticonvulsants: Salicylate can displace protein-bound phenytoin and valproic acid, leading to a decrease in the total concentration of phenytoin and an increase in serum valproic acid levels.

Beta Blockers: The hypotensive effects of beta blockers may be diminished by the concomitant administration of aspirin due to inhibition of renal prostaglandins, leading to decreased renal blood flow, and salt and fluid retention.

Diuretics: The effectiveness of diuretics in patients with underlying renal or cardiovascular disease may be diminished by the concomitant administration of aspirin due to inhibition of renal prostaglandins, leading to decreased renal blood flow and salt and fluid retention.

Methotrexate: Salicylate can inhibit renal clearance of methotrexate, leading to bone marrow toxicity, especially in the elderly or renal impaired.

Nonsteroidal Anti-inflammatory Drugs (NSAID's): The concurrent use of aspirin with other NSAID's should be avoided because this may increase bleeding or lead to decreased renal function.

Oral Hypoglycemics: Moderate doses of aspirin may increase the effectiveness of oral hypoglycemic drugs, leading to hypoglycemia.

Uricosuric Agents (Probenecid and Sulfinpyrazone): Salicylates antagonize the uricosuric action of uricosuric agents.

*Continued on next page*

## Ecotrin—Cont.

Carcinogenesis, Mutagenesis, Impairment of Fertility: Administration of aspirin for 68 weeks at 0.5 percent in the feed of rats was not carcinogenic. In the Ames Salmonella assay, aspirin was not mutagenic; however, aspirin did induce chromosome aberrations in cultured human fibroblasts. Aspirin inhibits ovulation in rats. (See Pregnancy.)

Pregnancy: Pregnant women should only take aspirin if clearly needed. Because of the known effects of NSAID's on the fetal cardiovascular system (closure of the ductus arteriosus), use during the third trimester of pregnancy should be avoided. Salicylate products have also been associated with alterations in maternal and neonatal hemostasis mechanisms, decreased birth weight, and with perinatal mortality.

Labor and Delivery: Aspirin should be avoided 1 week prior to and during labor and delivery because it can result in excessive blood loss at delivery. Prolonged gestation and prolonged labor due to prostaglandin inhibition have been reported.

Nursing Mothers: Nursing mothers should avoid using aspirin because salicylate is excreted in breast milk. Use of high doses may lead to rashes, platelet abnormalities, and bleeding in nursing infants.

Pediatric Use: Pediatric dosing recommendations for juvenile rheumatoid arthritis are based on well-controlled clinical studies. An initial dose of 90–130 mg/kg/day in divided doses, with an increase as needed for anti-inflammatory efficacy (target plasma salicylate levels of 150–300 mcg/mL) are effective. At high doses (i.e., plasma levels of greater than 200 mg/mL), the incidence of toxicity increases.

**Adverse Reactions:** Many adverse reactions due to aspirin ingestion are dose-related. The following is a list of adverse reactions that have been reported in the literature. (See Warnings.)

Body as a Whole: Fever, hypothermia, thirst.

Cardiovascular: Dysrhythmias, hypotension, tachycardia.

Central Nervous System: Agitation, cerebral edema, coma, confusion, dizziness, headache, subdural or intracranial hemorrhage, lethargy, seizures.

Fluid and Electrolyte: Dehydration, hyperkalemia, metabolic acidosis, respiratory alkalosis.

Gastrointestinal: Dyspepsia, GI bleeding, ulceration and perforation, nausea, vomiting, transient elevations of hepatic enzymes, hepatitis, Reye's Syndrome, pancreatitis.

Hematologic: Prolongation of the prothrombin time, disseminated intravascular coagulation, coagulopathy, thrombocytopenia.

Hypersensitivity: Acute anaphylaxis, angioedema, asthma, bronchospasm, laryngeal edema, urticaria.

Musculoskeletal: Rhabdomyolysis.

Metabolism: Hypoglycemia (in children), hyperglycemia.

Reproductive: Prolonged pregnancy and labor, stillbirths, lower birth weight infants, antepartum and postpartum bleeding.

Respiratory: Hyperpnea, pulmonary edema, tachypnea.

Special Senses: Hearing loss, tinnitus. Patients with high frequency hearing loss may have difficulty perceiving tinnitus. In these patients, tinnitus cannot be used as a clinical indicator of salicylism.

Urogenital: Interstitial nephritis, papillary necrosis, proteinuria, renal insufficiency and failure.

**Drug Abuse and Dependence:** Aspirin is non-narcotic. There is no known potential for addiction associated with the use of aspirin.

**Overdosage:** Salicylate toxicity may result from acute ingestion (overdose) or chronic intoxication. The early signs of salicylic overdose (salicylism), including tinnitus (ringing in the ears), occur at plasma concentrations approaching 200 mcg/mL. Plasma concentrations of aspirin above 300 mcg/mL are clearly toxic. Severe toxic effects are associated with levels above 400 mcg/mL. (See Clinical Pharmacology.) A single lethal dose of aspirin in adults is not known with certainty but death may be expected at 30 g. For real or suspected overdose, a Poison Control Center should be contacted immediately. Careful medical management is essential.

Signs and Symptoms: In acute overdose, severe acid-base and electrolyte disturbances may occur and are complicated by hyperthermia and dehydration. Respiratory alkalosis occurs early while hyperventilation is present, but is quickly followed by metabolic acidosis.

Treatment: Treatment consists primarily of supporting vital functions, increasing salicylate elimination, and correcting the acid-base disturbance. Gastric emptying and/or lavage is recommended as soon as possible after ingestion, even if the patient has vomited spontaneously. After lavage and/or emesis, administration of activated charcoal, as a slurry, is beneficial, if less than 3 hours have passed since ingestion. Charcoal adsorption should not be employed prior to emesis and lavage.

Severity of aspirin intoxication is determined by measuring the blood salicylate level. Acid-base status should be closely followed with serial blood gas and serum pH measurements. Fluid and electrolyte balance should be maintained.

In severe cases, hyperthermia and hypovolemia are the major immediate threats to life. Children should be sponged with tepid water. Replacement fluid should be administered intravenously and augmented with correction of acidosis. Plasma electrolytes and pH should be monitored to promote alkaline diuresis

of salicylate if renal function is normal. Infusion of glucose may be required to control hypoglycemia.

Hemodialysis and peritoneal dialysis can be performed to reduce the body drug content. In patients with renal insufficiency or in cases of life-threatening intoxication, dialysis is usually required. Exchange transfusion may be indicated in infants and young children.

**Dosage and Administration:** Each dose of aspirin should be taken with a full glass of water unless patient is fluid restricted. Anti-inflammatory and analgesic dosages should be individualized. When aspirin is used in high doses, the development of tinnitus may be used as a clinical sign of elevated plasma salicylate levels except in patients with high frequency hearing loss.

Ischemic Stroke and TIA: 50–325 mg once a day. Continue therapy indefinitely.

Suspected Acute MI: The initial dose of 160–162.5 mg is administered as soon as an MI is suspected. The maintenance dose of 160–162.5 mg a day is continued for 30 days post infarction. After 30 days, consider further therapy based on dosage and administration for prevention of recurrent MI.

Prevention of Recurrent MI: 75–325 mg once a day. Continue therapy indefinitely.

Unstable Angina Pectoris: 75–325 mg once a day. Continue therapy indefinitely.

Chronic Stable Angina Pectoris: 75–325 mg once a day. Continue therapy indefinitely.

CABG: 325 mg daily starting 6 hours post-procedure. Continue therapy for 1 year post-procedure.

PTCA: The initial dose of 325 mg should be given 2 hours pre-surgery. Maintenance dose is 160–325 mg daily. Continue therapy indefinitely.

Carotid Endarterectomy: Doses of 80 mg once daily to 650 mg twice daily, started presurgery, are recommended. Continue therapy indefinitely.

Rheumatoid Arthritis: The initial dose is 3 g a day in divided doses. Increase as needed for anti-inflammatory efficacy with target plasma salicylate levels of 150–300 mcg/mL. At high doses (i.e., plasma levels of greater than 200 mg/mL), the incidence of toxicity increases.

Juvenile Rheumatoid Arthritis: Initial dose is 90–130 mg/kg/day in divided doses. Increase as needed for anti-inflammatory efficacy with target plasma salicylate levels of 150–300 mcg/mL. At high doses (i.e., plasma levels of greater than 200 mg/mL), the incidence of toxicity increases.

Spondyloarthropathies: Up to 4 g per day in divided doses.

Osteoarthritis: Up to 3 g per day in divided doses.

Arthritis and Pleurisy of SLE: The initial dose is 3 g a day in divided doses. Increase as needed for anti-inflammatory efficacy with target plasma salicylate levels of 150–300 mcg/mL. At high doses (i.e., plasma levels of greater than 200 mg/mL), the incidence of toxicity increases.

**How Supplied:** 81 mg convex orange film coated tablet with ECOTRIN LOW printed in black ink on one side of the tablet. Available as follows
NDC 0108-0117-82 Bottle of 36 tablets
NDC 0108-0117-83 Bottle of 120 tablets
325 mg convex orange film coated tablet with ECOTRIN REG printed in black ink on one side of the tablet. Available as follows:
NDC 0108-0014-26 Bottle of 100 tablets
NDC 0108-0014-29 Bottle of 250 tablets
500 mg convex orange film coated tablet with ECOTRIN MAX printed in black ink on one side of the tablet. Available as follows:
NDC 0108-0016-23 Bottle of 60 tablets
NDC 0108-0016-27 Bottle of 150 tablets
Store in a tight container at 25°C (77° F); excursions permitted to 15–30° C (59–86° F).
*Shown in Product Identification Guide, page 507*

---

### GAVISCON® Regular Strength Antacid Tablets
[găv 'ĭs-kŏn ]

**Composition:** Each chewable tablet contains the following active ingredients:
Aluminum hydroxide dried gel... 80 mg
Magnesium trisilicate .................. 20 mg
and the following inactive ingredients: alginic acid, calcium stearate, flavor, sodium bicarbonate, starch (may contain corn starch), and sucrose.

**Actions:** Unique formulation produces soothing foam which floats on stomach contents. Foam containing antacid precedes stomach contents into the esophagus when reflux occurs to help protect the sensitive mucosa from further irritation. GAVISCON® acts locally without neutralizing entire stomach contents to help maintain integrity of the digestive process. Endoscopic studies indicate that GAVISCON Antacid Tablets are equally as effective in the erect or supine patient.

**Indications:** GAVISCON is specifically formulated for the temporary relief of heartburn (acid indigestion) due to acid reflux. GAVISCON is not indicated for the treatment of peptic ulcers.

**Directions:** Chew 2 to 4 tablets four times a day or as directed by a physician. Tablets should be taken after meals and at bedtime or as needed. For best results follow by a half glass of water or other liquid. DO NOT SWALLOW WHOLE.

**Warnings:** Do not take more than 16 tablets in a 24-hour period or 16 tablets daily for more than 2 weeks, except under the advice and supervision of a physician. Do not use this product except under the advice and supervision of a phy-

sician if you are on a sodium-restricted diet. Each GAVISCON Tablet contains approximately 0.8 mEq sodium.

**Drug Interaction Precaution:** Antacids may interact with certain prescription drugs. If you are presently taking a prescription drug, do not take this product without checking with your physician or other health professional.
Store at a controlled room temperature in a dry place.

Keep this and all drugs out of the reach of children. In case of accidental overdose, seek professional assistance or contact a poison control center immediately.

**How Supplied:** Bottles of 100 tablets and in foil-wrapped 2s in boxes of 30 tablets.
*Shown in Product Identification Guide, page 507*

---

### GAVISCON® EXTRA STRENGTH Antacid Tablets
[găv 'ĭs-kŏn ]

**Composition:** Each chewable tablet contains the following active ingredients:
Aluminum hydroxide ............... 160 mg
Magnesium carbonate ............. 105 mg
and the following inactive ingredients: alginic acid, calcium stearate, flavor, sodium bicarbonate, and sucrose. May contain stearic acid. Contains sorbitol or mannitol. May contain starch.

**Actions:** Gavison's unique antacid foam barrier neutralizes stomach acid.

**Indications:** For the relief of heartburn, sour stomach, acid indigestion and upset stomach associated with these conditions.

**Directions:** Chew 2 to 4 tablets four times a day or as directed by a physician. Tablets should be taken after meals and at bedtime or as needed. For best results follow by a half glass of water or other liquid. DO NOT SWALLOW WHOLE.

**Warnings:** Do not take more than 16 tablets in a 24-hour period or 16 tablets daily for more than 2 weeks, except under the advice and supervision of a physician. Do not use this product except under the advice and supervision of a physician if you are on a sodium-restricted diet. Each Extra Strength Gaviscon tablet contains approximately 1.3 mEq sodium.

**Drug Interaction Precaution:** Antacids may interact with certain prescription drugs. If you are presently taking a prescription drug, do not take this product without checking with your physician or other health professional.

Store at a controlled room temperature in a dry place.

Keep this and all drugs out of the reach of children. In case of accidental overdose, seek professional assistance or contact a poison control center immediately.

**How Supplied:** Bottles of 100 tablets and in foil-wrapped 2s in boxes of 6 and 30 tablets.
*Shown in Product Identification Guide, page 507*

---

### GAVISCON® Regular Strength Liquid Antacid
[găv 'ĭs-kŏn ]

**Composition:** Each tablespoonful (15 ml) contains the following active ingredients:
Aluminum hydroxide .................. 95 mg
Magnesium carbonate ............. 358 mg
and the following inactive ingredients: Benzyl alcohol, D&C Yellow #10, edetate disodium, FD&C Blue #1, flavor, glycerin, saccharin sodium, sodium alginate, sorbitol solution, water, and xanthan gum.

**Actions:** Gaviscon's unique antacid foam barrier neutralizes stomach acid.

**Indications:** For the relief of heartburn, sour stomach, acid indigestion and upset stomach associated with these conditions.

**Directions:** SHAKE WELL BEFORE USING. Take 1 or 2 tablespoonfuls four times a day or as directed by a physician. GAVISCON Regular Strength Liquid should be taken after meals and at bedtime. Dispense product only by spoon or other measuring device.

**Warnings:** Except under the advice and supervision of a physician, do not take more than 8 tablespoonfuls in a 24-hour period or 8 tablespoonfuls daily for more than 2 weeks. May have laxative effect. Do not use this product if you have a kidney disease. Do not use this product if you are on a sodium-restricted diet except under the advice and supervision of a physician. Each tablespoonful of GAVISCON Regular Strength Liquid contains approximately 1.7 mEq sodium. Keep this and all drugs out of the reach of children. In case of accidental overdose, seek professional assistance or contact a poison control center immediately.

**Drug Interaction Precaution:** Antacids may interact with certain prescription drugs. If you are presently taking a prescription drug, do not take this product without checking with your physician or other health professional.

Keep tightly closed. Avoid freezing. Store at a controlled room temperature.

**How Supplied:** 12 fluid oz (355 ml) bottles.
*Shown in Product Identification Guide, page 507*

---

### GAVISCON® EXTRA STRENGTH Liquid Antacid
[găv 'ĭs-kŏn ]

**Composition:** Each 2 teaspoonfuls (10 mL) contains the following active ingredients:

*Continued on next page*

## Gaviscon E. S. Liquid—Cont.

Aluminum hydroxide .................. 508 mg
Magnesium carbonate ............... 475 mg
and the following inactive ingredients: Benzyl alcohol, edetate disodium, flavor, glycerin, saccharin sodium, simethicone emulsion, sodium alginate, sorbitol solution, water, and xanthan gum.

**Actions:** Gaviscon's unique antacid foam barrier neutralizes stomach acid.

**Indications:** For the relief of heartburn, sour stomach, acid indigestion and upset stomach associated with these conditions.

**Directions:** SHAKE WELL BEFORE USING. Take 2 to 4 teaspoonfuls four times a day or as directed by a physician. GAVISCON Extra Strength Liquid should be taken after meals and at bedtime. Dispense product only by spoon or other measuring device.

**Warnings:** Except under the advice and supervision of a physician, do not take more than 16 teaspoonfuls in a 24-hour period or 16 teaspoonfuls daily for more than 2 weeks. May have laxative effect. Do not use this product if you have a kidney disease. Do not use this product if you are on a sodium-restricted diet except under the advice and supervision of a physician. Each teaspoonful contains approximately 0.9 mEq sodium.

Keep this and all drugs out of the reach of children. In case of accidental overdose, seek professional assistance or contact a poison control center immediately.

**Drug Interaction Precaution:** Antacids may interact with certain prescription drugs. If you are presently taking a prescription drug, do not take this product without checking with your physician or other health professional.

Keep tightly closed. Avoid freezing. Store at a controlled room temperature.

**How Supplied:** 12 fl oz (355 mL) bottles.

*Shown in Product Identification Guide, page 507*

---

## GLY–OXIDE® Liquid

**Description/Active Ingredient:** GLY-OXIDE® Liquid contains carbamide peroxide 10%.

**Actions:** GLY-OXIDE® Liquid has an oxygen-rich formula that works to relieve the pain of canker sores by cleaning and debriding damaged tissue so natural healing can occur. GLY-OXIDE Liquid's dense oxygenating microfoam helps destroy odor-forming germs and flushes out food particles that ordinary brushing can miss.

**Indications For Temporary Use:** Gly-Oxide liquid is for temporary use in cleansing canker sores and minor wound or gum inflammation resulting from mi-

nor dental procedures, dentures, orthodontic appliances, accidental injury, or other irritations of the mouth and gums. Gly-Oxide can also be used to guard against the risk of infections in the mouth and gums.

**Everyday Uses:** Gly-Oxide may be used routinely to improve oral hygiene as an aid to regular brushing or when regular brushing is inadequate or impossible such as total care geriatrics, etc. Gly-Oxide kills germs to reduce mouth odors and/or odors on dental appliances. Gly-Oxide penetrates between teeth and other areas of the mouth to flush out food particles ordinary brushing can miss. This can be especially useful when brushing is made more difficult by the presence of orthodontics or other dental appliances. Plus, Gly-Oxide helps remove stains on dental appliances to improve appearance.

**Directions For Temporary Use:** Do not dilute. Replace tip on bottle when not in use. **Adults and children 2 years of age and older:** Apply several drops directly from bottle onto affected area; spit out after 2 to 3 minutes. Use up to four times daily after meals and at bedtime or as directed by dentist or doctor. OR place 10 drops on tongue, mix with saliva, swish for several minutes, and then spit out. Use by children under 12 years of age should be supervised. **Children under 2 years of age:** Consult a dentist or doctor.

**Directions For Everyday Use:** The product may be used following the temporary use directions above. OR apply Gly-Oxide to the toothbrush (it will sink into the brush), cover with toothpaste, brush normally, and spit out.

**Warnings:** Severe or persistent oral inflammation, denture irritation, or gingivitis may be serious. If sore mouth symptoms do not improve in 7 days, or if irritation, pain, or redness persists or worsens, or if swelling, rash, or fever develops, discontinue use of product and see your dentist or doctor promptly. Avoid contact with eyes. **KEEP THIS AND ALL DRUGS OUT OF THE REACH OF CHILDREN.** In case of accidental overdose, seek professional assistance or contact a poison control center immediately.

**Inactive Ingredients:** Citric Acid, Flavor, Glycerin, Propylene Glycol, Sodium Stannate, Water, and Other Ingredients.

Protect from excessive heat and direct sunlight.

**How Supplied:** GLY-OXIDE® Liquid is available in $1/2$-fl-oz and 2-fl-oz plastic squeeze bottles with applicator spouts.

Comments or Questions? Call Toll-free 1-800-245-1040 Weekdays

SmithKline Beecham Consumer Healthcare, L.P.

Pittsburgh, PA 15230    Made in U.S.A.

*Shown in Product Identification Guide, page 507*

## GOODY'S
### Body Pain Formula Powder

**Indications:** FOR TEMPORARY RELIEF OF MINOR BODY ACHES & PAINS DUE TO MUSCULAR ACHES, ARTHRITIS & HEADACHES.

**Directions:** Adults: Place one powder on tongue and follow with liquid, or stir powder into a glass of water or other liquid. May be repeated in 4 to 6 hours. Do not take more than 4 powders in any 24-hour period. Children under 12 years of age: Consult a doctor.

**Warnings: Children and teenagers should not use this medicine for chicken pox or flu symptoms before a doctor is consulted about Reye's Syndrome, a rare but serious illness reported to be associated with aspirin.** As with any drug, if you are pregnant, or nursing a baby, seek the advice of a health professional before using this product.
**IT IS ESPECIALLY IMPORTANT NOT TO USE ASPIRIN DURING THE LAST 3 MONTHS OF PREGNANCY UNLESS SPECIFICALLY DIRECTED TO DO SO BY A DOCTOR BECAUSE IT MAY CAUSE PROBLEMS IN THE UNBORN CHILD OR COMPLICATIONS DURING DELIVERY.**
**Alcohol Warning:** If you consume 3 or more alcoholic drinks every day, ask your doctor whether you should take acetaminophen and aspirin or other pain relievers/fever reducers. Acetaminophen and aspirin may cause liver damage and stomach bleeding.
**Keep this and all medicines out of the reach of children. In case of accidental overdose, contact a doctor or poison control center immediately.**
This product contains aspirin and should not be taken by individuals who are sensitive to aspirin. If pain persists for more than 10 days, or if redness is present, consult a physician immediately.

**Active ingredients:** Each powder contains: 500 mg. aspirin and 325 mg. acetaminophen.

**Inactive Ingredients:** Each powder contains: Lactose and Potassium Chloride.

---

## GOODY'S®
### Extra Strength Headache Powder

**Indications:** For Temporary Relief of Minor Aches & Pains Due to Headaches, Arthritis, Colds & Fever

**Directions:** Adults: Place one powder on tongue and follow with liquid or stir powder into a glass of water or other liquid. May be repeated in 4 to 6 hours. Do not take more than 4 powders in any 24-hour period. Children under 12 years of age: Consult a doctor.

**Warnings: Children and teenagers should not use this medicine for chicken pox or flu symptoms before**

a doctor is consulted about Reye's Syndrome, a rare but serious illness reported to be associated with aspirin. As with any drug, if you are pregnant, or nursing a baby, seek the advice of a health professional before using this product. **IT IS ESPECIALLY IMPORTANT NOT TO USE ASPIRIN DURING THE LAST 3 MONTHS OF PREGNANCY UNLESS SPECIFICALLY DIRECTED TO DO SO BY A DOCTOR BECAUSE IT MAY CAUSE PROBLEMS IN THE UNBORN CHILD OR COMPLICATIONS DURING DELIVERY.** Alcohol Warning: If you consume 3 or more alcoholic drinks every day, ask your doctor whether you should take acetaminophen and aspirin or other pain relievers/fever reducers. Acetaminophen and aspirin may cause liver damage and stomach bleeding. **Keep this and all medicines out of the reach of children. In case of accidental overdose, contact a doctor or poison control center immediately.** This product contains aspirin and should not be taken by individuals who are sensitive to aspirin. If pain persists for more than 10 days or redness is present, consult a physician immediately.

**Active Ingredients:** Each Powder contains 520 mg. aspirin in combination with 260 mg. acetaminophen and 32.5 mg. caffeine.

**Inactive Ingredients:** Lactose and Potassium Chloride.

---

## GOODY'S®
### Extra Strength Pain Relief Tablets

**Indications:** Goody's EXTRA STRENGTH tablets are a specially developed pain reliever that provide fast & effective temporary relief from minor aches & pain due to headaches, arthritis, colds or "flu," muscle strain, backache & menstrual discomfort. It is recommended for temporary relief of toothaches and to reduce fever.

**Dosage:** Adults: Two tablets with water or other liquid. May be repeated in 4 to 6 hours. Do not take more than 8 tablets in any 24-hour period. Children under 12 years of age: Consult a doctor.

**Warnings: Children and teenagers should not use this medicine for chicken pox or flu symptoms before a doctor is consulted about Reye's Syndrome, a rare but serious illness reported to be associated with aspirin.** As with any drug, if you are pregnant, or nursing a baby, seek the advice of a health professional before using this product. IT IS ESPECIALLY IMPORTANT NOT TO USE ASPIRIN DURING THE LAST 3 MONTHS OF PREGNANCY UNLESS SPECIFICALLY DIRECTED TO DO SO BY A DOCTOR BECAUSE IT MAY CAUSE PROBLEMS IN THE UNBORN CHILD OR COMPLICATIONS DURING DELIVERY. Alcohol

**Warning:** If you consume 3 or more alcoholic drinks every day, ask your doctor whether you should take acetaminophen and aspirin or other pain relievers/fever reducers. Acetaminophen and aspirin may cause liver damage and stomach bleeding. **Keep this and all medicines out of the reach of children. In case of accidental overdose, contact a doctor or poison control center immediately.** This product contains aspirin and should not be taken by individuals who are sensitive to aspirin. If pain persists for more than 10 days, or redness is present, consult a physician immediately.

**Active Ingredients:** Each tablet contains 260 mg. aspirin in combination with 130 mg. acetaminophen and 16.25 mg. caffeine. **Inactive Ingredients:** Corn Starch, Crospovidone, Povidone, Pregelatinized Starch and Stearic Acid.

---

## GOODY'S PM® POWDER
### For Pain with Sleeplessness

**Indications:** For temporary relief of occasional headaches and minor aches and pains with accompanying sleeplessness.

**Directions:** Adults and children 12 years of age and older: One dose (2 powders). Take both powders at bedtime, if needed, or as directed by a doctor. Place powders on tongue and follow with liquid. If you prefer, stir powders into glass of water or other liquid.

**Warnings: KEEP THIS AND ALL MEDICINES OUT OF THE REACH OF CHILDREN. IN CASE OF ACCIDENTAL OVERDOSE, CONTACT A DOCTOR OR POISON CONTROL CENTER IMMEDIATELY. PROMPT MEDICAL ATTENTION IS CRITICAL FOR ADULTS AS WELL AS FOR CHILDREN EVEN IF YOU DO NOT NOTICE ANY SIGNS OR SYMPTOMS.** As with any drug, if you are pregnant or nursing a baby, seek the advice of a health professional before using this product. Do not give this product to children under 12 years of age. Do not use for more than 10 days or for fever for more than 3 days unless directed by a doctor. Consult your doctor if symptoms persist or get worse or new ones occur. If sleeplessness persists continuously for more than 2 weeks consult your doctor. Insomnia may be a symptom of serious underlying medical illness. Do not take this product, unless directed by a doctor, if you have a breathing problem such as emphysema or chronic bronchitis or if you have glaucoma or difficulty in urination due to enlargement of the prostate gland. **Do Not Use** with any other product containing diphenhydramine, including one applied topically. Avoid alcoholic beverages while taking this product. Do not use this product if you are taking sedatives or tranquilizers without first consulting your doctor. **Alcohol**

---

**Warning:** If you consume 3 or more alcoholic drinks every day, ask your doctor whether you should take acetaminophen or other pain relievers/fever reducers. Acetaminophen may cause liver damage.

**Caution:** This product will cause drowsiness. Do not drive a motor vehicle or operate machinery after use.

**Active Ingredients:** Each powder contains 500 mg. Acetaminophen and 38 mg. Diphenhydramine Citrate.

**Inactive Ingredients:** Citric Acid, Docusate Sodium, Fumaric Acid, Glycine, Lactose, Magnesium Stearate, Potassium Chloride, Silica Gel, Sodium Citrate Dihydrate.

---

## MASSENGILL® Douches, Towelettes and Cleansing Wash
[mas 'sen-gil ]

### PRODUCT OVERVIEW

**Key Facts:** Massengill is the brand name for a line of feminine hygiene products which are recommended for routine cleansing and for temporary relief of minor vaginal itching and irritation. Massengill disposable douches are available in two Vinegar & Water formulas (Extra Mild and Extra Cleansing), and other cosmetic solutions (Country Flowers, Fresh Baby Powder Scent, Fresh Mountain Breeze, and Spring Rain Freshness), and a Medicated formula (with povidone-iodine). Massengill also has products specially designed to safely and gently cleanse the external vaginal area: Baby Powder Soft Cloth Towelettes, Medicated Soft Cloth Towelettes and Feminine Cleansing Wash.

**Major Uses:** Massengill's Vinegar & Water, and other cosmetic douches are recommended for routine douching, or for cleansing following menstruation, prescribed use of vaginal medication or use of contraceptive creams or jellies. Massengill Medicated is recommended in a seven day regimen for the symptomatic relief of minor vaginal itching and irritation associated with vaginitis due to Candida albicans, Trichomonas vaginalis, and Gardnerella vaginalis. Massengill Feminine Cleansing Wash is a gentle soapfree way to clean the external vaginal area. Massengill Non-medicated Soft Cloth Towelettes are a convenient and portable way to cleanse the external vaginal area and wash odor away. Massengill Medicated Soft Cloth Towelettes provide temporary relief of minor external itching associated with irritation or skin rashes.

**Safety Information:** Do not douche during pregnancy unless directed by a physician. Douching does not prevent pregnancy. Do not use this product and consult your physician if you are experiencing any of the following symptoms:

*Continued on next page*

## Massengill Products—Cont.

unusual vaginal discharge, vaginal bleeding, painful and/or frequent urination, lower abdominal/pelvis pain, nausea or fever, or you or your sex partner have genital sores or ulcers.

If vaginal dryness or irritation occurs, discontinue use.

Massengill Medicated — Women with iodine-sensitivity should not use this product. If symptoms persist after seven days, or if redness, swelling or pain develop, consult a physician. Do not use while nursing unless directed by a physician.

### PRODUCT INFORMATION
#### MASSENGILL®
[mas 'sen-gil ]
**Disposable Douches**

**Ingredients:** DISPOSABLES: Extra Mild Vinegar and Water—Purified Water, Sodium Citrate, Citric Acid, and Vinegar.

Extra Cleansing Vinegar and Water—Purified Water, Sodium Citrate, Citric Acid, Vinegar, Diazolidinyl Urea, Octoxynol-9, Cetylpyridinium Chloride, Edetate Disodium.

Fresh Baby Powder Scent—Purified Water, Sodium Citrate, Citric Acid, SD Alcohol 40, Diazolidinyl Urea, Octoxynol-9, Fragrance, Cetylpyridinium Chloride, Edetate Disodium, FD&C Blue #1.

Country Flowers—Purified Water, Sodium Citrate, Citric Acid, SD Alcohol 40, Diazolidinyl Urea, Octoxynol-9, Fragrance, Cetylpyridinium Chloride, Edetate Disodium, D&C Red #28, FD&C Blue #1.

Fresh Mountain Breeze—Purified Water, SD Alcohol 40, Diazolidinyl Urea, Citric Acid, Sodium Citrate, Octoxynol-9, Fragrance, Cetylpyridinium Chloride, Edetate Disodium, FD&C Blue #1, D&C Yellow #10.

Spring Rain Freshness—Purified Water, SD Alcohol 40, Diazolidinyl Urea, Citric Acid, Sodium Citrate, Octoxynol-9, Fragrance, Cetylpyridinium Chloride, Edetate Disodium.

**Indications:** Recommended for routine cleansing, at the end of menstruation, after use of contraceptive creams or jellies (check the contraceptive package instructions first) or to rinse out the residue of prescribed vaginal medication (as directed by physician).

**Actions:** The buffered acid solutions of Massengill Douches can be valuable adjuncts to specific vaginal therapy following the prescribed use of vaginal medication or contraceptives and in feminine hygiene.

**Directions:** DISPOSABLES: Twist off flat tab from bottle containing premixed solution, attach nozzle supplied and use. The unit is completely disposable.

**Warning:** Douching does not prevent pregnancy. Do not use during pregnancy except under the advice and supervision of your physician. If vaginal dryness or irritation occurs, discontinue use. Use this product only as directed for routine cleansing. You should douche no more than twice a week except on the advice of your doctor.

**An association has been reported between douching and pelvic inflammatory disease (PID), a serious infection of your reproductive system which can lead to sterility and/or ectopic (tubal) pregnancy. PID requires immediate medical attention.**

**PID's most common symptoms are pain and/or tenderness in the lower part of the abdomen and pelvis. You may also experience a vaginal discharge, vaginal bleeding, nausea or fever. Other sexually transmitted diseases (STDs) have similar symptoms and/or frequent urination, genital sores, or ulcers. Douches should not be used for the self treatment of any STDs or PID. If you suspect you have one of these infections or PID, stop using this product and see your doctor immediately.**

**See the enclosed insert for important health information concerning sexually transmitted diseases and PID.**

**How Supplied:** Disposable—6 oz. plastic bottle.

---

#### MASSENGILL®
[mas 'sen-gil ]
**Baby Powder Scent Soft Cloth Towelette**

**Ingredients:** Purified Water, Lactic Acid, Sodium Lactate, Potassium Sorbate, Octoxynol-9, Disodium EDTA, Cetylpyridinium Chloride, and Fragrance.

**Indications:** For cleansing and refreshing the external vaginal area.

**Actions:** Massengill Baby Powder Scent Soft Cloth Towelette safely cleanse the external vaginal area. The towelette delivery system makes the application soft and gentle.

**Directions:** Remove towelette from foil packet, unfold, and gently wipe from front to back. Throw away towelette after it has been used once. Safe to use daily. For external use only.

**How Supplied:** Sixteen individually wrapped, disposable towelettes per carton.

---

#### MASSENGILL Feminine Cleansing Wash, Floral
[mas 'sen-gil ]

**Ingredients:** Purified Water, sodium laureth sulfate, magnesium laureth sulfate, sodium laureth-8 sulfate, magnesium laureth-8 sulfate, sodium oleth sulfate, magnesium oleth sulfate, lauramidopropyl betaine, myristamine oxide, lactic acid, PEG-120 methyl glucose di-

oleate, fragrance, sodium methylparaben, sodium ethylparaben, sodium propylparaben, methylchloroisothiazolinone, methylisothiazolinone, D&C Red #33.

**Indications:** For cleansing and refreshing of external vaginal area.

**Actions:** Massengill feminine cleansing wash safely and gently cleanses the external vaginal area.

**Directions:** Pour small amount into palm of hand or wash cloth and lather into wet skin. Rinse clean. Safe to use daily. For external use only.

**How Supplied:** 8 fl. oz plastic flip-top bottle.

---

#### MASSENGILL® Medicated
[mas 'sen-gil ]
**Disposable Douche**

**Active Ingredient:** Povidone-iodine: When mixed as directed a 0.30% solution is formed (Cepticin™).

**Indications:** For symptomatic relief of minor vaginal irritation or itching associated with vaginitis due to Candida albicans, Trichomonas vaginalis, and Gardnerella vaginalis.

**Action:** Povidone-iodine is widely recognized as an effective broad spectrum microbicide against both gram negative and gram positive bacteria, fungi, yeasts and protozoa. While remaining active in the presence of blood, serum or bodily secretions, it possesses virtually none of the irritating properties of iodine.

**Warning:** Douching does not prevent pregnancy. Do not use during pregnancy or while nursing except under the advice and supervision of your physician. If vaginal dryness or irritation occurs discontinue use. Use this product only as directed. Do not use this product for routine cleansing.

**An association has been reported between douching and pelvic inflammatory disease (PID), a serious infection of your reproductive system, which can lead to sterility and/or ectopic (tubal) pregnancy. PID requires immediate medical attention.**

**PID's most common symptoms are pain and/or tenderness in the lower part of the abdomen and pelvis. You may also experience a vaginal discharge, vaginal bleeding, nausea or fever. Other sexually transmitted diseases (STDs) have similar symptoms and/or frequent urination, genital sores, or ulcers. Douches should not be used for self-treatment of any STDs or PID. If you suspect you have one of these infections or PID, stop using this product and see your doctor immediately.**

**See the enclosed insert for important health information concerning sexually transmitted diseases and PID.**

**Women with iodine sensitivity should not use this product.**
**Keep out of the reach of children.**
Avoid storing at high temperature (greater than 100°F).
Protect from freezing.

**Dosage and Administration:** Dosage is provided as a single unit concentrate to be added to 6 oz. of sanitized water supplied in a disposable bottle. A specially designed nozzle is provided. After use, the unit is discarded. Use one bottle a day for seven days. Although symptoms may be relieved earlier, for maximum relief, treatment should be continued for the full seven days.

**How Supplied:** 6 oz. bottle of sanitized water with 0.17 oz. vial of povidone-iodine and nozzle.

*Shown in Product Identification Guide, page 507*

---

**MASSENGILL® Medicated**
[*mas 'sen-gil* ]
**Soft Cloth Towelette**

**Active Ingredient:** Hydrocortisone (0.5%).

**Inactive Ingredients:** Diazolidinyl Urea, DMDM Hydantoin, Isopropyl Myristate, Methylparaben, Polysorbate 60, Propylene Glycol, Propylparaben, Purified Water, Sorbitan Stearate, Steareth-2, Steareth-21.
Also available in non-medicated (Baby Powder Scent) to freshen and cleanse the external vaginal area.

**Indications:** For temporary, soothing relief of minor external feminine itching or other itching associated with minor skin irritations, and rashes. Other uses of this product should be only under the advice and supervision of a physician.

**Action:** Massengill Medicated Soft Cloth Towelettes contain hydrocortisone, a proven anti-inflammatory, anti-pruritic ingredient. The towelette delivery system makes the application soothing, soft, and gentle.

**Warnings:** For external use only. Avoid contact with eyes. If condition worsens, or if symptoms persist for more than seven days or symptoms recur within a few days, do not use this or any other hydrocortisone product unless you have consulted a physician. Do not use if you are experiencing a vaginal discharge, see a physician. Do not use this product for the treatment of diaper rash, see a physician.
Keep this and all drugs out of the reach of children. As with any drug, if you are pregnant or nursing a baby, seek the advice of a health professional before using this product. In case of accidental ingestion, seek professional assistance or contact a Poison Control Center immediately.

**Directions:** Adults and Children two years of age and older—apply to the af-

fected area not more than four times daily. Remove towelette from foil packet and gently wipe from front to back. Throw away towelette after it has been used once. Children under 2 years of age: DO NOT USE.

**How Supplied:** Ten individually wrapped, disposable towelettes per carton.

---

| | |
|---|---|
| Adults and children 12 years of age and over | 2 Tablets once or twice daily with water, not to exceed 4 tablets twice a day |
| Children 6 to under 12 years of age | 1 Tablet once or twice daily with water, not to exceed 2 tablets twice a day |
| Children 2 to under 6 years of age | 1/2 Tablet once or twice daily with water, not to exceed 1 tablet twice a day |
| Children under 2 years of age | Consult a doctor |

EDUCATIONAL MATERIAL

**"The facts about Vaginal Infections and STDs"**
A guide for women on vaginal infections and sexually transmitted diseases (STDs).
Free to physicians, pharmacists and patients in limited quantities by writing GlaxoSmithKline Consumer Healthcare, L.P. PO Box 1469, Pittsburgh, PA 15230 or calling 1-800-233-2426.

---

**NATURE'S REMEDY®**
**Nature's Gentle Laxative**

**Description:** Nature's Remedy® is a stimulant laxative with an active ingredient, Sennosides, that gently stimulates the body's natural function.

**Indication:** For relief of occasional constipation. Nature's Remedy tablets generally produce bowel movement in 6 to 12 hours.

**Active Ingredients:**
(in each tablet):                    **Purpose:**
Sennosides, USP,
   8.6 mg ...................... Stimulant laxative

**Inactive Ingredients:** FD&C blue #2 aluminum lake, FD&C yellow #6 aluminum lake, hydroxypropyl cellulose, hydroxypropyl methylcellulose, lactose, microcrystalline cellulose, polyethylene glycol, pregelatinized starch, silicon dioxide stearic acid, titanium dioxide

**Directions:**
[See table above]

**Warnings: Keep out of reach of children.** Do not use laxative products when abdominal pain, nausea, or vomiting are present unless directed by a doctor. If you have noticed a sudden change in bowel habits that persists over a period of 2 weeks, consult a doctor before

using a laxative. Laxative products should not be used for a period longer than 1 week unless directed by a doctor. Rectal bleeding or failure to have a bowel movement after use of a laxative may indicate a serious condition. Discontinue use and consult your doctor. In case of accidental overdose, seek professional assistance or contact a Poison Control Center immediately. As with any drug, if you are pregnant or nursing a baby, seek the advice of a health professional before using this product.

Store at room temperature, avoid excessive heat (greater than 100°F) or high humidity.

**How Supplied:** Beige, film-coated tablets with foil-backed blister packaging in boxes of 15, 30 and 60.

*Shown in Product Identification Guide, page 507*

---

**NICODERM® CQ®**
**Nicotine Transdermal System/Stop Smoking Aid**

**Formerly available only by prescription**
**Available as:**
             **Step 1 - 21 mg/24 hours**
             **Step 2 - 14 mg/24 hours**
             **Step 3 - 7 mg/24 hours**
**If you smoke:**
**More than 10 Cigarettes per Day: Start with Step 1**
**10 Cigarettes a Day or Less: Start with Step 2**
**WHAT IS THE NICODERM CQ PATCH AND HOW IS IT USED?**
NicoDerm CQ is a small, nicotine containing patch. When you put on a NicoDerm CQ patch, nicotine passes through the skin and into your body. NicoDerm CQ is very thin and uses special material to control how fast nicotine passes through the skin. Unlike the sudden jolts of nicotine delivered by cigarettes, the amount of nicotine you receive remains relatively smooth throughout the 24 or 16 hours period you wear the NicoDerm CQ patch. This helps to reduce cravings you may have for nicotine.

**Active Ingredient:** Nicotine

**Purpose:** Stop Smoking Aid

**Use:** reduces withdrawal symptoms, including nicotine craving, associated with quitting smoking

*Continued on next page*

## Nicoderm CQ—Cont.

### Directions:
- **if you are under 18 years of age, ask a doctor before use**
- before using this product, read the enclosed user's guide for complete directions and other information
- stop smoking completely when you begin using the patch
- **if you smoke more than 10 cigarettes per day,** use according to the following 10 week schedule:

| STEP 1 | STEP 2 | STEP 3 |
|---|---|---|
| Use one 21 mg patch/day | Use one 14 mg patch/day | Use one 7 mg patch/day |
| Weeks 1–6 | Weeks 7–8 | Weeks 9–10 |

- if you smoke **10 or less cigarettes per day,** do not use **STEP 1 (21 mg)**. Start with **STEP 2 (14 mg)** for 6 weeks, then **STEP 3 (7 mg)** for two weeks and then stop.
- steps 2 and 3 allow you to gradually reduce your level of nicotine. Completing the full program will increase your chances of quitting successfully.
- apply one new patch every 24 hours on skin that is dry, clean and hairless
- remove backing from patch and immediately press onto skin. Hold for 10 seconds.
- wash hands after applying or removing patch. Throw away the patch in the enclosed disposal tray. See enclosed user's guide for safety and handling.
- you may wear the patch for 16 or 24 hours
- if you crave cigarettes when you wake up, wear the patch for 24 hours
- if you have vivid dreams or other sleep disturbances, you may remove the patch at bedtime and apply a new one in the morning
- the used patch should be removed and a new one applied to a different skin site at the same time each day
- do not wear more than one patch at a time
- do not cut patch in half or into smaller pieces
- do not leave patch on for more than 24 hours because it may irritate your skin and loses strength after 24 hours
- stop using the patch at the end of 10 weeks. If you started with **STEP 2**, stop using the patch at the end of 8 weeks. If you still feel the need to use the patch talk to your doctor.

### Warnings:
**If you are pregnant or breast-feeding, only use this medicine on the advice of your health care provider.** Smoking can seriously harm your child. Try to stop smoking without using any nicotine replacement medicine. This medicine is believed to be safer than smoking. However, the risks to your child from this medicine are not fully known.

**Do Not Use**
- if you continue to smoke, chew tobacco, use snuff, or use a nicotine gum or other nicotine containing products

**Ask a doctor before use if you have**
- heart disease, recent heart attack, or irregular heartbeat. Nicotine can increase your heart rate.

- high blood pressure not controlled with medication. Nicotine can increase your blood pressure.
- an allergy to adhesive tape or skin problems because you are more likely to get rashes

**Ask a doctor or pharmacist before use if you are**
- using a non-nicotine stop smoking drug
- taking a prescription medication for depression or asthma. Your prescription dose may need to be adjusted.

**When using this product**
- do not smoke even when not wearing the patch. The nicotine in your skin will still be entering your blood stream for several hours after you take off the patch.
- if you have vivid dreams or other sleep disturbances remove this patch at bedtime

**Stop use and ask a doctor if**
- skin redness caused by the patch does not go away after four days, or if skin swells, or you get a rash
- irregular heartbeat or palpitations occur
- you get symptoms of nicotine overdose such as nausea, vomiting, dizziness, weakness and rapid heartbeat

**Keep out of reach of children and pets.** Used patches have enough nicotine to poison children and pets. If swallowed, get medical help or contact a Poison Control Center right away. Dispose of the used patches by folding sticky ends together and inserting in disposal tray in this box.

**READ THE LABEL**
Read the carton and the User's Guide before using this product. Keep the carton and User's Guide. They contain important information.

**Inactive Ingredients:** Ethylene vinyl acetate-copolymer, polyisobutylene and high density polyethylene between pigmented and clear polyester backings. Store at 20–25°C (68–77°F)

**TO INCREASE YOUR SUCCESS IN QUITTING:**
1. You must be motivated to quit.
2. Complete the full treatment program, applying a new patch every day.
3. Use with a support program as described in the Users Guide.

### NicoDerm CQ User's Guide
**KEYS TO SUCCESS**
1) You must really want to quit smoking for **NicoDerm® CQ®** to help you.
2) Complete the full program, applying a new patch every day.
3) **NicoDerm CQ** works best when used together with a support program: See page 3 for details.
4) If you have trouble using **NicoDerm CQ**, ask your doctor or pharmacist or call GlaxoSmithKline 1-800-834-5895 weekdays (10:00 am 4:30 pm EST).

**SO, YOU'VE DECIDED TO QUIT.**
Congratulations. Your decision to stop smoking is one of the most important things you can do to improve your health. Quitting smoking is a two-part process that involves:
1) overcoming your physical need for nicotine, and
2) breaking your smoking habit.
NicoDerm CQ helps smokers quit by reducing nicotine withdrawal symptoms.

Many NicoDerm CQ users will be able to stop smoking for a few days but often will start smoking again. Most smokers have to try to quit several times before they completely stop.

Your own chances of quitting smoking depend on how strongly you are addicted to nicotine, how much you want to quit, and how closely you follow a quitting plan like the one that comes with NicoDerm CQ.

**QUITTING SMOKING IS HARD!**
If you find you cannot stop or if you start smoking again after using NicoDerm CQ please talk to a health care professional who can help you find a program that may work better for you. Breaking this addiction doesn't happen overnight.

Because NicoDerm CQ provides some nicotine, the NicoDerm CQ patch will help you stop smoking by reducing nicotine withdrawal symptoms such as nicotine craving, nervousness and irritability.

This User's Guide will give you support as you become a non-smoker. It will answer common questions about NicoDerm CQ and give tips to help you stop smoking, and should be referred to often.

**WHERE TO GET HELP.**
You are more likely to stop smoking by using NicoDerm CQ with a support program that helps you break your smoking habit. There may be support groups in your area for people trying to quit. Call your local chapter of the American Lung Association, American Cancer Society or American Heart Association for further information. Toll free phone numbers are printed on the wallet card on the back cover of this User's Guide.

If you find you cannot stop smoking or if you start smoking again after using NicoDerm CQ, remember breaking this addiction doesn't happen overnight. You may want to talk to a health care professional who can help you improve your chances of quitting the next time you try NicoDerm CQ or another method.

**LET'S GET ORGANIZED.**
Your reason for quitting may be a combination of concerns about health, the effect of smoking on your appearance, and pressure from your family and friends to stop smoking. Or maybe you're concerned about the dangerous effect of second-hand smoke on the people you care about.

All of these are good reasons. You probably have others. Decide your most important reasons, and write them down on the wallet card inside the back cover of this User's Guide. Carry this card with you. In difficult moments, when you want to smoke, the card will remind you why you are quitting.

**WHAT YOU'RE UP AGAINST.**
Smoking is addictive in two ways. Your need for nicotine has become both physical and mental. You must overcome both addictions to stop smoking. So while NicoDerm CQ will lessen your body's craving for nicotine, you've got to want to quit smoking to overcome the mental de-

pendence on cigarettes. Once you've decided that you're going to quit, it's time to get started. But first, there are some important cautions you should consider. **SOME IMPORTANT WARNINGS.**

This product is only for those who want to stop smoking.

**Do not use**

- if you continue to smoke, chew tobacco, use snuff or use a nicotine gum or other nicotine products.

**Ask a doctor before use if you have:**

- heart disease, recent heart attack, or irregular heartbeat, Nicotine can increase your heart rate.
- high blood pressure not controlled with medication. Nicotine can increase your blood pressure.
- an allergy to adhesive tape or have skin problems because you are more likely to get rashes.

**Ask a doctor or pharmacist before use if you are**

- using a non-nicotine stop smoking drug
- taking a prescription medication for asthma or depression. Your prescription dose may need to be adjusted.

**When using this product:**

- do not smoke even when not wearing the patch. The nicotine in your skin will still be entering your bloodstream for several hours after you take off the patch.
- you have vivid dreams or other sleep disturbances remove this patch at bedtime.

**Stop use and ask a doctor if:**

- skin redness caused by the patch does not go away after four days, or if your skin swells or you get a rash.
- irregular heartbeat or palpitations occur
- you get symptoms of nicotine overdose, such as nausea, vomiting, dizziness, weakness and rapid heartbeat.

**If you are pregnant or breast-feeding, only use this medicine on the advice of your health care provider.** Smoking can seriously harm your child. Try to stop smoking without using any nicotine replacement medicine. This medicine is believed to be safer than smoking. However, the risks to your child from this medicine are not fully known.

**Keep out of reach of children and pets.** Used patches have enough nicotine to poison children and pets. If swallowed, get medical help or contact a Poison Control Center right away. Dispose of the used patches by folding sticky ends together and inserting in the disposal tray in this box.

**LET'S GET STARTED.**

**If you are under 18 years of age, ask a doctor before use.**

Becoming a non-smoker starts today. Your first step is to read through this entire User's Guide carefully.

**First, check that you bought the right starting dose.**

If you smoke more than 10 cigarettes a day, begin with Step 1 (21 mg). As the carton indicates, people who smoke 10 or less cigarettes per day should not use Step 1 (21 mg). They should start with Step 2 (14 mg). Throughout this User's

Guide we will give specific instructions for people who smoke 10 or less cigarettes per day.

**Next, set your personalized quitting schedule.**

Take out a calendar that you can use to track your progress. Pick a quit date, and mark this on your calendar using the stickers in the middle of this User's Guide, as described below.

**DIRECTIONS: FOR PEOPLE WHO SMOKE MORE THAN 10 CIGARETTES PER DAY**

**STEP 1. (Weeks 1–6). Your quit date (and the day you'll start using NicoDerm CQ patch).**

Choose your quit date (it should be soon).

This is the day you will quit smoking cigarettes entirely and begin using NicoDerm CQ to reduce your cravings for nicotine. Place the Step 1 sticker on this date. For the first six weeks, you'll use the highest-strength (21 mg) NicoDerm CQ patches. Be sure to follow the directions on page 10.

Completing the full program will increase your chances of quitting successfully. This is done by changing over to the Step 1 (14mg) patch for 2 weeks followed by a final 2 weeks with the Step 3 (7mg) patch. The Step 2 and Step 3 treatment periods allow you to gradually reduce the amount of nicotine you get, rather than stopping suddenly, and will increase your chances of quitting.

**STEP 2. (Weeks 7–8). The day you'll start reducing your use of NicoDerm CQ patch.**

Switching to Step 2 (14mg) patches after 6 weeks begins to gradually reduce your nicotine usage. Place the Step 2 sticker on this date (the first day of week seven). Use the 14mg patches for two weeks.

**STEP 3. (Weeks 9–10). The day you'll further start reducing your use of NicoDerm CQ patch.**

After eight weeks, nicotine intake is further reduced by moving down to Step 3 (7mg) patches. Place the Step 3 sticker on this date (the first day of week nine). Use the 7 mg patches for two weeks.

**THE NICODERM CQ PROGRAM**

| STEP 1 | STEP 2 | STEP 3 |
|---|---|---|
| Use one | Use one | Use one |
| 21 mg | 14 mg | 7 mg |
| patch/day | patch/day | patch/day |
| Weeks 1–6 | Weeks 7–8 | Weeks 9–10 |

**STOP USING NICODERM CQ AT THE END OF WEEK 10.** If you still feel the need to use the patch after Week 10, talk with your doctor or health professional.

**DIRECTIONS: FOR PEOPLE WHO SMOKE 10 OR LESS CIGARETTES PER DAY**

**Do not use Step 1 (21 mg).**

**Begin with STEP 2 – Initial Treatment Period (Weeks 1–6): 14mg patches.**

Choose our quit date (it should be soon). This is the Day you will quit smoking cigarettes entirely and begin using NicoDerm CQ to reduce your cravings for nicotine. Place the Step 2 sticker on this date. For the first six weeks, you'll

use the Step 2 (14mg) NicoDerm CQ patches. Be sure to follow the directions on page 10.

**Continue with STEP 3 – Step Down Treatment Period (Weeks 7–8): 7mg patches.**

Completing the full program will increase your chances of quitting successfully. This is done by changing over to the Step 3 (7mg) patches for 2 weeks. The two week step down treatment period allows you to gradually reduce the amount of nicotine you get, rather than stopping suddenly, and will increase your chances of quitting. Place the Step 3 sticker on the first day of week seven. Use the 7mg patches for two weeks. People who smoke 10 or less cigarettes per day should not use NicoDerm CQ for longer than 8 weeks. If you still feel the need to use NicoDerm CQ after 8 weeks, talk with your doctor.

**PLAN AHEAD.**

Because smoking is an addiction, it is not easy to stop. After you've given up nicotine, you may still have a strong urge to smoke. Plan ahead NOW for these times, so you're not tempted to start smoking again in a moment of weakness. The following tips may help:

- Keep the phone numbers of supportive friends and family members handy.
- Keep a record of your quitting process. Track whether you feel a craving for cigarettes. In the event that you slip, immediately stop smoking and resume your quit attempt with the NicoDerm CQ patch. If you smoke at all, write down what you think caused the slip.
- Put together an Emergency Kit that includes items that will help take your mind off occasional urges to smoke. You might include cinnamon gum or lemon drops to suck on, a relaxing cassette tape, and something for your hands to play with, like a smooth rock, rubber band or small metal balls.
- Set aside some small rewards, like a new magazine or a gift certificate from your favorite store, which you'll "give" yourself after passing difficult hurdles.
- Think now about the times when you most often want a cigarette, and then plan what else you might do instead of smoking. For instance, you might plan to take your coffee break in a new location, or take a walk right after dinner, so you won't be tempted to smoke.

**HOW NICODERM CQ WORKS.**

NicoDerm CQ patches provide nicotine to your system. They work as a temporary aid to help you quit smoking by reducing nicotine withdrawal symptoms, including nicotine craving. NicoDerm CQ provides a lower level of nicotine to your blood than cigarettes, and allows you to gradually do away with your body's need for nicotine.

Because NicoDerm CQ does not contain the tar or carbon monoxide of cigarette smoke, it does not have the same health dangers as tobacco. However, it still delivers nicotine, the addictive part of cigarette smoke. Nicotine can cause side effects such as headache, nausea, upset stomach, and dizziness.

*Continued on next page*

## Nicoderm CQ—Cont.

### HOW TO USE NICODERM CQ PATCHES.

Read all the following instructions, and the instructions on the outer carton, before using NicoDerm CQ. Refer to them often to make sure you're using NicoDerm CQ correctly. Please refer to the CD for additional help.

1) Stop smoking completely before you start using NicoDerm CQ.

2) To reduce nicotine craving and other withdrawal symptoms, use NicoDerm CQ according to the directions on pages 6–8.

3) Insert used NicoDerm CQ patches in the child resistant disposal tray provided in the box – safely away from children and pets.

### When to apply and remove NicoDerm CQ patches.

Each day apply a new patch to a different place on skin that is dry, clean and hairless. **You can wear a NicoDerm CQ patch for either 16 or 24 hours.** If you crave cigarettes when you wake up, wear the patch for 24 hours. If you begin to have vivid dreams or other disruptions of your sleep while wearing the patch 24 hours, try taking the patch off at bedtime (after about 16 hours) and putting on a new one when you get up the next day.

### PLACE THESE STICKERS ON YOUR CALENDAR

| STEP 1 | STEP 2 |
|---|---|
| A new 21 mg patch every day AT THE BEGINNING OF WEEK #1 (QUIT DAY) | A new 14 mg patch every day AT THE BEGINNING OF WEEK #7 |

**For people who smoke 10 or less cigarettes per day:** Do not use STEP 1 (21 mg). Use STEP 2 (14 mg) at the beginning of week #1 and STEP 3 (7 mg) at the beginning of week #7.

### PLACE THESE STICKERS ON YOUR CALENDAR

| STEP 3 | EX-SMOKER |
|---|---|
| A new 7 mg patch every day AT THE BEGINNING OF WEEK #9 | WHEN YOU HAVE COMPLETED YOUR QUITTING PROGRAM |

**Do not smoke even when you are not wearing the patch.**

Remove the used patch and put on a new patch at the same time every day. Applying the patch at about the same time each day (first thing in the morning, for instance) will help you remember when to put on a new patch. Do not leave the same NicoDerm CQ patch on for more than 24 hours because it may irritate your skin and because it loses strength after 24 hours.

Do not use NicoDerm CQ continuously for more than 10 weeks (8 weeks for people who smoke 10 or less cigarettes per day).

### How to apply a NicoDerm CQ patch.

1. Do not remove the NicoDerm CQ patch from its sealed protective pouch until you are ready to use it. NicoDerm CQ patches will lose nicotine to the air if you store them out of the pouch.

2. Choose a non-hairy, clean, dry area of skin. Do not put a NicoDerm CQ patch on skin that is burned, broken out, cut, or irritated in any way. Make sure your skin is free of lotion and soap before applying a patch.

3. A clear, protective liner covers the sticky back side of the NicoDerm CQ patch—the side that will be put on your skin. The liner has a slit down the middle to help you remove it from the patch. With the sticky back side facing you, pull half the liner away from the NicoDerm CQ patch starting at the middle slit, as shown in the illustration above. Hold the NicoDerm CQ patch at one of the outside edges (touch the sticky side as little as possible), and pull off the other half of the protective liner.

Place this liner in the slot in the disposable tray provided in the NicoDerm CQ package where it will be out of reach of children and pets.

4. Immediately apply the sticky side of the NicoDerm CQ patch to your skin. **Press the patch firmly on your skin with the heel of your hand for at least 10 seconds.** Make sure it sticks well to your skin, especially around the edges.

5. Wash your hands when you have finished applying the NicoDerm CQ patch. Nicotine on your hands could get into your eyes and nose, and cause stinging, redness, or more serious problems.

6. After 24 or 16 hours, remove the patch you have been wearing. Fold the used NicoDerm CQ patch in half with the sticky side together. Carefully dispose of the used patch in the slot of the disposal tray provided in the NicoDerm CQ package where it will be out of the reach of children and pets. Even used patches have enough nicotine to poison children and pets. Wash your hands.

7. Chose a different place on your skin to apply the next NicoDerm CQ patch and repeat Steps 1 to 6. Do not apply a new patch to a previously used skin site for at least one week.

### If your NicoDerm CQ patch gets wet during wearing.

Water will not harm the NicoDerm CQ patch you are wearing if applied properly. You can bathe, swim, or shower for short periods while you are wearing the NicoDerm CQ patch.

### If your NicoDerm CQ patch comes off while wearing.

NicoDerm CQ patches generally stick well to most people's skin. However, a patch may occasionally come off. If your NicoDerm CQ patch falls off during the day, put on a new patch, making sure you select a non-hairy, non-irritated area of the skin that is clean and dry.

If the soap you use has lanolin or moisturizers, the patch may not stick well. Using a different soap may help. Body creams, lotions and sunscreens can also cause problems with keeping your patch on. Do not apply creams or lotions to the place on your skin where you will put the patch.

If you have followed the directions and the patch still does not stick to you, try using medical adhesive tape over the patch.

### Disposing of NicoDerm CQ patches.

Fold the used patch in half with the sticky side together.

Carefully dispose of the patch in the disposal slot of the tray provided in the NicoDerm CQ package where it will be out of the reach of children and pets. Small amounts of nicotine, even from a used patch, can poison children and pets. **Keep all nicotine patches away from children and pets.** Wash your hands after disposing of the patch.

### If your skin reacts to the NicoDerm CQ patch.

When you first put on a NicoDerm CQ patch, mild itching, burning, or tingling is normal and should go away within an hour. After you remove a NicoDerm CQ patch, the skin under the patch might be somewhat red. Your skin should not stay red for more than a day after removing the patch. **Stop use and ask a doctor if skin redness caused by the patch does not go away after four days, or if your skin swells, or you get a rash. Do not put on a new patch.**

### Storage Instructions

Keep each NicoDerm CQ patch in its protective pouch, unopened, until you are ready to use it, because the patch will lose nicotine to the air if it's outside the pouch.

Store NicoDerm CQ patches at 20–25 C (68–77 F) because they are sensitive to heat. Remember, the inside of your car can reach temperatures much higher than this. A slight yellowing of the sticky side of the patch is normal. Do not use NicoDerm CQ patches stored in pouches that are open or torn.

### TIPS TO MAKE QUITTING EASIER.

Within the first few weeks of giving up smoking, you may be tempted to smoke for pleasure, particularly after completing a difficult task, or at a party or bar. Hear are some tips to help get you through the important first stages of becoming a nonsmoker:

### On Your Quit Date:

Ask your family, friends and co-workers to support you in your efforts to stop smoking.

- Throw away all your cigarettes, matches, lighters, ashtrays, etc.
- Keep busy on your quit day. Exercise. Go to a movie. Take a walk. Get together with friends.
- Figure out how much money you'll save by not smoking. Most ex-smokers can save more than $1,000 a year on the price of cigarettes alone.
- Write down what you will do with the money you save.
- Know your high risk situations and plan ahead how you will deal with them.
- Visit your dentist and have your teeth cleaned to get rid of the tobacco stains.

### Right after Quitting:

- During the first few days after you've stopped smoking, spend as much time as possible at places where smoking is not allowed.

- Drink large quantities of water and fruit juices.
- Try to avoid alcohol, coffee and other beverages you associate with smoking.
- Remember that temporary urges to smoke will pass, even if you don't smoke a cigarette.
- Keep your hands busy with something like a pencil or a paper clip.
- Find other activities that help you relax without cigarettes. Swim, jog, take a walk, play basketball.

Don't worry too much about gaining weight. Watch what you eat, take time for daily exercise, and change your eating habits if you need to.

- Laughter helps. Watch or read something funny

## WHAT TO EXPECT.

### The First Few Days.

Your body is now coming back into balance. During the first few days after you stop smoking, you might feel edgy and nervous and have trouble concentrating. You might get headaches, feel dizzy and a little out of sorts, feel sweaty or have stomach upsets. You might even have trouble sleeping at first. These are typical nicotine withdrawal symptoms that will go away with time. Your smoker's cough will get worse before it gets better. But don't worry, that's a good sign. Coughing helps clear the tar deposits out of your lungs.

### After A Week Or Two.

By now you should be feeling more confident that you can handle those smoking urges. Many of your nicotine withdrawal symptoms have left by now, and you should be noticing some positive signs: less coughing, better breathing and an improved sense of taste and smell, to name a few.

### After A Month.

You probably have the urge to smoke much less often now. But urges may still occur, and when they do, they are likely to be powerful ones that come out of nowhere. Don't let them catch you off guard. Plan ahead for these difficult times.

Concentrate on the ways non-smokers are more attractive than smokers. Their skin is less likely to wrinkle. Their teeth are whiter, cleaner. Their breath is fresher.

Their hair and clothes smell better. That cough that seems to make even a laugh sound more like a rattle is a thing of the past. Their children and others around them are healthier, too.

### What To Do About Relapse.

What should you do if you slip and start smoking again? The answer is simple. A lapse of one or two or even a few cigarettes should not spoil your efforts! Throw away your cigarettes, forgive yourself and continue with the program. Listen to the CD again and re-read the User's Guide to ensure that you're using NicoDerm CQ correctly and following the other important tips for dealing with the mental and social dependence on nicotine. Your doctor, pharmacist or other health professional can also provide use-

ful counseling on the importance of stopping smoking. You should consider them partners in your quit attempt.

### What To Do About Relapse After a Successful Quit Attempt.

If you have taken up regular smoking again, don't be discouraged. Research shows that the best thing you can do is try again, since several quitting attempts may be needed before you're successful. And your chances of quitting successfully increase with each quit attempt.

The important thing is to learn from your last attempt.

- Admit that you've slipped, but don't treat yourself as a failure.
- Try to identify the "trigger" that caused you to slip, and prepare a better plan for dealing with this problem next time.
- Talk positively to yourself – tell yourself that you have learned something from this experience.
- Make sure you used NicoDerm CQ patches correctly
- Remember that it takes practice to do anything, and quitting smoking is no exception.

### WHEN THE STRUGGLE IS OVER.

Once you've stopped smoking, take a second and pat yourself on the back. Now do it again. You deserve it. Remember now why you decided to stop smoking in the first place. Look at your list of reasons. Read them again. And smile.

Now think about all the money you are saving and what you'll do with it. All the non-smoking places you can go, and what you might do there. All those years you may have added to your life, and what you'll do with them. Remember that temptation may not be gone forever. However, the hard part is behind you so look forward with a positive attitude, and enjoy your new life as a non-smoker.

### QUESTIONS & ANSWERS

### 1. How will I feel when I stop smoking and start using NicoDerm CQ?

You'll need to prepare yourself for some nicotine withdrawal symptoms. These begin almost immediately after you stop smoking, and are usually at their worst during the first three or four days. Understand that any of the following is possible:

- craving for nicotine
- anxiety, irritability, restlessness, mood changes, nervousness
- disruptions of your sleep
- drowsiness
- trouble concentrating
- increased appetite and weight gain headaches, muscular pain, constipation, fatigue.

NicoDerm CQ reduces nicotine withdrawal symptoms such as irritability and nervousness, as well as the craving for nicotine you used to satisfy by having a cigarette.

### 2. Is NicoDerm CQ just substituting one form of nicotine for another?

NicoDerm CQ does contain nicotine. The purpose of NicoDerm CQ is to provide you with enough nicotine to reduce the physical withdrawal symptoms so you can deal with the mental aspects of quitting.

### 3. Can I be hurt by using NicoDerm CQ?

For most adults, the amount of nicotine delivered from the patch is less than from smoking. If you believe you may be sensitive to even this amount of nicotine, you should not use this product without advice from your doctor. There are also some important warnings in this User's Guide (See page 4).

### 4. Will I gain weight?

Many people do tend to gain a few pounds the first 8–10 weeks after they stop smoking. This is a very small price to pay for the enormous gains that you will make in your overall health and attractiveness. If you continue to gain weight after the first two months, try to analyze what you're doing differently. Reduce your fat intake, choose healthy snacks, and increase your physical activity to burn off the extra calories. Drink lots of water. This is good for your body and skin, and also helps to reduce the amount you eat.

### 5. Is NicoDerm CQ more expensive than smoking?

The total cost of NicoDerm CQ program is similar to what a person who smokes one and a half packs of cigarettes a day would spend on cigarettes for the same period of time. Also, use of NicoDerm CQ is only a short-term cost, while the cost of smoking is a long-term cost, including the health problems smoking causes.

### 6. What if I slip up?

Discard your cigarettes, forgive yourself and then get back on track. Don't consider yourself a failure or punish yourself. In fact, people who have already tried to quit are more likely to be successful the next time.

### GOOD LUCK!

### WALLET CARD

My most important reasons to quit smoking are:

### WALLET CARD

Where to call for Help:

| American Lung Association | American Cancer Society | American Heart Association |
|---|---|---|
| 800-586-4872 | 800-227-2345 | 800-242-8721 |

**For people who smoke more than 10 cigarettes per day:**

| STEP 1 | STEP 2 | STEP 3 |
|---|---|---|
| Use one 21 mg patch/day Weeks 1–6 | Use one 14 mg patch/day Weeks 7–8 | Use one 7 mg patch/day Weeks 9–10 |

**People who smoke 10 or less cigarettes per day.** Do not use STEP 1 (21 mg). Use STEP 2 (14 mg) for six weeks and STEP 3 (7 mg) for two weeks and then stop.

Copyright © 1999 GlaxoSmithKline

**For your family's protection, NicoDerm CQ patches are supplied in child resistant pouches. Do not use if individual pouch is open or torn.**

Manufactured by ALZA Corporation, Mountain View, CA 94043 for GlaxoSmithKline Consumer Healthcare, L.P.

*Continued on next page*

## Nicoderm CQ—Cont.

Comments or Questions? Call 1–800–834–5895 Weekdays. (10 a.m.– 4:30 p.m. EST).

- **Not for sale to those under 18 years of age.**
- **Proof of age required.**
- **Not for sale in vending machines or from any source where proof of age cannot be verified.**

**Available as**

NicoDerm CQ Step 1 (21 mg/24 hours)–7 Patches*

NicoDerm CQ Step 1 (21 mg/24 hours)–14 Patches*

NicoDerm 7 mg, 14 patches

NicoDerm CQ Step 2 (14 mg/24 hours)–7 Patches*

NicoDerm CQ Step 2 (14 mg/24 hours)–14 Patches

NicoDerm 14 mg, 14 patches

NicoDerm CQ Step 3 (7 mg/24 hours)–7 Patches**

NicoDerm CQ Step 3 (7 mg/24 hours)–14 Patches

NicoDerm 21 mg, 14 patches

\* User's Guide, CD & Child Resistant Disposal Tray

\*\* User's Guide, & Child Resistant Disposal Tray

*Shown in Product Identification Guide, page 507*

---

## NICODERM® CQ® CLEAR
### Nicotine Transdermal System/Stop Smoking Aid

**Formerly available only by prescription**
**Available as:**

Step 1 - 21 mg/24 hours
Step 2 - 14 mg/24 hours
Step 3 - 7 mg/24 hours

**If you smoke:**
**More than 10 Cigarettes per Day: Start with Step 1**
**10 Cigarettes a Day or Less: Start with Step 2**

### WHAT IS THE NICODERM CQ PATCH AND HOW IS IT USED?

NicoDerm CQ is a small, nicotine containing patch. When you put on a NicoDerm CQ patch, nicotine passes through the skin and into your body. NicoDerm CQ is very thin and uses special material to control how fast nicotine passes through the skin. Unlike the sudden jolts of nicotine delivered by cigarettes, the amount of nicotine you receive remains relatively smooth throughout the 24 or 16 hours period you wear the NicoDerm CQ patch. This helps to reduce cravings you may have for nicotine.

**Active Ingredient:** Nicotine

**Purpose:** Stop Smoking Aid

**Use:** reduces withdrawal symptoms, including nicotine craving, associated with quitting smoking

**Directions:**
- **if you are under 18 years of age, ask a doctor before use**

- before using this product, read the enclosed user's guide for complete directions and other information
- stop smoking completely when you begin using the patch
- **if you smoke more than 10 cigarettes per day,** use according to the following 10 week schedule:

| STEP 1 | STEP 2 | STEP 3 |
|---|---|---|
| Use one 21 mg patch/day | Use one 14 mg patch/day | Use one 7 mg patch/day |
| Weeks 1–6 | Weeks 7–8 | Weeks 9–10 |

- if you smoke **10 or less cigarettes per day,** do not use **STEP 1 (21 mg).** Start with **STEP 2 (14 mg)** for 6 weeks, then **STEP 3 (7 mg)** for two weeks and then stop.
- steps 2 and 3 allow you to gradually reduce your level of nicotine. Completing the full program will increase your chances of quitting successfully.
- apply one new patch every 24 hours on skin that is dry, clean and hairless
- remove backing from patch and immediately press onto skin. Hold for 10 seconds.
- wash hands after applying or removing patch. Throw away the patch in the enclosed disposal tray. See enclosed user's guide for safety and handling.
- you may wear the patch for 16 or 24 hours
- if you crave cigarettes when you wake up, wear the patch for 24 hours
- if you have vivid dreams or other sleep disturbances, you may remove the patch at bedtime and apply a new one in the morning
- the used patch should be removed and a new one applied to a different skin site at the same time each day
- do not wear more than one patch at a time
- do not cut patch in half or into smaller pieces
- do not leave patch on for more than 24 hours because it may irritate your skin and loses strength after 24 hours
- stop using the patch at the end of 10 weeks. If you started with **STEP 2,** stop using the patch at the end of 8 weeks. If you still feel the need to use the patch talk to your doctor.

**Warnings:**
**If you are pregnant or breast-feeding, only use this medicine on the advice of your health care provider.** Smoking can seriously harm your child. Try to stop smoking without using any nicotine replacement medicine. This medicine is believed to be safer than smoking. However, the risks to your child from this medicine are not fully known.

**Do Not Use**
- if you continue to smoke, chew tobacco, use snuff, or use a nicotine gum or other nicotine containing products

**Ask a doctor before use if you have**
- heart disease, recent heart attack, or irregular heartbeat. Nicotine can increase your heart rate.
- high blood pressure not controlled with medication. Nicotine can increase your blood pressure.
- an allergy to adhesive tape or skin problems because you are more likely to get rashes

**Ask a doctor or pharmacist before use if you are**
- using a non-nicotine stop smoking drug
- taking a prescription medication for depression or asthma. Your prescription dose may need to be adjusted.

**When using this product**
- do not smoke even when not wearing the patch. The nicotine in your skin will still be entering your blood stream for several hours after you take off the patch.
- if you have vivid dreams or other sleep disturbances remove this patch at bedtime

**Stop use and ask a doctor if**
- skin redness caused by the patch does not go away after four days, or if skin swells, or you get a rash
- irregular heartbeat or palpitations occur
- you get symptoms of nicotine overdose such as nausea, vomiting, dizziness, weakness and rapid heartbeat

**Keep out of reach of children and pets.** Used patches have enough nicotine to poison children and pets. If swallowed, get medical help or contact a Poison Control Center right away. Dispose of the used patches by folding sticky ends together and inserting in disposal tray in this box.

**READ THE LABEL**
Read the carton and the User's Guide before using this product. Keep the carton and User's Guide. They contain important information.

**Inactive Ingredients:** Ethylene vinyl acetate-copolymer, polyisobutylene and high density polyethylene between clear polyester backings.

Store at 20–25°C (68–77°F)

**TO INCREASE YOUR SUCCESS IN QUITTING:**
1. You must be motivated to quit.
2. Complete the full treatment program, applying a new patch every day.
3. Use with a support program as described in the Users Guide.

**NicoDerm CQ User's Guide**
**KEYS TO SUCCESS**
1) You will most really want to quit smoking for **NicoDerm® CQ®** to help you.
2) Complete the full program, applying a new patch every day.
3) **NicoDerm CQ** works best when used together with a support program: See page 3 for details.
4) If you have trouble using **NicoDerm CQ**, ask your doctor or pharmacist or call GlaxoSmithKline 1-800-834-5895 weekdays (10:00 am 4:30 pm EST).

**SO, YOU'VE DECIDED TO QUIT.**
Congratulations. Your decision to stop smoking is one of the most important things you can do to improve your health. Quitting smoking is a two-part process that involves:
1) overcoming your physical need for nicotine, and
2) breaking your smoking habit.
NicoDerm CQ helps smokers quit by reducing nicotine withdrawal symptoms.
Many NicoDerm CQ users will be able to stop smoking for a few days but often will start smoking again. Most smokers have to try to quit several times before they completely stop.

Your own chances of quitting smoking depend on how strongly you are addicted to nicotine, how much you want to quit, and how closely you follow a quitting plan like the one that comes with NicoDerm CQ.

## QUITTING SMOKING IS HARD!

If you find that you cannot stop or if you start smoking again after using NicoDerm CQ please talk to a health care professional who can help you find a program that may work better for you. Breaking this addiction doesn't happen overnight.

Because NicoDerm CQ provides some nicotine, the NicoDerm CQ patch will help you stop smoking by reducing nicotine withdrawal symptoms such as nicotine craving, nervousness and irritability.

This User's Guide will give you support as you become a non-smoker. It will answer common questions about NicoDerm CQ and give tips to help you stop smoking, and should be referred to often.

## WHERE TO GET HELP.

You are more likely to stop smoking by using NicoDerm CQ with a support program that helps you break your smoking habit. There may be support groups in your area for people trying to quit. Call your local chapter of the American Lung Association, American Cancer Society or American Heart Association for further information. Toll free phone numbers are printed on the wallet card on the back cover of this User's Guide.

If you find you cannot stop smoking or if you start smoking again after using NicoDerm CQ, remember breaking this addiction doesn't happen overnight. You may want to talk to a health care professional who can help you improve your chances of quitting the next time you try NicoDerm CQ or another method.

## LET'S GET ORGANIZED.

Your reason for quitting may be a combination of concerns about health, the effect of smoking on your appearance, and pressure from your family and friends to stop smoking. Or maybe you're concerned about the dangerous effect of second-hand smoke on the people you care about.

All of these are good reasons. You probably have others. Decide your most important reasons, and write them down on the wallet card inside the back cover of this User's Guide. Carry this card with you. In difficult moments, when you want to smoke, the card will remind you why you are quitting.

## WHAT YOU'RE UP AGAINST.

Smoking is addictive in two ways. Your need for nicotine has become both physical and mental. You must overcome both addictions to stop smoking. So while NicoDerm CQ will lessen your body's craving for nicotine, you've got to want to quit smoking to overcome the mental dependence on cigarettes. Once you've decided that you're going to quit, it's time to get started. But first, there are some important cautions you should consider.

## SOME IMPORTANT WARNINGS.

This product is only for those who want to stop smoking.

## Do not use

- if you continue to smoke, chew tobacco, use snuff or use a nicotine gum or other nicotine products.

## Ask a doctor before use if you have:

- heart disease, recent heart attack, or irregular heartbeat. Nicotine can increase your heart rate.
- high blood pressure not controlled with medication. Nicotine can increase your blood pressure.
- an allergy to adhesive tape or have skin problems because you are more likely to get rashes.

## Ask a doctor or pharmacist before use if you are

- using a non-nicotine stop smoking drug
- taking a prescription medication for asthma or depression. Your prescription dose may need to be adjusted.

## When using this product:

- do not smoke even when not wearing the patch. The nicotine in your skin will still be entering your bloodstream for several hours after you take off the patch.
- you have vivid dreams or other sleep disturbances remove this patch at bedtime.

## Stop use and ask a doctor if:

- skin redness caused by the patch does not go away after four days, or if your skin swells or you get a rash.
- irregular heartbeat or palpitations occur
- you get symptoms of nicotine overdose, such as nausea, vomiting, dizziness, weakness and rapid heartbeat.

**If you are pregnant or breast-feeding, only use this medicine on the advice of your health care provider.** Smoking can seriously harm your child. Try to stop smoking without using any nicotine replacement medicine. This medicine is believed to be safer than smoking. However, the risks to your child from this medicine are not fully known.

**Keep out of reach of children and pets.** Used patches have enough nicotine to poison children and pets. If swallowed, get medical help or contact a Poison Control Center right away. Dispose of the used patches by folding sticky ends together and inserting in the disposal tray in this box.

## LET'S GET STARTED.

**If you are under 18 years of age, ask a doctor before use.**

Becoming a non-smoker starts today. Your first step is to read through this entire User's Guide carefully.

**First, check that you bought the right starting dose.**

If you smoke more than 10 cigarettes a day, begin with Step 1 (21 mg). As the carton indicates, people who smoke 10 or less cigarettes per day should not use Step 1 (21 mg). They should start with Step 2 (14 mg). Throughout this User's Guide we will give specific instructions for people who smoke 10 or less cigarettes per day.

**Next, set your personalized quitting schedule.**

Take out a calendar that you can use to track your progress. Pick a quit date, and mark this on your calendar using the stickers in the middle of this User's Guide, as described below.

## DIRECTIONS: FOR PEOPLE WHO SMOKE MORE THAN 10 CIGARETTES PER DAY

**STEP 1. (Weeks 1–6). Your quit date (and the day you'll start using NicoDerm CQ patch).**

Choose your quit date (it should be soon).

This is the day you will quit smoking cigarettes entirely and begin using NicoDerm CQ to reduce your cravings for nicotine. Place the Step 1 sticker on this date. For the first six weeks, you'll use the highest-strength (21 mg) NicoDerm CQ patches. Be sure to follow the directions on page 10.

Completing the full program will increase your chances of quitting successfully. This is done by changing over to the Step 1 (14mg) patch for 2 weeks followed by a final 2 weeks with the Step 3 (7mg) patch. The Step 2 and Step 3 treatment periods allow you to gradually reduce the amount of nicotine you get, rather than stopping suddenly, and will increase your chances of quitting.

**STEP 2. (Weeks 7–8). The day you'll start reducing your use of NicoDerm CQ patch.**

Switching to Step 2 (14mg) patches after 6 weeks begins to gradually reduce your nicotine usage. Place the Step 2 sticker on this date (the first day of week seven). Use the 14mg patches for two weeks.

**STEP 3. (Weeks 9–10). The day you'll further start reducing your use of NicoDerm CQ patch.**

After eight weeks, nicotine intake is further reduced by moving down to Step 3 (7mg) patches. Place the Step 3 sticker on this date (the first day of week nine). Use the 7 mg patches for two weeks.

## THE NICODERM CQ PROGRAM

| STEP 1 | STEP 2 | STEP 3 |
|---|---|---|
| Use one | Use one | Use one |
| 21 mg | 14 mg | 7 mg |
| patch/day | patch/day | patch/day |
| Weeks 1–6 | Weeks 7–8 | Weeks 9–10 |

**STOP USING NICODERM CQ AT THE END OF WEEK 10.** If you still feel the need to use the patch after Week 10, talk with your doctor or health professional.

## DIRECTIONS: FOR PEOPLE WHO SMOKE 10 OR LESS CIGARETTES PER DAY

**Do not use Step 1 (21 mg).**

**Begin with STEP 2 – Initial Treatment Period (Weeks 1–6): 14mg patches.**

Choose our quit date (it should be soon). This is the Day you will quit smoking cigarettes entirely and begin using NicoDerm CQ to reduce your cravings for nicotine. Place the Step 2 sticker on this date. For the first six weeks, you'll use the Step 2 (14mg) NicoDerm CQ patches. Be sure to follow the directions on page 10.

*Continued on next page*

## Nicoderm CQ Clear—Cont.

**Continue with STEP 3 – Step Down Treatment Period (Weeks 7–8): 7mg patches.**

Completing the full program will increase your chances of quitting successfully. This is done by changing over to the Step 3 (7mg) patches for 2 weeks. The two week step down treatment period allows you to gradually reduce the amount of nicotine you get, rather than stopping suddenly, and will increase your chances of quitting. Place the Step 3 sticker on the first day of week seven. Use the 7mg patches for two weeks. People who smoke 10 or less cigarettes per day should not use NicoDerm CQ for longer than 8 weeks. If you still feel the need to use NicoDerm CQ after 8 weeks, talk with your doctor.

**PLAN AHEAD.**

Because smoking is an addiction, it is not easy to stop. After you've given up nicotine, you may still have a strong urge to smoke. Plan ahead NOW for these times, so you're not tempted to start smoking again in a moment of weakness. The following tips may help:

- Keep the phone numbers of supportive friends and family members handy.
- Keep a record of your quitting process. Track whether you feel a craving for cigarettes. In the event that you slip, immediately stop smoking and resume your quit attempt with the NicoDerm CQ patch. If you smoke at all, write down what you think caused the slip.
- Put together an Emergency Kit that includes items that will help take your mind off occasional urges to smoke. You might include cinnamon gum or lemon drops to suck on, a relaxing cassette tape, and something for your hands to play with, like a smooth rock, rubber band or small metal balls.
- Set aside some small rewards, like a new magazine or a gift certificate from your favorite store, which you'll "give" yourself after passing difficult hurdles.
- Think now about the times when you most often want a cigarette, and then plan what else you might do instead of smoking. For instance, you might plan to take your coffee break in a new location, or take a walk right after dinner, so you won't be tempted to smoke.

**HOW NICODERM CQ WORKS.**

NicoDerm CQ patches provide nicotine to your system. They work as a temporary aid to help you quit smoking by reducing nicotine withdrawal symptoms, including nicotine craving. NicoDerm CQ provides a lower level of nicotine to your blood than cigarettes, and allows you to gradually do away with your body's need for nicotine.

Because NicoDerm CQ does not contain the tar or carbon monoxide of cigarette smoke, it does not have the same health dangers as tobacco. However, it still delivers nicotine, the addictive part of cigarette smoke. Nicotine can cause side effects such as headache, nausea, upset stomach, and dizziness.

**HOW TO USE NICODERM CQ PATCHES.**

Read all the following instructions, and the instructions on the outer carton, before using NicoDerm CQ. Refer to them often to make sure you're using NicoDerm CQ correctly. Please refer to the CD for additional help.

1) Stop smoking completely before you start using NicoDerm CQ.

2) To reduce nicotine craving and other withdrawal symptoms, use NicoDerm CQ according to the directions on pages 6–8.

3) Insert used NicoDerm CQ patches in the child resistant disposal tray provided in the box – safely away from children and pets.

**When to apply and remove NicoDerm CQ patches.**

Each day apply a new patch to a different place on skin that is dry, clean and hairless. **You can wear a NicoDerm CQ patch for either 16 or 24 hours.** If you crave cigarettes when you wake up, wear the patch for 24 hours. If you begin to have vivid dreams or other disruptions of your sleep while wearing the patch 24 hours, try taking the patch off at bedtime (after about 16 hours) and putting on a new one when you get up the next day.

**PLACE THESE STICKERS ON YOUR CALENDAR**

| STEP 1 | STEP 2 |
|---|---|
| A new 21 mg patch every day AT THE BEGINNING OF WEEK #1 (QUIT DAY) | A new 14 mg patch every day AT THE BEGINNING OF WEEK #7 |

**For people who smoke 10 or less cigarettes per day:** Do not use STEP 1 (21 mg). Use STEP 2 (14 mg) at the beginning of week #1 and STEP 3 (7 mg) at the beginning of week #7.

**PLACE THESE STICKERS ON YOUR CALENDAR**

| STEP 3 | EX-SMOKER |
|---|---|
| A new 7 mg patch every day AT THE BEGINNING OF WEEK #9 | WHEN YOU HAVE COMPLETED YOUR QUITTING PROGRAM |

**Do not smoke even when you are not wearing the patch.**

Remove the used patch and put on a new patch at the same time every day. Applying the patch at about the same time each day (first thing in the morning, for instance) will help you remember when to put on a new patch. Do not leave the same NicoDerm CQ patch on for more than 24 hours because it may irritate your skin and because it loses strength after 24 hours.

Do not use NicoDerm CQ continuously for more than 10 weeks (8 weeks for people who smoke 10 or less cigarettes per day).

**How to apply a NicoDerm CQ patch.**

1. Do not remove the NicoDerm CQ patch from its sealed protective pouch until you are ready to use it. NicoDerm CQ patches will lose nicotine to the air if you store them out of the pouch.

2. Choose a non-hairy, clean, dry area of skin. Do not put a NicoDerm CQ patch on skin that is burned, broken out, cut, or irritated in any way. Make sure your skin is free of lotion and soap before applying a patch.

3. A clear, protective liner covers the sticky back side of the NicoDerm CQ patch—the side that will be put on your skin. The liner has a slit down the middle to help you remove it from the patch. With the sticky back side facing you, pull half the liner away from the NicoDerm CQ patch starting at the middle slit, as shown in the illustration above. Hold the NicoDerm CQ patch at one of the outside edges (touch the sticky side as little as possible), and pull off the other half of the protective liner.

Place this liner in the slot in the disposable tray provided in the NicoDerm CQ package where it will be out of reach of children and pets.

4. Immediately apply the sticky side of the NicoDerm CQ patch to your skin. **Press the patch firmly on your skin with the heel of your hand for at least 10 seconds.** Make sure it sticks well to your skin, especially around the edges.

5. Wash your hands when you have finished applying the NicoDerm CQ patch. Nicotine on your hands could get into your eyes and nose, and cause stinging, redness, or more serious problems.

6. After 24 or 16 hours, remove the patch you have been wearing. Fold the used NicoDerm CQ patch in half with the sticky side together. Carefully dispose of the used patch in the slot of the disposal tray provided in the NicoDerm CQ package where it will be out of the reach of children and pets. Even used patches have enough nicotine to poison children and pets. Wash your hands.

7. Chose a different place on your skin to apply the next NicoDerm CQ patch and repeat Steps 1 to 6. Do not apply a new patch to a previously used skin site for at least one week.

**If your NicoDerm CQ patch gets wet during wearing.**

Water will not harm the NicoDerm CQ patch you are wearing if applied properly. You can bathe, swim, or shower for short periods while you are wearing the NicoDerm CQ patch.

**If your NicoDerm CQ patch comes off while wearing.**

NicoDerm CQ patches generally stick well to most people's skin. However, a patch may occasionally come off. If your NicoDerm CQ patch falls off during the day, put on a new patch, making sure you select a non-hairy, non-irritated area of the skin that is clean and dry.

If the soap you use has lanolin or moisturizers, the patch may not stick well. Using a different soap may help. Body creams, lotions and sunscreens can also cause problems with keeping your patch on. Do not apply creams or lotions to the place on your skin where you will put the patch.

If you have followed the directions and the patch still does not stick to you, try using medical adhesive tape over the patch.

**Disposing of NicoDerm CQ patches.**

Fold the used patch in half with the sticky side together.

Carefully dispose of the patch in the disposal slot of the tray provided in the NicoDerm CQ package where it will be out of the reach of children and pets. Small amounts of nicotine, even from a used patch, can poison children and pets. **Keep all nicotine patches away from children and pets.** Wash your hands after disposing of the patch.

**If your skin reacts to the NicoDerm CQ patch.**

When you first put on a NicoDerm CQ patch, mild itching, burning, or tingling is normal and should go away within an hour. After you remove a NicoDerm CQ patch, the skin under the patch might be somewhat red. Your skin should not stay red for more than a day after removing the patch. **Stop use and ask a doctor if skin redness caused by the patch does not go away after four days, or if your skin swells, or you get a rash. Do not put on a new patch.**

**Storage Instructions**

Keep each NicoDerm CQ patch in its protective pouch, unopened, until you are ready to use it, because the patch will lose nicotine to the air if it's outside the pouch.

Store NicoDerm CQ patches at 20–25 C (68–77 F) because they are sensitive to heat. Remember, the inside of your car can reach temperatures much higher than this. A slight yellowing of the sticky side of the patch is normal. Do not use NicoDerm CQ patches stored in pouches that are open or torn.

**TIPS TO MAKE QUITTING EASIER.**

Within the first few weeks of giving up smoking, you may be tempted to smoke for pleasure, particularly after completing a difficult task, or at a party or bar. Hear are some tips to help get you through the important first stages of becoming a nonsmoker:

**On Your Quit Date:**

Ask your family, friends and co-workers to support you in your efforts to stop smoking.
- Throw away all your cigarettes, matches, lighters, ashtrays, etc.
- Keep busy on your quit day. Exercise. Go to a movie. Take a walk. Get together with friends.
- Figure out how much money you'll save by not smoking. Most ex-smokers can save more than $1,000 a year on the price of cigarettes alone.
- Write down what you will do with the money you save.
- Know your high risk situations and plan ahead how you will deal with them.
- Visit your dentist and have your teeth cleaned to get rid of the tobacco stains.

**Right after Quitting:**
- During the first few days after you've stopped smoking, spend as much time as possible at places where smoking is not allowed.
- Drink large quantities of water and fruit juices.
- Try to avoid alcohol, coffee and other beverages you associate with smoking.
- Remember that temporary urges to smoke will pass, even if you don't smoke a cigarette.

- Keep your hands busy with something like a pencil or a paper clip.
- Find other activities that help you relax without cigarettes. Swim, jog, take a walk, play basketball.

Don't worry too much about gaining weight. Watch what you eat, take time for daily exercise, and change your eating habits if you need to.
- Laughter helps. Watch or read something funny

**WHAT TO EXPECT.**

**The First Few Days.**

Your body is now coming back into balance. During the first few days after you stop smoking, you might feel edgy and nervous and have trouble concentrating. You might get headaches, feel dizzy and a little out of sorts, feel sweaty or have stomach upsets. You might even have trouble sleeping at first. These are typical nicotine withdrawal symptoms that will go away with time. Your smoker's cough will get worse before it gets better. But don't worry, that's a good sign. Coughing helps clear the tar deposits out of your lungs.

**After A Week Or Two.**

By now you should be feeling more confident that you can handle those smoking urges. Many of your nicotine withdrawal symptoms have left by now, and you should be noticing some positive signs: less coughing, better breathing and an improved sense of taste and smell, to name a few.

**After A Month.**

You probably have the urge to smoke much less often now. But urges may still occur, and when they do, they are likely to be powerful ones that come out of nowhere. Don't let them catch you off guard. Plan ahead for these difficult times.

Concentrate on the ways non-smokers are more attractive than smokers. Their skin is less likely to wrinkle. Their teeth are whiter, cleaner. Their breath is fresher.

Their hair and clothes smell better. That cough that seems to make even a laugh sound more like a rattle is a thing of the past. Their children and others around them are healthier, too.

**What To Do About Relapse.**

What should you do if you slip and start smoking again? The answer is simple. A lapse of one or two or even a few cigarettes should not spoil your efforts! Throw away your cigarettes, forgive yourself and continue with the program. Listen to the CD again and re-read the User's Guide to ensure that you're using NicoDerm CQ correctly and following the other important tips for dealing with the mental and social dependence on nicotine. Your doctor, pharmacist or other health professional can also provide useful counseling on the importance of stopping smoking. You should consider them partners in your quit attempt.

**What To Do About Relapse After a Successful Quit Attempt.**

If you have taken up regular smoking again, don't be discouraged. Research

shows that the best thing you can do is try again, since several quitting attempts may be needed before you're successful. And your chances of quitting successfully increase with each quit attempt.

The important thing is to learn from your last attempt.
- Admit that you've slipped, but don't treat yourself as a failure.
- Try to identify the "trigger" that caused you to slip, and prepare a better plan for dealing with this problem next time.
- Talk positively to yourself – tell yourself that you have learned something from this experience.
- Make sure you used NicoDerm CQ patches correctly
- Remember that it takes practice to do anything, and quitting smoking is no exception.

**WHEN THE STRUGGLE IS OVER.**

Once you've stopped smoking, take a second and pat yourself on your back. Now do it again. You deserve it. Remember now why you decided to stop smoking in the first place. Look at your list of reasons. Read them again. And smile.

Now think about all the money you are saving and what you'll do with it. All the non-smoking places you can go, and what you might do there. All those years you may have added to your life, and what you'll do with them. Remember that temptation may not be gone forever. However, the hard part is behind you so look forward with a positive attitude, and enjoy your new life as a non-smoker.

**QUESTIONS & ANSWERS**

**1. How will I feel when I stop smoking and start using NicoDerm CQ?**
You'll need to prepare yourself for some nicotine withdrawal symptoms. These begin almost immediately after you stop smoking, and are usually at their worst during the first three or four days. Understand that any of the following is possible:
- craving for nicotine
- anxiety, irritability, restlessness, mood changes, nervousness
- disruptions of your sleep
- drowsiness
- trouble concentrating
- increased appetite and weight gain headaches, muscular pain, constipation, fatigue.

NicoDerm CQ reduces nicotine withdrawal symptoms such as irritability and nervousness, as well as the craving for nicotine you used to satisfy by having a cigarette.

**2. Is NicoDerm CQ just substituting one form of nicotine for another?**
NicoDerm CQ does contain nicotine. The purpose of NicoDerm CQ is to provide you with enough nicotine to reduce the physical withdrawal symptoms so you can deal with the mental aspects of quitting.

**3. Can I be hurt by using NicoDerm CQ?**
For most adults, the amount of nicotine delivered from the patch is less than from smoking. If you believe you may be sensitive to even this amount of nicotine,

*Continued on next page*

## Nicoderm CQ Clear—Cont.

you should not use this product without advice from your doctor. There are also some important warnings in this User's Guide (See page 4).

### 4. Will I gain weight?
Many people do tend to gain a few pounds the first 8–10 weeks after they stop smoking. This is a very small price to pay for the enormous gains that you will make in your overall health and attractiveness. If you continue to gain weight after the first two months, try to analyze what you're doing differently. Reduce your fat intake, choose healthy snacks, and increase your physical activity to burn off the extra calories. Drink lots of water. This is good for your body and skin, and also helps to reduce the amount you eat.

### 5. Is NicoDerm CQ more expensive than smoking?
The total cost of NicoDerm CQ program is similar to what a person who smokes one and a half packs of cigarettes a day would spend on cigarettes for the same period of time. Also, use of NicoDerm CQ is only a short-term cost, while the cost of smoking is a long-term cost, including the health problems smoking causes.

### 6. What if I slip up?
Discard your cigarettes, forgive yourself and then get back on track. Don't consider yourself a failure or punish yourself. In fact, people who have already tried to quit are more likely to be successful the next time.

### GOOD LUCK!
### WALLET CARD
My most important reasons to quit smoking are:
### WALLET CARD
Where to call for Help:

| American Lung Association 800-586-4872 | American Cancer Society 800-227-2345 | American Heart Association 800-242-8721 |

**For people who smoke more than 10 cigarettes per day:**

| STEP 1 | STEP 2 | STEP 3 |
| Use one 21 mg patch/day Weeks 1–6 | Use one 14 mg patch/day Weeks 7–8 | Use one 7 mg patch/day Weeks 9–10 |

**People who smoke 10 or less cigarettes per day.** Do not use STEP 1 (21 mg). Use STEP 2 (14 mg) for six weeks and STEP 3 (7 mg) for two weeks and then stop.
Copyright © 1999 GlaxoSmithKline
**For your family's protection, NicoDerm CQ patches are supplied in child resistant pouches. Do not use if individual pouch is open or torn.**
Manufactured by ALZA Corporation, Mountain View, CA 94043 for GlaxoSmithKline Consumer Healthcare, L.P. Comments or Questions? Call 1–800–834–5895 Weekdays. (10 a.m.–4:30 p.m. EST).

- **Not for sale to those under 18 years of age.**
- **Proof of age required.**
- **Not for sale in vending machines or from any source where proof of age cannot be verified.**

### Available as
NicoDerm CQ Step 1 (21 mg/24 hours)–7 Patches*
NicoDerm CQ Step 1 (21 mg/24 hours)–14 Patches*
NicoDerm 7 mg, 14 patches
NicoDerm CQ Step 2 (14 mg/24 hours)–7 Patches*
NicoDerm CQ Step 2 (14 mg/24 hours)–14 Patches
NicoDerm 14 mg, 14 patches
NicoDerm CQ Step 3 (7 mg/24 hours)–7 Patches**
NicoDerm CQ Step 3 (7 mg/24 hours)–14 Patches
NicoDerm 21 mg, 14 patches
\*   User's Guide, CD & Child Resistant Disposal Tray
\*\* User's Guide, & Child Resistant Disposal Tray

---

## NICORETTE®
**Nicotine Polacrilex Gum/Stop Smoking Aid**
**Available in Original 2mg and 4mg Strengths,**
**Mint 2mg and 4mg Strengths and Orange 2mg and 4mg Strengths**

**If you smoke:**
**LESS THAN 25 CIGARETTES A DAY: Use 2 mg**
**25 OR MORE CIGARETTES A DAY: Use 4 mg**

**Action:  Stop Smoking Aid**

**Drug Facts:**

**Active Ingredient:                Purpose:**
**(In each chewing piece)**
Nicotine polacrilex,
    2 or 4 mg .................. Stop smoking aid

**Use:**
- reduces withdrawal symptoms, including nicotine craving, associated with quitting smoking

**Warnings:**
- **If you are pregnant or breast-feeding, only use this medicine on the advice of your health care provider.** Smoking can seriously harm your child. Try to stop smoking without using any nicotine replacement medicine. This medicine is believed to be safer than smoking. However, the risks to your child from this medicine are not fully known.

**Do not use:**
- if you continue to smoke, chew tobacco, use snuff, or use a nicotine patch or other nicotine containing products

**Ask a doctor before use if you have:**
- heart disease, recent heart attack, or irregular heartbeat. Nicotine can increase your heart rate.
- high blood pressure not controlled with medication. Nicotine can increase blood pressure.
- stomach ulcer or diabetes

**Ask a doctor or pharmacist before use if you are:**
- using a non-nicotine stop smoking drug
- taking prescription medicine for depression or asthma. Your prescription dose may need to be adjusted.

**Stop use and ask a doctor if:**
- mouth, teeth or jaw problems occur
- irregular heartbeat or palpitations occur
- you get symptoms of nicotine overdose such as nausea, vomiting, dizziness, diarrhea, weakness and rapid heartbeat

**Keep out of reach of children and pets.** Pieces of nicotine gum may have enough nicotine to make children and pets sick. Wrap used pieces of gum in paper and throw away in the trash. In case of overdose, get medical help or contact a Poison Control Center right away.

**Directions:**
- **if you are under 18 years of age, ask a doctor before use**
- before using this product, read the enclosed User's Guide for complete directions and other important information
- stop smoking completely when you begin using the gum
- **if you smoke 25 or more cigarettes a day;** use 4 mg nicotine gum
- **if you smoke less than 25 cigarettes a day;** use according to the following 12 week schedule
[See table below]
- nicotine gum is a medicine and must be used a certain way to get the best results
- chew the gum slowly until it tingles. Then park it between your cheek and gum. When the tingle is gone, begin chewing again, until the tingle returns.
- repeat this process until most of the tingle is gone (about 30 minutes)
- do not eat or drink for 15 minutes before chewing the nicotine gum, or while chewing a piece
- to improve your chances of quitting, use at least 9 pieces per day for the first 6 weeks
- if you experience strong or frequent cravings, you may use a second piece within the hour. However, do not continuously use one piece after another since this may cause you hiccups, heartburn, nausea or other side effects.
- do not use more than 24 pieces a day
- stop using the nicotine gum at the end

| Weeks 1 to 6 | Weeks 7 to 9 | Weeks 10 to 12 |
| --- | --- | --- |
| 1 piece every 1 to 2 hours | 1 piece every 2 to 4 hours | 1 piece every 4 to 8 hours |

of 12 weeks. If you still feel the need to use nicotine gum, talk to your doctor.

To remove the gum, tear off single unit.

Peel off backing starting at corner with loose edge.

Push gum through foil.

## TO INCREASE YOUR SUCCESS IN QUITTING:

1. You must be motivated to quit.
2. **Use Enough**—Chew **at least 9 pieces** of Nicorette per day during the first six weeks.
3. **Use Long Enough**—Use Nicorette for the full 12 weeks.
4. **Use with a support program** as described in the enclosed User's Guide.

*GlaxoSmithKline Consumer Healthcare, L.P. makes an annual grant to the American Cancer Society for cancer research and education for the use of their seal.

## READ THE LABEL

**Read the carton and the User's Guide before taking this product. Do not discard carton or User's Guide. They contain important information.**

**Other Information:**
- store at 20–25°C (68–77°F)
- protect from light

**Inactive Ingredients:**
**Original [2 mg] Inactive Ingredients:** Flavors, glycerin, gum base, sodium carbonate, sorbitol, sodium bicarbonate.
**Original [4 mg] Inactive Ingredients:** Flavors, glycerin, gum base, sodium carbonate, sorbitol, D&C Yellow 10.
**Mint 2 mg Inactive Ingredients:** Gum base, magnesium oxide, menthol, peppermint oil, sodium bicarbonate, sodium carbonate, xylitol.

**Mint 4 mg Inactive Ingredients:** Gum base, magnesium oxide, menthol, peppermint oil, sodium carbonate, xylitol, D&C yellow #10 Al. lake.
Do not store above 86°F (30°C). Protect from light.
**Orange [2 mg] Inactive Ingredients:** Flavor, gum base, magnesium oxide, sodium bicarbonate, sodium carbonate, xylitol
**Orange [4 mg] Inactive Ingredients:** Flavor, gum base, magnesium oxide, sodium carbonate, xylitol, D&C Yellow #10 Al. lake.

**How Supplied:** Nicorette Original, Mint, and Orange are available in:
  2 mg or 4 mg Starter kit*—108 pieces
  2 mg or 4 mg Refill—48 pieces
Nicorette Original & Mint are also available in 168 & 192 count refills
*User's Guide and Audio Tape included in kit
Blister packaged for your protection. **Do not use if individual seals are open or torn.**
**Questions or comments?** call **1-800-419-4766** weekdays (10:00 a.m.– 4:30 p.m. EST)

---

- not for sale to those under 18 years of age
- proof of age required
- not for sale in vending machines or from any source where proof of age cannot be verified

Manufactured by Pharmacia AB, Stockholm, Sweden for
**GlaxoSmithKline** Consumer Healthcare, L.P.
Pittsburgh, PA 15230
©2001 GlaxoSmithKline

---

## USER'S GUIDE:
## HOW TO USE NICORETTE TO HELP YOU QUIT SMOKING
### KEYS TO SUCCESS:

1) You must really want to quit smoking for Nicorette to help you.
2) You can greatly increase your chances for success by using at least 9 to 12 pieces every day when you start using Nicorette.
3) You should continue to use Nicorette as explained in the User's Guide for 12 full weeks.
4) Nicorette works best when used together with a support program.
5) If you have trouble using Nicorette, ask your doctor or pharmacist or call GlaxoSmithKline at 1-800-419-4766 weekdays (10:00am–4:30pm EST).

### SO YOU DECIDED TO QUIT

Congratulations. Your decision to stop smoking is an important one. That's why you've made the right choice in choosing Nicorette gum. Your own chances of quitting smoking depend on how much you want to quit, how strongly you are addicted to tobacco, and how closely you follow a quitting program like the one that comes with Nicorette.

### QUITTING SMOKING IS HARD!

If you've tried to quit before and haven't succeeded, don't be discouraged! Quitting isn't easy. It takes time, and most people try a few times before they are successful. The important thing is to try again until you succeed. This User's Guide will give you support as you become a non-smoker. It will answer common questions about Nicorette and give tips to help you stop smoking, and should be referred to often.

### WHERE TO GET HELP

You are more likely to stop smoking by using Nicorette with a support program that helps you break your smoking habit. There may be support groups in your area for people trying to quit. Call your local chapter of the American Lung Association (1-800-586-4872), American Cancer Society (1-800-227-2345) or American Heart Association (1-800-242-8721) for further information. If you find you cannot stop smoking or if you start smoking again after using Nicorette, remember breaking this addiction doesn't happen overnight. You may want to talk to a health care professional who can help you improve your chances of quitting the next time you try Nicorette or another method.

### LET'S GET ORGANIZED

Your reason for quitting may be a combination of concerns about health, the effect of smoking on your appearance, and pressure from your family and friends to stop smoking. Or maybe you're concerned about the dangerous effect of second-hand smoke on the people you care about. All of these are good reasons. You probably have others. Decide your most important reasons, and write them down on the wallet card inside the back cover of the User's Guide. Carry this card with you. In difficult moments, when you want to smoke, the card will remind you why you are quitting.

### WHAT YOU'RE UP AGAINST

Smoking is addictive in two ways. Your need for nicotine has become both physical and mental. You must overcome both addictions to stop smoking. So while Nicorette will lessen your body's physical addiction to nicotine, you've got to want to quit smoking to overcome the mental dependence on cigarettes. Once you've decided that you're going to quit, it's time to get started. But first, there are some important cautions you should consider.
**SOME IMPORTANT WARNINGS.** This product is only for those who want to stop smoking.
**If you are pregnant or breast-feeding, only use this medicine on the advice of your health care provider.** Smoking can seriously harm your child. Try to stop smoking without using any nicotine replacement medicine. This medicine is believed to be safer than smoking. However, the risks to your child from this medicine are not fully known.

### Do not use
- if you continue to smoke, chew tobacco, use snuff, or use a nicotine patch or other nicotine containing products.

### Ask a doctor before use if you have
- heart disease, recent heart attack, or irregular heartbeat. Nicotine can increase your heart rate.
- high blood pressure not controlled with medication. Nicotine can increase your blood pressure.

*Continued on next page*

**Nicorette—Cont.**

• stomach ulcer or diabetes
**Ask a doctor or pharmacist before use if you are**
• using a non-nicotine stop smoking drug
• taking a prescription medicine for depression or asthma. Your prescription dose may need to be adjusted.
**Stop use and ask a doctor if**
• mouth, teeth or jaw problems occur
• irregular heartbeat or palpitations occur
• you get symptoms of nicotine overdose such as nausea, vomiting, dizziness, diarrhea, weakness and rapid heartbeat
**Keep out of reach of children and pets.** Pieces of nicotine gum may have enough nicotine to make children and pets sick. Wrap used pieces of gum in paper and throw away in the trash. In case of overdose, get medical help or contact a Poison Control Center right away.

**LET'S GET STARTED**
Becoming a non-smoker starts today. First, check that you bought the right starting dose next, read through the entire User's Guide carefully. **Then, set your personalized quitting schedule.** Take out a calendar that you can use to track your progress, and identify four dates, using the stickers in the User's Guide.
**STEP 1: (Weeks 1–6) Your quit date (and the day you'll start using Nicorette gum).** Choose your quit date (it should be soon). This is the day you will quit smoking cigarettes entirely and begin using Nicorette to satisfy your craving for nicotine. For the first six weeks, you'll use a piece of Nicorette every hour or two. Be sure to follow the directions on pages 8 and 11 of the User's Guide. Place the Step 1 sticker on this date.
**STEP 2: (Weeks 7–9) The day you'll start reducing your use of Nicorette.** After six weeks, you'll begin gradually reducing your Nicorette usage to one piece every two to four hours. Place the Step 2 sticker on this date (the first day of week seven).
**STEP 3: (Weeks 10–12) The day you'll further reduce your use of Nicorette.** Nine weeks after you begin using Nicorette, you will further reduce your nicotine intake by using one piece every four to eight hours. Place the Step 3 sticker on this date (the first day of week ten). For the next three weeks, you'll use a piece of Nicorette every four to eight hours. **End of treatment: The day you'll complete Nicorette therapy.**
**Nicorette** should not be used for longer than twelve weeks. Identify the date thirteen weeks after the date you chose in Step 1 and place the "EX-Smoker" sticker on your calendar.
**PLAN AHEAD**
Because smoking is an addiction, it is not easy to stop. After you've given up cigarettes, you will still have a strong urge to smoke. Plan ahead NOW for these times, so you're not defeated in a moment of weakness. The following tips may help:
• Keep the phone numbers of supportive friends and family members handy.

• Keep a record of your quitting process. Track the number of Nicorette pieces you use each day, and whether you feel a craving for cigarettes. If you smoke at all, write down what you think caused the slip.
• Put together an Emergency Kit that includes items that will help take your mind off occasional urges to smoke. Include cinnamon gum or lemon drops to suck on, a relaxing cassette tape and something for your hands to play with, like a smooth rock, rubber band or small metal balls.
• Set aside some small rewards, like a new magazine or a gift certificate from your favorite store, which you'll 'give' yourself after passing difficult hurdles.
• Think now about the times when you most often want a cigarette, and then plan what else you might do instead of smoking. For instance, you might plan to take your coffee break in a new location, or take a walk right after dinner, so you won't be tempted to smoke.

**HOW NICORETTE GUM WORKS**
Nicorette's sugar-free chewing pieces provide nicotine to your system—they work as a temporary aid to help you quit smoking by reducing nicotine withdrawal symptoms. Nicorette provides a lower level of nicotine to your blood than cigarettes, and allows you to gradually do away with your body's need for nicotine. Because Nicorette does not contain the tar or carbon monoxide of cigarette smoke, it does not have the same health dangers as tobacco. However, it still delivers nicotine, the addictive part of cigarette smoke. Nicotine can cause side effects such as headache, nausea, upset stomach and dizziness.

**HOW TO USE NICORETTE GUM**
**If you are under 18 years of age, ask a doctor before use.**
Before you can use Nicorette correctly, you have to practice! That sounds silly, but it isn't.
**Nicorette isn't like ordinary chewing gum.** It's a medicine, and must be chewed a certain way to work right. Chewed like ordinary gum, Nicorette won't work well and can cause side effects. An overdose can occur if you chew more than one piece of Nicorette at the same time, or if you chew many pieces one after another. Read all the following instructions before using Nicorette. Refer to them often to make sure you're using Nicorette gum correctly. If you chew too fast, or do not chew correctly, you may get hiccups, heartburn, or other stomach problems.
1. Stop smoking completely before you start using Nicorette.
2. To reduce craving and other withdrawal symptoms, use Nicorette according to the dosage schedule on page 11 of the User's Guide.

The following chart lists the recommended usage schedule for Nicorette:

| Weeks 1 through 6 | Weeks 7 through 9 | Weeks 10 through 12 |
|---|---|---|
| 1 piece every 1 to 2 hours | 1 piece every 2 to 4 hours | 1 piece every 4 to 8 hours |

**DO NOT USE MORE THAN 24 PIECES PER DAY.**

3. Chew each Nicorette piece <u>very slowly several times.</u>
4. Stop chewing when you notice a peppery taste, or a slight tingling in your mouth. (This usually happens after about 15 chews, but may vary from person to person.)
5. "PARK" the Nicorette piece between your cheek and gum and leave it there.
6. When the peppery taste or tingle is almost gone (in about a minute), start to chew a few times slowly again. When the taste or tingle returns, stop again.
7. Park the Nicorette piece again (in a different place in your mouth).
8. Repeat steps 3 to 7 (chew, chew, park) until most of the nicotine is gone from the Nicorette piece (usually happens in about half an hour; the peppery taste or tingle won't return).
9. Wrap the used Nicorette in paper and throw away in the trash.
See the chart in the **"DIRECTIONS"** section above for the recommended usage schedule for Nicorette.
[See table above]
To improve your chances of quitting, use at least 9 pieces of Nicorette a day. Heavier smokers may need more pieces to reduce their cravings. Don't eat or drink for 15 minutes before using Nicorette or while chewing a piece. The effectiveness of Nicorette may be reduced by some foods and drinks, such as coffee, juices, wine or soft drinks.

**HOW TO REDUCE YOUR NICORETTE USAGE**
The goal of using Nicorette is to slowly reduce your dependence on nicotine. The schedule for using Nicorette will help you reduce your nicotine craving gradually. Here are some tips to help you cut back during each step:
• After a while, start chewing each Nicorette piece for only 10 to 15 minutes, instead of half an hour. Then gradually begin to reduce the number of pieces used.
• Or, try chewing each piece for longer than half an hour, but reduce the number of pieces you use each day.
• Substitute ordinary chewing gum for some of the Nicorette pieces you would normally use. Increase the number of pieces of ordinary gum as you cut back on the Nicorette pieces.
**STOP USING NICORETTE AT THE END OF WEEK 12.** If you still feel the need to use Nicorette after Week 12, talk with your doctor.

**TIPS TO MAKE QUITTING EASIER**
Within the first few weeks of giving up smoking, you may be tempted to smoke for pleasure, particularly after completing a difficult task, or at a party or bar. Here are some tips to help get you through the important first stages of becoming a non-smoker:

**On your Quit Date:**
- Ask your family, friends, and co-workers to support you in your efforts to stop smoking.
- Throw away all your cigarettes, matches, lighters, ashtrays, etc.
- Keep busy on your quit day. Exercise. Go to a movie. Take a walk. Get together with friends.
- Figure out how much money you'll save by not smoking. Most ex-smokers can save more than $1,000 a year.
- Write down what you will do with the money you save.
- Know your high risk situations and plan ahead how you will deal with them.
- Keep Nicorette gum near your bed, so you'll be prepared for any nicotine cravings when you wake up in the morning.
- Visit your dentist and have your teeth cleaned to get rid of the tobacco stains.

**Right after Quitting:**
- During the first few days after you've stopped smoking, spend as much time as possible at places where smoking is not allowed.
- Drink large quantities of water and fruit juices.
- Try to avoid alcohol, coffee and other beverages you associate with smoking.
- Remember that temporary urges to smoke will pass, even if you don't smoke a cigarette.
- Keep your hands busy with something like a pencil or a paper clip.
- Find other activities which help you relax without cigarettes. Swim, jog, take a walk, play basketball.
- Don't worry too much about gaining weight. Watch what you eat, take time for daily exercise, and change your eating habits if you need to.
- Laughter helps. Watch or read something funny.

**WHAT TO EXPECT**

Your body is now coming back into balance. During the first few days after you stop smoking, you might feel edgy and nervous and have trouble concentrating. You might get headaches, feel dizzy and a little out of sorts, feel sweaty or have stomach upsets. You might even have trouble sleeping at first. These are typical withdrawal symptoms that will go away with time. Your smoker's cough will get worse before it gets better. But don't worry, that's a good sign. Coughing helps clear the tar deposits out of your lungs.

**After a Week or Two.**

By now you should be feeling more confident that you can handle those smoking urges. Many of your withdrawal symptoms have left by now, and you should be noticing some positive signs: less coughing, better breathing and an improved sense of taste and smell, to name a few.

**After a Month.**

You probably have the urge to smoke much less often now. But urges may still occur, and when they do, they are likely to be powerful ones that come out of nowhere. Don't let them catch you off guard. Plan ahead for these difficult times. Concentrate on the ways non-smokers are more attractive than smokers. Their skin is less likely to wrinkle.

Their teeth are whiter, cleaner. Their breath is fresher. Their hair and clothes smell better. That cough that seems to make even a laugh sound more like a rattle is a thing of the past. Their children and others around them are healthier, too.

**What To Do About Relapse.**

What should you do if you slip and start smoking again? The answer is simple. A lapse of one or two or even a few cigarettes has not spoiled your efforts! Discard your cigarettes, forgive yourself and try again. If you start smoking again, keep your box of Nicorette for your next quit attempt. If you have taken up regular smoking again, don't be discouraged. Research shows that the best thing you can do is to try again. The important thing is to learn from your last attempt.
- Admit that you've slipped, but don't treat yourself as a failure.
- Try to identify the 'trigger' that caused you to slip, and prepare a better plan for dealing with this problem next time.
- Talk positively to yourself—tell yourself that you have learned something from this experience.
- Make sure you used Nicorette gum correctly over the full 12 weeks to reduce your craving for nicotine.
- Remember that it takes practice to do anything, and quitting smoking is no exception.

**WHEN THE STRUGGLE IS OVER**

Once you've stopped smoking, take a second and pat yourself on the back. Now do it again. You deserve it. Remember now why you decided to stop smoking in the first place. Look at your list of reasons. Read them again. And smile. Now think about all the money you are saving and what you'll do with it. All the non-smoking places you can go, and what you might do there. All those years you may have added to your life, and what you'll do with them. Remember that temptation may not be gone forever. However, the hard part is behind you, so look forward with a positive attitude and enjoy your new life as a non-smoker.

**QUESTIONS & ANSWERS**

**1. How will I feel when I stop smoking and start using Nicorette?** You'll need to prepare yourself for some nicotine withdrawal symptoms. These begin almost immediately after you stop smoking, and are usually at their worst during the first three to four days. Understand that any of the following is possible:
- craving for cigarettes
- anxiety, irritability, restlessness, mood changes, nervousness
- drowsiness
- trouble concentrating
- increased appetite and weight gain
- headaches, muscular pain, constipation, fatigue.

Nicorette can help provide relief from withdrawal symptoms such as irritability and nervousness, as well as the craving for nicotine you used to satisfy by having a cigarette.

**2. Is Nicorette just substuting one form of nicotine for another?** Nicorette does contain nicotine. The purpose of Nicorette is to provide you with enough nicotine to help control the physical withdrawal symptoms so you can deal

with the mental aspects of quitting. During the 12 week program, you will gradually reduce your nicotine intake by switching to fewer pieces each day. Remember, don't use Nicorette together with nicotine patches or other nicotine containing products.

**3. Can I be hurt by using Nicorette?** For most adults, the amount of nicotine in the gum is less than from smoking. Some people will be sensitive to even this amount of nicotine and should not use this product without advice from their doctor. Because Nicorette is a gum-based product, chewing it can cause dental fillings to loosen and aggravate other mouth, tooth and jaw problems. Nicorette can also cause hiccups, heartburn and other stomach problems especially if chewed too quickly or not chewed correctly.

**4. Will I gain weight?** Many people do tend to gain a few pounds in the first 8–10 weeks after they stop smoking. This is a very small price to pay for the enormous gains that you will make in your overall health and attractiveness. If you continue to gain weight after the first two months, try to analyze what you're doing differently. Reduce your fat intake, choose healthy snacks, and increase your physical activity to burn off the extra calories.

**5. Is Nicorette more expensive than smoking?** The total cost of Nicorette for the twelve week program is about equal to what a person who smokes one and a half packs of cigarettes a day would spend on cigarettes for the same period of time. Also use of Nicorette is only a short-term cost, while the cost of smoking is a long-term cost, because of the health problems smoking causes.

**6. What if I slip up?** Discard your cigarettes, forgive yourself and then get back on track. Don't consider yourself a failure or punish yourself. In fact, people who have already tried to quit are more likely to be successful the next time.

**GOOD LUCK!**

[End User's Guide]

---

**To remove the gum, tear off a single unit.**

**Peel off backing starting at corner with loose edge.**

**Push gum through foil.**

Blister packaged for your protection. Do not use if individual seals are broken.

Manufactured by Pharmacia & Upjohn AB, Stockholm, Sweden for SmithKline Beecham Consumer Healthcare, LP Pittsburgh, PA 15230

Comments or Questions? Call 1-800-419-4766 weekdays.

(10 a.m.–4:30 p.m. EST).
- **Not for sale to those under 18 years of age.**
- **Proof of age required.**
- **Not for sale in vending machines or from any source where proof of age cannot be verified.**

Nicorette Original, Mint, and Orange are available in:

2 mg or 4 mg Starter kit*—108 pieces

2 mg or 4 mg Refill—48 pieces

*Continued on next page*

## Nicorette—Cont.

*User's Guide and Audio Tape included in kit
*Shown in Product Identification Guide, page 508*

---

**Maximum Strength**

## NYTOL® QUICKGELS® SOFTGELS

**Indication:** For relief of occasional sleeplessness.

**Directions:** Adults and children 12 years of age and over: oral dosage is one softgel (50 mg) at bedtime if needed, or as directed by a doctor.

**Warnings:** Do not give to children under 12 years of age. If sleeplessness persists continuously for more than two weeks, consult your doctor. Insomnia may be a symptom of serious underlying medical illness. **Do not take this product, unless directed by a doctor, if you have a breathing problem such as emphysema or chronic bronchitis, or if you have glaucoma or difficulty in urination due to enlargement of the prostate gland. Do not use** with any other product containing diphenhydramine, including one applied topically. Avoid alcoholic beverages while taking this product. Do not take this product if you are taking sedatives or tranquilizers, without first consulting your doctor. In case of accidental overdose, seek professional assistance or contact a Poison Control Center immediately. As with any drug, if you are pregnant or nursing a baby, seek the advice of a health professional before using this product. Keep out of reach of children.

**Drug Interactions:** Alcohol and other drugs which cause CNS depression will heighten the depressant effect of this product. Monoamine oxidase (MAO) inhibitors will prolong and intensify the anticholinergic effects of antihistamines.

**Symptoms and Treatment of Oral Overdosage:** In adults overdose may cause CNS depression resulting in hypnosis and coma. In children CNS hyperexcitability may follow sedation; the stimulant phase may bring tremor, delirium and convulsions. Gastrointestinal reactions may include dry mouth, appetite loss, nausea and/or vomiting. Respiratory distress and cardiovascular complications (hypotension) may be evident. Treatment includes inducing emesis and controlling symptoms.

**Active Ingredient:** Diphenhydramine Hydrochloride 50 mg per softgel.

**Inactive Ingredients:** Edible Ink, Gelatin, Glycerin, Polyethylene Glycol, Purified Water, Sorbitol.

**How Supplied:** Available in packages of 8 and 16 softgels.

## NYTOL® QUICK CAPS® CAPLETS

**Indication:** For relief of occasional sleeplessness.

**Directions:** Adults and children 12 years of age and over: oral dosage is two caplets (50 mg) at bedtime if needed, or as directed by a doctor.

**Warnings:** Do not give to children under 12 years of age. If sleeplessness persists continuously for more than two weeks, consult your doctor. Insomnia may be a symptom of serious underlying medical illness. **Do not take this product, unless directed by a doctor, if you have a breathing problem such as emphysema or chronic bronchitis, or if you have glaucoma or difficulty in urination due to enlargement of the prostate gland. Do not use** with any other product containing diphenhydramine, including one applied topically. Avoid alcoholic beverages while taking this product. Do not take this product if you are taking sedatives or tranquilizers, without first consulting your doctor. In case of accidental overdose, seek professional assistance or contact a Poison Control Center immediately. As with any drug, if you are pregnant or nursing a baby, seek the advice of a health professional before using this product. Keep out of reach of children.

**Drug Interactions:** Alcohol and other drugs which cause CNS depression will heighten the depressant effect of this product. Monoamine oxidase (MAO) inhibitors will prolong and intensify the anticholinergic effects of antihistamines.

**Symptoms and Treatment of Oral Overdosage:** In adults, overdose may cause CNS depression resulting in hypnosis and coma. In children, CNS hyperexcitability may follow sedation; the stimulant phase may bring tremor, delirium and convulsions. Gastrointestinal reactions may include dry mouth, appetite loss, nausea and/or vomiting. Respiratory distress and cardiovascular complications (hypotension) may be evident. Treatment includes inducing emesis and controlling symptoms.

**Active Ingredient:** Diphenhydramine Hydrochloride 25 mg per caplet.

**Inactive Ingredients:** Corn Starch, Lactose, Microcrystalline Cellulose, Silica, Stearic Acid.

**How supplied:** Available in tamper-evident packages of 16, 32 and 72 caplets.
*Shown in Product Identification Guide, page 508*

---

**Quick Dissolve**
## PHAZYME®-125 MG Chewable Tablets
[fay-zime]

**Description:** A great tasting, smooth cool mint chewable tablet containing simethicone, an antiflatulent to alleviate or relieve the symptoms referred to as gas. Uniquely formulated to dissolve quickly and completely in your mouth. It has no known side effects or drug interactions.

**Active Ingredient:** Each tablet contains simethicone 125 mg.

**Inactive Ingredients:** Aspartame, citricacid, colloidal silicon dioxide, crospovidone, dextrates, maltodextrin, mannitol, peppermint flavor, pregelatinized starch, sodium bicarbonate, sorbitol, talc, tribasic calcium phosphate.

**Actions:** Simethicone minimizes gas formation and relieves gas entrapment in both the stomach and the lower G.I. tract. This action combats the distress due to gastrointestinal gas.

**Other Information:** Each tablet contains sodium 8 mg. Phenylketonurics: contains phenylalanine 0.4 mg per tablet.

**Indication:** Relieves pressure, bloating or fullness commonly referred to as gas.

**Warnings:** Keep this and all drugs out of the reach of children. If condition persists, consult your physician.
Store at room temperature 59°–86°F (15°–30°C).

**Dosage:** Directions: Chew one or two tablets thoroughly, as needed after a meal]. Do not exceed four tablets per day except under the advice and supervision of a physician.

**How Supplied:** White, bevel-edged tablets imprinted with "Phazyme 125" in 18 count and 48 count bottles.
*Shown in Product Identification Guide, page 508*

---

**Ultra Strength**
## PHAZYME®-180 MG Softgels
[fay-zime]

**Description:** An orange, easy to swallow softgel, containing simethicone, an antiflatulent to alleviate or relieve the symptoms referred to as gas. It has no known side effects or drug interactions.

**Active Ingredient:** Each softgel contains simethicone 180 mg.

**Inactive Ingredients:** FD&C Yellow No. 6, gelatin, glycerin, and white edible ink.

**Actions:** Simethicone minimizes gas formation and relieves gas entrapment in both the stomach and the lower G.I. tract. This action combats the distress due to gastrointestinal gas.

**Indication:** Relieves pressure, bloating or fullness commonly referred to as gas.

**Warnings:** Keep this and all drugs out of the reach of children. If condition persists, consult your physician.
Store at room temperature 59°–86°F (15°–30°C).

**Dosage:** Directions: Swallow one or two softgels as needed after a meal. Do not exceed two softgels per day except under the advice and supervision of a physician.

**How Supplied:** Orange softgel imprinted with "PZ 180" in 12 count and 36 count blister pack, 60 count and 100 count bottles.

*Shown in Product Identification Guide, page 508*

---

## SENSODYNE® FRESH MINT
## SENSODYNE® COOL GEL
## SENSODYNE® WITH BAKING SODA
## SENSODYNE® TARTAR CONTROL
## SENSODYNE® TARTAR CONTROL PLUS WHITENING
## SENSODYNE® ORIGINAL FLAVOR
## SENSODYNE® EXTRA WHITENING
**Anticavity toothpaste for sensitive teeth**

**Active Ingredients:** 5% Potassium Nitrate and 0.15% w/v Sodium Monofluorophosphate (Extra Whitening) or Sodium Fluoride (Fresh Mint, 0.15% w/v; Baking Soda, 0.15% w/v; Cool Gel, 0.13% w/v; Tartar Control, 0.13% w/v; Tartar Control Plus Whitening 0.145% w/v; Original Flavor, 0.13% w/v). Sensodyne Fresh Mint, Sensodyne Cool Gel, Sensodyne with Baking Soda, Sensodyne Tartar Control, Sensodyne Tartar Control Plus Whitening, Sensodyne Original Flavor and Sensodyne Extra Whitening contain fluoride for cavity prevention and Potassium Nitrate clinically proven to reduce pain sensitivity for relief of dentinal hypersensitivity resulting from the exposure of tooth dentin due to periodontal surgery, cervical (gum line) erosion, abrasion or recession which causes pain on contact with hot, cold, or tactile stimuli.

**Inactive Ingredients:** *Baking Soda:* Flavor, Glycerin, Hydrated Silica, Hydroxyethylcellulose, Methylparaben, Propylparaben, Silica, Sodium Bicarbonate, Sodium Lauryl Sulfate, Sodium Saccharin, Titanium Dioxide, Water.
*Extra Whitening:* Calcium Peroxide, Flavor, Glycerin, Hydrated Silica, PEG-12, PEG-75, Silica, Sodium Carbonate, Sodium Lauryl Sulfate, Sodium Saccharin, Titanium Dioxide, Water.
*Tartar Control:* Cellulose Gum, Cocamidopropyl Betaine, Flavor, Glycerin, Hydrated Silica, Silica, Sodium Bicarbonate, Sodium Saccharin, Tetrapotassium Pyrophosphate, Titanium Dioxide, Water.
*Tartar Control Plus Whitening:* Cellulose Gum, Flavor, Glycerin, Polyethylene Glycol, Silica, Sodium Lauryl Sulfate, Sodium Saccharin, Tetrapotassium Pyrophosphate, Titanium Dioxide, Water.
*Cool Gel:* Cellulose Gum, FD&C Blue #1, Flavor, Glycerin, Hydrated Silica, Silica, Sodium Methyl Cocoyl Taurate, Sodium Saccharin, Sorbitol, Trisodium Phosphate, Water.

*Fresh Mint: Inactive Ingredients:* Carbomer, cellulose gum, D&C yellow #10, FD&C blue #1, flavor, glycerin, hydrated silica, octadecene/MA copolymer, poloxamer 407, potassium hydroxide, sodium lauroyl sarcosinate, sodium saccharin, sorbitol, titanium dioxide, water, xanthan gum.
*Original Flavor:* Cellulose Gum, D&C Red No. 28, Glycerin, Hydrated Silica, Peppermint Oil, Silica, Sodium Methyl Cocoyl Taurate, Sodium Saccharin, Sorbitol, Titanium Dioxide, Trisodium Phosphate, Water.

**Actions:** All Sensodyne Formulas significantly reduce tooth hypersensitivity, with response to therapy evident after two weeks of use. Controlled double-blind clinical studies provide substantial evidence of the safety and effectiveness of Potassium Nitrate. The current theory on mechanism of action is that potassium nitrate has an effect on neural transmission, interrupting the signal which would result in the sensation of pain. Fluorides are anticariogenic, forming fluoroapatite in the outer surface of the dental enamel which is resistant to acids and caries.

**Warnings:** Sensitive teeth may indicate a serious problem that may need prompt care by a dentist. See your dentist if the problem persists or worsens. Do not use this product longer than 4 weeks unless recommended by a dentist or physician. Keep this and all drugs out of the reach of children. If you accidentally swallow more than used for brushing, seek professional assistance or contact a Poison Control Center immediately.

**Dosage and Administration:** Adults and children 12 years of age and older: Apply a 1-inch strip of the product onto a soft bristle toothbrush. Brush teeth thoroughly for at least 1 minute twice a day (morning and evening) or as recommended by a dentist or physician. Make sure to brush all sensitive areas of the teeth. Children under 12 years of age: consult a dentist or physician.

**How Supplied:** All Sensodyne formulas are supplied in 2.1 oz. (60g), 4.0 oz. (113g) and 6.0 oz. (170g) tubes. Sensodyne Cool Gel is supplied in 4.0 oz. and 6.0 oz. tubes. Sensodyne Baking Soda is supplied in 4.0 oz and 6.0 oz. only.

---

## SINGLET® For Adults
## Nasal Decongestant/Antihistamine/ Analgesic (pain reliever)/Antipyretic (fever reducer)

**Indications:** For temporary relief of nasal congestion and sinus and headache pain associated with sinusitis or due to a cold, hay fever or other upper respiratory allergies. Also temporarily relieves nasal congestion, sinus headache, runny nose, sneezing, itching of the nose or throat, and itchy, watery eyes due to hay fever or other upper respiratory allergies. Also temporarily relieves fever due to the common cold.

**Directions:** Adults (12 years and older): 1 caplet every 4 to 6 hours, **not to exceed 4 caplets in any 24-hour period,** or as directed by a doctor. Children under 12 years of age: Consult a doctor.

**Warnings: Do not exceed recommended dosage.** If nervousness, dizziness, or sleeplessness occur, discontinue use and consult a doctor. Do not take this product for more than 10 days. If symptoms do not improve or are accompanied by fever that lasts for more than 3 days, or if new symptoms occur, consult a doctor. Do not take this product, unless directed by a doctor, if you have a breathing problem such as emphysema or chronic bronchitis, or if you have heart disease, high blood pressure, thyroid disease, diabetes, glaucoma or difficulty in urination due to enlargement of the prostate gland. May cause excitability especially in children. May cause drowsiness; alcohol, sedatives, and tranquilizers may increase the drowsiness effect. Avoid alcoholic beverages while taking this product. Do not take this product if you are taking sedatives or tranquilizers, without first consulting your doctor. Use caution when driving a motor vehicle or operating machinery. **KEEP THIS AND ALL DRUGS OUT OF THE REACH OF CHILDREN.** Prompt medical attention is critical for adults as well as for children even if you do not notice any signs or symptoms. In case of accidental overdose, seek professional assistance or contact a Poison Control Center immediately. As with any drug, if you are pregnant or nursing a baby, seek the advice of a health professional before using this product.

**Alcohol Warning:** If you consume 3 or more alcoholic drinks every day, ask your doctor whether you should take acetaminophen or other pain reliever/fever reducers. Acetaminophen may cause liver damage.

**Drug Interaction Precaution:** Do not use this product if you are now taking a prescription monoamine oxidase inhibitor (MAOI) (certain drugs for depression, psychiatric or emotional conditions, or Parkinson's disease), or for 2 weeks after stopping the MAOI drug. If you are uncertain whether your prescription drug contains an MAOI, consult a health professional before taking this product.

**Active Ingredients:** Each caplet contains: Pseudoephedrine Hydrochloride 60 mg, Chlorpheniramine Maleate 4 mg, Acetaminophen 650 mg.

**Inactive Ingredients:** D&C Red 27, D&C Yellow 10, FD&C Blue 1, Hydroxypropyl Cellulose, Hydroxypropyl Methylcellulose, Magnesium Stearate, Microcrystalline Cellulose, Polyethylene Glycol, Pregelatinized Corn Starch, Sodium Starch Glycolate, Sucrose and Titanium Dioxide.
Store at room temperature (59°–86°F). Avoid excessive heat and humidity.

*Continued on next page*

## Singlet—Cont.

Comments or Questions? Call toll-free 1-800-245-1040 weekdays
Distributed by: GlaxoSmithKline Consumer Healthcare, L.P.
Pittsburgh, PA 15230. Made in U.S.A.

## SOMINEX Original Formula
## Nighttime Sleep Aid
## Doctor-preferred sleep ingredient

**Indications:** Helps to reduce difficulty falling asleep.

**Directions:** Adults and children 12 years and over: Take 2 tablets at bedtime if needed, or as directed by a doctor. For best results, take recommended dose. This will provide approximately six to eight hours of restful sleep.

**Warnings:** Do not give to children under 12 years of age. If sleeplessness persists continually for more than 2 weeks, consult your doctor. Insomnia may be a symptom of serious underlying medical illness. Do not take this product, unless directed by a doctor, if you have a breathing problem such as emphysema or chronic bronchitis, or if you have glaucoma or difficulty in urination due to enlargement of the prostate gland. Avoid alcoholic beverages while taking this product. Do not take this product if you are taking sedatives or tranquilizers, without first consulting your doctor. As with any drug, if you are pregnant or nursing a baby, seek the advice of a health professional before using this product. **Keep this and all drugs out of the reach of children.** In case of accidental overdose, seek professional assistance or contact a poison control center immediately.

**Active Ingredients:** Each tablet contains 25 mg Diphenhydramine HCl.

**Inactive Ingredients:** Dibasic Calcium Phosphate, FD&C Blue #1, Magnesium Stearate, Microcrystalline Cellulose, Silicon Dioxide, Starch.
**Tamper Evident Feature:** Individually sealed in foil for your protection. Do not use if foil or plastic bubble is torn or punctured.
Store at room temperature, avoid excessive heat (greater than 100°F) or humidity.

**How Supplied:** Consumer Packages of 16, 32 and 72 tablets
Also Available in Maximum Strength Formula.
Comments or Questions? Call Toll-Free 1-800-245-1040 Weekdays.
GlaxoSmithKline Consumer Healthcare, L.P.
Pittsburgh, PA 15230. Made in U.S.A.

## TAGAMET HB® 200
## Cimetidine Tablets 200 mg/
## Acid Reducer

Tagamet HB® 200 relieves and prevents heartburn, acid indigestion and sour stomach when used as directed. It contains the same ingredient found in prescription strength Tagamet. Tagamet HB 200 reduces the production of stomach acid.
**ACTIVE        INGREDIENT** Cimetidine, 200 mg.
**INACTIVE INGREDIENTS** Cellulose, cornstarch, hydroxypropyl methylcellulose, magnesium stearate, polyethylene glycol, polysorbate 80, povidone, sodium lauryl sulfate, sodium starch glycolate, titanium dioxide.
**USES:**
- For relief of heartburn associated with acid indigestion and sour stomach.
- For prevention of heartburn associated with acid indigestion and sour stomach brought on by eating or drinking certain food and beverages.

**Directions:**
- For **relief** of symptoms, swallow 1 tablet with a glass of water.
- For **prevention** of symptoms, swallow 1 tablet with a glass of water **right before or anytime up to 30 minutes before** eating food or drinking beverages that cause heartburn.
- Tagamet HB 200 can be used up to twice daily (up to 2 tablets in 24 hours).
- This product should not be given to children under 12 years old unless directed by a doctor.

**Warnings:**
**Allergy Warning:** Do not use if you are allergic to Tagamet HB 200 (cimetidine) or other acid reducers.
**Ask a Doctor Before Use If You are Taking:**
- theophylline (oral asthma medicine)
- warfarin (blood thinning medicine)
- phenytoin (seizure medicine)
If you are not sure whether your medication contains one of these drugs or have any other questions about medicines you are taking, call our consumer affairs specialist at 1-800-482-4394.
- Do not take the maximum daily dosage for more than 2 weeks continuously except under the advice and supervision of a doctor.
- If you have trouble swallowing, or persistent abdominal pain, see your doctor promptly. You may have a serious condition that may need a different treatment.
- As with any drug, if you are pregnant or nursing a baby, seek the advice of a health professional before using this product.
- Keep this and all medications out of the reach of children.
- In case of accidental overdose, seek professional assistance or contact a poison control center immediately.
**READ THE LABEL**
**Read the directions and warnings before taking this medication.**
Store at 15°–30°C (59°–86°F).
Comments or questions? Call Toll-Free 1-800-482-4394 weekdays.
**PHARMACOKINETIC INTERACTIONS**
Cimetidine at prescription doses is known to inhibit various P450 metabolizing isoenzymes, which could affect metabolism of other drugs and increase their blood concentration. Investigation of pharmacokinetic interactions at the recommended OTC doses of cimetidine have thus far shown only small effects. A pharmacokinetic study conducted in 26 normal male subjects (mean age, 38 years) at steady state using the maximum recommended OTC dose level (200 mg twice a day), showed that Tagamet HB 200, on average, increased the 24 hour AUC of theophylline by 14% and increased peak theophylline levels by 15%. This interaction should be borne in mind in advising patients on the use of Tagamet HB 200. At the prescription doses of cimetidine, clinically significant pharmacokinetic interactions between cimetidine and warfarin, phenytoin, and theophylline have been reported. At prescription doses, pharmacokinetic interactions have been reported for a number of other drugs as well, such as with dihydropyridine calcium channel blockers or some short acting benzodiazepines. At the maximum recommended OTC dose level (200 mg twice a day), a pharmacokinetic study conducted in 21 normal male subjects (mean age, 38 years) showed that Tagamet HB 200, on average, increased the total AUC of triazolam by 26–28% and increased peak triazolam levels by 11–23%. Tagamet HB 200 did not alter the apparent terminal elimination half-life of triazolam.

**How Supplied:** Tagamet HB 200 (Cimetidine Tablets 200 mg) is available in boxes of blister packs in 6, 12, 18, 30, 50, 70 & 80 tablet sizes.
*Shown in Product Identification Guide, page 508*

## TAGAMET HB® 200
## Cimetidine Suspension 200 mg
## Acid Reducer

**Tagamet HB® 200 relieves and prevents heartburn, acid indigestion and sour stomach. When used as directed. It contains the same ingredient found in prescription strength Tagamet. Tagamet HB® 200 reduces the production of stomach acid.**

**Active        Ingredient** Cimetidine, 200 mg.

**Uses**
- relieves heartburn associated with acid indigestion and sour stomach
- prevents heartburn associated with acid indigestion and sour stomach brought on by eating or drinking certain food and beverages.

**Warnings**
**Allergy alert:** Do not use if you are allergic to cimetidine or other acid reducers.
**Do not use**
- in children under 12 years (see **Directions**)
- if you have trouble swallowing
- with other acid reducers
**Ask a doctor or pharmacist before use if you are taking**
- **theophylline (oral asthma medicine)**
- **warfarin (blood thinning medicine)**
- **phenytoin (seizure medicine)**

If you are not sure you are taking one of these medicines, talk to your doctor or pharmacist.

**Stop use and ask a doctor if**
• stomach pain continues
• you need to take this product for more than 14 days

**If pregnant or breast-feeding,** ask a health professional before use.

**Keep out of reach of children.**

In case of overdose, get medical help or contact a Poison Control Center right away.

**Directions**
• shake well
• adults and children 12 years and over:
  • to **relieve** symptoms, take 4 teaspoons (20 mL) in pre-measured dose cup provided, with a glass of water
  • to **prevent** symptoms, take 4 teaspoons (20 mL) in pre-measured dose cup provided, with a glass of water **right before or any time up to 30 minutes before** eating food or drinking beverages that cause heartburn
  • do not take more than 4 teaspoons twice in 24 hours
  • children under 12 years: **not for use in children under 12. The safety and effectiveness for use in children under 12 has not been proven**.

**Other Information**
• store at 20–30°C (68–86°F)

**Inactive Ingredients** butylparaben, FD&C blue #1, flavors, microcrystalline cellulose and carboxymethylcellulose sodium, propylene glycol, propylparaben, purified water, saccharin sodium, sucrose, xanthan gum

**Pharmacokinetic Interactions** Cimetidine at prescription doses is known to inhibit various P450 metabolizing isoenzymes, which could affect metabolism of other drugs and increase their blood concentration. Investigation of pharmacokinetic interactions at the recommended OTC does of cimetidine have thus far shown only small effects. A pharmacokinetic study conducted in 26 normal male subjects (mean age, 38 years) at steady state using the maximum recommended OTC dose level (200 mg twice a day), on average, increased the 24 hour AUC of theophylline by 14% and increased peak theophylline levels by 15%. This interaction should be borne in mind in advising patients on the use of Tagamet HB 200. At the prescription doses of cimetidine, clinically significant pharmacokinetic interactions between cimetidine and warfarin, phenytoin, and theophylline have been reported. At prescription doses, pharmacokinetic interactions have been reported for a number of other drugs as well, such as with dihydropyridine calcium channel blockers or some short acting benzodiazepines. At the maximum recommended OTC dose level (200 mg twice a day), a pharmacokinetic study conducted in 21 normal male subjects (mean age, 38 years) showed that Tagament HB 200, on average, increased the total AUC of triazolam by 26–28% and increased peak triazolam levels by 11–

23%. The apparent terminal elimination half life of triazolam was not altered at this dosage.

*Shown in Product Identification Guide, page 508*

## TEGRIN® DANDRUFF SHAMPOO – EXTRA CONDITIONING

**Description:** Tegrin® Dandruff Shampoo contains 7% Coal Tar Solution, USP, equivalent to 1.1% coal tar, in a pleasantly scented, high-foaming, cleansing shampoo base with emollients, conditioners and other formula components.

**Indications:** Tegrin® Dandruff Shampoo controls the flaking and itching of the scalp associated with dandruff, seborrheic dermatitis, and psoriasis.

**Directions:** Shake well. Wet hair. Lather, rinse, repeat. For best results use at least twice a week or as directed by a doctor.

**Warnings:** For external use only. Avoid contact with eyes. If contact occurs, rinse eyes thoroughly with water. If condition worsens or does not improve after regular use of this product as directed, consult a doctor. Use caution in exposing skin to sunlight after applying this product. It may increase tendency to sunburn for up to 24 hours after application. Do not use for prolonged periods without consulting a doctor. Do not use this product with other forms of psoriasis therapy, such as ultraviolet radiation or prescription drugs, unless directed by a doctor. Keep out of reach of children. In case of accidental ingestion, seek professional assistance or contact a Poison Control Center immediately.

**Active Ingredient:** 7% Coal Tar Solution, USP, Equivalent to 1.1% Coal Tar. Coal Tar is obtained in the destructive distillation of bituminous coal and is a highly effective agent for controlling the flaking and itching of the scalp associated with dandruff, seborrheic dermatitis, and psoriasis. The action of coal tar is believed to be keratolytic, antiseptic, antipruritic, and astringent. The coal tar solution used in Tegrin® Dandruff Shampoo is prepared in such a way as to reduce the pitch and other irritant components found in crude coal tar without reduction in therapeutic potency.
Coal Tar Solution has been used clinically for many years as a remedy for dandruff and for scaling associated with scalp disorders such as seborrhea and psoriasis. Its mechanism of action has not been fully established, but it is believed to retard the rate of turnover of epidermal cells with regular use. A number of clinical studies have demonstrated the performance attributes of Tegrin® Dandruff Shampoo against dandruff and seborrheic dermatitis. In addition to relieving the above symptoms, Tegrin® Dandruff Shampoo, used regularly, maintains scalp and hair cleanliness and leaves the hair lustrous and manageable.

**Inactive Ingredients for:**
Tegrin® Dandruff Shampoo – Extra Conditioning
Alcohol (7.0%), Ammonium Lauryl Sulfate, Citric Acid, FD&C Blue #1, Fragrance, Glycol Stearate (and) Sodium Laureth Sulfate (and) Hexylene Glycol, Guar Hydroxypropyltrimonium Chloride, Hydroxypropyl Methylcellulose, Lauramide DEA, Methylparaben, Propylparaben, Sodium Lauryl Sulfate, Water.

**How supplied:** Tegrin® Dandruff Shampoo is available in Extra Conditioning and Fresh Herbal formulas and supplied in 7 fl. oz. (207 ml) plastic bottles.

## TEGRIN® DANDRUFF SHAMPOO-FRESH HERBAL

**Description:** Tegrin® Dandruff Shampoo contains 7% Coal Tar Solution, USP, equivalent to 1.1% coal tar, in a pleasantly scented, high-foaming, cleansing shampoo base with emollients, conditioners and other formula components.

**Indications:** Tegrin® Dandruff Shampoo controls the flaking and itching of the scalp associated with dandruff, seborrheic dermatitis, and psoriasis.

**Directions:** Shake well. Wet hair. Lather, rinse, repeat. For best results use at least twice a week or as directed by a doctor.

**Warnings:** For external use only. Avoid contact with eyes. If contact occurs, rinse eyes thoroughly with water. If condition worsens or does not improve after regular use of this product as directed, consult a doctor. Use caution in exposing skin to sunlight after applying this product. It may increase tendency to sunburn for up to 24 hours after application. Do not use for prolonged periods without consulting a doctor. Do not use this product with other forms of psoriasis therapy, such as ultraviolet radiation or prescription drugs, unless directed by a doctor. Keep out of reach of children. In case of accidental ingestion, seek professional assistance or contact a Poison Control Center immediately.

**Active Ingredient:** 7% Coal Tar Solution, USP, Equivalent to 1.1% Coal Tar. Coal Tar is obtained in the destructive distillation of bituminous coal and is a highly effective agent for controlling the flaking and itching of the scalp associated with dandruff, seborrheic dermatitis and psoriasis. The action of coal tar is believed to be keratolytic, antiseptic, antipruritic, and astringent. The coal tar solution used in Tegrin® Dandruff Shampoo is prepared in such a way as to reduce the pitch and other irritant components found in crude coal tar without reduction in therapeutic potency.
Coal Tar Solution has been used clinically for many years as a remedy for

*Continued on next page*

## Tegrin Herbal—Cont.

dandruff and for scaling associated with scalp disorders such as seborrhea and psoriasis. Its mechanism of action has not been fully established, but it is believed to retard the rate of turnover of epidermal cells with regular use. A number of clinical studies have demonstrated the performance attributes of Tegrin® Dandruff Shampoo against dandruff and seborrheic dermatitis. In addition to relieving the above symptoms, Tegrin® Dandruff Shampoo, used regularly, maintains scalp and hair cleanliness and leaves the hair lustrous and manageable.

**Inactive Ingredients For:**
Tegrin® Dandruff Shampoo–Fresh Herbal
Alcohol (7.0%), Citric Acid, Cocamide DEA, FD&C Blue #1, Fragrance, Glycol Stearate (and) Sodium Laureth Sulfate (and) Hexylene Glycol, Hydroxypropyl Methylcellulose, Methylparaben, Propylparaben, Sodium Lauryl Sulfate, Water.

**How Supplied:** Tegrin® Dandruff Shampoo is available in Extra Conditioning and Fresh Herbal formulas and supplied in 7 fl. oz. (207 ml) plastic bottles.
*Shown in Product Identification Guide, page 508*

---

## TEGRIN® SKIN CREAM FOR PSORIASIS

**Description:** Tegrin® Skin Cream for Psoriasis contains 5% Coal Tar Solution, USP, equivalent to 0.8% Coal Tar and alcohol of 4.7%.

**Indications:** For relief of itching, flaking and irritation of the skin associated with psoriasis and seborrheic dermatitis.

**Directions:** Apply to affected areas one to four times daily or as directed by a doctor.

**Warnings:** For external use only. Avoid contact with eyes. If contact occurs, rinse eyes thoroughly with water. If condition worsens or does not improve after regular use of this product as directed, consult a doctor. Use caution in exposing skin to sunlight after applying this product. It may increase tendency to sunburn for up to 24 hours after application. Do not use for prolonged periods without consulting a doctor. Do not use this product with other forms of psoriasis therapy, such as ultra-violet radiation or prescription drugs, unless directed by a doctor. If the condition covers a large area of the body, consult your doctor before using this product. Keep out of reach of children. In case of accidental ingestion, seek professional assistance or contact a Poison Control Center immediately.

**Active Ingredient:** 5% Coal Tar Solution, USP, equivalent to 0.8% Coal Tar.

**Inactive Ingredients:** Acetylated Lanolin Alcohol, Alcohol (4.7%), Carbomer-934P, Ceteth-2, Ceteth-16, Cetyl Acetate, Cetyl Alcohol, D&C Red No. 28, Fragrance, Glyceryl Tribehenate, Laneth-16, Lanolin Alcohol, Laureth-23, Methyl Gluceth-20, Methylchloroisothiazolinone, Methylisothiazolinone, Mineral Oil, Octyldodecanol, Oleth-16, Petrolatum, Potassium Hydroxide, Purified Water, Steareth-16, Stearyl Alcohol, Titanium Dioxide.

**How Supplied:** Tegrin® Skin Cream for Psoriasis is available in a 2 oz (57g) tube.
*Shown in Product Identification Guide, page 508*

---

## TUMS® Regular Antacid/Calcium Supplement Tablets
## TUMS E–X® and TUMS E–X® Sugar Free Antacid/Calcium Supplement Tablets
## TUMS ULTRA® Antacid/Calcium Supplement Tablets

**Professional Labeling:** Indicated for the symptomatic relief of hyperacidity associated with the diagnosis of peptic ulcer, gastritis, peptic esophagitis, gastric hyperacidity, and hiatal hernia.

**Indications:** For fast relief of acid indigestion, heartburn, sour stomach, and upset stomach associated with these symptoms.

**Active Ingredient:**
**Tums,** Calcium Carbonate 500 mg
**Tums E-X,** Calcium Carbonate 750 mg
**Tums ULTRA,** Calcium Carbonate 1000 mg

**Actions:** Tums provides rapid neutralization of stomach acid. Each Tums tablet has an acid-neutralizing capacity (ANC) of 10 mEq. Each Tums E-X tablet has an ANC of 15 mEq and each Tums ULTRA tablet, an ANC of 20 mEq. This high neutralization capacity makes Tums tablets an ideal antacid for management of conditions associated with hyperacidity. It effectively neutralizes free acid yet does not cause systemic alkalosis in the presence of normal renal function. A double-blind placebo-controlled clinical study demonstrated that calcium carbonate taken at a dosage of 16 Tums tablets daily for a two-week period was non-constipating/non-laxative.

**Warnings: Tums:** Do not take more than 15 tablets in a 24-hour period or use the maximum dosage of this product for more than 2 weeks, except under the advice and supervision of a physician. If symptoms persist for 2 weeks, stop using this product and see a physician. Keep this and all drugs out of the reach of children.

**Tums E-X:** Do not take more than 10 tablets in a 24-hour period or use the maximum dosage of this product for more than two weeks, except under the advice and supervision of a physician. If symptoms persist for two weeks, stop using this product and see a physician. Keep this and all drugs out of the reach of children.

Additionally, for Tums Ex Sugar Free: Phenylketonurics: Contains phenylalanine, less than 1 mg per tablet.

**Tums ULTRA:** Do not take more than 7 tablets in 24-hour period or use the maximum dosage of this product for more than two weeks, except under the advice and supervision of a physician. If symptoms persist for two weeks, stop using and see a physician. Keep this and all drugs out of the reach of children.

**Drug Interaction Precaution:** Antacids may interact with certain prescription drugs. If you are presently taking a prescription drug, do not take this product without checking with your physician or other health professional.

**Dosage and Administration:**
**Tums:** Chew 2-4 tablets as symptoms occur. Repeat hourly if symptoms return, or as directed by physician.
**Tums E-X:** Chew 2-4 tablets as symptoms occur. Repeat hourly if symptoms return, or as directed by a physician.
**Tums ULTRA:** Chew 2-3 tablets as symptoms occur. Repeat hourly if symptoms return, or as directed by a physician.

**AS A DIETARY SUPPLEMENT:**
**Calcium Supplement Directions**
Tums, Tums E-X, & Tums ULTRA:
**USES:** As a daily source of extra calcium. Tums is recommended by the National Osteoporosis Foundation.

**IMPORTANT INFORMATION ON OSTEOPOROSIS:** Research shows that certain ethnic, age and other groups are at higher risk for developing osteoporosis, including Caucasian and Asian teen and young adult women, menopausal women, older persons and those persons with a family history of fragile bones. **A balanced diet with enough calcium and regular exercise throughout life will help you to build and maintain**

| | Tums | Tums E-X | Tums E-X Sugar Free | Tums Ultra |
|---|---|---|---|---|
| Serving Size | 2 Tablets | 2 Tablets | 2 Tablets | 2 Tablets |
| **Amount Per Serving** | | | | |
| Calories | 5 | 10 | 5 | 10 |
| Sorbitol (g) | — | — | 1 | — |
| Sugars (g) | 1 | 2 | — | 3 |
| Calcium (mg) | 400 | 600 | 600 | 800 |
| % Daily Value | 40 | 60 | 60 | 80 |
| Sodium (mg) | — | 5 | — | 10 |
| % Daily Value | | <1% | | <1% |

Supplement Facts

**healthy bones and may reduce your risk of developing osteoporosis.** Adequate calcium intake is important, but daily intakes above 2,000 mg are not likely to provide any additional benefit.

**DIRECTIONS:** Chew 2 tablets twice daily.
[See table at bottom of previous page]

**Ingredients (all variants except sugar free):** Sucrose, Corn Starch, Talc, Mineral Oil, Flavors (natural and/or artificial), Sodium Polyphosphate. May also contain 1% or less of Adipic Acid, Blue 1 Lake, Yellow 6 Lake, Yellow 5 Lake, Red 40 Lake.

**Ingredients (Sugar Free):** Sorbitol, Acacia, Natural and Artificial Flavors, Calcium Stearate, Adipic Acid, Yellow 6 Lake, Aspartame.

**How Supplied:**
**Tums: Peppermint flavor** is available in 12-tablet rolls, 3-roll wraps, and bottles of 75, 150, and 180. **Assorted Flavors** (Cherry, Lemon, Orange, and Lime), are available in 12-tablet rolls, 3-roll wraps, and bottles of 75, 150, 180, and 400.
**Tums E-X: Wintergreen** 3-roll wraps and bottles of 48, 96, and 116.
**Tums E-X: Assorted Fruit, Assorted Tropical Fruit, and Assorted Berries, Fresh Blend** 8 tablet rolls, 3-roll wraps, 6-roll wraps, and bottles of 48, 96, and 116. Assorted Tropical Fruit and Assorted Berries are also available in bottles of 250 tablets.
**Tums EX Sugar Free:** Orange Cream; bottles of 48 and 96 tablets.
**Tums ULTRA: Assorted Berries,** and **Spearmint** bottles of 160 tablets. **Assorted Fruit** and **Assorted Mint** bottles of 36, 72, and 86 tablets. Assorted Fruit also available in bottles of 160 tablets.
**Tropical Fruit** bottles of 160 tablets.
*Shown in Product Identification Guide, page 508*

---

**VIVARIN Tablets & Caplets**
**Alertness Aid with Caffeine**
**Maximum Strength**

Each Tablet or Caplet Contains 200 mg. Caffeine, Equal to About Two Cups of Coffee
Take Vivarin for a safe, fast pick up anytime you feel drowsy and need to be alert. The caffeine in Vivarin is less irritating to your stomach than coffee, according to a government appointed panel of experts.

**FDA APPROVED USES:** Helps restore mental alertness or wakefulness when experiencing fatigue or drowsiness.

**Active Ingredients:** Caffeine 200 mg.

**Inactive Ingredients:** Tablet: Colloidal Silicon Dioxide, D&C Yellow #10 Al. Lake, Dextrose, FD&C Yellow #6 Al. Lake, Magnesium Stearate, Microcrystalline Cellulose, Starch.
Caplet: Carnauba Wax, Colloidal Silicon Dioxide, D&C Yellow #10 Al Lake, Dextrose, FD&C Yellow #6 Al Lake, Hydroxypropyl Methylcellulose, Magnesium Stearate, Microcrystalline Cellulose, Polyethylene Glycol, Polysorbate 80, Starch, Titanium Dioxide.

**Directions:** Adults and children 12 years and over: Take 1 tablet (200 mg) not more often than every 3 to 4 hours.

**Warnings:** The recommended dose of this product contains about as much caffeine as two cups of coffee. Limit the use of caffeine containing medications, foods, or beverages while taking this product because too much caffeine may cause nervousness, irritability, sleeplessness, and occasionally, rapid heartbeat. For occasional use only. Not intended for use as a substitute for sleep. If fatigue or drowsiness persists or continues to recur, consult a doctor. Do not give to children under 12 years of age. As with any drug, if you are pregnant or nursing a baby, seek the advice of a health professional before using this product. In case of accidental overdose, seek professional assistance or contact a poison control center immediately. Keep this and all drugs out of the reach of children.

Tamper Evident Feature: Individually sealed in foil for your protection. Do not use if foil or plastic bubble is torn or punctured.

Store at room temperature, avoid excessive heat (greater than 100°F) or humidity.

**How Supplied:**
Tablets: Consumer packages of 16, 40 and 80 tablets
Caplets: Consumer packages of 24 and 48 caplets

Comments or Questions? Call Toll-Free 1-800-245-1040 Weekdays.
SmithKline Beecham Consumer Healthcare, L.P.
Pittsburgh, PA 15230. Made in U.S.A.
©1996 SmithKline Beecham
*Shown in Product Identification Guide, page 509*

---

**IF YOU SUSPECT**
**AN INTERACTION. . .**
The 1,800-page
*PDR Companion Guide*™ can help.
Use the order form
in the front of this book.

---

**A.C. Grace Co.**
**1100 QUITMAN ROAD**
**P.O. BOX 570**
**BIG SANDY, TX 75755**

**Direct Inquiries to:**
Inquiries: (903) 636-4368
Orders Only: 800-833-4368

---

**UNIQUE E®**
**NATURAL VITAMIN E COMPLEX**
**MIXED TOCOPHEROL CONCENTRATE**

**Description:**
*Established 1962...* OUR ONLY PRODUCT.
WHY UNIQUE?
All NATURAL VITAMIN E COMPLEX. *NOT* the *dl* SYNTHETIC CHEMICAL form, *NOT ESTER*IFIED TOCOPHERYL ACETATE (OR SUCCINATE), *NOT* the ORDINARY SOY OIL DILUTED MIXED TOCOPHEROLS OR ADULTERATED FORMS.

Each soft easy-to-swallow high quality pure **VEGETABLE GEL CAPSULE** contains **ALL NATURAL** *UN*ESTERIFIED **VITAMIN E COMPLEX** providing **400 I.U. ANTI***THROMBIC* function d-alpha tocopherol with other naturally occuring **ANTI***OX*IDANT tocopherols, **d-beta, d GAMMA, d-delta** for maximum protection against harmful free radical damage and inhibiting peroxynitrites damaging to brain cells.

*NO* SOY or other OIL FILLER additives which can turn rancid and cause harmful free radical damage even in sealed gel capsules.

NO ALLERGY CAUSING PRESERVATIVES, COLORS OR FLAVORINGS.

UNIQUE E® capsule potency is stabilized and Certified by Assay.

**Dosage:** Up to 6 capsules daily as directed by your physician according to individual weight or need, usually 1 capsule per each 40 lbs. of total body weight. Best results when ENTIRE daily dose is taken just before or with the morning meal.

**How Supplied:**
Bottles of 180 and 90 easy-to-swallow high quality pure vegetable gel capsules in safety sealed light protected bottles.

---

**UNKNOWN DRUG?**
Consult the
Product Identification Guide
(Gray Pages)
for full-color photos of
leading over-the-counter
medications

# Hyland's, Inc.
See Standard Homeopathic Company

---

# Johnson & Johnson • MERCK

Consumer Pharmaceuticals Co.
7050 CAMP HILL ROAD
FORT WASHINGTON, PA 19034

**Direct Inquiries to:**
Consumer Affairs Department
Fort Washington, PA 19034
(215) 273-7000
**For Medical Information Contact:**
**In Emergencies:**
(215) 273-7000

## PEPCID AC®
### TABLETS, Chewable Tablets and Gelcaps

**Description:**
**Active Ingredient:** Famotidine 10 mg per tablet.
**Inactive Ingredients:** TABLETS: Hydroxypropyl cellulose, hydroxypropyl methylcellulose, red iron oxide, magnesium stearate, microcrystalline cellulose, starch, talc, titanium dioxide.
CHEWABLE TABLETS: aspartame, cellulose acetate, flavors, hydroxypropyl cellulose, hydroxypropyl methylcellulose, lactose, magnesium stearate, mannitol, microcrystalline cellulose, red ferric oxide.
GELCAPS: benzyl alcohol, black iron oxide, butylparaben, castor oil, edetate calcium disodium, FD&C red #40, gelatin, hydroxypropyl methylcellulose, magnesium stearate, methylparaben, microcrystalline cellulose, pregelatinized corn starch, propylene glycol, propylparaben, sodium lauryl sulfate, sodium propionate, talc, titanium dioxide.

**Product Benefits:**
• **1 Tablet, Chewable Tablet or Gelcap** relieves heartburn and acid indigestion.
• Pepcid AC prevents heartburn and acid indigestion brought on by consuming food and beverages.
It contains famotidine, a prescription-proven medicine.
The ingredient in PEPCID AC, famotidine, has been prescribed by doctors for years to treat millions of patients safely and effectively. The active ingredient in PEPCID AC has been taken safely with many frequently prescribed medications.

**Action:**
It is normal for the stomach to produce acid, especially after consuming food and beverages. However, acid in the wrong place (the esophagus), or too much acid, can cause burning pain and discomfort that interfere with everyday activities.

• **Heartburn—Caused by acid in the esophagus**

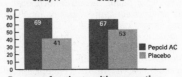

A valve-like muscle called the lower esophageal sphincter (LES) is relaxed in an open position

Burning pain/discomfort

Excess acid moves up into esophagus

**In clinical studies, PEPCID AC was significantly better than placebo pills in relieving and preventing heartburn.**

Percent of heartburn episodes completely relieved

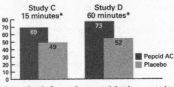

*Time taken before eating a meal that is expected to cause symptoms.

**Uses:**
• **For Relief** of heartburn, associated with acid indigestion, and sour stomach;
• **For Prevention** of heartburn associated with acid indigestion and sour stomach brought on by consuming food and beverages.

**Tips for Managing Heartburn:**
• Do not lie flat or bend over soon after eating.
• Do not eat late at night, or just before bedtime.
• Avoid food or drinks that are more likely to cause heartburn, such as rich, spicy, fatty, and fried foods, chocolate, caffeine, alcohol, and even some fruits and vegetables.
• Eat slowly and do not eat big meals.
• If you are overweight, lose weight.
• If you smoke, quit smoking.
• Raise the head of your bed.
• Wear loose fitting clothing around your stomach.

**Warnings:**
**Allergy alert** Do not use if you are allergic to famotidine or other acid reducers
**Do not use:**
• if you have trouble swallowing
• with other acid reducers
**Stop use and ask a doctor if:**
• stomach pain continues
• you need to take this product for more than 14 days
**If pregnant or breast-feeding,** ask a health professional before use.
**Keep out of reach of children.** In case of overdose, get medical help or contact a Poison Control Center right away.

**Directions:**
• Tablet: To relieve symptoms, swallow 1 tablet with a glass of water.

Chewable Tablet: To relieve symptoms, chew one tablet thoroughly
Gelcap: To relieve symptoms, swallow one gelcap with a glass of water.
• Tablet & Gelcap: To prevent symptoms, swallow one tablet or gelcap with a glass of water any time from 15 to 60 minutes before eating food or drinking beverages that cause heartburn.
• Chewable Tablet: To prevent symptoms, chew one chewable tablet before swallowing any time from 15 to 60 minutes before eating food or drinking beverages that cause heartburn.
• Can be used up to twice daily (up to 2 tablets or gelcaps in 24 hours).
• This product should not be given to children under 12 years old unless directed by a doctor.
**Other Information:**
• read the directions and warnings before use
• protect from moisture
• keep the carton and package insert, they contain important information
• store at 25°–33°C (77°–86°F)
in addition to the above the following also applies to the chewable tablet
• do not use if individual pouch is open or torn
• phenylketonurics: contains phenylalanine 1.4 mg per chewable tablet

**How Supplied:**
Pepcid AC Tablet is available as a rose-colored tablet identified as 'PEPCID AC'. NDC 16837-872
Pepcid AC Gelcap is available as a rose and white gelatin coated, capsule shaped tablet identified as 'PEPCID AC'. NDC 16837-856
Pepcid AC Chewable Tablet is available as a rose-colored chewable tablet identified as 'PEPCID AC'. NDC 16837-873
*Shown in Product Identification Guide, page 509*

---

## PEPCID® COMPLETE
**Acid Reducer + Antacid**
**with DUAL ACTION**
**Reduces and Neutralizes Acid**

**Description:** Pepcid Complete combines an acid reducer (famotidine) with antacids (calcium carbonate and magnesium hydroxide) to relieve heartburn in two different ways: Acid reducers decrease the production of new stomach acid; antacids neutralize acid that is already in the stomach. The active ingredients in PEPCID COMPLETE have been used for years to treat acid-related problems in millions of people safely and effectively.

**Uses:** To relieve heartburn associated with acid indigestion and sour stomach.

| Active Ingredients: (in each chewablet tablet) | Purpose: |
| --- | --- |
| Famotidine 10mg | Acid Reducer |
| Calcium Carbonate 800 mg | Antacid |
| Magnesium Hydroxide 165 mg | Antacid |

In clinical studies, PEPCID COMPLETE was significantly better than placebo pills in relieving heartburn.

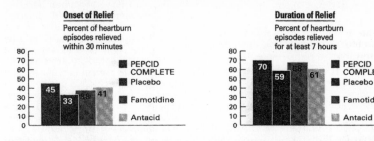

**Onset of Relief**

Percent of heartburn episodes relieved within 30 minutes

- PEPCID COMPLETE
- Placebo
- Famotidine
- Antacid

45 33 38 41

**Duration of Relief**

Percent of heartburn episodes relieved for at least 7 hours

- PEPCID COMPLETE
- Placebo
- Famotidine
- Antacid

70 59 68 61

### Inactive Ingredients:
Cellulose acetate, corn starch, dextrates, flavors, hydroxypropyl cellulose, hydroxypropyl methylcellulose, lactose, magnesium stearate, pregelatinized starch, red iron oxide, sodium lauryl sulfate, sugar

### Sodium Content:
Each chewable tablet contains 0.5 mg of sodium.

### Acid Neutralizing Capacity:
Each chewable tablet contains 21.7 mEq of acid neutralizing capacity.

### Action:
It is normal for the stomach to produce acid, especially after consuming food and beverages. However, acid in the stomach may move up into the wrong place (the esophagus), causing burning pain and discomfort that interfere with everyday activities.

**Heartburn—Caused by acid in the esophagus**
- Burning pain/discomfort in esophagus
- A valve-like muscle called the lower esophageal sphincter (LES) is relaxed in an open position
- Acid moves up from stomach

### PROVEN EFFECTIVE IN CLINICAL STUDIES
[See figure at top of page]

### Directions:
- Adults and children 12 years and over:
  - **do not swallow tablet whole; chew completely.**
  - to relieve symptoms, chew 1 tablet before swallowing.
  - do not use more than 2 chewable tablets in 24 hours.
- Children under 12 years: ask a doctor.

### Warnings:
- **Allergy alert:** Do not use if you are allergic to famotidine or other acid reducers.
- **Do not use:** if you have trouble swallowing.
- With other famotidine products or acid reducers.
- **Ask a doctor or pharmacist before use if you are** taking a prescription drug. Antacids may interact with certain prescription drugs.
- **Stop use and ask a doctor if** stomach pain continues
- You need to take this product for more than 14 days.
- **If pregnant or breast-feeding,** ask a health professional before use.
- **Keep out of reach of children.** In case of overdose, get medical help or contact a poison control center right away.

### Tips For Managing Heartburn
- Do not lie flat or bend over soon after eating.
- Do not eat late at night, or just before bedtime.
- Certain foods or drinks are more likely to cause heartburn, such as rich, spicy, fatty, and fried foods, chocolate, caffeine, alcohol, and even some fruits and vegetables.
- Eat slowly and do not eat big meals.
- If you are overweight, lose weight.
- If you smoke, quit smoking.
- Raise the head of your bed.
- Wear loose fitting clothing around your stomach.

### Other Information:
- read the directions and warnings before use.
- keep the carton and package insert. They contain important information.
- store at 25°–30°C (77—86 F).
- protect from moisture.

### How Supplied:
Pepcid Complete is available as a rose-colored chewable tablet identified by 'P'. NDC 16837-888

*Shown in Product Identification Guide, page 509*

---

## Lederle Consumer Health

**A Division of Whitehall-Robins Healthcare**
**FIVE GIRALDA FARMS**
**MADISON, NJ 07940**

**Direct Inquiries to:**
Lederle Consumer Product Information
(800) 282-8805

### FIBERCON®
*[fī-bĕr-cŏn ]*
**Calcium Polycarbophil**
**Bulk-Forming Laxative**

### Active ingredient
**(in each caplet):**
Calcium polycarbophil 625 mg (eqivalent to 500 mg polycarbophil)

### Inactive ingredients:
calcium carbonate, caramel, crospovidone, hydroxypropyl methylcellulose, magnesium stearate, microcrystalline cellulose, mineral oil, povidone, silica gel and sodium lauryl sulfate

### Uses:
- relieves constipation to help restore and maintain regularity
- this product generally produces bowel movement in 12 to 72 hours

### Directions:
- take this product (child or adult dose) with at least 8 ounces (a full glass) of water or other fluid Taking this product without enough liquid may cause choking See choking warning
- FiberCon works naturally so continued use for one to three days is normally required to provide full benefit Dosage may vary according to diet, exercise, previous laxative use or severity of constipation
[See table below]

### Warnings:
**Choking:** Taking this product without adequate fluid may cause it to swell and block your throat or esophagus and may cause choking. Do not take this product if you have difficulty in swallowing. If you experience chest pain, vomiting, or difficulty in swallowing or breathing after taking this product, seek immediate medical attention.

**Ask a doctor before use if you have:**
- abdominal pain, nausea, or vomiting
- a sudden change in bowel habits that persists over a period of 2 weeks

**When using this product:**
- do not use for more than 7 days unless directed by a doctor
- do not take caplets more than 4 times in a 24 hour period unless directed by a doctor

**Stop use and ask a doctor if** rectal bleeding occurs or if you fail to have a bowel movement after use of this or any other laxative These could be signs of a serious condition

**Drug Interaction precaution:** Each caplet contains 122mg calcium. If you are taking any form of tetracycline antibiotic, FiberCon should be taken at least 1 hour before or 2 hours after you have taken the antibiotic

**Keep out of reach of children.** In case of overdose, get medical help or contact a Poison Control Center right away

**Storage:** Protect contents from moisture. Store at 20–25°C (68–77°F)

**How Supplied:** Film-coated scored caplets.

Package of 36 caplets, and

Bottles of 60, 90 and 150 caplets.

| Age | Recommended dose | Daily maximum |
|---|---|---|
| adults & children over 12 | 2 caplets once a day | up to 4 times a day |
| children 6 to 12 years | 1 caplet once a day | up to 4 times a day |
| children under 6 years | consult a physician | |

# McNeil Consumer and Specialty Pharmaceuticals

### Division of McNeil-PPC, Inc.
### FORT WASHINGTON, PA 19034

**Direct Inquiries to:**
Consumer Relationship Center
Fort Washington, PA 19034
(215) 273-7000

## Maximum Strength GAS AID Softgels

**Description:** Each softgel of Maximum Strength GasAid contains simethicone 125 mg.

**Actions:** Simethicone acts in the stomach and intestines by altering the surface tension of gas bubbles enabling them to coalesce, thereby freeing and eliminating the gas more easily by belching or passing flatus.

**Uses:** Relieves bloating, pressure, fullness or stuffed feeling commonly referred to as gas.

**Directions:** Adults and children 12 years and over: take 1–2 softgels as needed after meals and at bedtime. Do not take more than 4 softgels in 24 hours unless directed by a doctor.

**Warnings**
Keep out of reach of children.

**Other Information:**
- do not use if carton or any blister unit is open or broken
- store at room temperature. Avoid high humidity and excessive heat (40°C).

**Inactive Ingredients:** D&C yellow #10, FD&C blue #1, FD&C red #40, gelatin, glycerin, peppermint oil, titanium dioxide.

**How Supplied:** Softgels in 12s, 24s, and 48s blister packaging. Each Maximum Strength GasAid softgel is oval, green in color, and imprinted with "I-G" on one side.

*Shown in Product Identification Guide, page 510*

## IMODIUM® A–D Liquid and Caplets
### (loperamide hydrochloride)

**Description:** Each 5 mL (teaspoon) of *IMODIUM® A-D* liquid contains loperamide hydrochloride 1 mg. *IMODIUM® A-D* liquid is stable, cherry-mint flavored, and clear in color.
Each caplet of *IMODIUM® A-D* contains 2 mg of loperamide and is scored and colored green.

**Actions:** *IMODIUM® A-D* contains a clinically proven antidiarrheal medication. Loperamide HCl acts by slowing intestinal motility and by affecting water and electrolyte movement through the bowel.

**Indication:** *IMODIUM® A-D* controls the symptoms of diarrhea, including Traveler's Diarrhea.

**Directions:** Use the enclosed cup to accurately measure Imodium® A-D Liquid. Drink plenty of clear fluids to help prevent dehydration, which may accompany diarrhea.
**ADULTS AND CHILDREN 12 YEARS OF AGE AND OLDER:** Take 4 teaspoonfuls (1 dosage cup) or 2 caplets after the first loose bowel movement and 2 teaspoonfuls or 1 caplet after each subsequent loose bowel movement but no more than 8 teaspoonfuls or 4 caplets a day for no more than 2 days.
**CHILDREN 9–11 YEARS OLD (60–95 LBS):** Take 2 teaspoonfuls (1/2 dosage cup) or 1 caplet after the first loose bowel movement and 1 teaspoonful or 1/2 caplet after each subsequent loose bowel movement but no more than 6 teaspoonfuls or 3 caplets a day for no more than 2 days.
**CHILDREN 6–8 YEARS OLD (48–59 LBS):** Take 2 teaspoonfuls (1/2 dosage cup) or 1 caplet after the first loose bowel movement and 1 teaspoonful or 1/2 caplet after each subsequent loose bowel movement but no more than 4 teaspoonfuls or 2 caplets a day for no more than 2 days. Professional Dosage Schedule for children 2–5 years old (24–47 lbs): 1 teaspoonful after first loose bowel movement, followed by 1 after each subsequent loose bowel movement. Do not exceed 3 teaspoonfuls a day.

**Warnings: KEEP THIS AND ALL DRUGS OUT OF THE REACH OF CHILDREN.** Do not use for more than two days unless directed by a physician. **DO NOT USE IF DIARRHEA IS ACCOMPANIED BY HIGH FEVER (GREATER THAN 101°F), OR IF BLOOD OR MUCUS IS PRESENT IN THE STOOL, OR IF YOU HAVE HAD A RASH OR OTHER ALLERGIC REACTION TO LOPERAMIDE HCl.** If you are taking antibiotics or have a history of liver disease, consult a physician before using this product. As with any drug, if you are pregnant or nursing a baby, seek the advice of a health professional before using this product. In case of accidental overdose, seek professional assistance or contact a poison control center immediately.

**Professional Information:**
**Overdosage Information** Overdosage of loperamide HCl in man may result in constipation, CNS depression and nausea. A slurry of activated charcoal administered promptly after ingestion of loperamide hydrochloride can reduce the amount of drug which is absorbed. If vomiting occurs spontaneously upon ingestion, a slurry of 100 grams of activated charcoal should be administered orally as soon as fluids can be retained. If vomiting has not occurred, and CNS depression is evident, gastric lavage should be performed followed by administration of 100 gms of the activated charcoal slurry through the gastric tube. In the event of overdosage, patients should be monitored for signs of CNS depression for at least 24 hours. Children may be more sensitive to central nervous system effects than adults. If CNS depression is observed, naloxone may be administered. If responsive to naloxone, vital signs must be monitored carefully for recurrence of symptoms of drug overdose for at least 24 hours after the last dose of naloxone.

**Inactive Ingredients:**
**Liquid:** Benzoic acid, citric acid, flavors, glycerin, propylene glycol, purified water, sodium benzoate, sorbitol, sucrose, contains 0.5% alcohol.
**Caplets:** Dibasic calcium phosphate, magnesium stearate, microcrystalline cellulose, colloidal silicon dioxide, FD&C Blue #1 and D&C Yellow #10.

**How Supplied: Liquid:** Cherry-mint flavored liquid (clear) 2 fl. oz. and 4 fl. oz. tamper evident bottles with child resistant safety caps and special dosage cups. Store between 20–25 °C (68–77 °F). Avoid excessive heat.
**Caplets:** Green scored caplets in 6s, 12s, 18s, 24s, 48s and 72s blister packaging which is tamper evident and child resistant. Store at 15–30°C (59–86°F)

*Shown in Product Identification Guide, page 510*

## IMODIUM® ADVANCED
### Caplets & Chewable Tablets
### (loperamide HCl/simethicone)

**Description:** Each easy to swallow caplet and mint-flavored chewable tablet of *Imodium® Advanced* contains loperamide HCl 2 mg/simethicone 125 mg.

**Actions:** *Imodium® Advanced* combines original prescription strength Imodium® to control the symptoms of diarrhea plus simethicone to relieve bloating, pressure and cramps commonly referred to as gas. Loperamide HCl acts by slowing intestinal motility and by affecting water and electrolyte movement through the bowel. Simethicone acts in the stomach and intestines by altering the surface tension of gas bubbles enabling them to coalesce, thereby freeing and eliminating the gas more easily by belching or passing flatus.

**Uses:** Controls the symptoms of diarrhea plus bloating, pressure, and cramps commonly referred to as gas.

**Directions:** Swallow (caplet)/chew (tablet) the first dose and take with water after the first loose stool. If needed, swallow/chew the next dose and take with water after the next loose stool. Drink plenty of clear liquids to prevent dehydration.

**Adults aged 12 years and over:** Swallow (caplet)/chew (tablet) 2 caplets/tablets and take with water after the first loose stool. If needed, swallow/chew 1 caplet/tablet and take with water after the next loose stool. Do not exceed 4 caplets/tablets a day.

**Children 9-11 years (60-95 lbs):** Swallow (caplet)/chew (tablet) 1 caplet/tablet and take with water after the first loose stool. If needed, swallow/chew 1/2 tablet and take with water after the next loose stool. Do not exceed 3 caplets/tablets a day.

**Children 6-8 years (48-59 lbs):** Swallow (caplet)/chew (tablet) 1 caplet/tablet and take with water after the first loose stool. If needed, swallow/chew 1/2 caplet/tablet and take with water after the next loose stool. Do not exceed 2 caplets/tablets a day.

**Children under 6 years old (up to 47 lbs):** Consult a physician. Not intended for use in children under 6 years old.

**Warnings:**
**Do Not Use If:**
• You have a high fever (over 101° F)
• Blood or mucus is in your stool
• You have had a rash or other allergic reaction to Loperamide HCl
**Do Not Use Without Asking A Doctor:**
• For more than 2 days
• If you are taking antibiotics
• If you have a history of liver disease
As with any drug, If you are pregnant or nursing a baby, seek the advice of a health professional before using this product.
• **Keep this and all drugs out of the reach of children.**
• In case of accidental overdose, seek professional assistance or call a poison control center immediately.

**Professional Information:**
**Overdosage Information** Overdosage of loperamide HCl in man may result in constipation, CNS depression and nausea. A slurry of activated charcoal administered promptly after ingestion of loperamide hydrochloride can reduce the amount of drug which is absorbed. If vomiting occurs spontaneously upon ingestion, a slurry of 100 grams of activated charcoal should be administered orally as soon as fluids can be retained. If vomiting has not occurred, and CNS depression is evident, gastric lavage should be performed followed by administration of 100 gms of the activated charcoal slurry through the gastric tube. In the event of overdosage, patients should be monitored for signs of CNS depression for at least 24 hours. Children may be more sensitive to central nervous system effects than adults. If CNS depression is observed, naloxone may be administered. If responsive to naloxone, vital signs must be monitored carefully for recurrence of symptoms of drug overdose for at least 24 hours after the last dose of naloxone. No treatment is necessary for the simethicone ingestion in this circumstance.

**Inactive Ingredients:**
**Caplets:** acesulfame K, cellulose, dibasic calcium phosphate, flavor, sodium starch glycolate, stearic acid **Chewable Tablets:** Cellulose acetate, corn starch, D&C Yellow No. 10, dextrates, FD&C Blue No. 1, flavors, microcrystalline cellulose, polymethacrylates, saccharin sodium, sorbitol, stearic acid, sucrose, tribasic calcium phosphate.

**How Supplied:**
Mint Chewable Tablets in 6's, 12's, 18's, 30's, and 42's blister packaging which is tamper evident and child resistant. Each Imodium® Advanced tablet is round, light green in color and has "IMODIUM" embossed on one side and "2/125" on the other side.
Store at 15–30°C (59–86°F). Imodium Advanced Caplets are available in blister packs of 12's and 18's and bottles of 30's and 42's.

*Shown in Product Identification Guide, page 510*

---

**MOTRIN® IB ibuprofen Pain Reliever/Fever Reducer**

**Tablets, Caplets and Gelcaps**

**Description:** Each *MOTRIN® IB Tablet, Caplet and Gelcap* contains ibuprofen 200 mg.

**Indications:** *MOTRIN® IB Tablets, Caplets and Gelcaps:* For the temporary relief of headache, muscular aches, the minor pain of arthritis, toothache, backache, minor aches and pains associated with the common cold, the pain of menstrual cramps, and for reduction of fever.

**Directions:** **Do not take more than directed. Adults:** Take 1 tablet, caplet or gelcap every 4 to 6 hours while symptoms persist. If pain or fever does not respond to 1 tablet, caplet or gelcap, 2 tablets, caplets or gelcaps may be used, but do not exceed 6 tablets, caplets or gelcaps in 24 hours, unless directed by a doctor. The smallest effective dose should be used. Take with food or milk if occasional and mild heartburn, upset stomach or stomach pain occurs with use. Consult a doctor if these symptoms are more than mild or if they persist. **Children:** Do not give this product to children under 12 except under the advice and supervision of a doctor.

**Warnings:** Do not take for pain for more than 10 days or for fever for more than 3 days unless directed by a doctor. If pain or fever persists or gets worse, if new symptoms occur, or if the painful area is red or swollen, consult a doctor. These could be signs of a serious illness. If you are under a doctor's care for any serious condition, consult a doctor before taking this product. As with aspirin and acetaminophen, if you have any condition which requires you to take prescription drugs, or if you have had any problems or serious side effects from taking any non-prescription pain reliever, do not take MOTRIN® IB without first discussing it with your doctor. If you experience any symptoms which are unusual or seem unrelated to the condition for which you took ibuprofen, consult a doctor before taking any more of it. Although ibuprofen is indicated for the same conditions as aspirin and acetaminophen, it should not be taken with them except under a doctor's direction. Do not combine this product with any other ibuprofen-containing product. Keep this and all drugs out of the reach of children. In case of accidental overdose, seek professional assistance or contact a poison control center immediately. As with any drug, if you are pregnant or nursing a baby, seek the advice of a health professional before using this product. IT IS ESPECIALLY IMPORTANT NOT TO USE IBUPROFEN DURING THE LAST 3 MONTHS OF PREGNANCY UNLESS SPECIFICALLY DIRECTED TO DO SO BY A DOCTOR BECAUSE IT MAY CAUSE PROBLEMS IN THE UNBORN CHILD OR COMPLICATIONS DURING DELIVERY.
**Allergy Alert:** ibuprofen may cause a severe allergic reaction which may include:
• hives • facial swelling
• asthma (wheezing) • shock
**Do not use** if you have ever had an allergic reaction to any other pain reliever/fever reducer.
**Stop use and ask a doctor if** an allergic reaction occurs. Seek medical help right away.

**Alcohol Warning:** If you consume 3 or more alcoholic drinks every day, ask your doctor whether you should take ibuprofen or other pain relievers/fever reducers. Ibuprofen may cause stomach bleeding.

**Professional Information:**
**Overdosage Information for Adult Motrin®**
**IBUPROFEN**
The *toxicity of ibuprofen* overdose is dependent upon the amount of drug ingested and the time elapsed since ingestion, though individual response may vary, which makes it necessary to evaluate each case individually. Although uncommon, serious toxicity and death have been reported in the medical literature with ibuprofen overdosage. The most frequently reported symptoms of ibuprofen overdose include abdominal pain, nausea, vomiting, lethargy and drowsiness. Other central nervous system symptoms include headache, tinnitus, CNS depression and seizures. Metabolic acidosis, coma, acute renal failure and apnea (primarily in very young children) may rarely occur. Cardiovascular toxicity, including hypotension, bradycardia, tachycardia and atrial fibrillation, also have been reported. The *treatment of acute ibuprofen overdose* is primarily supportive. Management of hypotension, acidosis and gastrointestinal bleeding may be necessary. In cases of acute overdose, the stomach should be emptied through ipe-

*Continued on next page*

## Motrin IB—Cont.

cac-induced emesis or lavage. Emesis is most effective if initiated within 30 minutes of ingestion. Orally administered activated charcoal may help in reducing the absorption and reabsorption of ibuprofen. In children, the estimated amount of ibuprofen ingested per body weight may be helpful to predict the potential for development of toxicity although each case must be evaluated. Ingestion of less than 100 mg/kg is unlikely to produce toxicity. Children ingesting 100 to 200 mg/kg may be managed with induced emesis and a minimal observation time of four hours. Children ingesting 200 to 400 mg/kg of ibuprofen should have immediate gastric emptying and at least four hours observation in a health care facility. Children ingesting greater than 400 mg/kg require immediate medical referral, careful observation and appropriate supportive therapy. Ipecac-induced emesis is not recommended in overdoses greater than 400 mg/kg because of the risk of convulsions and the potential for aspiration of gastric contents. In adult patients the history of the dose reportedly ingested does not appear to be predictive of toxicity. The need for referral and follow-up must be judged by the circumstances at the time of the overdose ingestion. Symptomatic adults should be admitted to a health care facility for observation.

**Our Adult MOTRIN® combination products contain pseudoephedrine in addition to ibuprofen. For basic overdose information regarding pseudoephedrine, please see below. For additional emergency information, please contact your local poison control center.**

**PSEUDOEPHEDRINE**

Symptoms from pseudoephedrine overdose consist most often of mild anxiety, tachycardia and/or mild hypertension. Symptoms usually appear within 4 to 8 hours and are transient, usually requiring no treatment.

**Inactive Ingredients: Tablets and Caplets**: Carnauba wax, corn starch, FD&C Yellow #6, hydroxypropyl methylcellulose, iron oxide, polydextrose, polyethylene glycol, silicon dioxide, stearic acid, titanium dioxide.

**Gelcaps:** Benzyl alcohol, butylparaben, butyl alcohol, castor oil, colloidal silicon dioxide, cornstarch, edetate calcium disodium, FDC Yellow No. 6, gelatin, hydroxypropyl methylcellulose, iron oxide black, magnesium stearate, methylparaben, microcrystalline cellulose, povidone, pregelatinized starch, propylene glycol, propylparaben, SDA 3A alcohol, sodium lauryl sulfate, sodium propionate, sodium starch glycolate, and titanium dioxide.

**How Supplied: Tablets**: (orange, printed "MOTRIN IB" in black) in tamper evident packaging of 24, 50, 100, and 165. Store between 20°–25° C (68°–77° F)

**Caplets:** (orange, printed "MOTRIN IB" in black) in tamper evident packaging of 24, 50, 60, 100, 130, 165, 250, 300 and 500. Store between 20°–25° C (68°–77° F)

**Gelcaps:** (colored orange and white, printed "MOTRIN IB" in black) in tamper evident packaging of 24, 50 and 100. Store between 20–25° C (68–77° F)

*Shown in Product Identification Guide, page 511*

---

## MOTRIN® Sinus/Headache Caplets

**Description:** Each MOTRIN® Sinus/Headache Caplet contains ibuprofen 200 mg and pseudoephedrine HCl 30 mg.

**Uses:** temporarily relieves these symptoms associated with sinusitis, the common cold or flu:
• nasal congestion • headache
• body aches and pains • fever

**Directions:**
• **Do not take more than directed. Adults and children 12 years and older:**
• take 1 caplet every 4 to 6 hours while symptoms persist
• if symptoms do not respond to 1 caplet, 2 caplets may be used, but do not take more than 6 caplets in 24 hours, unless directed by a doctor
• the smallest effective dose should be used
**Children under 12 years:** ask a doctor.

**Warnings: Allergy alert:** Ibuprofen may cause a severe allergic reaction which may include:
• hives • facial swelling
• asthma (wheezing) • shock
**Alcohol warning:** If you consume 3 or more alcoholic drinks every day, ask your doctor whether you should take ibuprofen or other pain relievers/fever reducers. Ibuprofen may cause stomach bleeding.
**Do not use**
• if you are now taking a prescription monoamine oxidase inhibitor (MAOI) (certain drugs for depression, psychiatric or emotional conditions, or Parkinson's disease), or for 2 weeks after stopping the MAOI drug. If you do not know if your prescription drug contains an MAOI, ask a doctor or pharmacist before taking this product.
• if you have ever had an allergic reaction to any other pain reliever/fever reducer
**Ask a doctor before use if you have**
• heart disease • high blood pressure
• thyroid disease • diabetes
• trouble urinating due to an enlarged prostate gland
• stomach pain • problems or serious side effects from taking pain relievers or fever reducers
**Ask a doctor or pharmacist before use if you are**
• under a doctor's care for any serious condition
• taking any other drug
• taking any other product that contains ibuprofen, or any other pain reliever/fever reducer

**When using this product**
• do not exceed recommended dosage
• give with food or milk of stomach upset occurs
**Stop use and ask a doctor if**
• an allergic reaction occurs. Seek medical help right away.
• any new symptoms appear
• redness or swelling is present in the painful area
• you get nervous, dizzy or sleepless
• stomach pain or upset gets worse or lasts
• pain gets worse or lasts more than 7 days
• fever gets worse or lasts more than 3 days
**If pregnant or breast-feeding,** ask a health professional before use. It is especially important not to use ibuprofen during the last 3 months of pregnancy unless definitely directed to do so by a doctor because it may cause problems in the unborn child or complications during delivery.
**Keep out of reach of children.** In case of overdose, get medical help or contact a Poison Control Center right away.
**Other Information:**
• do not use if blister unit is broken or open
• Store at 20–25°C (68–77°F). Avoid excessive heat.

**Professional Information:**
**Overdosage Information**
For overdosage information, please refer to pgs. 667–668.

**Inactive Ingredients: Caplets:** carnauba wax, cellulose, corn starch, FD&C Red #40, hydroxypropyl methylcellulose, silicon dioxide, sodium lauryl sulfate, sodium starch glycolate, stearic acid, titanium dioxide, triacetin.

**How Supplied: Caplets:** (white, printed "Motrin Sinus/Headache" in red) in blister packs of 20 and 40.

*Shown in Product Identification Guide, page 511*

---

**Infants' MOTRIN® ibuprofen Concentrated Drops**

**Children's MOTRIN® ibuprofen Oral Suspension and Chewable Tablets**

**Junior Strength MOTRIN® ibuprofen Caplets and Chewable Tablets**

Product information for all dosages of Children's MOTRIN have been combined under this heading

**Description:** *Infants' MOTRIN® Concentrated Drops* are available in an alcohol-free, berry-flavored suspension and a non-staining, dye-free, berry-flavored suspension. Each 1.25 mL contains ibuprofen 50 mg. *Children's MOTRIN® Oral Suspension* is available as an alcohol-free, berry, dye-free berry, bubblegum or grape-flavored suspension. Each 5 mL (teaspoon) of *Children's MOTRIN® Oral Suspension* contains ibuprofen 100 mg. Each *Children's MOTRIN® Chewable Tablet* contains 50 mg of ibuprofen and is available as orange or grape-flavored chewable tablets. *Junior Strength MOTRIN® Chewable Tablets* and *Junior Strength MOTRIN® Caplets* contain ibuprofen 100 mg. *Junior Strength MOTRIN® Chewable Tablets* are available in orange or grape flavors. *Junior Strength MOTRIN® Caplets* are available as easy-to-swallow caplets (capsule-shaped tablet).

**Uses:** temporarily:
• reduces fever
• relieves minor aches and pains due to the common cold, flu, sore throat, headaches and toothaches

**Directions:** See Table 2: Children's Motrin Dosing Chart on pg. 671.

**Warnings:**
**Allergy alert:** Ibuprofen may cause a severe allergic reaction which may include:
• hives • facial swelling
• asthma (wheezing) • shock
**Sore throat warning:** Severe or persistent sore throat or sore throat accompanied by high fever, headache, nausea, and vomiting may be serious. Consult doctor promptly. Do not use more than 2 days or administer to children under 3 years of age unless directed by doctor.
**Do not use** if the child has ever had an allergic reaction to any other fever reducer/pain reliever
**Ask a doctor before use if the child has**
• not been drinking fluids
• lost a lot of fluid due to continued vomiting or diarrhea
• stomach pain
• problems or serious side effects from taking fever reducers or pain relievers
**Ask a doctor or pharmacist before use if the child**
• under a doctor's care for any serious condition
• taking any other drug
• taking any other product that contains ibuprofen, or any other fever reducer/pain reliever
**When using this product**
• mouth or throat burning may occur; give with food or water (*Children's MOTRIN® Chewable Tablets and Junior Strength MOTRIN® Chewable Tablets* only)
• give with food or milk if stomach upset occurs
**Stop use and ask a doctor if**
• an allergic reaction occurs. Seek medical help right away.
• fever or pain gets worse or lasts more than 3 days
• the child does not get any relief within first day (24 hours) of treatment
• stomach pain or upset gets worse or lasts
• redness or swelling is present in the painful area
• any new symptoms appear
**Keep out of reach of children.** In case of overdose, get medical help or contact a Poison Control Center right away.

**Other Information:**
*Infants', Children's and Junior Strength MOTRIN® products:*
• Store at 20–25°C (68–77°F)

*Infants' MOTRIN® Concentrated Drops:*
• **do not use if plastic carton wrap or bottle wrap imprinted "Safety Seal®" is broken or missing.**
*Children's MOTRIN® Suspension Liquid:*
• **do not use if plastic carton wrap or bottle wrap imprinted "Safety Seal®" is broken or missing**
*Children's MOTRIN® Chewable Tablets:*
• Phenylketonurics: Contains phenylalanine 1.4 mg per tablet
• **do not use if neck wrap or foil inner seal imprinted "Safety Seal®" is broken or missing**
*Junior Strength MOTRIN® Caplets and Chewable Tablets:*
• phenylketonurics: contains phenylalanine 2.8 mg per tablet (tablet only)
• **do not use if neck wrap or foil inner seal imprinted "Safety Seal®" is broken or missing**

**Professional Information:**
**Overdosage Information for all Infants', Children's & Junior Strength Motrin® Products**
**IBUPROFEN:** The *toxicity of ibuprofen* overdose is dependent upon the amount of drug ingested and the time elapsed since ingestion, though individual response may vary, which makes it necessary to evaluate each case individually. Although uncommon, serious toxicity and death have been reported in the medical literature with ibuprofen overdosage. The most frequently reported symptoms of ibuprofen overdose include abdominal pain, nausea, vomiting, lethargy and drowsiness. Other central nervous system symptoms include headache, tinnitus, CNS depression and seizures. Metabolic acidosis, coma, acute renal failure and apnea (primarily in very young children) may rarely occur. Cardiovascular toxicity, including hypotension, bradycardia, tachycardia and atrial fibrillation, also have been reported.
The *treatment of acute ibuprofen overdose* is primarily supportive. Management of hypotension, acidosis and gastrointestinal bleeding may be necessary. In cases of acute overdose, the stomach should be emptied through ipecac-induced emesis or lavage. Emesis is most effective if initiated within 30 minutes of ingestion. Orally administered activated charcoal may help in reducing the absorption and reabsorption of ibuprofen. In children, the estimated amount of ibuprofen ingested per body weight may be helpful to predict the potential for development of toxicity although each case must be evaluated. Ingestion of less than 100 mg/kg is unlikely to produce toxicity. Children ingesting 100 to 200 mg/kg may be managed with induced emesis and a minimal observation time of four hours. Children ingesting 200 to 400 mg/kg of ibuprofen should have immediate gastric emptying and at least four hours observation in a health care facility. Children ingesting greater than 400 mg/kg require immediate medical referral, careful observation and appropriate supportive therapy. Ipecac-induced emesis is not recommended in overdoses greater than 400 mg/kg because of the risk of convulsions and the

potential for aspiration of gastric contents.
In adults patients the history of the dose reportedly ingested does not appear to be predictive of toxicity. The need for referral and follow-up must be judged by the circumstances at the time of the overdose ingestion. Symptomatic adults should be admitted to a health care facility for observation.
**Our Children's MOTRIN® Cold products contain pseudoephedrine in addition to ibuprofen. The following is basic overdose information regarding pseudoephedrine.**
**PSEUDOEPHEDRINE:** Symptoms from pseudoephedrine overdose consist most often of mild anxiety, tachycardia and/or mild hypertension. Symptoms usually appear within 4 to 8 hours of ingestion and are transient, usually requiring no treatment.
**For additional emergency information, please contact your local poison control center.**

**Inactive Ingredients:** *Infants' MOTRIN® Concentrated Drops:* Berry-Flavored: citric acid, corn starch, FD&C Red #40, flavors, glycerin polysorbate 80, purified water, sodium benzoate, sorbitol, sucrose, xanthan gum. **Dye-Free Berry-Flavored:** artificial flavors, citric acid, corn starch, glycerin, polysorbate 80, purified water, sodium benzoate, sorbitol, sucrose, xanthan gum.
*Children's MOTRIN® Oral Suspension:* **Berry-Flavored:** acesulfame potassium, citric acid, corn starch, D&C Yellow #10, FD&C Red #40, glycerin, natural and artificial flavors, polysorbate 80, purified water, sodium benzoate, sucrose, xanthan gum. **Dye-Free Berry-Flavored:** acesulfame potassium, citric acid, corn starch, glycerin, natural and artificial flavors, polysorbate 80, purified water, sodium benzoate, sucrose, xanthan gum. **Bubble Gum-Flavored:** acesulfame potassium, citric acid, corn starch, FD&C Red #40, glycerin, natural and artificial flavors, polysorbate 80, purified water, sodium benzoate, sucrose, xanthan gum. **Grape-Flavored:** acesulfame potassium, citric acid, corn starch, D&C Red #33, FD&C Blue #1, FD&C Red #40, glycerin, natural and artificial flavors, polysorbate 80, purified water, sodium benzoate, sucrose, xanthan gum.
*Children's MOTRIN® Chewable Tablets:* **Orange-Flavored:** acesulfame K, aspartame, cellulose, citric acid, FD&C Yellow #6, flavor, fumaric acid, hydroxyethyl cellulose, hydroxypropyl methylcellulose, magnesium stearate, mannitol, povidone, sodium lauryl sulfate, sodium starch glycolate. **Grape-Flavored:** acesulfame K, aspartame, cellulose, citric acid, D&C Red #7, D&C Red #30, FD&C Blue #1, flavor, fumaric acid, hydroxyethyl cellulose, hydroxypropyl methylcellulose, magnesium stearate, mannitol, povidone, sodium lauryl sulfate, sodium starch glycolate.
*Junior Strength MOTRIN® Chewable Tablets:* **Orange-Flavored:** acesulfame K, aspartame, cellulose, citric acid,

*Continued on next page*

## Motrin Infants'—Cont.

FD&C yellow #6, flavor, fumaric acid, hydroxyethyl cellulose, hydroxypropyl methylcellulose, magnesium stearate, mannitol, povidone, sodium lauryl sulfate, sodium starch glycolate. **Grape-Flavored:** acesulfame K, aspartame, cellulose, citric acid, D&C Red #7, D&C Red #30, FD&C Blue #1, flavor, fumaric acid, hydroxyethyl cellulose, hydroxypropyl methylcellulose, magnesium stearate, mannitol, povidone, sodium lauryl sulfate, sodium starch glycolate. **Easy-To-Swallow Caplets:** carnauba wax, cellulose, corn starch, D&C Yellow #10, FD&C Yellow #6, hydroxypropyl methylcellulose, polydextrose, polyethylene glycol, propylene glycol, silicon dioxide, sodium starch glycolate, titanium dioxide, triacetin.

**How Supplied:** *Infants' MOTRIN® Concentrated Drops:* Berry-flavored, pink-colored liquid and Berry-Flavored, Dye-Free, white-colored liquid in ½ fl. oz. bottles.
*Children's MOTRIN® Oral Suspension:* Berry-flavored, pink-colored; Berry-Flavored, Dye-Free white-colored, Bubble Gum-flavored, pink-colored and Grape-flavored, purple-colored liquid in tamper evident bottles of 2 and 4 fl. oz.
*Children's MOTRIN® Chewable Tablets:* Orange-flavored, orange-colored and Grape-flavored, purple-colored chewable tablets in 24 count bottles.
*Junior Strength MOTRIN® Chewable Tablets:* Orange-flavored, orange-colored chewable tablets or Grape-flavored, purple-colored chewable tablets in 24 count bottles.
*Junior Strength MOTRIN® Caplets:* Easy-to-swallow caplets (capsule shaped tablets) in 24 count bottles.
*Shown in Product Identification Guide, page 510*

## Children's MOTRIN® Cold ibuprofen/pseudoephedrine HCl Oral Suspension

**Description:** *Children's MOTRIN® Cold Oral Suspension* is an alcohol-free berry, dye-free berry, or grape-flavored suspension. Each 5 mL (teaspoonful) contains the pain reliever/fever reducer ibuprofen 100 mg and the nasal decongestant pseudoephedrine HCl 15 mg.

**Uses:** temporarily relieves these cold, sinus and flu symptoms:
•nasal and sinus congestion
•stuffy nose •headache •sore throat
•minor body aches and pains •fever

**Directions:** See Table 2: Children's Motrin Dosing Chart on pg. 671.

**Warnings: Allergy alert:** Ibuprofen may cause a severe allergic reaction which may include:
•hives •facial swelling
•asthma (wheezing) •shock
**Sore throat warning:** Severe or persistent sore throat or sore throat accompanied by high fever, headache, nausea, and vomiting may be serious. Consult a doctor promptly. Do not use more than

2 days or administer to children under 3 years of age unless directed by doctor.
**Do not use**
• if the child has ever had an allergic reaction to any other pain reliever/fever reducer and/or nasal decongestant
• in a child who is taking a prescription monoamine oxidase inhibitor [MAOI] (certain drugs for depression, psychiatric or emotional conditions, or Parkinson's disease), or for 2 weeks after stopping the MAOI drug. If you do not know if your child's prescription drug contains an MAOI, ask a doctor or pharmacist before giving this product.
**Ask a doctor before use if the child has**
• not been drinking fluids
• lost a lot of fluid due to continued vomiting or diarrhea
• problems or serious side effects from taking pain relievers, fever reducers or nasal decongestants
• stomach pain
• heart disease
• high blood pressure
• thyroid disease
• diabetes
**Ask a doctor or pharmacist before use if the child is**
• under a doctor's care for any continuing medical condition
• taking any other drug
• taking any other product that contains ibuprofen or pseudoephedrine
• taking any other pain reliever/fever reducer and/or nasal decongestant
**When using this product**
• **do not exceed recommended dosage**
• give with food or milk if stomach upset occurs
**Stop use and ask a doctor if**
• an allergic reaction occurs. Seek medical help right away.
• the child does not get any relief within first day (24 hours) of treatment
• fever, pain or nasal congestion gets worse, or lasts for more than 3 days
• stomach pain or upset gets worse or lasts
• symptoms continue or get worse
• redness or swelling is present in the painful area
• the child gets nervous, dizzy, sleepless or sleepy
• any new symptoms appear
**Keep out of reach of children.** In case of overdose, get medical help or contact a Poison Control Center right away.
**Other Information:**
• **do not use if plastic carton wrap or bottle wrap imprinted "Safety Seal®" is broken or missing.**
• Store at 20–25°C (68–77°F)

**Professional Information:**
**Overdosage Information**
For overdosage information, please refer to pg. 669.

**Inactive Ingredients: Berry Flavor:** acesulfame potassium, citric acid, corn starch, D&C yellow #10, FD&C red #40, flavors, glycerin, polysorbate 80, purified water, sodium benzoate, sucrose, xanthan gum. **Dye-Free Berry Flavor:** acesulfame potassium, citric acid, corn starch, flavors, glycerin, polysorbate 80, purified water, sodium benzoate, sucrose, xanthan gum. **Grape Flavor:** acesulfame potassium, citric acid, corn starch, D&C red #33, FD&C blue #1, FD&C red #40, flavors, glycerin, polysorbate 80, purified water, sodium benzoate, sucrose, xanthan gum.

**How Supplied:** Berry-flavored, pink-colored, Grape-flavored, purple-colored, and Dye-Free Berry-flavored, white-colored liquid in tamper evident bottles of 4 fl. oz.
*Shown in Product Identification Guide, page 510*

## Children's Motrin® Dosing Chart
[See table at top of next page]

## MOTRIN® MIGRAINE PAIN CAPLETS

**Description:** Each *Motrin® Migraine Pain Caplet* contains ibuprofen 200 mg.

**Use:** treats pain of migraine headache

**Directions:**
Adults:
• take 1 or 2 caplets with a glass of water
• the smallest effective dose should be used
• if symptoms persist or worsen, ask your doctor
• do not take more than 2 caplets in 24 hours for pain of migraine unless directed by a doctor
Under 18 years of age:
• ask a doctor

**Warnings:**
**Allergy alert:** ibuprofen may cause a severe allergic reaction which may include:
• hives • facial swelling
• asthma (wheezing) • shock
**Alcohol warning:** If you consume 3 or more alcoholic drinks every day, ask your doctor whether you should take ibuprofen or other pain relievers/fever reducers. Ibuprofen may cause stomach bleeding.
**Do not use** if you have ever had an allergic reaction to any other pain relievers/fever reducer
**Ask a doctor before use if you have**
• never had migraines diagnosed by a health professional
• a headache that is different from your usual migraines
• the worst headache of your life
• fever and stiff neck
• headaches beginning after or caused by head injury, exertion, coughing or bending
• experienced your first headache after the age of 50
• daily headaches
• a migraine headache so severe as to require bed rest
• problems or serious side effects from taking pain relievers or fever reducers
• stomach pain
• vomiting with your migraine headache
**Ask a doctor or pharmacist before use if you are**
• under a doctor's care for any serious condition
• taking any other drug
• taking any other product that contains ibuprofen, or any other pain reliever/fever reducer
**Stop use and ask a doctor if**
• an allergic reaction occurs. Seek medical help right away.
• migraine headache pain is not relieved or gets worse after first dose

Table 2. Children's Motrin Dosing Chart

| PRODUCT FORM | INGREDIENTS | 0-5 mos* | 6-11 mos | 12-23 mos | 2-3 yrs | 4-5 yrs | 6-8 yrs | 9-10 yrs | 11 yrs | Maximum doses/ 24 hrs |
|---|---|---|---|---|---|---|---|---|---|---|
| **AGE GROUP*** | | 0-5 mos* | 6-11 mos | 12-23 mos | 2-3 yrs | 4-5 yrs | 6-8 yrs | 9-10 yrs | 11 yrs | Maximum doses/ 24 hrs |
| **WEIGHT** | (if possible use weight to dose; otherwise use age) | 6-11 lbs | 12-17 lbs | 18-23 lbs | 24-35 lbs | 36-47 lbs | 48-59 lbs | 60-71 lbs | 72-95 lbs | |
| **INGREDIENTS** Dose to be administered based on weight or age† | | | | | | | | | | |
| **Infants' Drops** Per 1.25 mL | | | | | | | | | | |
| **Infants' Motrin** Concentrated Drops Berry Flavor & Dye-Free Berry Flavor | Ibuprofen 50 mg | — | 1.25 mL | 1.875 mL | — | — | — | — | — | 4 times in 24 hrs |
| **Children's Liquid** Per 5 mL teaspoonful (TSP) | | | | | | | | | | |
| **Children's Motrin** Suspension | Ibuprofen 100 mg | — | — | — | 1 TSP | 1 ½ TSP | 2 TSP | 2 ½ TSP | 3 TSP | 4 times in 24 hrs |
| **Children's Motrin Cold** Suspension Liquid† | Ibuprofen 100 mg Pseudoephedrine 15 mg | — | — | — | 1 TSP | 1 TSP | 2 TSP | 2 TSP | 2 TSP | 4 times in 24 hrs |
| **Children's Tablets & Caplets** Per tablet/ caplet | | | | | | | | | | |
| **Children's Motrin** Chewable Tablets | Ibuprofen 50 mg | — | — | — | 2 tablets | 3 tablets | 4 tablets | 5 tablets | 6 tablets | 4 times in 24 hrs |
| **Junior Strength Motrin** Chewable Tablets | Ibuprofen 100 mg | — | — | — | — | — | 2 tablets | 2 ½ tablets | 3 tablets | 4 times in 24 hrs |
| **Junior Strength Motrin Caplets** | Ibuprofen 100 mg | — | — | — | — | — | 2 caplets | 2 ½ caplets | 3 caplets | 4 times in 24 hrs |

†Do not give, take or chew more than directed. If needed, repeat dose every 6-8 hours; except for Children's Motrin Cold which is every 6 hours.
* Under 6 mos, call a doctor.
- Infants' Motrin Drops are more concentrated than Children's Motrin Liquids. The Infants' Concentrated Drops have been specifically designed for use only with enclosed dosing device. Do not use any other dosing device with this product.
- Children's Motrin Liquids are less concentrated than Infants' Motrin Drops. The Children's Motrin Liquids have been specifically designed for use with the enclosed measuring cup. Use only enclosed measuring cup to dose this product.
- Children's Motrin Chewable Tablets are not the same concentration as Junior Strength Motrin Chewable Tablets.
- Junior Strength Motrin Chewable Tablets contain twice as much medicine as Children's Motrin Chewable Tablets.

## Motrin Migraine—Cont.

- stomach pain or upset gets worse or lasts
- new or unexpected symptoms occur

**If pregnant or breast-feeding,** ask a health professional before use. It is especially important not to use ibuprofen during the last 3 months of pregnancy unless definitely directed to do so by a doctor because it may cause problems in the unborn child or complications during delivery.

**Keep out of reach of children.** In case of overdose, get medical help or contact a Poison Control Center right away.

### Other Information:
- do not use if neck wrap or foil inner seal imprinted **"Safety Seal"** is broken or missing
- store at 20–25°C (68–77°F)

### Professional Information:
### Overdosage Information
For overdosage information, please refer to pgs. 667–668.

**Inactive Ingredients:** carnauba wax, corn starch, hydroxypropyl methylcellulose, iron oxide black, pregelatinized starch, propylene glycol, silicon dioxide, stearic acid, titanium dioxide

### How Supplied:
Caplets (white printed "Motrin M" in black) in tamper evident packaging of 24, 50, and 100.
*Shown in Product Identification Guide, page 511*

---

## NIZORAL® A-D
## KETOCONAZOLE SHAMPOO 1%

**Description:** *Nizoral® A-D (Ketoconazole Shampoo 1%) Anti-Dandruff Shampoo* is a light-blue liquid for topical application, containing the broad spectrum synthetic antifungal agent Ketoconazole in a concentration of 1%.

**Use:** Controls the flaking, scaling, and itching associated with dandruff.

### Directions:
**Adults and children 12 years and over:**
- wet hair thoroughly
- apply shampoo, generously lather, rinse thoroughly. Repeat.
- use every 3–4 days for up to 8 weeks or as directed by a doctor. Then use only as needed to control dandruff.

Children under 12 years. Ask a doctor.

### Warnings:
### Do Not Use
- on scalp that is broken or inflamed
- if you are allergic to ingredients in this product

### When Using This Product
- avoid contact with eyes
- if product gets into eyes, rinse thoroughly with water

### Stop use and ask a doctor if
- rash appears
- condition worsens or does not improve in 2–4 weeks

**If pregnant or breast-feeding,** ask a doctor before use.

**Keep out of the reach of children.** If swallowed get medical help or contact a Poison Control Center right away.

### Other Information
- store between 35° and 86°F (2° and 30°C)
- protect from light • protect from freezing

### Professional Information:
**Overdosage Information** *Nizoral® A-D (Ketoconazole) 1% Shampoo* is intended for external use only. In the event of accidental ingestion, supportive measures should be employed. Induced emesis and gastric lavage should usually be avoided.

**Inactive Ingredients:** acrylic acid polymer (carbomer 1342), butylated hydroxytoluene, cocamide MEA, FD&C Blue #1, fragrance, glycol distearate, polyquaternium-7, quaternium-15, sodium chloride, sodium cocoyl sarcosinate, sodium hydroxide and/or hydrochloric acid, sodium laureth sulfate, tetrasodium EDTA, water.

**How Supplied:** Available in 4 and 7 fl oz bottles and Travel size packets - 10 packets 0.2 fl oz (6 mL) each.
*Shown in Product Identification Guide, page 511*

---

## SIMPLY SLEEP™
## Nighttime Sleep Aid

**Description:** *SIMPLY SLEEP™* is a non habit-forming nighttime sleep aid. Each *SIMPLY SLEEP™* Caplet contains diphenhydramine HCl 25 mg.

**Actions:** *SIMPLY SLEEP™* contains an antihistamine (diphenhydramine HCl) which has sedative properties.

**Use:** relief of occasional sleeplessness

**Directions: adults and children 12 years and over:** take 2 caplets at bedtime if needed or as directed by a doctor. **children under 12 years:** do not use

**Precautions:** If a rare sensitivity reaction occurs, the drug should be discontinued.

### Warnings:
### Do not use
- in children under 12 years of age

### Ask a doctor before use if you have
- a breathing problem such as emphysema or chronic bronchitis
- trouble urinating due to an enlarged prostate gland
- glaucoma

**Ask a doctor before use if you are** taking sedatives or tranquilizers

### When using this product
- drowsiness may occur
- avoid alcoholic drinks
- do not drive a motor vehicle or operate machinery

### Stop use and ask a doctor if
- sleeplessness persists continuously for more than 2 weeks

Insomnia may be a symptom of serious underlying medical illness.

**If pregnant or breast-feeding,** ask a health professional before use.

**Keep out of reach of children.** In case of overdose, get medical help or contact a Poison Control Center right away.

### Other Information:
- **Do not use if blister carton is opened or if blister unit is broken.**
- Store at room temperature

**Inactive Ingredients:** cellulose, croscarmellose sodium, dibasic calcium phosphate, dihydrate, FD&C Blue #1, hydroxypropyl methylcellulose, magnesium stearate, polyethylene glycol, polysorbate 80, titanium dioxide.

**How Supplied:** Light blue mini-caplets embossed with "SL" on one side in blister packs of 24 and 48.
*Shown in Product Identification Guide, page 511*

---

## Regular Strength TYLENOL® acetaminophen Tablets
## Extra Strength TYLENOL® acetaminophen Gelcaps, Geltabs, Caplets, Tablets
## Extra Strength TYLENOL® acetaminophen Adult Liquid Pain Reliever
## TYLENOL® acetaminophen Arthritis Pain Extended Relief Caplets

**Product information for all dosage forms of Adult TYLENOL actaminophen have been combined under this heading.**

**Description:** *Each Regular Strength TYLENOL® Tablet contains acetaminophen 325 mg. Each Extra Strength TYLENOL® Gelcap, Geltab, Caplet, or Tablet contains acetaminophen 500 mg. Extra Strength TYLENOL® Adult Liquid is alcohol-free and each 15 mL (1/2 fl oz or one tablespoonful) contains 500 mg acetaminophen. Each TYLENOL® Arthritis Pain Extended Relief Caplet contains acetaminophen 650 mg.*

**Actions:** Acetaminophen is a clinically proven analgesic/antipyretic. Acetaminophen produces analgesia by elevation of the pain threshold and antipyresis through action on the hypothalamic heat-regulating center. Acetaminophen is equal to aspirin in analgesic and antipyretic effectiveness and it is unlikely to produce many of the side effects associated with aspirin and aspirin-containing products. *Tylenol Arthritis Pain Extended Relief* uses a unique, patented bilayer caplet. The first layer dissolves quickly to provide prompt relief while the second layer is time released to provide up to 8 hours of relief.

**Uses:** *Regular Strength TYLENOL® Tablets, Extra Strength TYLENOL® Gelcaps, Geltabs, Caplets, or Tablets:* For the temporary relief of minor aches and pains associated with headache, muscular aches, backache, minor arthritis pain, common cold, toothache, menstrual cramps and for the reduction of fever. *Extra Strength TYLENOL® Adult Liquid:* temporarily relieves minor aches and pains due to:
- headache • muscular aches
- backache • arthritis
- the common cold • toothache
- menstrual cramps

reduces fever
*TYLENOL® Arthritis Pain Extended Relief Caplets:* temporarily relieves minor aches and pains due to:
- arthritis
- the common cold

- headache
- toothache
- muscular aches
- backache
- menstrual cramps

**Directions:** *Regular Strength TYLENOL® Tablets:* **Adults and children 12 years of age and older:** Take 2 tablets every 4 to 6 hours as needed. Do not take more than 12 tablets in 24 hours, or as directed by a doctor. **Children 6–11 years of age:** Take 1 tablet every 4 to 6 hours as needed. Do not take more than 5 tablets in 24 hours **Children under 6 years of age:** Do not use this adult Regular Strength product in children under 6 years of age. This will provide more than the recommended dose (overdose) of TYLENOL® and could cause serious health problems.
*Extra Strength TYLENOL® Gelcaps, Geltabs, Caplets, or Tablets:* **Adults and Children 12 years of age and older:** Take 2 gelcaps, geltabs, caplets, or tablets every 4 to 6 hours as needed. Do not take more than 8 gelcaps, geltabs, caplets or tablets in 24 hours, or as directed by a doctor. **Children under 12 years:** Do not use this adult Extra Strength product in children under 12 years of age. This will provide more than the recommended dose (overdose) of TYLENOL® and could cause serious health problems.
*Extra Strength TYLENOL® Adult Liquid:* **Adults and children 12 years and over:**
- take 2 tablespoons (tbsp.) in dose cup provided every 4 to 6 hours as needed
- do not take more than 8 tablespoons in 24 hours

**children under 12 years:** do not use this adult Extra Strength product in children under 12 years of age; this will provide more than the recommended dose (overdose) of TYLENOL® and could cause serious health problems.
*TYLENOL® Arthritis Pain Extended Relief Caplets:*
- do not take more than directed

**adults:**
- take 2 caplets every 8 hours with water
- swallow whole – do not crush, chew or dissolve
- do not take more than 6 caplets in 24 hours
- do not use for more than 10 days unless directed by a doctor

**under 18 years of age:**
- ask a doctor

**Precautions:** If a rare sensitivity reaction occurs, the drug should be discontinued.

**Warnings:** *Regular Strength TYLENOL® Tablets, Extra Strength TYLENOL® Gelcaps, Geltabs, Caplets, or Tablets:*
**Alcohol Warning:** If you consume 3 or more alcoholic drinks every day, ask your doctor whether you should take acetaminophen or other pain relievers/fever reducers. Acetaminophen may cause liver damage. **Do not use if carton is opened or red neck wrap or foil inner seal imprinted with "Safety Seal®" is broken.**
**Do not Use:**
- with any other product containing acetaminophen.

- for more than 10 days for pain unless directed by doctor.
- for more than 3 days for fever unless directed by a doctor.

**Stop Using And Ask a Doctor If:**
- symptoms do not improve
- new symptoms occur
- pain or fever persists or gets worse
- redness or swelling is present

**Do not exceed recommended dose.** Keep this and all drugs out of the reach of children. In case of accidental overdose, contact a physician or poison control center immediately. Prompt medical attention is critical for adults as well as for children even if you do not notice any signs or symptoms. As with any drug, if you are pregnant or nursing a baby, seek the advise of a health professional before using this product.
*Extra Strength TYLENOL® Adult Liquid and TYLENOL® Arthritis Pain Extended Relief Caplets:* **Alcohol Warning:** If you consume 3 or more alcoholic drinks every day, ask your doctor whether you should take acetaminophen or other pain relievers/fever reducers. Acetaminophen may cause liver damage.
**Do not Use**
- with any other product containing acetaminophen.

**Stop use and ask a doctor if**
- New symptoms occur
- Redness or swelling is present
- Pain gets worse or lasts for more than 10 days
- fever gets worse or lasts for more than 3 days (*Extra Strength TYLENOL® Adult Liquid only*)

**If pregnant or breast-feeding,** ask a health professional before use.
**Keep out of the reach of children.** In case of overdose, get medical help or contact a Poison Control Center right away. Quick medical attention is critical for adults as well as for children even if you do not notice signs or symptoms.

**Other information**
*Extra Strength TYLENOL® Adult Liquid*
- **do not use if carton is opened, or if bottle wrap or foil inner seal imprinted "Safety Seal®" is broken or missing.**
- Store at room temperature

*TYLENOL® Arthritis Pain Extended Relief Caplets*
- **do not use if carton is opened or red neck wrap or foil inner seal with "Safety Seal®" is broken**
- store at 20–25°C (68–77°F)
- avoid excessive heat at 40°C (104°F)

**Professional Information:**
**Overdosage Information for all Adult Tylenol products**

**ACETAMINOPHEN:** Acetaminophen in massive overdosage may cause hepatic toxicity in some patients. In adults and adolescents ($\geq$ 12 years of age), hepatic toxicity may occur following ingestion of greater than 7.5 to 10 grams over a period of 8 hours or less. Fatalities are infrequent (less than 3–4% of untreated cases) and have rarely been reported with overdoses of less than 15 grams. In children (<12 years of age), an acute overdosage of less than 150 mg/kg has not been associated with hepatic toxicity. Early symptoms following a potentially hepatotoxic overdose may include: nausea, vomiting, diaphoresis and general

malaise. Clinical and laboratory evidence of hepatic toxicity may not be apparent until 48 to 72 hours postingestion. In adults and adolescents, any individual presenting with an unknown amount of acetaminophen ingested or with a questionable or unreliable history about the time of ingestion should have a plasma acetaminophen level drawn and be treated with N-acetylcysteine. For full prescribing information, refer to the N-acetylcysteine package insert. Do not await results of assays for plasma acetaminophen levels before initiating treatment with N-acetylcysteine. The following additional procedures are recommended: Promptly initiate gastric decontamination of the stomach. A plasma acetaminophen assay should be obtained as early as possible, but no sooner than four hours following ingestion. If an acetaminophen *extended release* product is involved, it may be appropriate to obtain an additional plasma acetaminophen level 4–6 hours following the initial acetaminophen level. If either acetaminophen level plots above the treatment line on the acetaminophen overdose nomogram, N-acetylcysteine treatment should be continued for a full course of therapy. Liver function studies should be obtained initially and repeated at 24-hour intervals. Serious toxicity or fatalities have been extremely infrequent following an acute acetaminophen overdose in young children, possibly because of differences in the way they metabolize acetaminophen. In children, the maximum potential amount ingested can be more easily estimated. If more than 150 mg/kg or an unknown amount was ingested, obtain a plasma acetaminophen level as soon as possible, but no sooner than 4 hours following ingestion. If an acetaminophen *extended release* product is involved, it may be appropriate to obtain an additional plasma acetaminophen level 4–6 hours following the initial acetaminophen level. If either acetaminophen level plots above the treatment line on the acetaminophen overdose nomogram, N-acetylcysteine treatment should be initiated and continued for a full course of therapy. If an assay cannot be obtained and the estimated acetaminophen ingestion exceeds 150 mg/kg, dosing with N-acetylcysteine should be initiated and continued for a full course of therapy. For additional emergency information, call your regional poison center or call the Rocky Mountain Poison Center toll-free, (1-800-525-6115).
**Our adult Tylenol® combination products contain active ingredients in addition to acetaminophen. The following is basic overdose information regarding those ingredients.**
**CHLORPHENIRAMINE:** Chlorpheniramine toxicity should be treated as you would an anthihistamine/anticholinergic overdose and is likely to be present within a few hours after acute ingestion.
**DEXTROMETHORPHAN:** Acute dextromethorphan overdose usually does not result in serious signs and symptoms unless massive amounts have been in-

*Continued on next page*

## Tylenol—Cont.

gested. Signs and symptoms of a substantial overdose may include nausea and vomiting, visual disturbances, CNS disturbances and urinary retention

**DIPHENHYDRAMINE:** Diphenhydramine toxicity should be treated as you would an antihistamine/anticholinergic overdose and is likely to be present within a few hours after acute ingestion.

**DOXYLAMINE:** Doxylamine toxicity should be treated as you would an antihistamine/anticholinergic overdose and is likely to be present within a few hours after acute ingestion.

**GUAIFENESIN:** Guaifenesin should be treated as a nontoxic ingestion.

**PAMABROM:** Acute overexposure of diuretics is primarily associated with fluid and electrolyte loss. Fluid loss should be treated with the appropriate intravenous and/or oral fluids.

**PSEUDOEPHEDRINE:** Symptoms from pseudoephedrine overdose consist most often of mild anxiety, tachycardia and/or mild hypertension. Symptoms usually appear within 4 to 8 hours of ingestion and are transient, usually requiring no treatment.

**For additional emergency information, please contact your local poison control center.**

**Alcohol Information:** Chronic heavy alcohol abusers may be at increased risk of liver toxicity from excessive acetaminophen use, although reports of this event are rare. Reports usually involve cases of severe chronic alcoholics and the dosages of acetaminophen most often exceed recommended doses and often involve substantial overdose. Healthcare professionals should alert their patients who regularly consume large amounts of alcohol not to exceed recommended doses of acetaminophen.

**Inactive Ingredients:** *Regular Strength TYLENOL® Tablets:* Cellulose, Corn Starch, Magnesium Stearate, Sodium Starch Glycolate.

*Extra Strength TYLENOL® Tablets:* Cellulose, Corn Starch, Magnesium Stearate, Sodium Starch Glycolate. *Caplets:* Cellulose, Corn Starch, FD&C Red No. 40, Hydroxypropyl Methylcellulose, Magnesium Stearate, Polyethylene Glycol, Sodium Starch Glycolate. *Gelcaps:* benzyl alcohol, butylparaben, castor oil, cellulose, corn starch, D&C Yellow #10, edetate calcium disodium, FD&C Blue #1, FD&C Blue #2, FD&C Red #40, gelatin, hydroxypropyl methylcellulose, magnesium stearate, methylparaben, propylparaben, sodium lauryl sulfate, sodium propionate, sodium starch glycolate, titanium dioxide. *Geltabs:* benzyl alcohol, butylparaben, castor oil, cellulose, corn starch, D&C Yellow #10, edetate calcium disodium, FD&C Blue #1, FD&C Blue #2, FD&C Red #40, gelatin, hydroxypropyl methylcellulose, magnesium stearate, methylparaben, propyl-

paraben, sodium lauryl sulfate, sodium propionate, sodium starch glycolate, titanium dioxide.

*Extra Strength TYLENOL® Adult Liquid:* citric acid, D&C Red #33, FD&C Red #40, flavor, high fructose corn syrup, polyethylene glycol, propylene glycol, purified water, saccharin sodium, sodium benzoate, sorbitol

*TYLENOL® Arthritis Pain Extended Relief Caplets:* corn starch, hydroxyethyl cellulose, hydroxypropyl methylcellulose, magnesium stearate, microcrystalline cellulose, povidone, powdered cellulose, pregelatinized starch, sodium starch glycolate, titanium dioxide, triacetin.

**How Supplied:** *Regular Strength TYLENOL® Tablets:* (colored white, scored, imprinted "TYLENOL" and "325")—tamper-evident bottles of 100. Store at room temperature.

*Extra Strength TYLENOL® Tablets:* (colored white, imprinted "TYLENOL" and "500")—tamper-evident bottles of 30, 60, 100, and 200. Store at room temperature. *Caplets* (colored white, imprinted "TYLENOL 500 mg")—vials of 10, 10 blister packs, and tamper-evident bottles of 24, 50, 100, 175, and 250. Store at room temperature. *Gelcaps* (colored yellow and red, imprinted "Tylenol 500") tamper-evident bottles of 24, 50, 100, and 225. Store at room temperature; avoid high humidity and excessive heat 40°C (104°F). *Geltabs* (colored yellow and red, imprinted "Tylenol 500") tamper-evident bottles of 24, 50, and 100. Store at room temperature; avoid high humidity and excessive heat 40°C (104°F).

*Extra Strength TYLENOL® Adult Liquid:* Cherry-flavored liquid (colored red) 8 fl. oz. tamper-evident bottle with child resistant safety cap and special dosage cup.

*TYLENOL® Arthritis Pain Extended Relief Caplets:* (colored white, engraved "TYLENOL ER") tamper-evident bottles of 24, 50, and 100, 150, 250 and 290's.

*Shown in Product Identification Guide, page 512, 513*

---

**TYLENOL® Severe Allergy Caplets**

**Maximum Strength**

**TYLENOL® Allergy Sinus NightTime Caplets**

**Maximum Strength**

**TYLENOL® Allergy Sinus Caplets, Gelcaps and Geltabs**

**Product information for all dosage forms of TYLENOL Allergy have been combined under this heading.**

**Description:** Each *TYLENOL® Severe Allergy Caplet* contains acetaminophen 500 mg and diphenhydramine HCl 12.5 mg. Each *Maximum Strength TYLENOL® Allergy Sinus NightTime Caplet* contains acetaminophen 500 mg,

diphenhydramine HCl 25 mg, and pseudoephedrine HCl 30 mg. Each *Maximum Strength TYLENOL® Allergy Sinus Caplet Gelcap and Geltab* contains acetaminophen 500 mg, chlorpheniramine maleate 2 mg, and pseudoephedrine HCl 30 mg.

**Actions:** *TYLENOL® Severe Allergy Caplets* contain a clinically proven analgesic-antipyretic and antihistamine. Acetaminophen produces analgesia by elevation of the pain threshold and antipyresis through action on the hypothalamic heat regulating center. Acetaminophen is equal to aspirin in analgesic and antipyretic effectiveness, and it is unlikely to produce many of the side effects associated with aspirin and aspirin-containing products.

Diphenhydramine HCl is an antihistamine which helps provide temporary relief of itchy, watery eyes, runny nose, sneezing, itching of the nose or throat due to hay fever or other respiratory allergies.

*Maximum Strength TYLENOL® Allergy Sinus NightTime Caplets* contain, in addition to the above ingredients, a decongestant, pseudoephedrine HCl. Pseudoephedrine is a sympathomimetic amine which provides temporary relief of nasal and sinus congestion.

*Maximum Strength TYLENOL® Allergy Sinus Caplets, Gelcaps and Geltabs* contain acetaminophen, pseudoephedrine HCl and the antihistamine, chlorpheniramine maleate. Chlorpheniramine is an antihistamine which helps provide temporary relief of runny nose, sneezing and watery and itchy eyes.

**Uses:** *TYLENOL® Severe Allergy:* temporarily relieves these symptoms due to hay fever or other respiratory allergies:
• itchy, watery eyes • runny nose
• sneezing • sore throat
• itching of nose or throat

*Maximum Strength TYLENOL® Allergy Sinus NightTime and TYLENOL® Allergy Sinus:* temporarily relieves these symptoms due to hay fever or other respiratory allergies:
• nasal congestion • sinus pressure
• sinus pain • headache
• runny nose • sneezing
• itchy, watery eyes • itchy throat

**Precautions:** If a rare sensitivity reaction occurs, the drug should be discontinued.

**Directions:** *TYLENOL® Severe Allergy:*
• do not take more than directed
**adults and children 12 years and over:**
• take 2 caplets every 4 to 6 hours as needed
• do not take more than 8 caplets in 24 hours
**children under 12 years:** do not use this adult product in children under 12 years of age; this will provide more than the recommended dose (overdose) and could cause serious health problems
*Maximum Strength TYLENOL® Allergy Sinus NightTime:*
• do not take more than directed

**adults and children 12 years and over:**
- take 2 caplets every 4 to 6 hours as needed
- do not take more than 8 caplets in 24 hours

**children under 12 years:** do not use this adult product in children under 12 years of age; this will provide more than the recommended dose (overdose) and could cause serious health problems.

*Maximum Strength TYLENOL® Allergy Sinus:*
- do not take more than directed

**adults and children 12 years and over:**
- take two every 4 to 6 hours as needed
- do not take more than 8 caplets in 24 hours

**children under 12 years:** do not use this adult product in children under 12 years of age; this will provide more than the recommended dose (overdose) and could cause serious health problems.

**Warnings: Alcohol warning:** If you consume 3 or more alcoholic drinks every day, ask your doctor whether your should take acetaminophen or other pain relievers/fever reducers. Acetaminophen may cause liver damage.

**Sore throat warning:** If sore throat is severe, persists for more than 2 days, is accompanied or followed by fever, headache, rash, nausea or vomiting, consult a doctor promptly.

**Do not use**
- if you are now taking a prescription monoamine oxidase inhibitor (MAOI) (certain drugs for depression, psychiatric or emotional conditions, or Parkinson's disease) or for 2 weeks after stopping the MAOI drug. If you do not know if your prescription drug contains an MAOI, ask a doctor or pharmacist before taking this product (does not apply to *TYLENOL® Severe Allergy*)
- with any other product containing acetaminophen

**Ask a doctor or pharmacist before use if you are** taking sedatives or tranquilizers

**Stop use and ask a doctor if**
- new symptoms occur
- redness or swelling is present
- pain gets worse or lasts for more than 7 days
- fever gets worse or lasts for more than 3 days
- you get nervous, dizzy or sleepless (does not apply to TYLENOL® Severe Allergy)

**If pregnant or breast feeding,** ask a health professional before use.

**Keep out of reach of children.** In case of overdose, get medical help or contact a Poison Control Center right away. Quick medical attention is critical for adults as well as children even if you do not notice any signs or symptoms.

**When using this product**
- marked drowsiness may occur
- avoid alcoholic drinks
- alcohol, sedatives and tranquilizers may increase drowsiness
- be careful when driving a motor vehicle or operating machinery
- excitability may occur, especially in children

*TYLENOL® Severe Allergy*

**Ask a doctor before use if you have**
- glaucoma
- trouble urinating due to an enlarged prostate gland

- a breathing problem such as emphysema or chronic bronchitis

*Maximum Strength TYLENOL® Allergy Sinus NightTime and Maximum Strength TYLENOL® Allergy Sinus*

**Ask a doctor before use if you have**
- heart disease • glaucoma • diabetes
- thyroid disease • high blood pressure
- trouble urinating due to an enlarged prostate gland
- a breathing problem such as emphysema or chronic bronchitis

**Other information**
- **do not use if carton is opened or if blister unit is broken**

*TYLENOL® Allergy Sinus Caplet and TYLENOL® Allergy Sinus NightTime Caplet:*
- store at room temperature

*TYLENOL® Allergy Sinus Gelcap & Geltabs*
- store at room temperature; avoid high humidity and excessive heat 40°C (104°F)

**Professional Information:**
**Overdosage Information:**
For overdosage information, please refer to pgs. 673–674.

**Inactive Ingredients:** *TYLENOL® Severe Allergy:* **Caplets:** carnauba wax, cellulose, corn starch, D&C Yellow #10, FD&C Yellow #6, hydroxpropyl cellulose, hydroxypropyl methylcellulose, iron oxide, magnesium stearate, polyethylene glycol, sodium citrate, sodium starch glycolate, titanium dioxide.

*Maximum Strength TYLENOL® Allergy Sinus NightTime:* **Caplets:** carnauba wax, cellulose, corn starch, D&C Yellow #10, FD&C Blue #1, hydroxypropyl methylcellulose, iron oxide, magnesium stearate, polyethylene glycol, polysorbate 80, sodium citrate, sodium starch glycolate, titanium dioxide.

*Maximum Strength TYLENOL® Allergy Sinus:* **Caplets:** carnauba wax, cellulose, corn starch, D&C Yellow #10, FD&C Blue #1, FD&C Yellow #6, hydroxypropyl cellulose, hydroxypropyl methylcellulose, iron oxide, magnesium stearate, polyethylene glycol, sodium starch glycolate, titanium dioxide. **Gelcaps and Geltabs:** benzyl alcohol, butylparaben, castor oil, cellulose, corn starch, D&C Yellow #10, edetate calcium disodium, FD&C Blue #1, FD&C Blue #2, gelatin, hydroxypropyl methylcellulose, magnesium stearate, methylparaben, propylparaben, sodium lauryl sulfate, sodium propionate, sodium starch glycolate, titanium dioxide.

**How Supplied:** *TYLENOL® Severe Allergy:* **Caplets:** Yellow film-coated, imprinted with "TYLENOL Severe Allergy" on one side—blister packs of 24.

*Maximum Strength TYLENOL® Allergy Sinus NightTime:* **Caplets:** Light blue film-coated, imprinted with "TYLENOL A/S NightTime" on one side—blister packs of 24.

*Maximum Strength TYLENOL® Allergy Sinus:* **Caplets:** Yellow film-coated, imprinted with "TYLENOL Allergy Sinus" on one side—blister packs of 24.

**Gelcaps and Geltabs:** Green and yellow-colored, imprinted with "TYLENOL A/S"—blister packs of 24 and 48.
*Shown in Product Identification Guide, page 512, 513*

---

**Multi-Symptom TYLENOL® Cold Non-Drowsy Caplets and Gelcaps**

**Multi-Symptom TYLENOL® Cold Complete Formula Caplets**

**Product information for all dosage forms of TYLENOL Cold have been combined under this heading.**

**Description:** Each *Multi-Symptom TYLENOL® Cold Non-Drowsy Caplet and Gelcap* contains acetaminophen 325 mg, dextromethorphan HBr 15 mg, and pseudoephedrine HCl 30 mg. Each *Multi-Symptom TYLENOL® Cold Complete Formula Caplet* contains acetaminophen 325 mg, chlorpheniramine maleate 2 mg, dextromethorphan HBr 15 mg, and pseudoephedrine HCl 30 mg.

**Actions:** *Multi-Symptom TYLENOL® Cold Non-Drowsy* contains a clinically proven analgesic-antipyretic, a decongestant and a cough suppressant. Acetaminophen produces analgesia by elevation of the pain threshold and antipyresis through action on the hypothalamic heat regulating center. Acetaminophen is equal to aspirin in analgesic and antipyretic effectiveness and it is unlikely to produce many of the side effects associated with aspirin and aspirin-containing products. Pseudoephedrine is a sympathomimetic amine which provides temporary relief of nasal congestion. Dextromethorphan is a cough suppressant which provides temporary relief of coughs due to minor throat irritations that may occur with the common cold. *Multi-Symptom TYLENOL® Cold Complete Formula Caplets* contain, in addition to the above ingredients, an antihistamine. Chlorpheniramine is an antihistamine which helps provide temporary relief of runny nose, sneezing and watery and itchy eyes.

**Uses:** *Multi-Symptom TYLENOL® Cold Non-Drowsy:* temporarily relieves these cold symptoms:
- cough • sore throat • minor aches and pains • headaches • nasal congestion
- temporarily reduces fever

*Multi-Symptom TYLENOL® Cold Complete Formula:* For the temporary relief of these cold symptoms: minor aches and pains, headaches, sore throat, nasal congestion, runny nose, coughs, sneezing, watery and itchy eyes. For the reduction of fever.

**Directions:** *Multi-Symptom TYLENOL® Cold Non Drowsy and Multi-Symptom TYLENOL® Cold Complete Formula:* **do not take more than directed**

*Continued on next page*

## Tylenol Cold—Cont.

**Adults and children 12 years and over:**
• take 2 every 6 hours as needed
• do not take more than 8 in 24 hours
**Children 6–11 years:**
• take 1 every 6 hours
• do not take more than 4 in 24 hours
**Children under 6 years** do not use this product in children under 6 years of age; this will provide more than the recommended dose (overdose) and could cause serious health problems.

**Precautions:** If a rare sensitivity reaction occurs, the drug should be discontinued.

**Warnings: Alcohol Warning:** If you consume 3 or more alcoholic drinks every day, ask your doctor whether you should take acetaminophen or other pain relievers/fever reducers. Acetaminophen may cause liver damage.

**Sore throat warning:** If sore throat is severe, persists for more than 2 days, is accompanied or followed by fever, headache, rash, nausea or vomiting, consult a doctor promptly.

**Do not use**
• if you are now taking a prescription monoamine oxidase inhibitor (MAOI) (certain drugs for depression, psychiatric, emotional conditions or Parkinson's disease), or for 2 weeks after stopping the MAOI drug. If you do not know if your prescription drug contains an MAOI, ask a doctor or pharmacist before taking this product.
• with any other product containing acetaminophen

**Stop use and ask a doctor if**
• new symptoms occur
• pain gets worse or lasts for more than 7 days
• fever gets worse or lasts for more than 3 days
• you get nervous, dizzy or sleepless
• cough lasts more than 7 days, comes back or occurs with fever, rash or headache that lasts. These could be signs of a serious condition.

**If pregnant or breast-feeding**, ask a health professional before use.

**Keep out of reach of children.** In case of overdose, get medical help or contact a Poison Control Center right away. Quick medical attention is critical for adults as well as for children even if you don't notice any signs or symptoms.

**Ask a doctor before use if you have**
• heart disease • diabetes • thyroid disease • cough that occurs with too much phlegm (mucus) • high blood pressure • trouble urinating due to an enlarged prostate gland • chronic cough that lasts as occurs with smoking, asthma, chronic bronchitis or emphysema

**When using this product**
• do not exceed recommended dosage
*Multi-Symptom TYLENOL® Cold Complete Formula:*
**Ask a doctor before use if you have**
• heart disease • glaucoma • diabetes • thyroid disease • cough that occurs with too much phlegm (mucus) • high blood pressure • a breathing problem or chronic cough that lasts as occurs with

smoking, asthma, chronic bronchitis or emphysema • trouble urinating due to an enlarged prostate gland
**Ask a doctor or pharmacist before use if you are** taking sedatives or tranquilizers
**When using this product**
• do not exceed recommended dosage
• drowsiness may occur • avoid alcoholic drinks • alcohol, sedatives and tranquilizers may increase drowsiness • be careful when driving a motor vehicle or operating machinery • excitability may occur, especially in children
**Other information**
• do not use if carton is opened or if blister unit is broken
• store at room temperature (avoid high humidity and excessive heat 40°C (104°F)—applies to TYLENOL® Cold Non-Drowsy Gelcap only)

### Professional Information:
**Overdosage Information**
For overdosage information, please refer to pgs. 673–674.

**Inactive Ingredients:** *Multi-Symptom TYLENOL® Cold Non Drowsy Formula:* **Caplets:** carnauba wax, cellulose, corn starch, D&C Yellow #10, FD&C Blue #1, hydroxypropyl methylcellulose, iron oxide, magnesium stearate, sodium starch glycolate, titanium dioxide, triacetin.
**Gelcaps:** benzyl alcohol, butylparaben, castor oil, cellulose, corn starch, D&C Yellow #10, edetate calcium disodium, FD&C Red #40, gelatin, hydroxypropyl methylcellulose, iron oxide, magnesium stearate, methylparaben, propylparaben, sodium lauryl sulfate, sodium propionate, sodium starch glycolate, titanium dioxide.
*Multi-Symptom TYLENOL® Cold Complete Formula:* **Caplets:** carnauba wax, cellulose, corn starch, D&C Yellow #10, FD&C Blue #1, FD&C Yellow #6, hydroxypropyl methylcellulose, iron oxide, magnesium stearate, sodium starch glycolate, titanium dioxide, triacetin.

**How Supplied:** *Multi-Symptom TYLENOL® Cold Non Drowsy:* **Caplets:** White-colored, imprinted with "TYLENOL Cold"—blister packs of 24.
**Gelcaps:** Red- and tan-colored, imprinted with "TYLENOL COLD"—blister packs of 24.
*Multi-Symptom TYLENOL® Cold Complete Formula:* **Caplets:** Yellow-colored, imprinted with "TYLENOL Cold"—blister packs of 24.
*Shown in Product Identification Guide, page 513*

### Multi-Symptom
### TYLENOL® Cold
### Severe Congestion Non-Drowsy

**Description:** Each *Multi-Symptom TYLENOL® Cold Severe Congestion Non-Drowsy Caplet* contains acetaminophen 325 mg, dextromethorphan HBr 15 mg, guaifenesin 200 mg and pseudoephedrine HCl 30 mg.

**Actions:** *Multi-Symptom TYLENOL® Cold Severe Congestion Non-Drowsy Caplets* contain a clinically proven analgesic-antipyretic, decongestant, expectorant and cough suppressant. Acetaminophen produces analgesia by elevation of the pain threshold and antipyresis through action on the hypothalamic heat regulating center. Acetaminophen is equal to aspirin in analgesic and antipyretic effectiveness and is unlikely to produce many of the side effects associated with aspirin and aspirin-containing products. Pseudoephedrine is a sympathomimetic amine which provides temporary relief of nasal congestion. Guaifenesin is an expectorant which helps loosen phlegm (mucus) and thin bronchial secretions to make coughs more productive. Dextromethorphan is a cough suppressant which provides temporary relief of coughs due to minor throat irritations that may occur with the common cold.

**Uses:** temporarily relieves these cold symptoms:
• cough • sore throat • minor aches and pains • headaches • nasal congestion
• helps loosen phlegm (mucus) and thin bronchial secretions to make coughs more productive
• temporarily reduces fever

**Directions:**
• do not take more than directed
**adults and children 12 years and over:**
• take 2 caplets every 6–8 hours as needed
• do not take more than 8 caplets in 24 hours
**children 6–11 years:**
• take 1 caplet every 6–8 hours
• do not take more than 4 caplets in 24 hours
**children under 6 years:** do not use this product in children under 6 years of age; this will provide more than the recommended dose (overdose) and could cause serious health problems.

**Precautions:** If a rare sensitivity reaction occurs, the drug should be discontinued.

**Warnings: Alcohol warning:** If you consume 3 or more alcoholic drinks every day, ask your doctor whether you should take acetaminophen or other pain relievers/fever reducers. Acetaminophen may cause liver damage.

**Sore throat warning:** If sore throat is severe, persists for more than 2 days, is accompanied or followed by fever, headache, rash, nausea or vomiting, consult a doctor promptly.

**Do not use**
• if you are now taking a prescription monoamine oxidase inhibitor (MAOI) (certain drugs for depression, psychiatric, emotional conditions or Parkinson's disease), or for 2 weeks after stopping the MAOI drug. If you do not know if your prescription drug contains an MAOI, ask a doctor or pharmacist before taking this product.
• with any other product containing acetaminophen

### Ask a doctor before use if you have

- heart disease • diabetes • thyroid disease • cough that occurs with too much phlegm (mucus) • high blood pressure
- trouble urinating due to an enlarged prostate gland • chronic cough that lasts as occurs with smoking, asthma, chronic bronchitis or emphysema

### When using this product

- **do not exceed recommended dosage**

### Stop use and ask a doctor if

- new symptoms occur
- redness or swelling is present
- pain gets worse or lasts for more than 7 days
- fever gets worse or lasts for more than 3 days
- you get nervous, dizzy or sleepless
- cough lasts more than 7 days, comes back or occurs with fever, rash or headache that lasts. These could be signs of a serious condition.

**If pregnant or breast-feeding,** ask a health professional before use.

**Keep out of reach of children.** In case of overdose, get medical help or contact a Poison Control Center right away. Quick medical attention is critical for adults as well as for children even if you do not notice any signs or symptoms.

### Other Information:

- **do not use if carton is opened or if blister unit is broken**
- Store at room temperature. Avoid high humidity and excess heat.

### Professional Information:
### Overdosage Information

For overdosage information, please refer to pgs. 673–674.

**Inactive Ingredients:** carnauba wax, cellulose, corn starch, D&C Yellow #10, FD&C Blue #1, FD&C Yellow #6, hydroxypropyl methylcellulose, iron oxide, povidone, silicon dioxide, sodium starch glycolate, stearic acid, titanium dioxide, triacetin.

**How Supplied: Caplets:** Buttery-tan-colored, imprinted with *"TYLENOL COLD SC"* in green ink—blister packs of 24.

*Shown in Product Identification Guide, page 513*

---

### Maximum Strength TYLENOL® Flu Non-Drowsy Gelcaps

### Maximum Strength TYLENOL® Flu NightTime Gelcaps

### Maximum Strength TYLENOL® Flu NightTime Liquid

**Product information for all dosage forms of TYLENOL Flu have been combined under this heading.**

**Description:** Each *Maximum Strength TYLENOL® Flu Non-Drowsy Gelcap* contains acetaminophen 500 mg, dextromethorphan HBr 15 mg and pseudoephedrine HCl 30 mg. Each *Maximum Strength TYLENOL® Flu NightTime Gelcap* contains acetaminophen 500 mg, diphenhydramine HCl 25 mg and pseudoephedrine HCl 30 mg. *Maximum Strength TYLENOL® Flu NightTime Liquid:* Each 30 mL (2 tablespoonsful) contains acetaminophen 1000 mg, dextromethorphan HBr 30 mg, doxylamine succinate 12.5 mg, and pseudoephedrine HCl 60 mg.

**Actions:** *Maximum Strength TYLENOL® Flu Non-Drowsy Gelcaps* contain a clinically proven analgesic-antipyretic, a decongestant and a cough suppressant. Acetaminophen produces analgesia by elevation of the pain threshold and antipyresis through action on the hypothalamic heat regulating center. Acetaminophen is equal to aspirin in analgesic and antipyretic effectiveness and it is unlikely to produce many of the side effects associated with aspirin and aspirin-containing products. Pseudoephedrine hydrochloride is a sympathomimetic amine which provides temporary relief of nasal congestion. Dextromethorphan is a cough suppressant which provides temporary relief of coughs due to minor throat irritations that may occur with the common cold. *Maximum Strength TYLENOL® Flu NightTime Gelcaps* contains the same clinically proven analgesic-antipyretic and decongestant as *Maximum Strength TYLENOL Flu Non-Drowsy Gelcaps* along with an antihistamine. Diphenhydramine is an antihistamine which helps provide temporary relief of runny nose and sneezing. *Maximum Strength TYLENOL® Flu NightTime Liquid* contains the same clinically proven analgesic-antipyretic, decongestant and cough suppressant as *Maximum Strength TYLENOL Flu Non-Drowsy Gelcaps* along with an antihistamine. Doxylamine succinate is an antihistamine which helps provide temporary relief of runny nose and sneezing.

**Uses:** *Maximum Strength TYLENOL® Flu Non-Drowsy Gelcaps:* temporarily relieves these cold and flu symptoms:

- minor aches and pains • headaches
- sore throat • nasal congestion
- coughs
- temporarily reduces fever

*Maximum Strength TYLENOL® Flu NightTime Gelcaps:* temporarily relieves these cold and flu symptoms:

- minor aches and pains • headaches
- sore throat • nasal congestion • runny nose • sneezing
- temporarily reduces fever

*Maximum Strength TYLENOL® Flu NightTime Liquid:* temporarily relieves these cold and flu symptoms:

- body aches and headaches • coughs
- nasal congestion • sore throat • runny nose • sneezing
- temporarily reduces fever

**Directions:** *Maximum Strength TYLENOL® Flu Non-Drowsy Gelcaps:*

- do not take more than directed

**adults and children 12 years and over:**

- take 2 gelcaps every 6 hours as needed
- do not take more than 8 gelcaps in 24 hours

**children under 12 years:** do not use this adult product in children under 12 years of age; this will provide more than the recommended dose (overdose) and could cause serious health problems.

*Maximum Strength TYLENOL® Flu NightTime Gelcaps:*

- do not take more than directed

**adults and children 12 years and over:**

- take 2 gelcaps at bedtime
- may repeat every 6 hours
- do not take more than 8 gelcaps in 24 hours

**children under 12 years:** do not use this adult product in children under 12 years of age; this will provide more than the recommended dose (overdose) and could cause serious health problems.

*Maximum Strength TYLENOL® Flu NightTime Liquid:*

- do not take more than directed

**adults and children 12 years and over:**

- take 2 tablespoons (tbsp) in dose cap provided every 6 hours as needed
- do not take more than 8 tablespoons in 24 hours

**children under 12 years:** do not use this adult product in children under 12 years of age; this will provide more than the recommended dose (overdose) and could cause serious health problems.

**Precautions:** If a rare sensitivity reaction occurs, the drug should be discontinued.

**Warnings: Alcohol Warning:** If you consume 3 or more alcoholic drinks every day, ask your doctor whether you should take acetaminophen or other pain relievers/fever reducers. Acetaminophen may cause liver damage.

**Sore throat warning:** If sore throat is severe, persists for more than 2 days, is accompanied or followed by fever, headache, rash, nausea or vomiting, consult a doctor promptly.

### Do not use

- if you are now taking a prescription monoamine-oxidase inhibitor (MAOI) (certain drugs for depression, psychiatric, emotional conditions or Parkinson's disease or for 2 weeks after stopping the MAOI drug. If you do not know if your prescription drug contains an MAOI, ask a doctor or pharmacist before taking this product.
- with any other product containing acetaminophen

**If pregnant or breast-feeding,** ask a health professional before use.

**Keep out of reach of children.** In case of overdose, get medical help or contact a Poison Control Center right away. Quick medical attention is critical for adults as well as for children even if you do not notice any signs or symptoms.

*Maximum Strength TYLENOL® Flu Non-Drowsy Gelcaps*

### Ask a doctor before use if you have

- heart disease • diabetes • thyroid disease • cough that occurs with too much phlegm (mucus) • high blood pressure • trouble urinating due to an enlarged prostate gland • chronic cough that lasts as occurs with smoking, asthma, chronic bronchitis or emphysema

*Continued on next page*

## Tylenol Flu—Cont.

**When using this product**
- **do not exceed recommended dosage**

**Stop use and ask a doctor if**
- new symptoms occur
- redness or swelling is present
- pain gets worse or lasts for more than 7 days
- fever gets worse or lasts for more than 3 days
- you get nervous, dizzy or sleepless
- cough lasts more than 7 days, comes back or occurs with fever, rash or headache that lasts. These could be signs of a serious condition.

*Maximum Strength TYLENOL® Flu NightTime Gelcaps*

**Ask a doctor before use if you have**
- heart disease • glaucoma • diabetes
- thyroid disease • high blood pressure
- trouble urinating due to an enlarged prostate gland • a breathing problem such as emphysema or chronic bronchitis

**Ask a doctor or pharmacist before use if you are** taking sedatives or tranquilizers

**When using this product**
- **do not exceed recommended dosage**
- marked drowsiness may occur
- avoid alcoholic drinks
- alcohol, sedatives and tranquilizers may increase drowsiness.
- be careful when driving a motor vehicle or operating machinery
- excitability may occur especially in children

**Stop use and ask a doctor if**
- new symptoms occur
- redness or swelling is present
- pain gets worse or lasts for more than 7 days
- fever gets worse or lasts for more than 3 days
- you get nervous, dizzy or sleepless

*Maximum Strength TYLENOL® Flu NightTime Liquid*

**Ask a doctor before use if you have**
- heart disease • glaucoma • diabetes
- thyroid disease • cough that occurs with too much phlegm (mucus)
- high blood pressure • a breathing problem such as emphysema or chronic bronchitis • trouble urinating due to an enlarged prostate gland

**Ask a doctor or pharmacist before use if you are** taking sedatives or tranquilizers

**When using this product**
- **do not exceed recommended dosage**
- marked drowsiness may occur
- avoid alcoholic drinks
- alcohol, sedatives and tranquilizers may increase drowsiness
- be careful when driving a motor vehicle or operating machinery
- excitability may occur, especially in children

**Stop use and ask a doctor if**
- new symptoms occur
- redness or swelling is present
- pain gets worse or lasts for more than 7 days
- fever gets worse or lasts for more than 3 days
- you get nervous, dizzy or sleepless
- cough lasts for more than 7 days, comes back or occurs with fever, rash or headache that lasts. These could be signs of a serious condition.

**Other Information:**

*Maximum Strength TYLENOL® Flu Non-Drowsy Gelcaps and Maximum Strength TYLENOL® Flu NightTime Gelcaps:*
- **do not use if carton is opened or if blister unit is broken**
- Store at room temperature; avoid high humidity and excessive heat 40°C (104°F)

*Maximum Strength TYLENOL® Flu NightTime Liquid*
- **do not use if carton is opened or if bottle wrap or foil inner seal imprinted "Safety Seal®" is broken or missing**
- Store at room temperature

**Professional Information:**
**Overdosage Information**
For overdosage information, please refer to pgs. 673–674.

**Inactive Ingredients:** *Maximum Strength TYLENOL® Flu Non-Drowsy Gelcaps:* benzyl alcohol, butylparaben, castor oil, cellulose, corn starch, edetate calcium disodium, FD&C Blue #1, FD&C Red #40, gelatin, hydroxypropyl methylcellulose, iron oxide, magnesium stearate, methylparaben, propylparaben, sodium lauryl sulfate, sodium propionate, sodium starch glycolate, titanium dioxide.

*Maximum Strength TYLENOL® Flu NightTime Gelcaps:* benzyl alcohol, butylparaben, castor oil, cellulose, corn starch, D&C Red #28, edetate calcium disodium, FD&C Blue #1, gelatin, hydroxypropyl methylcellulose, iron oxide, magnesium stearate, methylparaben, propylparaben, sodium citrate, sodium lauryl sulfate, sodium propionate, sodium starch glycolate, titanium dioxide.

*Maximum Strength TYLENOL® Flu NightTime Liquid:* citric acid, corn syrup, D&C Red #33, FD&C Red #40, flavors, polyethylene glycol, propylene glycol, purified water, saccharin sodium, sodium benzoate, sorbitol.

**How Supplied:** *Maximum Strength TYLENOL® Flu Non-Drowsy* Gelcaps: Burgundy- and white-colored gelcap, imprinted with "TYLENOL FLU" in gray ink—blister packs of 24.

*Maximum Strength TYLENOL® Flu NightTime:* **Gelcaps:** Blue and white-colored gelcap, imprinted with "TYLENOL FLU NT" gray ink—blister packs of 12 and 24. **Liquid:** Red-colored—bottles of 8 fl. oz with child resistant safety cap and tamper evident packaging.

*Shown in Product Identification Guide, page 513*

---

**Extra Strength**
**TYLENOL® PM**
**Pain Reliever/Sleep Aid Caplets, Geltabs and Gelcaps**

**Description:** Each *Extra Strength TYLENOL® PM Caplet, Geltab* or *Gelcap* contains acetaminophen 500 mg and diphenhydramine HCl 25 mg.

**Actions:** *Extra Strength TYLENOL® PM Caplets, Geltabs* and *Gelcaps* contain a clinically proven analgesic-antipyretic and an antihistamine. Maximum allowable non-prescription levels of acetaminophen and diphenhydramine provide temporary relief of occasional headaches and minor aches and pains accompanying sleeplessness. Acetaminophen is equal to aspirin in analgesic and antipyretic effectiveness and it is unlikely to produce many of the side effects associated with aspirin containing products. Acetaminophen produces analgesia by elevation of the pain threshold. Diphenhydramine HCl is an antihistamine with sedative properties.

**Uses:** For the temporary relief of occasional headaches and minor aches and pains with accompanying sleeplessness.

**Directions: Adults and children 12 years of age and older:** Take 2 caplets, geltabs or gelcaps at bedtime or as directed by a doctor. **Children under 12 years of age:** Do not use this adult product in children under 12 years of age. This will provide more than the recommended dose (overdose) and could cause serious health problems.

**Precautions:** If a rare sensitivity reaction occurs, the drug should be discontinued.

**Warnings: Alcohol Warning:** If you consume 3 or more alcoholic drinks every day, ask your doctor whether you should take acetaminophen or other pain relievers/fever reducers. Acetaminophen may cause liver damage.

**Do not use if carton is opened or neck wrap or foil inner seal imprinted with "Safety Seal®" is broken.** If sleeplessness persists continuously for more than 2 weeks, consult your doctor. Insomnia may be a symptom of serious underlying medical illness. Do not take for pain for more than 10 days or for fever for more than 3 days unless directed by a doctor. If pain or fever persists, or gets worse, if new symptoms occur, or if redness or swelling is present, consult a doctor because these could be signs of a serious condition. Do not take this product, unless directed by a doctor, if you have a breathing problem such as emphysema or chronic bronchitis, or if you have glaucoma or difficulty in urination due to enlargement of the prostate gland. Avoid alcoholic beverages while taking this product. Do not take this product if your are taking sedatives or tranquilizers without first consulting your doctor. **Do not exceed recommended dose.** Keep this and all drugs out of the reach of children. In case of accidental overdose, contact a physician or poison control center immediately. Prompt medical attention is critical for adults as well as for children even if you do not notice any signs or symptoms. As with any drug, if you are pregnant or nursing a baby, seek the advice of a health professional before using this product. Do not use with other products containing acetaminophen.

**CAUTION: This product will cause drowsiness. Do not drive a motor vehicle or operate machinery after use.**

## Professional Information:
### Overdosage Information
For overdosage information, please refer to pgs. 673–674.

**Inactive Ingredients: Caplets:** Carnauba Wax, Cellulose, Cornstarch, FD&C Blue #1, FD&C Blue #2, Hydroxypropyl Methylcellulose, Magnesium Stearate, Polyethylene Glycol, Polysorbate 80, Sodium Citrate, Sodium Starch Glycolate, Titanium Dioxide.

**Geltabs/Gelcaps:** Benzyl Alcohol, Butylparaben, Castor Oil, Cellulose, Corn Starch, D&C Red #28, Edetate Calcium Disodium, FD&C Blue #1, Gelatin, Hydroxypropyl Methylcellulose, Magnesium Stearate, Methylparaben, Propylparaben, Sodium Citrate, Sodium Lauryl Sulfate, Sodium Propionate, Sodium Starch Glycolate, Titanium Dioxide.

**How Supplied: Caplets** (colored light blue imprinted "Tylenol PM") tamper-evident bottles of 24, 50, 100, and 150. Store at room temperature.

**Gelcaps** (colored blue and white imprinted "TYLENOL PM") tamper-evident bottles of 24 and 50. Store at room temperature; avoid high humidity and excessive heat 40°C (104°F).

**Geltabs** (colored blue and white imprinted "TYLENOL PM") tamper-evident bottles of 24, 50, and 100. Store at room temperature; avoid high humidity and excessive heat 40°C (104°F).

*Shown in Product Identification Guide, page 513*

---

**Maximum Strength TYLENOL® Sinus Non-Drowsy Geltabs, Gelcaps and Caplets**

**Maximum Strength TYLENOL® Sinus NightTime Caplets**

**Product information for all dosage forms of TYLENOL Sinus have been combined under this heading.**

**Description:** Each *Maximum Strength TYLENOL® Sinus Non-Drowsy Geltab, Gelcap, or Caplet* contains acetaminophen 500 mg and pseudoephedrine HCl 30 mg. Each *Maximum Strength TYLENOL® Sinus NightTime Caplet* contains acetaminophen 500 mg, doxylamine succinate 6.25 mg and pseudoephedrine HCl 30 mg.

**Actions:** *Maximum Strength TYLENOL® Sinus Non-Drowsy* is a clinically proven analgesic-antipyretic and a decongestant. Maximum allowable non-prescription levels of acetaminophen and pseudoephedrine provide temporary relief of sinus pain and headache and congestion. Acetaminophen is equal to aspirin in analgesic and antipyretic effectiveness and it is unlikely to produce many of the side effects associated with aspirin and aspirin-containing products. Acetaminophen produces analgesia by elevation of the pain threshold and antipyresis through action on the hypothalamic heat regulating center. Pseudoephedrine hydrochloride is a sympathomimetic amine which promotes sinus cavity drainage by reducing nasopharyngeal mucosal congestion.
*Maximum Strength TYLENOL® Sinus NightTime Caplets* contain, in addition to the above ingredients, an antihistamine which provides temporary relief of runny nose and itching of the nose or throat.

**Uses:** *Maximum Strength TYLENOL® Sinus Non-Drowsy:* temporarily relieves:
• sinus pain • headache • nasal and sinus congestion
*Maximum Strength TYLENOL® Sinus NightTime:* temporarily relieves:
• nasal congestion • sinus pressure
• sinus pain • headache • runny nose • sneezing • itchy, watery eyes • itching of the nose or throat

**Precautions:** If a rare sensitivity reaction occurs, the drug should be discontinued.

**Directions:** *Maximum Strength TYLENOL® Sinus Non-Drowsy:*
• do not take more than directed
**adults and children 12 years and over:**
• take 2 every 4–6 hours.
• do not take more than 8 in 24 hours, or as directed by a doctor.
**children under 12 years:**
• do not use this adult product in children under 12 years of age; this will provide more than the recommended dose (overdose) and could cause serious health problems.
*Maximum Strength TYLENOL® Sinus NightTime:*
• do not take more than directed
**adults and children 12 years and over:**
• take 2 caplets every 4 to 6 hours as needed
• do not take more than 8 caplets in 24 hours.
**children under 12 years:**
• do not use this adult product in children under 12 years of age; this will provide more than the recommended dose (overdose) and could cause serious health problems.

**Warnings: Alcohol warning:** If you consume 3 or more alcoholic drinks every day, ask your doctor whether you should take acetaminophen or other pain relievers/fever reducers. Acetaminophen may cause liver damage.
**Do not use**
• if you are now taking a prescription monamine oxidase inhibitor (MAOI) (certain drugs for depression, psychic or emotional conditions or Parkinson's disease), or for weeks after stopping the MAOI drug. If you do not know if your prescription drug contains an MAOI, ask a doctor or pharmacist before taking this product
**Stop use and ask a doctor if**
• new symptoms occur
• redness or swelling is present
• pains gets worse or last for more than 7 days
• fever gets worse or lasts for more than 3 days

• you get nervous, dizzy or sleepless
**If pregnant or breast feeding,** ask a health professional before use.
**Keep out of reach of children.** In case of overdose get medical help or contact a Poison Control Center right away. Quick medical attention is critical for adults as well as for children even if you do not notice any signs or symptoms.
*Maximum Strength TYLENOL® Sinus Non-Drowsy Geltabs, Gelcaps and Caplets*
**Ask a doctor if you have**
• heart disease • high blood pressure
• thyroid disease • diabetes
• trouble urinating due to an enlarged prostate gland
**When using this product**
• do not exceed recommend dosage
*Maximum Strength TYLENOL® Sinus NightTime Caplets*
**Ask a doctor before use if you have**
• heart disease • glaucoma • diabetes
• thyroid disease • high blood pressure • trouble urinating due to an enlarged prostate gland
• a breathing problem such as emphysema or chronic bronchitis
**Ask a doctor or pharmacist before use if you are** taking sedatives or tranquilizers
**When using this product**
• do not exceed recommended dosage
• marked drowsiness may occur
• avoid alcoholic drinks
• alcohol, sedatives and tranquilizers may increase drowsiness
• be careful when driving a motor vehicle or operating machinery
• excitability may occur, especially in children
**Other Information**
• do not use if carton is opened or if blister unit is broken
*Maximum Strength TYLENOL® Sinus Geltabs and Gelcaps*
• store at room temperature; avoid high humidity and excessive heat 40°C (104°F)
*Maximum Strength TYLENOL® Sinus Caplets and Maximum Strength TYLENOL® Sinus NightTime Caplets*
• store at room temperature

## Professional Information:
### Overdosage Information
For overdosage information, please refer to pgs. 673–674.

**Inactive Ingredients:** *Maximum Strength TYLENOL® Sinus Non-Drowsy Formula:* **Caplets:** carnauba wax, cellulose, corn starch, D&C Yellow #10, FD&C Blue #1, FD&C Red #40, hydroxypropyl methylcellulose, iron oxide, magnesium stearate, polyethylene glycol, polysorbate 80, sodium starch glycolate, titanium dioxide.

**Gelcaps and Geltabs:** benzyl alcohol, butylparaben, castor oil, cellulose, corn starch, D&C Yellow #10, edetate calcium disodium, FD&C Blue #1, gelatin, hydroxypropyl methylcellulose, iron oxide, magnesium stearate, methylparaben, propylparaben, sodium lauryl sulfate, sodium propionate, sodium starch glycolate, titanium dioxide.
*Maximum Strength TYLENOL® Sinus NightTime Caplets:* cellulose, corn

*Continued on next page*

## Tylenol Sinus—Cont.

starch, FD&C Blue #1, FD&C Blue #2, hydroxypropyl methylcellulose, iron oxide, silicon dioxide, sodium starch glycolate, stearic acid, titanium dioxide, triacetin.

**How Supplied:** *Maximum Strength TYLENOL® Sinus Non-Drowsy Formula:*
**Caplets:** Light green-colored, imprinted with "TYLENOL Sinus" in green ink—blister packs of 24 and 48.
**Gelcaps:** Green- and white-colored, imprinted with "TYLENOL Sinus" in dark green ink—blister packs of 24 and 48.
**Geltabs:** Green-colored on one side and white-colored on opposite side, imprinted with "TYLENOL Sinus" in gray ink—blister packs of 24 and 48.
*Maximum Strength TYLENOL® Sinus NightTime Caplets:* Green-colored, imprinted with "Tylenol Sinus NT"—blister packs of 24.

*Shown in Product Identification Guide, page 513*

---

## Maximum Strength TYLENOL® Sore Throat Adult Liquid

**Description:** *Maximum Strength TYLENOL® Sore Throat Liquid* is available in Honey Lemon Flavor or Cherry Flavor and contains acetaminophen 1000 mg in each 30 mL (2 Tablespoonsful).

**Actions:** Acetaminophen is a clinically proven analgesic/antipyretic. Acetaminophen produces analgesia by elevation of the pain threshold and antipyresis through action on the hypothalamic heat regulating center. Acetaminophen is equal to aspirin in analgesic and antipyretic effectiveness and it is unlikely to produce many of the side effects associated with aspirin and aspirin-containing products.

**Uses:** temporarily relieves minor aches and pains due to:
• sore throat • headache • muscular aches • the common cold
• temporarily reduces fever

**Directions:**
• do not take more than directed
**adults and children 12 years of age and over:**
• take 2 tablespoons (tbsp) in dose cup provided every 4 to 6 hours as needed
• do not use more than 8 tablespoons in 24 hours
**children under 12 years:** do not use this adult product in children under 12 years of age; this will provide more than the recommended dose (overdose) of TYLENOL® and could cause serious health problems.

**Precautions:** If a rare sensitivity reaction occurs, the drug should be discontinued.

**Warnings: Alcohol warning:** If you consume 3 or more alcoholic drinks every day, ask your doctor whether you should take acetaminophen or other pain relievers/fever reducers. Acetaminophen may cause liver damage.
**Sore throat warning:** If sore throat is severe, persists for more than 2 days, is accompanied or followed by fever, headache, rash, nausea or vomiting, consult a doctor promptly.
**Do Not Use:**
• with any other product containing acetaminophen
**Stop Use and Ask a Doctor if**
• new symptoms occur
• redness or swelling is present
• pain gets worse or lasts for more than 10 days
• fever gets worse or lasts for more than 3 days
**If pregnant or breast-feeding,** ask a health professional before use.
**Keep out of the reach of children.** In case of overdose, get medical help or contact a Poison Control Center right away. Quick medical attention is critical for adults as well as for children even if you do not notice any signs or symptoms.

**Other Information**
• **do not use if carton is opened or if bottle wrap or foil inner seal imprinted "Safety Seal©" is broken or missing**
• store at room temperature

**Professional Information:**
**Overdosage Information**
For overdosage information, please refer to pgs. 673–674.

**Inactive Ingredients:** *Maximum Strength TYLENOL® Sore Throat Honey-Lemon-Flavored Adult Liquid:* carmel color, citric acid, flavor, high fructose corn syrup, polyethylene glycol, propylene glycol, purified water, saccharin sodium, sodium benzoate, sorbitol
*Maximum Strength TYLENOL® Sore Throat Cherry-Flavored Adult Liquid:* citric acid, D&C Red # 33, FD&C Red # 40, flavor, high fructose corn syrup, polyethylene glycol, propylene glycol, purified water, saccharin sodium, sodium benzoate, sorbitol

**How Supplied:** Honey lemon-flavored or cherry-flavored liquid in child-resistant tamper-evident bottles of 8 fl. oz.

*Shown in Product Identification Guide, page 513*

---

## Women's TYLENOL® Menstrual Relief Pain Reliever/ Diuretic Caplets

**Description:** Each *Women's Tylenol® Menstrual Relief Caplet* contains acetaminophen 500 mg and pamabrom 25 mg.

**Actions:** *Women's TYLENOL® Menstrual Relief Caplets* contain a clinically proven analgesic-antipyretic and a diuretic. Maximum allowable non-prescription levels of acetaminophen and pamabrom provide temporary relief of minor aches and pains due to cramps, headache, and backache and water retention, weight gain, bloating, swelling and full feeling associated with the premenstrual and menstrual periods. Acetaminophen is equal to aspirin in analgesic and antipyretic effectiveness and it is unlikely to produce many of the side effects associated with aspirin containing products. Acetaminophen produces analgesia by elevation of the pain threshold. Pamabrom is a diuretic which relieves water retention.

**Uses:**
• temporarily relieves minor aches and pains due to:
  • cramps • headache • backache
• temporarily relieves water-weight gain, bloating, swelling and full feeling associated with the premenstrual and menstrual periods

**Directions:**
• **do not take more than directed**
**adults and children 12 years and over:** take 2 caplets every 4 to 6 hours; do not take more than 8 caplets in 24 hours, or as directed by a doctor
**children under 12 years:** do not use this adult product in children under 12 years of age; this will provide more than the recommended dose (overdose) and could cause serious health problems

**Precautions:** If a rare sensitivity reaction occurs, the drug should be discontinued.

**Warnings: Alcohol warning:** If you consume 3 or more alcoholic drinks every day, ask your doctor whether you should take acetaminophen or other pain relievers/fever reducers. Acetaminophen may cause liver damage.

**Do not use**
• with any other product containing acetaminophen
**Stop use and ask a doctor if**
• new symptoms occur
• redness or swelling is present
• pain gets worse or lasts for more than 10 days
**If pregnant or breast-feeding,** ask a health professional before use.
**Keep out of reach of children.** In case of overdose, get medical help or contact a Poison Control Center right away. Prompt medical attention is critical for adults as well as for children even if you do not notice any signs or symptoms.

**Other Information**
• **do not use if carton is opened, or if neck wrap or foil inner seal imprinted "Safety Seal®" is broken or missing**
• store at room temperature, avoid excessive heat 104°F (40°C)

**Professional Information:**
**Overdosage Information**
For overdosage information, please refer to pgs. 673–674.

**Inactive Ingredients:** cellulose, corn starch, hydroxypropyl methylcellulose, magnesium stearate, polydextrose, polyethylene glycol, sodium starch glycolate, titanium dioxide, triacetin.

**How Supplied:** White capsule shaped caplets with TYME printed on one side in tamper-evident bottles of 24 and 40.

*Shown in Product Identification Guide, page 514*

---

**Infants' TYLENOL®**
**acetaminophen Concentrated Drops**

**Children's TYLENOL®**
**acetaminophen Suspension Liquid and Soft Chews Chewable Tablets**

**Junior Strength TYLENOL®**
**acetaminophen Soft Chews Chewable Tablets**

**Product information for all dosages of Children's TYLENOL have been combined under this heading**

**Description:** *Infants' TYLENOL® Concentrated Drops* are stable, alcohol-free, grape-flavored and purple in color or cherry-flavored and red in color. Each 1.6 mL (2 dropperfuls) contains 160 mg acetaminophen. *Infants' TYLENOL® Concentrated Drops* features the SAFE-TY-LOCK™ Bottle. The SAFE-TY-LOCK™ Bottle has a unique safety barrier inside the bottle which helps make administration easier. The integrated dropper promotes proper administration. The innovative design eliminates excess product on dropper. The star-shaped barrier inside the bottle minimizes spills and discourages pouring into a spoon. *Children's TYLENOL® Suspension Liquid* is stable, alcohol-free, cherry-flavored and red in color, or bubble gum-flavored and pink in color, or grape-flavored and purple in color. Each 5 mL (one teaspoonful) contains 160 mg acetaminophen. Each *Children's TYLENOL® Soft Chews Chewable Tablet* contains 80 mg acetaminophen in a grape, bubble gum, or fruit flavor. *Each Junior Strength TYLENOL® Soft Chews Chewable Tablet* contains 160 mg acetaminophen in a grape or fruit-flavored chewable tablet.

**Actions:** Acetaminophen is a clinically proven analgesic/antipyretic. Acetaminophen produces analgesia by elevation of the pain threshold and antipyresis through action on the hypothalamic heat-regulating center. Acetaminophen is equal to aspirin in analgesic and antipyretic effectiveness and it is unlikely to produce many of the side effects associated with aspirin and aspirin-containing products.

**Uses:** *Infants' TYLENOL® Concentrated Drops:* temporarily:
• reduces fever
• relieves minor aches and pains due to:
  • the common cold • flu • headaches
  • sore throat • immunizations • toothaches
*Children's TYLENOL® Suspension Liquid and Children's TYLENOL® Soft Chews Chewable Tablets:* temporarily relieves minor aches and pains due to:
• the common cold • flu • headaches
  • sore throat • immunizations
• toothaches

• reduces fever
*Junior Strength TYLENOL® Soft Chews Chewable Tablets:* temporarily relieves minor aches and pains due to: • the common cold • flu • headache • muscle aches • sprains • overexertion
• reduces fever

**Directions:** See Table 1: Children's Tylenol Dosing Chart on pgs. 684–686.

**Precautions:** If a rare sensitivity reaction occurs, the drug should be discontinued.

**Warnings:**
**Sore throat warning:** if sore throat is severe, persists for more than 2 days, is accompanied or followed by fever, headache, rash, nausea, or vomiting, consult a doctor promptly (excluding *Junior Strength TYLENOL® Soft Chews Chewable Tablets*).
**Do not use**
• with any other product containing acetaminophen
**When using this product**
• **do not exceed recommended dose;** taking more than the recommended dose (overdose) may not provide more relief and could cause serious health problems
**Stop use and ask a doctor if**
• new symptoms occur
• redness or swelling is present
• pain gets worse or lasts for more than 5 days
• fever gets worse or lasts for more than 3 days
**Keep out of the reach of children.** In case of overdose, get medical help or contact a Poison Control Center right away. Quick medical attention is critical even if you do not notice any signs or symptoms.
**Other Information:**
*Infants' TYLENOL® Concentrated Drops:*
• **Do not use if carton wrap or bottle wrap imprinted "Safety Seal®" is broken or missing.**
• Store at room temperature
*Children's TYLENOL® Suspension Liquid:*
• **Do not use if bottle wrap, or foil inner seal imprinted "Safety Seal®" is broken or missing**
• Store at room temperature
*Children's TYLENOL® Soft Chews Chewable Tablets:*
• phenylketonurics: fruit and grape contain phenylalanine 3 mg per tablet, bubble gum contains phenylalanine 6 mg per tablet
• **Do not use if carton is opened or if neck wrap or foil inner seal imprinted "Safety Seal®" is broken or missing.**
*Junior Strength TYLENOL® Soft Chews Chewable Tablets:*
• Phenylketonurics: contains phenylalanine 6 mg per tablet

**Professional Information:**
**Overdosage Information for all Infants', Children's & Junior Strength Tylenol® Products**

**ACETAMINOPHEN:** Acetaminophen in massive overdosage may cause hepatic toxicity in some patients. In adults and adolescents ($\geq$ 12 years of age), hepatic toxicity may occur following ingestion of greater than 7.5 to 10 grams over a period of 8 hours or less. Fatalities are infrequent (less than 3–4% of untreated cases) and have rarely been reported with overdoses of less than 15 grams. In children (<12 years of age), an acute overdosage of less than 150 mg/kghas not been associated with hepatic toxicity. Early symptoms following a potentially hepatotoxic overdose may include: nausea, vomiting, diaphoresis and general malaise. Clinical and laboratory evidence of hepatic toxicity may not be apparent until 48 to 72 hours postingestion. In adults and adolescents, any individual presenting with an unknown amount of acetaminophen ingested or with a questionable or unreliable history about the time of ingestion should have a plasma acetaminophen level drawn and be treated with *N*-acetylcysteine. For full prescribing information, refer to the *N*-acetylcysteine package insert. Do not await results of assays for plasma acetaminophen levels before initiating treatment with *N*-acetylcysteine. The following additional procedures are recommended: Promptly initiate gastric decontamination of the stomach. A plasma acetaminophen assay should be obtained as early as possible, but no sooner than four hours following ingestion. If an acetaminophen *extended release* product is involved, it may be appropriate to obtain an additional plasma acetaminophen level 4–6 hours following the initial acetaminophen level. If either acetaminophen level plots above the treatment line on the acetaminophen overdose nomogram, *N*-acetylcysteine treatment should be continued for a full course of therapy. Liver function studies should be obtained initially and repeated at 24-hour intervals. Serious toxicity or fatalities have been extremely infrequent following an acute acetaminophen overdose in young children, possibly because of differences in the way they metabolize acetaminophen. In children, the maximum potential amount ingested can be more easily estimated. If more than 150 mg/kg or an unknown amount was ingested, obtain a plasma acetaminophen level as soon as possible, but no sooner than 4 hours following ingestion. If an acetaminophen *extended release* product is involved, it may be appropriate to obtain an additional plasma acetaminophen level 4–6 hours following the initial acetaminophen level. If either acetaminophen level plots above the treatment line on the acetaminophen overdose nomogram, *N*-acetylcysteine treatment should be initiated and continued for a full course of therapy. If an assay cannot be obtained and the estimated acetaminophen ingestion exceeds 150 mg/kg, dosing with *N*-acetylcysteine should be initiated and continued for a full course of therapy. For additional emer-

*Continued on next page*

## Tylenol Infants—Cont.

gency information, call your regional poison center or call the Rocky Mountain Poison Center toll-free, (1-800-525-6115). **Our pediatric Tylenol® combination products contain active ingredients in addition to acetaminophen. The following is basic overdose information regarding those ingredients.**
**CHLORPHENIRAMINE:** Chlorpheniramine toxicity should be treated as you would an antihistamine/anticholinergic overdose and is likely to be present within a few hours after acute ingestion.
**DEXTROMETHORPHAN:** Acute dextromethorphan overdose usually does not result in serious signs and symptoms unless massive amounts have been ingested. Signs and symptoms of a substantial overdose may include nausea and vomiting, visual disturbances, CNS disturbances and urinary retention.
**DIPHENHYDRAMINE:** Diphenhydramine toxicity should be treated as you would an antihistamine/anticholinergic overdose and is likely to be present within a few hours after acute ingestion.
**PSEUDOEPHEDRINE:** Symptoms from pseudoephedrine overdose consist most often of mild anxiety, tachycardia and/or mild hypertension. Symptoms usually appear within 4 to 8 hours of ingestion and are transient, usually requiring no treatment.
**For additional emergency information, please contact your local poison control center.**

**Inactive Ingredients:** *Infants' TYLENOL® Concentrated Drops:* Cherry-Flavored: butylparaben, cellulose, citric acid, corn syrup, FD&C Red #40, flavors, glycerin, propylene glycol, purified water, sodium benzoate, sorbitol, xanthan gum. **Grape-Flavored:** butylparaben, cellulose, citric acid, corn syrup, D&C Red #33, FD&C Blue #1, flavors, glycerin, propylene glycol, purified water, sodium benzoate, sorbitol, xanthan gum.
*Children's TYLENOL® Suspension Liquid:* butylparaben, cellulose, citric acid, corn syrup, flavors, glycerin, propylene glycol, purified water, sodium benzoate, sorbitol, xanthan gum. In addition to the above ingredients cherry-flavored suspension contains FD&C Red #40, bubble gum-flavored suspension contains D&C Red #33 and FD&C Red #40, and grape-flavored suspension contains D&C Red #33 and FD&C Blue #1.
*Children's TYLENOL® Soft Chews Chewable Tablets:* **Fruit-Flavored**: aspartame, cellulose, cellulose acetate citric acid, D&C Red #7, flavors, magnesium stearate, mannitol, povidone. **Grape-Flavored:** aspartame, cellulose, cellulose acetate, citric acid, D&C Red #7, D&C Red #30, FD&C Blue #1, flavors, magnesium stearate, mannitol, povidone. **Bubble Gum-Flavored:** aspartame, cellulose, cellulose acetate, D&C Red #7, flavors, magnesium stearate, mannitol, povidone.

*Junior Strength TYLENOL® Soft Chews Chewable Tablets:* **Fruit-Flavored**: aspartame, cellulose, citric acid, D&C Red #7, flavors, magnesium stearate, mannitol, povidone. **Grape-Flavored:** aspartame, cellulose, citric acid, D&C Red #7, D&C Red #30, FD&C Blue #1, flavors, magnesium stearate, mannitol, povidone.

**How Supplied:** *Infants' TYLENOL® Concentrated Drops:* (purple-colored grape): bottles of ½ oz (15 mL) and 1 oz (30 mL); (red-colored cherry): bottles of ½ oz and 1 oz, each with calibrated plastic dropper.
*Children's TYLENOL® Suspension Liquid:* (red-colored cherry): bottles of 2 and 4 fl oz. (pink-colored bubble gum and purple-colored grape): bottles of 4 fl. oz.
*Children's TYLENOL® Soft Chews Chewable Tablets:* (pink-colored fruit, purple-colored grape, pink-colored bubble gum, scored, imprinted "TY80"). Bottles of 30 and also blister packaged 60's and 96's (fruit).
*Junior Strength TYLENOL® Soft Chews Chewable Tablets:* (purple-colored grape or pink-colored fruit, imprinted "TY 160") Package of 24. All packages listed above are safety sealed and use child-resistant safety caps or blisters.

*Shown in Product Identification Guide, page 511, 512*

## CHILDREN'S TYLENOL® Allergy-D Liquid

**Description:** *Children's TYLENOL® Allergy-D Liquid* is Bubble Gum Blast-flavored and contains no alcohol or aspirin. Each teaspoonful (5 mL) contains acetaminophen 160 mg, diphenhydramine HCl 12.5 mg and pseudoephedrine HCl 15 mg.

**Actions:** *Children's TYLENOL® Allergy-D Liquid* combines the analgesic-antipyretic acetaminophen with the antihistamine diphenhydramine hydrochloride and the decongestant pseudoephedrine hydrochloride to provide fast, effective, temporary relief of all your child's symptoms associated with hay fever and other respiratory allergies including sneezing, sore throat, itchy throat, itchy/watery eyes, runny nose, stuffy nose and nasal congestion. Acetaminophen is equal to aspirin in analgesic and antipyretic effectiveness and it is unlikely to produce the side effects often associated with aspirin or aspirin-containing products.

**Uses:** temporarily relieves these hay fever and upper respiratory allergy symptoms:
• nasal congestion • sore throat
• runny nose • sneezing
• stuffy nose • minor aches and pains
• itchy, watery eyes
• temporarily reduces fever

**Directions:** See Table 1: Children's Tylenol Dosing Chart on pgs. 684–686.

**Precautions:** If a rare sensitivity reaction occurs, the drug should be discontinued.

**Warnings: Sore throat warning:** If sore throat is severe, persists for more than 2 days, is accompanied or followed by fever, headache, rash, nausea or vomiting, consult a doctor promptly.

**Do not use**
• in a child who is taking a prescription monoamine oxidase inhibitor (MAOI) (certain drugs for depression, psychiatric, emotional conditions or Parkinson's disease) or for 2 weeks after stopping the MAOI drug. If you do not know if your child's prescription drug contains an MAOI, ask a doctor or pharmacist before giving this product.
• with any other product containing acetaminophen.

**Ask a doctor before use if the child has**
• heart disease • high blood pressure
• thyroid disease • diabetes
• glaucoma • a breathing problem such as chronic bronchitis

**When using this product**
• do not exceed recommended dosage; taking more than the recommended dose (overdose) may not provide more relief and could cause serious health problems.
• marked drowsiness may occur
• excitability may occur, especially in children

**Stop use and ask a doctor if**
• new symptoms occur
• redness or swelling is present
• pain gets worse or lasts for more than 5 days
• fever gets worse or lasts for more than 3 days
• nervousness, dizziness or sleeplessness occurs

**Keep out of reach of children.** In case of overdose, get medical help or contact a Poison Control Center right away. Quick medical attention is critical even if you do not notice any signs or symptoms

**Other Information:**
• do not use if plastic carton wrap, bottle wrap, or foil inner seal imprinted "Safety Seal®" is broken or missing.
• Store at room temperature

**Professional Information:**
**Overdosage Information**

For overdosage information, please refer to pgs. 681–682.

**Inactive Ingredients:** benzoic acid, citric acid, corn syrup, D&C Red #33, FD&C Red #40, flavors, polyethylene glycol, propylene glycol, purified water, sodium benzoate, sorbitol.

**How Supplied:** Pink-colored–child-resistant bottles of 4 fl. oz.

*Shown in Product Identification Guide, page 511*

## Infants' TYLENOL® Cold Decongestant & Fever Reducer Concentrated Drops

## Infants' TYLENOL® Cold Decongestant & Fever Reducer Concentrated Drops Plus Cough

## Children's TYLENOL® Cold Suspension Liquid and Chewable Tablets

## Children's TYLENOL® Cold Plus Cough Suspension Liquid and Chewable Tablets

**Description:** *Infants' TYLENOL® Cold Decongestant & Fever Reducer Concentrated Drops* are alcohol-free, aspirin-free, BubbleGum Blast-flavored and red in color. Each 1.6 mL (2 dropperfuls) contains acetaminophen 160 mg and pseudoephedrine HCl 15 mg. *Infants' TYLENOL® Cold Decongestant & Fever Reducer Concentrated Drops Plus Cough* are alcohol-free, aspirin-free, Wild-Cherry-flavored and red in color. Each 1.6 mL (2 dropperfuls) contains acetaminophen 160 mg, dextromethorphan HBr 5 mg, and pseudoephedrine HCl 15 mg. *Children's TYLENOL® Cold Suspension Liquid* is Great Grape-flavored and contains no alcohol or aspirin. Each teaspoonful (5 mL) contains acetaminophen 160 mg, chlorpheniramine maleate 1 mg and pseudoephedrine HCl 15 mg. *Children's TYLENOL® Cold Chewable Tablets* are Great Grape-flavored and each tablet contains acetaminophen 80 mg, chlorpheniramine maleate 0.5 mg and pseudoephedrine HCl 7.5 mg. *Children's TYLENOL® Cold Plus Cough Suspension Liquid* is Wild-Cherry-flavored and contains no alcohol or aspirin. Each teaspoonful (5 mL) contains acetaminophen 160 mg, chlorpheniramine maleate 1 mg, dextromethorphan HBr 5 mg and pseudoephedrine HCl 15 mg. *Children's TYLENOL® Cold Plus Cough Chewable Tablets* are Wild-Cherry-flavored and each tablet contains acetaminophen 80 mg, chlorpheniramine maleate 0.5 mg, dextromethorphan HBr 2.5 mg, and pseudoephedrine HCl 7.5 mg.

**Actions:** Acetaminophen is a clinically proven analgesic/antipyretic. Acetaminophen produces analgesia by elevation of the pain threshold and antipyresis through action on the hypothalamic heat-regulating center. Acetaminophen is equal to aspirin in analgesic and antipyretic effectiveness and it is unlikely to produce many of the side effects associated with aspirin and aspirin-containing products.
Pseudoephedrine hydrochloride is a sympathomimetic amine which provides temporary relief of nasal congestion.
Chlorpheniramine maleate is an antihistamine that provides temporary relief of runny nose, sneezing and watery and itchy eyes.
Dextromethorphan hydrobromide is a cough suppressant which helps relieve coughs.

**Uses:** *Infants' TYLENOL® Cold Decongestant & Fever Reducer Concentrated Drops:* temporarily relieves these cold symptoms:
• minor aches and pains
• nasal congestion • headaches
• temporarily reduces fever
*Infants' TYLENOL® Cold Decongestant & Fever Reducer Concentrated Drops Plus Cough:* temporarily relieves these cold symptoms:
• coughs • nasal congestion
• minor aches and pains
• sore throat • headaches
• temporarily reduces fever
*Children's TYLENOL® Cold Suspension Liquid* and *Chewable Tablets:* temporarily relieves these cold symptoms:
• nasal congestion • sore throat • runny nose • sneezing • headache • minor aches and pains
• temporarily reduces fever
*Children's TYLENOL® Cold Plus Cough Suspension Liquid* and *Chewable Tablets:* temporarily relieves these cold symptoms:
• nasal congestion • sore throat • runny nose • sneezing • headache • minor aches and pains • coughs
• temporarily reduces fever

**Directions:** See Table 1: Children's Tylenol Dosing Chart on pgs. 684–686.

**Precautions:** If a rare sensitivity reaction occurs, the drug should be discontinued.

**Warnings: Sore throat warning:** If sore throat is severe, persists for more than 2 days, is accompanied by or followed by fever, headache, rash, nausea or vomiting, consult a doctor promptly (does not apply to *Infants' TYLENOL® Cold Decongestant and Fever Reducer Drops*)
Do not use
• in a child who is taking a prescription monoamine oxidase inhibitor (MAOI) (certain drugs for depression, psychiatric, emotional conditions or Parkinson's disease), or for 2 weeks after stopping the MAOI drug. If you do not know if your child's prescription drug contains an MAOI, ask a doctor or pharmacist before giving this product.
• with any products containing acetaminophen
**Keep out of the reach of children.** In case of overdose, get medical help or contact a Poison Control Center right away. Quick medical attention is critical even if you do not notice any signs or symptoms.
**Stop use and ask a doctor if**
• new symptoms occur
• redness or swelling is present
• pain gets worse or lasts for more than 5 days
• fever gets worse or lasts for more than 3 days
• nervousness, dizziness or sleeplessness occurs
• cough lasts for more than 7 days, comes back or occurs with fever, rash or headache that lasts. These could be signs of a serious condition. (*Infants' TYLENOL® Cold Decongestant and Fever Reducer Drops Plus Cough and Children's TYLENOL® Cold Plus Cough Products* only)

*Infants' TYLENOL® Cold Decongestant and Fever Reducer Drops*
**Ask a doctor before use if the child has**
• heart disease • high blood pressure
• thyroid disease • diabetes
**When using this product**
• **do not exceed recommended dosage;** taking more than the recommended dose (overdose) may not provide more relief and could cause serious health problems
*Infants' TYLENOL® Cold Decongestant and Fever Reducer Drops Plus Cough*
**Ask a doctor before use if the child has**
• heart disease • high blood pressure
• cough that occurs with too much phlegm (mucus) • thyroid disease • diabetes • chronic cough that lasts as occurs with asthma
**When using this product**
• **do not exceed recommended dosage;** taking more than the recommended dose (overdose) may not provide more relief and could cause serious health problems.
*Children's TYLENOL® Cold Suspension Liquid and Chewable Tablets*
**Ask a doctor before use if the child has**
• heart disease • thyroid disease • glaucoma • high blood pressure • diabetes
• a breathing problem such as chronic bronchitis
**When using this product**
• **do not exceed recommended dosage;** taking more than the recommended dose (overdose) may not provide more relief and could cause serious health problems.
• drowsiness may occur
• excitability may occur, especially in children
*Children's TYLENOL® Cold Plus Cough Suspension Liquid and Chewable Tablets*
**Ask a doctor before use if the child has**
• heart disease • thyroid disease • glaucoma • high blood pressure • diabetes
• cough that occurs with too much phlegm (mucus) • chronic cough that lasts as occurs with asthma
**When using this product**
• **do not exceed recommended dosage;** taking more than the recommended dose (overdose) may not provide more relief and could cause serious health problems.
• drowsiness may occur
• excitability may occur, especially in children
**Other Information**
*Infants' TYLENOL® Cold Decongestant & Fever Reducer Drops, Infants' TYLENOL® Cold Decongestant & Fever Reducer Drops Plus Cough, Children's TYLENOL® Cold Suspension Liquid & Children's TYLENOL® Cold Plus Cough Suspension Liquid*
• **do not use if plastic carton wrap or bottle wrap imprinted "Safety Seal®" is broken or missing**
• Store at room temperature
*Children's TYLENOL® Cold Chewable Tablets*
• phenylketonurics: contains phenylalanine 6 mg per tablet
• **do not use if carton is opened or if blister unit is broken**
• Store at room temperature

*Continued on next page*

**TABLE 1**
Children's Tylenol® Dosing Chart

| PRODUCT FORM | INGREDIENTS | 0–3 mos / 6–11 lbs | 4–11 mos / 12–17 lbs | 12–23 mos / 18–23 lbs | 2–3 yrs / 24–35 lbs | 4–5 yrs / 36–47 lbs | 6–8 yrs / 48–59 lbs | 9–10 yrs / 60–71 lbs | 11 yrs / 72–95 lbs | 12 yrs / Over 96 lbs | Maximum doses/24 hrs |
|---|---|---|---|---|---|---|---|---|---|---|---|
| **AGE GROUP** / **WEIGHT** | (if possible use weight to dose; otherwise use age) | | | | | | | | | | |
| | Dose to be administered based on weight or age† | | | | | | | | | | |
| **Infants' Drops** | Per dropperful (0.8 mL) | | | | | | | | | | |
| **Infants' Tylenol** Concentrated Drops | Acetaminophen 80 mg | ½ dropperful (0.4 mL)* | 1 dropperful (0.8 mL)* | 1½ dropperfuls (0.8 + 0.4 mL)* | 2 dropperfuls (0.8 + 0.8 mL) | — | — | — | — | — | 5 times in 24 hrs |
| **Infants' Tylenol Cold** Decongestant & Fever Reducer Concentrated Drops | Acetaminophen 80 mg Pseudoephedrine HCl 7.5 mg | ½ dropperful (0.4 mL)* | 1 dropperful (0.8 mL)* | 1½ dropperfuls (0.8 + 0.4 mL)* | 2 dropperfuls (0.8 + 0.8 mL) | — | — | — | — | — | 4 times in 24 hrs |
| **Infants' Tylenol Cold** Decongestant & Fever Reducer Concentrated Drops **Plus** Cough | Acetaminophen 80 mg Dextromethorphan HBr 2.5 mg Pseudoephedrine HCl 7.5 mg | ½ dropperful (0.4 mL)* | 1 dropperful (0.8 mL)* | 1½ dropperfuls (0.8 + 0.4 mL)* | 2 dropperfuls (0.8 + 0.8 mL) | — | — | — | — | — | 4 times in 24 hrs |
| **Children's Liquids** | Per 5 mL teaspoonful (TSP) | | | | | | | | | | |
| **Children's Tylenol** Suspension Liquid | Acetaminophen 160 mg | — | ½ TSP* | ¾ TSP* | 1 TSP | 1½ TSP | 2 TSP | 2½ TSP | 3 TSP | — | 5 times in 24 hrs |
| **Children's Tylenol Cold** Suspension Liquid | Acetaminophen 160 mg Chlorpheniramine Maleate 1 mg Pseudoephedrine HCl 15 mg | — | ½ TSP** | ¾ TSP** | 1 TSP** | 1½ TSP** | 2 TSP | 2½ TSP | 3 TSP | — | 4 times in 24 hrs |

| Product | Ingredients | | | | | | | | | | Frequency |
|---|---|---|---|---|---|---|---|---|---|---|---|
| **Children's Tylenol Cold Plus Cough** Suspension Liquid | Acetaminophen 160 mg Chlorpheniramine Maleate 1 mg Dextromethorphan HBr 5 mg Pseudoephedrine HCl 15 mg | — | ½ TSP** | ¾ TSP** | 1 TSP** | 1 ½ TSP** | 2 TSP | 2 ½ TSP | 3 TSP | — | 4 times in 24 hrs |
| **Children's Tylenol Flu** Suspension Liquid† | Acetaminophen 160 mg Chlorpheniramine Maleate 1 mg Dextromethorphan HBr 7.5 mg Pseudoephedrine HCl 15 mg | — | ½ TSP** | ¾ TSP** | 1 TSP** | 1 ½ TSP** | 2 TSP | 2 ½ TSP | 3 TSP | — | 4 times in 24 hrs |
| **Children's Tylenol Sinus** Suspension Liquid | Acetaminophen 160 mg Pseudoephedrine HCl 15 mg | — | ½ TSP* | ¾ TSP* | 1 TSP | 1 ½ TSP | 2 TSP | 2 ½ TSP | 3 TSP | — | 4 times in 24 hrs |
| **Children's Tylenol Allergy-D** Liquid | Acetaminophen 160 mg Diphenhydramine HCl 12.5 mg Pseudoephedrine HCl 15 mg | — | ½ TSP** | ¾ TSP** | 1 TSP** | 1 ½ TSP** | 2 TSP | 2 ½ TSP | 3 TSP | — | 4 times in 24 hrs |

† All products may be dosed every 4 hours, if needed; except for Children's Tylenol Flu which is dosed every 6–8 hrs, if needed.
* Under 2 years (under 24 lbs), consult a doctor.
** Under 6 years (under 48 lbs), consult a doctor.
• Infants' Tylenol Drops are more concentrated than Children's Tylenol Liquids. The Infants' Concentrated Drops have been specifically designed for use only with enclosed dropper. Do not use any other dosing device with this product.
• Children's Tylenol Liquids are less concentrated than Infants' Tylenol Concentrated Drops. The Children's Tylenol Liquids have been specifically designed for use with the enclosed measuring cup. Use only enclosed measuring cup to dose this product.
• Children's Tylenol Soft Chews Chewable Tablets are not the same concentration as Junior Strength Tylenol Soft Chews Chewable Tablets.
• Junior Strength Tylenol Soft Chews Chewable Tablets contain twice as much medicine as Children's Tylenol Soft Chews Chewable Tablets.

*Table continued on next page*

**TABLE 1**
**Children's Tylenol® Dosing Chart (continued)**

| AGE GROUP | 0–3 mos | 4–11 mos | 12–23 mos | 2–3 yrs | 4–5 yrs | 6–8 yrs | 9–10 yrs | 11 yrs | 12 yrs | Maximum doses/24 hrs |
|---|---|---|---|---|---|---|---|---|---|---|
| **WEIGHT** (if possible use weight to dose; otherwise use age) | 6–11 lbs | 12–17 lbs | 18–23 lbs | 24–35 lbs | 36–47 lbs | 48–59 lbs | 60–71 lbs | 72–95 lbs | Over 96 lbs | |
| **PRODUCT FORM / INGREDIENTS** Dose to be administered based on weight or age† / **Per tablet** | | | | | | | | | | |
| **Children's Tylenol** Soft Chews Chewable Tablets — Acetaminophen 80 mg | — | — | — | 2 tablets | 3 tablets | 4 tablets | 5 tablets | 6 tablets | — | 5 times in 24 hrs |
| **Children's Tylenol Cold** Chewable Tablets — Acetaminophen 80 mg, Chlorpheniramine Maleate 0.5 mg, Pseudoephedrine HCl 7.5 mg | — | — | — | 2 tablets** | 3 tablets** | 4 tablets | 5 tablets | 6 tablets | — | 4 times in 24 hrs |
| **Children's Tylenol Cold Plus Cough** Chewable Tablets — Acetaminophen 80 mg, Chlorpheniramine Maleate 0.5 mg, Dextromethorphan HBr 2.5 mg, Pseudoephedrine HCl 7.5 mg | — | — | — | 2 tablets** | 3 tablets** | 4 tablets | 5 tablets | 6 tablets | — | 4 times in 24 hrs |
| **Junior Strength Tylenol** Soft Chews Chewable Tablets — Acetaminophen 160 mg | — | — | — | — | — | 2 tablets | 2½ tablets | 3 tablets | 4 tablets | 5 times in 24 hrs |

† All products may be dosed every 4 hours, if needed; except for Children's Tylenol Flu which is dosed every 6–8 hrs, if needed.
* Under 2 years (under 24 lbs), consult a doctor.                                    ** Under 6 years (under 48 lbs), consult a doctor.
• Infants' Tylenol Drops are more concentrated than Children's Tylenol Liquids. The Infants' Concentrated Drops have been specifically designed for use only with enclosed dropper. Do not use any other dosing device with this product.
• Children's Tylenol Liquids are less concentrated than Infants' Tylenol Concentrated Drops. The Children's Tylenol Liquids have been specifically designed for use with the enclosed measuring cup. Use only enclosed measuring cup to dose this product.
• Children's Tylenol Soft Chews Chewable Tablets are not the same concentration as Junior Strength Tylenol Soft Chews Chewable Tablets.
• Junior Strength Tylenol Soft Chews Chewable Tablets contain twice as much medicine as Children's Tylenol Soft Chews Chewable Tablets.

*Children's TYLENOL® Cold Plus Cough Chewable Tablets*
- phenylketonurics: contains phenylalanine 4 mg per tablet
- **do not use if carton is opened or if blister unit is broken**
- Store at room temperature

### Professional Information: Overdosage Information

For overdosage information, please refer to pgs. 681–682.

### Inactive Ingredients:

*Infants' TYLENOL® Cold Decongestant & Fever Reducer Concentrated Drops:* citric acid, corn syrup, FD&C Red #40, flavors, polyethylene glycol, propylene glycol, saccharin, sodium benzoate.

*Infants' TYLENOL® Cold Decongestant & Fever Reducer Concentrated Drops Plus Cough:* acesulfame potassium, citric acid, corn syrup, FD&C Red #40, flavors, polyethylene glycol, propylene glycol, sodium benzoate.

*Children's       TYLENOL®      Cold:* **Suspension Liquid:** acesulfame potassium, butylparaben, cellulose, citric acid, corn syrup, D&C Red #33, FD&C Blue #1, FD&C Red #40, flavors, glycerin, propylene glycol, purified water, sodium benzoate, sodium carboxymethylcellulose, sorbitol, xanthan gum. **Chewable Tablets:** aspartame, basic polymethacrylate, cellulose, cellulose acetate, citric acid, D&C Red #7, FD&C Blue #1, flavors, hydroxypropyl methylcellulose, magnesium stearate, mannitol.

*Children's TYLENOL® Cold Plus Cough:* **Suspension Liquid:** acesulfame potassium, butylparaben, cellulose, citric acid, corn syrup, D&C Red #33, FD&C Red #40, flavors, glycerin, propylene glycol, sodium benzoate, sorbitol, xanthan gum. **Chewable Tablets:** aspartame, basic polymethacrylate, cellulose, cellulose acetate, D&C Red #7, flavors, hydroxypropyl methylcellulose, magnesium stearate, mannitol.

### How Supplied: *Infants' TYLENOL® Cold Decongestant & Fever Reducer Concentrated Drops, Infants' TYLENOL® Cold Decongestant & Fever Reducer Concentrated Drops Plus Cough:* Red-colored drops in bottles of ¹⁄₂ fl. oz.

*Children's      TYLENOL®      Cold:* **Suspension Liquid:** Purple-colored-bottles of 4 fl. oz. Store at room temperature. **Chewable Tablets:** Purple-colored, imprinted "TYLENOL COLD" on one side and "TC" on opposite side- blisters of 24.

*Children's TYLENOL® Cold Plus Cough:* **Suspension Liquid:** Red-colored suspension-bottles of 4 fl. oz.

**Chewable Tablets:** Red-colored, imprinted TYLENOL C/C" on one side and "TC/C" on the opposite side- blisters of 24.

*Shown in Product Identification Guide, page 511, 512*

## Children's TYLENOL® Flu Suspension Liquid

**Description:** *Children's TYLENOL® Flu Suspension Liquid* is Bubble Gum Blast-flavored and contains no alcohol or aspirin. Each teaspoonful (5 mL) contains acetaminophen 160 mg, chlorpheniramine maleate 1 mg, dextromethorphan HBr 7.5 mg and pseudoephedrine HCl 15 mg.

**Actions:** *Children's TYLENOL® Flu Suspension Liquid* combines the analgesic-antipyretic acetaminophen with the decongestant pseudoephedrine hydrochloride, the cough suppressant dextromethorphan hydrobromide and the antihistamine chlorpheniramine maleate to provide fast, effective, temporary relief of all your child's symptoms associated with flu including fever, body aches, headache, stuffy nose, runny nose, sore throat and coughs. Acetaminophen is equal to aspirin in analgesic and antipyretic effectiveness and it is unlikely to produce the side effects often associated with aspirin or aspirin-containing products.

**Uses:**   temporarily relieves these cold and flu symptoms:
- nasal congestion • sore throat
- runny nose • sneezing
- headache • minor aches and pains
- coughs
- temporarily reduces fever

**Directions:** See Table 1: Children's Tylenol Dosing Chart on pgs. 684–686.

**Precautions:**   If a rare sensitivity reaction occurs, the drug should be discontinued.

**Warnings:   Sore throat warning:** If sore throat is severe, persists for more than 2 days, is accompanied or followed by fever, headache, rash, nausea or vomiting, consult a doctor promptly.

**Do not use**
- in a child who is taking a monoamine oxidase inhibitor (MAOI) (certain drugs for depression, psychiatric or emotional conditions, or Parkinson's disease), or for 2 weeks after stopping the MAOI drug. If you do not know if your child's prescription drug contains an MAOI, ask a doctor or pharmacist before giving this product.
- with any other product containing acetaminophen.

**Ask a doctor before use if the child has**
- heart disease • thyroid disease
- glaucoma • high blood pressure
- diabetes • cough that occurs with too much phlegm (mucus)
- chronic cough that lasts as occurs with asthma

**When using this product**
- **do not exceed recommended dosage:** taking more than the recommended dose (overdose) may not provide more relief and could cause serious health problems.
- drowsiness may occur
- excitability may occur, especially in children

**Stop use and ask a doctor if**
- new symptoms occur
- redness or swelling is present
- pain gets worse or lasts for more than 5 days

- fever gets worse or lasts for more than 3 days
- nervousness, dizziness or sleeplessness occurs
- cough lasts more than 7 days, comes back or occurs with fever, rash or headache that lasts. These could be signs of a serious condition.

**Keep out of reach of children.** In case of overdose, get medical help or contact a Poison Control Center right away. Quick medical attention is critical even if you do not notice any signs or symptoms.

**Other Information:**
- **do not use if bottle wrap or foil inner seal imprinted "Safety Seal®" is broken or missing.**
- store at room temperature

### Professional Information: Overdosage Information

For overdosage information, please refer to pgs. 681–682.

**Inactive Ingredients:** acesulfame potassium, butylparaben, cellulose, citric acid, corn syrup, D&C Red #33, FD&C Red #40, flavors, glycerin, propylene glycol, purified water, sodium benzoate, sorbitol, xanthan gum.

**How Supplied:** Pinkish-red-colored suspension liquid in bottles of 4 fl. oz.

*Shown in Product Identification Guide, page 512*

---

## Children's TYLENOL® Sinus Suspension Liquid

**Description:** *Children's TYLENOL® Sinus Suspension Liquid* is Fruit Burst-flavored and contains no alcohol or aspirin. Each teaspoonful (5 mL) contains acetaminophen 160 mg and pseudoephedrine HCl 15 mg.

**Actions:** *Children's       TYLENOL® Sinus Suspension Liquid* combines the analgesic-antipyretic    acetaminophen with the decongestant pseudoephedrine hydrochloride to provide fast, effective, temporary relief of all your child's sinus symptoms including stuffy nose, sinus headache, sinus pressure, sinus pain, and nasal congestion. Acetaminophen is equal to aspirin in analgesic and antipyretic effectiveness and is unlikely to produce the side effects often associated with aspirin or aspirin-containing products.

**Uses:**   temporarily relieves:
- sinus congestion
- stuffy nose
- sinus pressure
- minor aches, pains and headache
- temporarily reduces fever

**Directions:** See Table 1: Children's Tylenol Dosing Chart on pgs. 684–686.

**Precautions:**   If a rare sensitivity reaction occurs, the drug should be discontinued.

**Warnings:   Do not use**
- in a child who is taking a prescription monoamine oxidase inhibitor (MAOI)

*Continued on next page*

## Tylenol Children's Sinus—Cont.

(certain drugs for depression, psychiatric, emotional conditions or Parkinson's disease), or for 2 weeks after stopping the MAOI drug. If you do not know if your child's prescription drug contains an MAOI, ask a doctor or pharmacist before giving this product.
- with any products containing acetaminophen

**Ask a doctor before use if the child has**
- heart disease
- high blood pressure
- thyroid disease
- diabetes

**When using this product**
- **do not exceed recommended dosage;** taking more than the recommended dose (overdose) may not provide more relief and could cause serious health problems.

**Stop use and ask a doctor if**
- new symptoms occur
- fever gets worse or lasts for more than 3 days
- redness or swelling is present
- nervousness, dizziness or sleeplessness occurs
- pain gets worse or lasts for more than 5 days

**Keep out of reach of children.**
In case of overdose, get medical help or contact a Poison Control Center right away. Prompt medical attention is critical even if you do not notice any signs or symptoms.

**Other Information:**
- do not use if plastic carton wrap, bottle wrap, or foil inner seal imprinted "Safety Seal®" is broken or missing
- store at room temperature

**Professional Information:**
**Overdosage Information**
For overdosage information, please refer to pgs. 681–682.

**Inactive Ingredients:** acesulfame potassium, butylparaben, cellulose, citric acid, corn syrup, D&C Red #33, FD&C Red #40, flavors, glycerin, propylene glycol, purified water, sodium benzoate, sorbitol, xanthan gum.

**How Supplied:** Red-colored–child resistant bottles of 4 fl. oz.

*Shown in Product Identification Guide, page 512*

---

### UNKNOWN DRUG?
Consult the
Product Identification Guide
(Gray Pages)
for full-color photos of
leading over-the-counter
medications

### Children's Tylenol® Dosing Chart

[See table on pages 684, 685 and 686]

---

## Medtech
**488 MAIN AVENUE
NORWALK, CT 06851**

**Address Questions and Comments to:**
(800) 443-4908

**Other Medtech Products:**
APF Arthritis Pain Formula
Freezone Corn & Callus Liquid
Heet Pain Relieving Liniment
Mosco One Step Corn Remover Pads
Mosco Liquid Corn Remover
Oxipor Psoriasis Lotion
Zincon Medicated Dandruff Shampoo

### COMPOUND W® One Step Wart Remover Pads
### COMPOUND W® One Step Plantar Pads
### COMPOUND W® One Step Pads For Kids
Salicylic Acid

**Indications:** Compound W® One Step and One Step Pads for Kids: For the removal of common warts. The common wart is easily recognized by the rough "cauliflower like" appearance of the surface.

**Active Ingredient:**          **Purpose:**
40% Salicylic Acid in a
plaster vehicle ... Plantar/Wart Remover

**Indications:** Compound W® One Step Plantar Pads: For the removal of plantar warts on the bottom of the foot. The plantar wart is recognized by its location only on the bottom of the foot, its tenderness, and the interruption of the footprint pattern.

**Warnings:**
**Do Not Use If:**
- you are diabetic • you have poor blood circulation.

**Do Not Use On:**
- irritated skin • any area that is infected or reddened • moles • birthmarks
- warts with hair growing from them • genital warts • warts on the face • warts on mucous membranes, such as inside mouth, nose, anus, genitals, lips

**Stop Using This Product and See Your Doctor If:**
- discomfort persists.

**For external use only.** Keep this and all drugs out of the reach of children. In case of accidental ingestion, seek professional assistance or contact a poison control center immediately.

**Directions:** Wash affected area. May soak wart in warm water for 5 minutes. Dry area thoroughly. Remove medicated pad from backing paper by pulling from center of pad. Then apply. Repeat procedure every 48 hours as needed (until wart is removed) for up to 12 weeks.

**Adult Supervision of Compound W Pads For Kids recommended.**

---

**Inactive Ingredients:** Lanolin, Polybutene, Rosin Ester, Rubber.
Store at room temperature. Avoid excessive heat (37°C, 99°F).

**How Supplied:** Compound W One Step Pads: 14 Medicated One Step Pads **Compound W One Step Plantar Warts:** 20 Medicated One Step Pads **Compound W One Step Pads for Kids:** 12 Medicated Pads
Mfg. for Medtech, Jackson WY 83001 USA, Made in Japan, Questions? 1-800-443-4908

©Medtech R 2/99

---

### COMPOUND W® Wart Remover
**LIQUID & GEL**
**Maximum Strength**
**Salicylic Acid**

**Active Ingredient**          **Purpose**
Salicylic Acid 17% w/w....Wart Remover

**Indications:** For the removal of common warts. The common wart is easily recognized by the rough "cauliflower-like" appearance of the surface.

**Warnings: LIQUID**
**Do Not Use If:**
- you are diabetic • you have poor blood circulation.

**Do Not Use On:**
- irritated skin • any area that is infected or reddened • moles • birthmarks
- warts with hair growing from them • genital warts • warts on the face
- warts on mucous membranes, such as inside mouth, nose, anus, genitals, lips.

**When Using This Product:**
- avoid contact with eyes. If product gets into eyes, flush with water for 15 minutes.

**Stop Using This Product and See Your Doctor If:**
- discomfort persists.

**Extremely flammable.** Keep away from fire or flame. Cap bottle tightly and store at room temperature away from heat. Avoid inhaling vapors. **For external use only.** Keep this and all drugs out of the reach of children. In case of accidental ingestion, seek professional assistance or contact a poison control center immediately.

**Warnings: GEL**
**Do Not Use If:**
- you are diabetic • you have poor blood circulation.

**Do Not Use On:**
- irritated skin • any area that is infected or reddened • moles • birthmarks
- warts with hair growing from them • genital warts • warts on the face • warts on mucous membranes, such as inside mouth, nose, anus, genitals, lips.

**When Using This Product:**
- avoid contact with eyes. If product gets into eyes, flush with water for 15 minutes.

# PRODUCT INFORMATION

**Stop Using This Product and See Your Doctor If:**
• discomfort persists.

**Extremely flammable.** Keep away from fire or flame. Cap tube tightly and store at room temperature away from heat. Avoid inhaling vapors. **For external use only.** Keep this and all drugs out of the reach of children. In case of accidental ingestion, seek professional assistance or contact a poison control center immediately.

**Directions:**
**LIQUID:** Wash affected area. May soak wart in warm water for 5 minutes. Dry area thoroughly. Using the applicator apply Compound W Liquid to each wart. Let dry. Repeat procedure once or twice daily as needed (until wart is removed) for up to 12 weeks.
**GEL:** Wash affected area. May soak wart in warm water for 5 minutes. Dry area thoroughly. By squeezing the tube gently, apply one drop at a time to sufficiently cover each wart. Let dry. Repeat procedure once or twice daily as needed (until wart is removed) for up to 12 weeks.

**Inactive Ingredients:**
**LIQUID:** Alcohol 21.2%, Camphor, Castor Oil, Collodion, Ether 63.6%, Ethylcellulose, Hypophosphorous Acid, Menthol, Polysorbate 80
**GEL:** Alcohol 67.5% by vol., Camphor, Castor Oil, Collodion, Colloidal Silicon Dioxide, Hydroxypropyl Cellulose, Hypophosphorous Acid, Polysorbate 80

**How Supplied:**
**LIQUID:** .31 FL OZ
**GEL:** Net Wt .25 oz (7g)
Mfg. for Medtech, Jackson WY 83001 USA

Question? 1-800-443-4908
LIQUID: © Medtech, R5/99
GEL: © Medtech, R6/99

---

**PERCOGESIC®
EXTRA STRENGTH**
• **PAIN RELIEVER**
• **FEVER REDUCER**
• **ANTIHISTAMINE**
**Aspirin Free**

**Active Ingredient Per Coated Caplet**      **Purpose**
Acetaminophen
500 mg .............................. Pain Reliever, Fever Reducer
Diphenhydramine HCl 12.5 mg .... Antihistamine

**Indications:** For the temporary relief of minor aches and pains associated with headaches, muscular aches, backaches, premenstrual and menstrual discomfort, colds, the flu, toothaches, minor pain from arthritis, to reduce fever, as well as temporary relief of runny nose, sneezing, itching of the nose or throat, and itchy, watery eyes due to hayfever.

**Directions:** Adults (12 years and over): 2 caplets every 6 hours while symptoms persist. Maximum daily dose 8 caplets. Children under 12 years of age: consult a doctor.
Store at room temperature. Avoid excessive heat.

**Inactive Ingredients:** Corn Starch, FD&C Yellow #6 Aluminum Lake, Hydroxypropylmethylcellulose, Magnesium Stearate, Microcrystalline Cellulose, Polydextrose, Polyethylene Glycol, Povidone, Silicon Dioxide, Stearic Acid, Titanium Dioxide, Triacetin.

**Warnings:** May cause marked drowsiness; alcohol, sedatives, and tranquilizers may increase the drowsiness effect. Avoid alcoholic beverages while taking this product. Use caution when driving a motor vehicle or operating machinery. May cause excitability, especially in children. Do not give to children for arthritis pain, unless directed by a doctor. **Do Not Use (unless directed by a doctor): If you are:** • taking sedatives or tranquilizers **If you have:** • a breathing problem such as emphysema or chronic bronchitis • glaucoma • difficulty in urination due to enlargement of the prostate gland **Stop Using This Product and Consult a Doctor If:** pain persists for more than 10 days (adults) or 5 days (children) • fever persists more than 3 days (unless directed by a doctor) • condition worsens or new symptoms occur • redness or swelling is present. **These may be signs of a serious condition.** As with any drug, if you are pregnant or nursing a baby, seek the advice of a health professional before using this product. **Keep this and all drugs out of the reach of children.** In case of accidental overdose, contact a physician or poison control center immediately. Prompt medical attention is critical for adults as well as for children even if you do not notice any signs or symptoms.

**Alcohol Warning:** If you consume 3 or more alcoholic drinks every day, ask your doctor whether you should take acetaminophen or other pain relievers/fever reducers. Acetaminophen may cause liver damage.

**How Supplied** 40 Coated caplets
Mfg. for Medtech, Jackson, WY 83001 USA
Questions? 800-443-4908 © Medtech, R10/98

---

**DERMOPLAST®**
**Hospital Strength**
**Pain Relieving Spray**

**Active Ingredients:**      **Purpose:**
Benzocaine USP 20% ...... Topical Anesthetic
Menthol 0.5% ....................... Antipruritic

**Indications:** For temporary relief of pain and itching associated with •sunburn •insect bites •minor cuts •scrapes •minor burns •minor skin irritations

**Warnings:**
When Using This Product: •use only as directed •avoid contact with eyes Stop Using This Product If: •condition worsens •symptoms persist for more than 7 days •symptoms clear up and recur within a few days. **Consult a physician.** For external use only. Contents under pressure. Do not puncture or incinerate. Do not expose to heat or temperature above 120° F. Do not use near open flame. **Keep this and all drugs out of reach of children.** If accidentally ingested, seek professional assistance or contact a poison control center immediately. Intentional misuse by deliberately concentrating and inhaling the contents can be harmful or fatal.

**Directions:** Children under 2 years of age: do not use. Consult physician. Adults and children 2 years and older: clean and apply to affected area not more than 3 to 4 times daily. Hold can 6 to 12 inches away from affected area. Point spray nozzle and press button. To apply to face, spray in palm of hand.

**Other information:** Store at room temperature (approximately 25° C, 77° F).

**Inactive Ingredients:** Acetylated Lanolin Alcohol, Aloe Vera Oil, Butane, Cetyl Acetate, Hydrofluorocarbon, Methylparaben, PEG-8 Laurate, Polysorbate 85.

**How Supplied:** NET WT. 2¾ FL OZ (81 ml)
Manufactured for Medtech, Jackson WY 83001 USA
Questions? 1-800-443-4908

---

**DERMOPLAST® Antibacterial Spray**
**Hospital Strength**
**Antiseptic * Anesthetic**

**Active Ingredients:**      **Purpose:**
Benzethonium Chloride USP 0.2% ......................... Antibacterial.
Benzocaine USP 20% ........ Topical Anesthetic

**Indications:** First aid to help prevent infection and provide temporary relief of pain and itching associated with •sunburn •insect bites •minor cuts •scrapes •minor burns •minor skin irritations

**Warnings:**
Do Not Use: •in eyes •on deep or puncture wounds, animal bites or serious burns. Consult a doctor
When Using This Product: •use only as directed •do not apply over large areas of the body •do not use longer than 1 week, unless directed by a doctor
Stop Using This Product and Consult A Doctor If: •condition worsens •symptoms persist for more than 7 days •symptoms clear up and recur within a few days.

*Continued on next page*

## Dermoplast Antibac.—Cont.

For external use only. Contents under pressure. Do not puncture or incinerate. Do not expose to heat or temperature above 120 F. Do not use near open flame. **Keep this and all drugs out of reach of children.** If accidentally ingested, seek professional assistance or contact a poison control center immediately. Intentional misuse by deliberately concentrating and inhaling the contents can be harmful or fatal.

**Directions:** Children under 2 years of age: do not use. Consult a doctor. Adults and children 2 years and older: clean and apply to affected area not more than 3 times daily. Hold can 6 to 12 inches away from affected area. Point spray nozzle and press button. May be covered with a sterile bandage. If bandaged, let dry first **Other information:** Store at room temperature (approximately 25° C, 77° F).

**Inactive Ingredients:** Acetulan, Aloe Vera Oil, Menthol, Methyl Paraben USP, N-Butane/P152a (65:35), PEG 400, Monolaurate, Polysorbate 85.

**How Supplied:** 2¾ FL OZ (81 ml) Manufactured for Medtech, Jackson WY 83001 USA Questions? 1-800-443-4908

---

## MOMENTUM® Bachache Relief
**Magnesium Salicylate**
**Extra Strength Analgesic**

**Active Ingredient Per Caplet:** Magnesium Salicylate Tetrahydrate 580mg (Equivalent to 467mg of Magnesium Salicylate Anhydrous).
**Purpose:** Analgesic

**Uses:** For temporary relief of minor aches and pains associated with:
• Backache and muscular aches
• Back pain due to muscle strain or spasm
• Muscle stiffness
Provides maximum dosage of Magnesium Salicylate back pain medicine available without a prescription

**Warnings:**
• Do not take this product if you are taking a prescription drug for anticoagulation (thinning of the blood), diabetes, gout, or arthritis unless directed by a doctor.
• Do not take for pain for more than 10 days unless directed by a doctor.
• Children or teenagers should not use this product for chicken pox or flu symptoms before a doctor is consulted about Reye Syndrone, a rare but serious illness.

**Alcohol Warning:** If you consume 3 or more alcoholic drinks every day, ask your doctor whether you should take magnesium salicylate or other pain relievers/fever reducers. Magnesium salicylate may cause stomach bleeding.

**Ask a Doctor Before Use:**
**If you are:**
• Allergic to salicylates (including aspirin)

**If you have:**
• Recurring stomach problems such as heartburn, nausea, pain
• Ulcers or bleeding problems
**Consult a Doctor After Use If:**
• Pain persists or gets worse
• Redness or swelling is present
• New or unexpected symptoms occur
• You experience ringing in the ears or a loss of hearing
**These could be signs of a serious condition**
As with any drug, if you are pregnant or nursing a baby, seek the advice of a health professional before using this product.
**Keep this and all drugs out of reach of children.** In case of accidental overdose, seek professional assistance or contact a poison control center immediately.

**Directions:**

| Adults: | Take with a full glass of water. Take 2 caplets every 6 hours while symptoms persist. Do not take more than 8 caplets in 24 hours. |
|---|---|
| Children under 12 yrs: | Consult a doctor. |

**How Supplied:** 48 Coated Caplets Do not use if imprinted foil seal under cap is broken or missing. Store at room temperature between 15°–30°C (59°–86°F).

**Inactive Ingredients:** Hydrogenated Vegetable Oil, Hydroxypropyl Methylcellulose Microcrystalline Cellulose, Polyethylene Glycol, Polysorbate 80, Titanium Dioxide
**Manufactured for Medtech, Jackson, WY 83001 USA • Questions? 800-443-4908**

---

## NEW-SKIN® Liquid Bandage
**Antiseptic For Minor Cuts & Scrapes**

**Description:** New-Skin dries rapidly to form a tough protective cover that is antiseptic, flexible, waterproof and lets skin breathe. Completely covers the entire wound to keep out dirt and germs. New-Skin Liquid is suited for smaller areas. Try New-Skin Spray for large areas on legs and arms.

**Uses:** • **Protects cuts and scrapes** • **Prevents and protects blisters** • **Helps prevent the formation of calluses** • **Covers painful hangnails** • **Particularly useful for bowlers, golfers, tennis players, fisherman and musicans**
**Caution:** For use on minor cuts and abrasions only. Do not apply to infected areas or wounds that are draining. Consult physician for: deep cuts, serious bleeding, puncture wounds, or application over sutures; if diabetic or have poor circulation; if redness, swelling or pain

persists or increases; if infection occurs. Intentional misuse by deliberately concentrating and inhaling contents can be harmful or fatal. For topical external use only. Keep away from eyes and other mucous membranes.

**Directions:** Thoroughly clean affected area with soap and water. Dry. Apply a coating of New-Skin. Let dry. A second coating may be applied for extra protection. New-Skin may be applied as necessary. A standard coating will last 24–48 hours. Do not apply in conjunction with other first aid products, lotions, drugs, or creams. May temporarily sting upon application.
**TO REMOVE:** Apply more New-Skin and quickly wipe off. Finger nail polish remover may dissolve New-Skin.

**Warning:** **FLAMMABLE: Do not use or store near heat or open flame • Keep this and all drugs out of the reach of children • In case of accidental ingestion, seek medical assistance or contact your poison control center immediately • Do not allow to come in contact with floors, countertops or other finished surfaces - will stain.**

**Contains:** Pyroxylin Solution, Alcohol 6.7%, Oil of Cloves, 8-hydroxyquinoline

**How Supplied:** .3 FL. OZ. also available in 1 FL OZ and 1 FL OZ SPRAY
**Mfg. for Medtech, Jackson WY 83001 USA Questions? 800-443-4908 © Medtech, R5/99**

---

## PERCOGESIC®
**Aspirin-Free Pain Reliever**

**Active Ingredient per caplet:**
                                        **Purpose:**
Acetaminophen 325 mg,
Phenyltoloxamine Citrate
30 mg ............................................ Analgesic

**Indications:** For the temporary relief of minor aches and pains associated with headaches, muscular aches, backaches, premenstrual and menstrual periods, colds, the flu, toothaches, as well as for minor pain from arthritis, and to reduce fever.

**Directions:** Adults (12 years and over) – 1 or 2 tablets every 4 hours. Maximum daily dose – 8 tablets. Children (6 to under 12 years) – 1 tablet every 4 hours. Maximum daily dose – 4 tablets. Children under 6 years of age: Consult a doctor.

**Warnings:** Do not take this product for pain for more than 10 days (adults) or 5 days (children), and do not take for fever for more than 3 days unless directed by a doctor. If pain or fever persists or worsens, new symptoms occur or redness or swelling is present, consult a doctor, as these could be signs of a serious condition. Do not give to children for arthritis pain unless directed by a doctor. May cause excitability, especially in children. Do not take this product, unless directed by a doctor, if you have a breathing problem such as emphysema or chronic bronchitis, or if you have glaucoma or difficulty in urination due to enlargement of the prostate gland. May cause marked drowsiness; alcohol, sedatives, and tranquilizers may increase the drowsiness effect. Avoid alcoholic beverages while taking this product. Do not take this product if you are taking sedatives or tranquilizers without first consulting your doctor. Use caution when driving a motor vehicle or operating machinery.

**Alcohol Warning:** If you consume 3 or more alcoholic drinks every day, ask your doctor whether you should take acetaminophen or other pain relievers/fever reducers. Acetaminophen may cause liver damage.
**KEEP THIS AND ALL DRUGS OUT OF THE REACH OF CHILDREN.** In case of accidental overdose, seek professional assistance or contact a poison control center immediately. Prompt medical attention is critical for adults as well as for children even if you do not notice any signs or symptoms. As with any drug, if you are pregnant or nursing a baby, seek the advice of a health professional before using this product.

**How Supplied:** 24 Coated Tablets; 50 coated tablets*; 90 coated tablets **STORE AT ROOM TEMPERATURE. AVOID EXCESSIVE HEAT.**

---

*Percogesic Aspirin Free Analgesic 50 tablets package is for Households without young children.

**Active Ingredients:** Each tablet contains Acetaminophen 325 mg, Phenyltoloxamine Citrate 30 mg.

**Inactive Ingredients:** Cellulose, FD&C Yellow No. 6, Flavor, Hydroxypropyl Methylcellulose, Magnesium Stearate, Polyethylene Glycol, Povidone, Silica Gel, Starch, Stearic Acid, Sucrose. Mfg. for Medtech Jackson, WY 83001 U.S.A.

---

## Mission Pharmacal Company
**10999 IH 10 WEST
SUITE 1000
SAN ANTONIO, TX 78230-1355**

**Direct Inquiries to:**
PO Box 786099
San Antonio, TX 78278-6099
TOLL FREE: (800) 292-7364
(210) 696-8400
FAX: (210) 696-6010
**For Medical Information Contact:**
**In Emergencies:**
George Alexandrides
(830) 249-9822
FAX: (830) 816-2545

### THERA-GESIC®
[thĕr'ə-jē-zik]
**(Methyl Salicylate 15%, Menthol 1%)
Topical Therapeutic Analgesic Creme**

**Description:** THERA-GESIC® contains methyl salicylate and menthol in a rapidly absorbed greaseless base containing carbomer 934, dimethicone, glycerine, methylparaben, propylparaben, sodium lauryl sulfate, trolamine, and water.

**Indications:** For the temporary relief of minor aches and pains of muscles and joints associated with arthritis, simple backache, strains, sprains and sports injuries.

**Warnings: FOR EXTERNAL USE ONLY. Use only as directed. Keep away from children to avoid accidental poisoning. Keep away from eyes, mucous membranes, broken or irritated skin. Do not use THERA-GESIC® if you have skin sensitive to oil of wintergreen (methyl salicylate).** If skin irritation develops, if pain lasts 7 days or more, or if redness is present, discontinue use and consult a physician immediately. DO NOT SWALLOW. If swallowed induce vomiting, call a physician. Contact a physician before applying this medicine to children, including teenagers, with chicken pox or flu.

**Directions:** ADULTS AND CHILDREN 12 OR MORE YEARS OF AGE: An application of THERA-GESIC® is the gentle massaging of several thin layers of creme into and around the sore or painful area. The number of thin layers controls the intensity of the action. One thin layer provides a mild effect, two thin layers provide a strong effect and three thin layers provide a very strong effect. Do not apply more than 3 to 4 times daily. Once THERA-GESIC® has penetrated the skin, the area may be washed, leaving it dry, clean and fragrance-free without decreasing the effectiveness of the product. IF YOU INTEND TO WRAP, BANDAGE OR COVER THE AREA WHERE YOU HAVE APPLIED THERA-GESIC®, IT MUST BE WASHED THOROUGHLY TO AVOID EXCESSIVE IRRITATION. DO NOT USE A HEATING PAD AFTER APPLICATION OF THERA-GESIC®.

**How Supplied:**
NDC 0178-0320-03          3 oz. tube
NDC 0178-0320-05          5 oz. tube
Store at room temperature.

---

**FACED WITH AN
Rx SIDE EFFECT?**
Turn to the
Companion Drug Index
for products that
provide symptomatic
relief.

---

## Novartis Consumer Health, Inc.
**200 KIMBALL DRIVE
PARSIPPANY, NJ 07054-0622**

**Direct Product Inquiries to:**
Consumer & Professional Affairs
(800) 452-0051
Fax: (800) 635-2801

**Or write to above address.**

### DESENEX® ANTIFUNGALS

All products are Prescription Strength
*Shake Powder*
*Liquid Spray*
*Spray Powder*
*Jock Itch Spray Powder*

**Indications:** Cures most athlete's foot (tinea pedis), jock itch (tinea cruris) and ringworm (tinea corporis). For effective relief of the itching, burning, cracking and scaling which can accompany these conditions. Desenex powders also help keep feet dry.

**Active Ingredient:** *Shake Powder, Liquid Spray, Spray Powder,* and *Jock Itch Spray Powder*—Miconazole nitrate 2%.

**Inactive Ingredients:**
*SHAKE POWDER*—Corn starch, corn starch/acrylamide/sodium acrylate polymer, fragrance, talc.
*LIQUID SPRAY*—Polyethylene glycol 300, polysorbate 20, SD alcohol 40-B (15% w/w). Propellant: Dimethyl ether.
*SPRAY POWDER*—Aloe vera gel, aluminum starch octenyl succinate, isopropyl myristate, propylene carbonate, SD alcohol 40-B (10% w/w), sorbitan monooleate, stearalkonium hectorite. Propellant: Isobutane/propane.
*JOCK ITCH SPRAY POWDER*—Aloe vera gel, aluminum starch octenyl succinate, isopropyl myristate, propylene carbonate, SD alcohol 40-B (10% w/w), sorbitan monooleate, stearalkonium hectorite. Propellant: Isobutane/propane.

**Warnings:** Do not use on children under 2 years of age unless directed by a doctor. For external use only. Avoid contact with the eyes. If irritation occurs, or if there is no improvement within 4 weeks (for athlete's foot or ringworm) or within 2 weeks for jock itch, discontinue use and consult a doctor. **Keep this and all drugs out of the reach of children.** In case of accidental ingestion, seek professional assistance or contact a

*Continued on next page*

---

*Information on Novartis Consumer Health, Inc., products appearing on these pages is effective as of November 2001.*

## Desenex—Cont.

poison control center immediately. Use only as directed. *For Spray Powders and Liquid Spray*—Avoid inhaling. Avoid contact with the eyes or other mucous membranes. Contents under pressure. Do not puncture or incinerate. Flammable mixture, do not use near fire or flame. Do not expose to heat or temperatures above 49°C (120°F). Use only as directed. Intentional misuse by deliberately concentrating and inhaling the contents can be harmful or fatal.

**Directions:** Clean the affected area and dry thoroughly. Apply a thin layer of the product over affected area twice daily (morning and night) or as directed by a doctor. (For Sprays: **Shake Spray can well,** and hold 4″ to 6″ from skin when applying.) For athlete's foot, pay special attention to the spaces between the toes. Wear well-fitting, ventilated shoes and change shoes and socks at least once daily. For athlete's foot or ringworm, use daily for 4 weeks. For jock itch, use daily for 2 weeks. If condition persists longer, consult a doctor. Supervise children in the use of this product. This product is not effective on the scalp or nails.

**How Supplied:**
*Shake Powder*—1.5 oz, 3 oz, 4 oz. plastic bottles.
*Spray Powder*—3 oz, 4 oz. cans.
*Liquid Spray*—3.5 oz, 4.6 oz. cans.
Store **powders/spray powders** and **liquid sprays** at room temperature, 15°–30°C (59°–86°F). See container bottom for lot number and expiration date. Spray powders: Tamper-resistant aerosol can for your protection. If clogging occurs, remove button and clean nozzle with pin.

*DesenexMax® Cream*
**Active Ingredient:** Terbinafine hydrochloride 1%
**Inactive Ingredients:** benzyl alcohol, cetyl alcohol, cetyl palmitate, isopropyl myristate, polysorbate 60, purified water, sodium hydroxide, sorbitan monostearate, stearyl alcohol.

**Warnings:** For external use only. **Do not use:**
• On nails or scalp
• In or near the mouth or the eyes
• For vaginal yeast infections
When using this produt do not get into the eyes. If eye contact occurs, rinse thoroughly with water. Stop use and ask a doctor if too much irritaiton occurs or gets worse. Keep out of reach of children. Of swallowed, get medical help or contact a poison control center right away.

**Directions: Adults and children** 12 years and over:
• Use the tip of the cap to break the seal and open the tube
• Wash the affected skin with soap and water and dry completely before applying
• For athlete's foot wear well-fitting, ventilated shoes. Change shoes and socks at least once daily.

• **Between the toes only:** apply twice a day (morning and night) for 1 week or as directed by a doctor.

1 week between the toes

• **on the bottom or sides of the foot:** apply twice a day (morning and night) for 2 weeks or as directed by a doctor.

2 weeks on the bottom or sides of the foot

• **for jock itch and ringworm:** apply once a day (morning or night) for 1 week or as directed by a doctor.
• wash hands after each use
• children under 12 years: ask a doctor

**How Supplied:** 0.42 oz. (12 gram) and 0.85 oz. (24 gram) cartons.
Do not use if seal on tube is broken or is not visible. Store between 5° and 30° C (41° and 86° F).
**Questions:** Call **1-800-452-0051** 24 hours a day, 7 days a week
**Novartis Consumer Health Inc.**
Parsippany, NJ 07054-0622
©2002
*Shown in Product Identification Guide, page 514*

---

## EX–LAX® Chocolated Laxative Pieces

**Active Ingredient:** Sennosides, USP, 15mg

**Use: For Relief of**
• OCCASIONAL CONSTIPATION (IRREGULARITY). This product generally produces bowel movement in 6 to 12 hours.

**Directions:** Adults and children 12 years of age and over: chew 2 chocolated pieces once or twice daily. Children 6 to under 12 years of age: chew 1 chocolated piece once or twice daily. Children under 6 years of age: consult a doctor.

**Warnings:**
• as with any drug, if you are pregnant or nursing a baby, seek the advice of a health professional before using the product.
**Unless directed by a doctor, do not use**
• laxative products when abdominal pain, nausea, or vomiting is present.
• laxative products for a period longer than 1 week.
**Consult a doctor before using a laxative if**
• you have noticed a sudden change in bowel habits that persists over a period of 2 weeks.
**Consult a doctor and stop using a laxative if**
• rectal bleeding occurs or you fail to have a bowel movement after use be-

cause this may indicate a serious condition.
**Keep this and all drugs out of the reach of children**
In case of accidental overdose, seek professional assistance or contact a poison control center immediately.

**Inactive Ingredients:** cocoa, confectioners sugar, hydrogenated palm kernel oil, lecithin, non-fat dry milk, vanillin. Store at controlled room temperature 20–25°C (68–77°F)

**How Supplied:** Available in boxes of 18 and 48 chewable chocolated pieces.
*Shown in Product Identification Guide, page 514*

---

**EX–LAX® Laxative Pills**
**Regular Strength Ex-Lax®**
**Laxative Pills**
**Maximum Strength Ex-Lax®**
**Laxative Pills**

**Active Ingredients:** *Regular Strength Ex-Lax Laxative Pills:* Sennosides, USP, 15 mg. *Maximum Relief Formula Ex-Lax Laxative Pills:* Sennosides, USP, 25 mg.

**Use: For Relief of**
• OCCASIONAL CONSTIPATION (IRREGULARITY). This product generally produces bowel movement in 6 to 12 hours.

**Warnings:**
• as with any drug, if you are pregnant or nursing a baby, seek the advice of a health professional before using this product.
**Unless directed by a doctor, do not use:**
• laxative products when abdominal pain, nausea, or vomiting is present.
• laxative products for a period longer than 1 week.
**Consult a doctor before using a laxative if:**
• you have noticed a sudden change in bowel habits that persists over a period of 2 weeks.
**Consult a doctor and stop using a laxative if:**
• rectal bleeding occurs or you fail to have a bowel movement after use because this may indicate a serious condition.
**Keep this and all drugs out of the reach of children.** In case of accidental overdose, seek professional assistance or contact a poison control center immediately.

**Dosage and Administration:** *Regular Strength Ex-Lax Laxative Pills, and Maximum Strength Ex-Lax Laxative Pills*—Adults and children 12 years of age and over: take 2 pills once or twice daily with a glass of water. Children 6 to under 12 years of age: take 1 pill once or twice daily with a glass of water. Children under 6 years of age: consult a doctor.

**Inactive Ingredients:** *Regular Strength Ex-Lax Laxative Pills*—acacia, alginic acid, carnauba wax, colloidal silicon dioxide, dibasic calcium phosphate, iron oxides, magnesium stearate, microcrystalline cellulose, sodium benzoate, sodium lauryl sulfate, starch, stearic acid, sucrose, talc, titanium dioxide. Sodium-free. **Maximum Strength Ex-Lax Laxative Pills:** acacia, alginic acid, FD&C Blue No. 1 aluminum lake, carnauba wax, colloidal silicon dioxide, dibasic calcium phosphate, magnesium stearate, microcrystalline cellulose, povidone, sodium benzoate, sodium lauryl sulfate, starch, stearic acid, sucrose, talc, titanium dioxide. Very low sodium.

Store at controlled room temperature 20–25°C (68–77°F)

**How Supplied:** *Regular Strength Ex-Lax Laxative Pills*—Available in boxes of 8 and 30 pills. *Maximum Strength Ex-Lax Laxative Pills*—Available in boxes of 24, 48, and 90 pills.

*Shown in Product Identification Guide, page 514*

---

### Ex-Lax® Milk of Magnesia STIMULANT FREE Liquid: Laxative/Antacid, Chocolate Creme, Mint, Raspberry Creme

**Indications:** As a Laxative: To relieve occasional constipation (irregularity). This saline laxative product generally produces bowel movement in ½ to 6 hours.
As an Antacid: To relieve acid indigestion, sour stomach and heartburn.

**Active Ingredient:** Magnesium hydroxide – 400 mg per teaspoon (5 ml)

**Inactive Ingredients:**
*Chocolate Creme:* Carboxymethylcellulose sodium, flavors, glycerin, hydroxypropyl methylcellulose, microcrystalline cellulose, purified water, saccharin sodium, simethicone, sorbitol.
*Mint:* Carboxymethylcellulose sodium, flavor, glycerin, hydroxypropyl methylcellulose, microcrystalline cellulose, purified water, saccharin sodium, simethicone, sorbitol.
*Raspberry Creme:* Carboxymethylcellulose sodium, flavor, glycerin, hydroxypropyl methylcellulose, microcrystalline cellulose, purified water, saccharin sodium, simethicone, sorbitol.

**Directions: Shake well before using.**
Keep tightly closed and avoid freezing.
**For Laxative Use: Adults/Children – 12 years and older:** 2–4 tablespoonsful (TBSP) at bedtime or upon arising, followed by a full glass (8 oz.) of liquid.
**Children: DO NOT USE DOSAGE CUP – 6–11 years:** 1–2 tablespoonsful (TBSP), followed by a full glass (8 oz.) of liquid.
**2–5 years:** 1–3 teaspoonsful, followed by a full glass (8 oz.) of liquid.
**Under 2 years:** Consult a doctor.
**FOR ANTACID USE: DO NOT USE DOSAGE CUP – Adults/Children - 12 years and older:** 1–3 teaspoonsful with a little water, up to four times a day or as directed by a doctor.

**Drug Interaction Precaution:** Antacids may interact with certain prescription drugs. If you are presently taking a prescription drug, do not take this product without checking with your doctor or other health professional.

**Laxative Warnings:** Do not take any laxative if abdominal pain, nausea, vomiting or kidney disease are present unless directed by a doctor. If you have noticed a sudden change in bowel habits persisting for over 2 weeks, consult a doctor before using a laxative. Laxative products should not be used for a period longer than 1 week, unless directed by a doctor. Rectal bleeding or failure to have a bowel movement after use of a laxative may indicate a serious condition. Discontinue use and consult your doctor.

**Antacid Warnings:** Do not take more than the maximum recommended daily dosage in a 24 hour period (See Directions), or use the maximum dosage of this product for more than two weeks, or use this product if you have kidney disease, except under the advice and supervision of a doctor. May have laxative effect.

As with any drug, if you are pregnant or nursing a baby, seek the advice of a health professional before using this product. Keep this and all drugs out of the reach of children. In case of accidental overdose, seek professional assistance or contact a poison control central immediately.

**How Supplied:** EX-LAX MILK OF MAGNESIA is available in chocolate creme, mint and raspberry creme flavors and comes in 12 oz (355 ml) and 26 oz (769 ml) bottles.
Store at controlled room temperature 20–25°C (68–77°F).
Distributed by:
**NOVARTIS**
Novartis Consumer Health, Inc.
Parsippany, NJ 07901-1312

*Shown in Product Identification Guide, page 514*

---

### GAS-X® REGULAR STRENGTH GAS-X® EXTRA STRENGTH GAS-X® MAXIMUM STRENGTH Antigas Softgels and Chewable Tablets GAS-X® WITH MAALOX® Antigas/Antacid Chewable Tablets

**Active Ingredients:**
Regular Strength—Each chewable tablet contains simethicone 80 mg.
Extra Strength—Each chewable tablet and swallowable softgel contains simethicone, 125 mg.
Maximum Strength—Each Swallowable softgel contains sinethicone, 166 mg.
Gas-X with Maalox—Each extra strength chewable tablet contains simethicone 125 mg and calcium carbonate 500 mg.

**Inactive Ingredients:**
Regular Strength Peppermint Creme: calcium carbonate, dextrose, flavors, maltodextrin, starch.

Regular Strength Cherry Creme: calcium carbonate, D&C Red 30, aluminum lake, dextrose, flavors, maltodextrin, starch.
Extra Strength Peppermint Creme: calcium phosphate tribasic, colloidal silicon dioxide, D&C Yellow 10 aluminum lake, D&C Red 30 aluminum lake, dextrose, flavors, maltodextrin, starch.
Extra Strength Cherry Creme: calcium phosphate tribasic, colloidal silicon dioxide, D&C Red 30 aluminum lake, dextrose, flavors, maltodextrin, starch.
Extra Strength Softgels: D&C Yellow 10, FD&C Blue 1, FD&C Red 40, gelatin, glycerin, peppermint oil, purified water, sorbitol, titanium dioxide.
Maximum Strength Softgels: D&C Red 33, FD&C Blue 1, FD&C Red 40, gelatin, glycerin, peppermint oil, purified water, sorbitol.
Gas-X With Maalox Wildberry: colloidal silicon dioxide, D&C Red 30, dextrose, flavors, maltodextrin, mannitol, pregelatinized starch, talc, tribasic calcium phosphate
Gas-X With Maalox Orange: colloidal silicon dioxide, dextrose, FD&C yellow 6 aluminum lake, flavors, maltodextrin, mannitol, pregelatinized starch, talc, tribasic calcium phosphate

**Use:**
Gas-X: For the relief of pressure and bloating commonly referred to as gas.
Gas-X with Maalox: Relief of the concurrent symptoms of gas associated with heartburn, sour stomach or acid indigestion.

**Warning: Keep out of reach of children.**

**Drug Interaction Precautions:** No known drug interaction.

**Warnings:**
**Ask a doctor or pharmacist before use** if you are now taking a prescription drug. Antacids may interact with certain prescription drugs.
Keep out of reach of children.

**Dosage and Administration:** For Chewable Tablets: Adults: Chew one or two tablets as needed after meals or at bedtime. Do not exceed six Regular Strength chewable tablets or four Extra Strength chewable tablets in 24 hours except under the advice and supervision of a physician.
For Extra Strength Softgels: Adults: Swallow with water 1 or 2 softgels as needed after meals or at bedtime. Do not exceed 4 softgels in 24 hours unless recommended by your physician.
For Maximum Strength Softgels: Adults: Swallow with water one or two softgels as needed after meals or at bedtime. Do

*Continued on next page*

---

*Information on Novartis Consumer Health, Inc., products appearing on these pages is effective as of November 2001.*

## Gas-X—Cont.

not exceed 3 softgels in 24 hours except under the advice and supervision of a physician.

Under Gas-X with Maalox: Chew 1 to 2 tablets as symptoms occur or as directed by a physician. Do not take more than 4 tablets in a 24-hour period or use the maximum dosage for more than 2 weeks under the advice and supervision of a physician.

**Professional Labeling:** Gas-X may be used in the alleviation of postoperative bloating/pressure, and for use in endoscopic examination.

**How Supplied:**
Regular Strength Chewable tablets are available in peppermint creme and cherry creme flavored, chewable, scored tablets in boxes of 12 tablets and 36 tablets.
Extra Strength Chewable tablets are available in peppermint creme and cherry creme flavored, chewable, scored tablets in boxes of 18 tablets and 48 tablets.
Easy-to-swallow, tasteless/Extra Strength Softgels are available in boxes of 10 pills, 30 pills, 50 pills and 60 pills.
Easy-to-swallow, tasteless/Maximum Strength Softgels are available in box of 50 pills.
Gas-X With Maalox Orange 8's 24's, Wildberry 8's 24's, Chewable Tablets
*Shown in Product Identification Guide, page 514*

---

## LAMISIL AT® ANTIFUNGAL
**TERBINAFINE HYDROCHLORIDE
CREAM 1%
CURES MOST ATHLETE'S FOOT
CURES MOST JOCK ITCH
CURES MOST RINGWORM**

**Description:** For effective relief of itching and burning. Full prescription strength.

**Active ingredient:**
Terbinafine hydrochloride 1%
*Purpose:* Antifungal

**Inactive ingredients:** benzyl alcohol, cetyl alcohol, cetyl palmitate, isopropyl myristate, polysorbate 60, purified water, sodium hydroxide, sorbitan monostearate, stearyl alcohol.

**Uses:**
**For Athlete's Foot:**
•cures most athlete's foot (tinea pedis) •cures most jock itch (tinea cruris) and ringworm (tinea corporis) •relieves itching, burning, cracking and scaling which accompany these conditions
**For Jock Itch:**
•cures most jock itch (tinea cruris) •relieves itching, burning, cracking and scaling which accompany this condition

**Warnings:**
**For external use only**

**Do not use** on nails or scalp, in or near the mouth or the eyes, for vaginal yeast infections.
**When using this product** do not get into the eyes. If eye contact occurs, rinse thoroughly with water.
**Stop use and ask a doctor if** too much irritation occurs or gets worse.
**Keep out of reach of children.** If swallowed, get medical help or contact a poison control center right away.

**Directions:**
• adults and children 12 years and over:
  • use the tip of the cap to break the seal and open the tube
  • wash the affected skin with soap and water and dry completely before applying
  • **for athlete's foot** wear well-fitting, ventilated shoes. Change shoes and socks at least once daily.
    • **between the toes only:** apply twice a day (morning and night) for **1 week** or as directed by a doctor.

1 week between the toes

  • **on the bottom or sides of the foot:** apply twice a day (morning and night) for **2 weeks** or as directed by a doctor.

2 weeks on the bottom or sides of the foot

  • wash hands after each use
• children under 12 years: ask a doctor
**For Jock Itch and Ringworm**
• adults and children 12 years and over
  • use the tip of the cap to break the seal and open the tube
  • wash the affected skin with soap and water and dry completely before applying
  • apply once a day (morning **or** night) for **1 week** or as directed by a doctor.
  • wash hands after each use
• children under 12 years: ask a doctor

**How Supplied:** Athlete's Foot — Net wt. 12g (.42 oz.) tube and 24g (.85 oz.) tube, Jock Itch — Net wt. 12g (.42 oz.) tube.
**Other information:** •do not use if seal on tube is broken or is not visible
•store between 5° and 30° C (41° and 86° F)
**Questions?**
**Call 1-800-452-0051**
**24 hours a day, 7 days a week.**
**Novartis Consumer Health, Inc.**
Parsippany, NJ 07054-0622
©2002
*Shown in Product Identification Guide, page 515*

---

## LAMISIL AT® ANTIFUNGAL
**TERBINAFINE HYDROCHLORIDE
SOLUTION 1%
CURES MOST ATHLETE'S FOOT
CURES MOST JOCK ITCH
CURES MOST RING WORM**

**Description:** For effective relief of itching and burning. Full prescription strength. Dries fast. Not greasy.

**Active Ingredient:** Terbinafine Hydrochloride 1%.
**Purpose:** Antifungal

**Inactive Ingredients:** Cetomacrogol, Ethanol, Propylene Glycol, Purified Water USP

**Uses:**
**Lamisil AT® Solution Dropper** and **Lamisil AT® Spray Pump**
**For Athlete's Foot and Jock Itch:**
• Cures most athlete's foot (tinea pedis) between the toes. Effectiveness on the bottom or sides of foot is unknown.
• Cures most jock itch (tinea cruris) and ringworm (tinea corporis)
• Relieves itching, burning, cracking, and scaling which accompany these conditions

**Warnings:**
**For external use only:**
**Do not use:**
• on nails or scalp
• in or near the mouth or the eyes
• for vaginal yeast infections
**When using this product** do not get into eyes. If contact occurs, rinse eyes thoroughly with water.
**Stop use and ask a doctor** if too much irritation occurs or gets worse.
**Keep out of reach of children.** If swallowed, get medical help or contact a poison control center right away.

**Directions:**
• adults and children 12 years and older
  • wash the affected skin with soap and water and dry completely before applying
  • **for athlete's foot between the toes** apply twice a day (morning and night) for 1 week or as directed by a doctor. Wear well-fitting, ventilated shoes. Change shoes and socks at least once daily.
  • **for jock itch and ringworm** apply to affected area once a day (morning **or** night) for 1 week or as directed by a doctor

1 week between the toes

  • wash hands after each use
• children under 12 years: ask a doctor
• spray affected area once a day (morning **or** night) for 1 week or as directed by a doctor. (spray pump only)
**How Supplied:** Bottle of 30 ml (1 fl. oz.). Solution Dropper or Spray Pump
**Other Information:** Store at 8°–25°C (46°–77°F).
**Questions?**
Call **1-800-452-0051** 24 hours a day, 7 days a week.
**Novartis Consumer Health, Inc.**
Parsippany, NJ 07054-0622 ©2002
*Shown in Product Identification Guide, page 515*

## MAALOX® MAX MAXIMUM STRENGTH ANTACID/ANTI-GAS Liquid
Oral Suspension Antacid/Anti-Gas

**Liquids**
☐ **Lemon**
☐ **Cherry**
☐ **Mint**
☐ **Vanilla Crème**
☐ **Peaches n' Crème**
☐ **Wild Berry**

**Description:** MAALOX® Max Maximum Strength Antacid/Anti-Gas, a balanced combination of magnesium and aluminum hydroxides plus simethicone, is an antacid/anti-gas product to provide symptomatic relief of acid indigestion, heartburn, sour stomach, upset stomach associated with these symptoms and relief of pressure and bloating commonly referred to as gas.

**Composition:** To provide symptomatic relief of hyperacidity plus alleviation of gas symptoms, each teaspoonful contains:
[See table above]

**Inactive Ingredients:** Butylparaben, Carboxymethylcellulose Sodium, D&C Yellow #10 (Lemon Flavor only), Flavor, Hydroxypropyl Methylcellulose, Microcrystalline Cellulose, Potassium Citrate, Propylparaben, Purified Water, Saccharin Sodium, Sorbitol.

**Warnings**
**Ask a doctor before use if** you have kidney disease.
**Ask a doctor or pharmacist before use if** you are taking a prescription drug. Antacids may interact with certain prescription drugs.
**Stop use and ask a doctor if** symptoms last for more than 2 weeks
**Keep out of reach of children.**

**Directions**
• shake well before using
• Adults/children 12 years and older: take 2 to 4 teaspoons four times a day or as directed by a physician
• do not take more than 12 teaspoonsful in 24 hours or use the maximum dosage for more than 2 weeks.
• Children under 12 years: consult a physician
To aid in establishing proper dosage schedules, the following information is provided:

**MAALOX® Max Maximum Strength Antacid/Anti-Gas**

| | Per 2 Tsp. (10 mL) (Minimum Recommended Dosage) |
|---|---|
| Acid neutralizing capacity | 38.8 mEq |

**Professional Labeling**
**Indications:** As an antacid for symptomatic relief of hyperacidity associated with the diagnosis of peptic ulcer, gastritis, peptic esophagitis, gastric hyperacidity, or hiatal hernia. As an antiflatulent to alleviate the symptoms of gas, including postoperative gas pain.

| Active Ingredients | Maximum Strength Maalox® Antacid/Anti-Gas Per Tsp. (5 mL) | Purpose |
|---|---|---|
| Aluminum Hydroxide (equivalent to dried gel, USP) | 400 mg | antacid |
| Magnesium Hydroxide | 400 mg | antacid |
| Simethicone | 40 mg | antigas |

**Warnings:** Prolonged use of aluminum-containing antacids in patients with renal failure may result in or worsen dialysis osteomalacia. Elevated tissue aluminum levels contribute to the development of the dialysis encephalopathy and osteomalacia syndromes. Small amounts of aluminum are absorbed from the gastrointestinal tract and renal excretion of aluminum is impaired in renal failure. Aluminum is not well removed by dialysis because it is bound to albumin and transferrin, which do not cross dialysis membranes. As a result, aluminum is deposited in bone, and dialysis osteomalacia may develop when large amounts of aluminum are ingested orally by patients with impaired renal function. Aluminum forms insoluble complexes with phosphate in the gastrointestinal tract, thus decreasing phosphate absorption. Prolonged use of aluminum-containing antacids by normophosphatemic patients may result in hypophosphatemia if phosphate intake is not adequate. In its more severe forms, hypophosphatemia can lead to anorexia, malaise, muscle weakness, and osteomalacia.

**Advantages:** In addition to the fast acting antacid ingredients, Aluminum Hydroxide and Magnesium Hydroxide, MAALOX® Max Maximum Strength Antacid/Antigas contains the powerful antigas ingredient, simethicone, to provide concurrent fast relief from discomfort associated with gas.

**How Supplied:**
**MAALOX® MAX MAXIMUM STRENGTH ANTACID/ANTI-GAS Liquid**
**Oral Suspension Antacid/Anti-Gas**
**Lemon** is available in plastic bottles of 5 fl. oz. (148 mL), 12 fl. oz. (355 mL), and 26 fl. oz. (769 mL).
**Cherry** is available in plastic bottles of 12 fl. oz. (355 mL) and 26 fl. oz. (769 mL).
**Mint** is available in plastic bottles of 12 fl. oz. (355 mL) and 26 fl. oz. (769 mL).
**Peaches n' Crème** is available in Plastic Bottles of 12 fl. oz. (355 mL).
**Vanilla Crème** is available in Plastic Bottles of 12 fl. oz. (355 mL).

**Wild Berry** is available in Plastic Bottles of 12 fl. oz. (355 mL).
*Shown in Product Identification Guide, page 515*

---

## MAALOX®
**Regular Strength**
**Liquid Antacid/Anti-Gas**

**Liquids**
• Cooling Mint
• Smooth Cherry

**Description:** Maalox® Antacid/Anti-Gas, a balanced combination of magnesium and aluminum hydroxides plus simethicone, is an Antacid/Anti-Gas product to provide relief of acid indigestion, heartburn, sour stomach, upset stomach associated with these symptoms, and relief of pressure and bloating commonly referred to as gas.
[See table at top of next page]

**Inactive Ingredients:** Butylparaben, Carboxymethylcellulose Sodium, D&C Yellow #10 (Lemon flavor only), Flavor, Hydroxypropyl Methylcellulose, Microcrystalline Cellulose, Propylparaben, Purified Water, Saccharin Sodium, Sorbitol.

| Maalox Suspension Per 2 Tsp. (10 mL) (Minimum Recommended Dosage) | |
|---|---|
| Acid neutralizing capacity | 19.4 mEq |

**Warnings**
**Ask a doctor before use** if you have kidney disease
**Ask a doctor or pharmacist before use** if you are taking a prescription drug. Antacids may interact with certain prescription drugs.
**Stop use and ask a doctor** if symptoms last for more than 2 weeks
**Keep out of reach of children.**

*Continued on next page*

*Information on Novartis Consumer Health, Inc., products appearing on these pages is effective as of November 2001.*

| Active Ingredients | Maalox Suspension 5 mL teaspoon | Purpose |
|---|---|---|
| Aluminum Hydroxide (equivalent to dried gel, USP) | 200 mg | Antacid |
| Magnesium Hydroxide | 200 mg | Antacid |
| Simethicone | 20 mg | Antigas |

## Maalox Antacid Liquid—Cont.

### Directions
- shake well before using
- Adults/children 12 years and older: take 2 to 4 teaspoons four times a day or as directed by a physician
- do not take more than 16 teaspoonsful in 24 hours or use the maximum dosage for more than 2 weeks.
- Children under 12 years: consult a physician

### Professional Labeling

**Indications:** As an antacid for symptomatic relief of hyperacidity associated with the diagnosis of peptic ulcer, gastritis, peptic esophagitis, gastric hyperacidity, or hiatal hernia. As an antiflatulent to alleviate the symptoms of gas, including postoperative gas pain.

**Warnings:** Prolonged use of aluminum-containing antacids in patients with renal failure may result in or worsen dialysis osteomalacia. Elevated tissue aluminum levels contribute to the development of the dialysis encephalopathy and osteomalacia syndromes. Small amounts of aluminum are absorbed from the gastrointestinal tract and renal excretion of aluminum is impaired in renal failure. Aluminum is not well removed by dialysis because it is bound to albumin and transferrin, which do not cross dialysis membranes. As a result, aluminum is deposited in bone, and dialysis osteomalacia may develop when large amounts of aluminum are ingested orally by patients with impaired renal function. Aluminum forms insoluble complexes with phosphate in the gastrointestinal tract, thus decreasing phosphate absorption. Prolonged use of aluminum-containing antacids by normophosphatemic patients may result in hypophosphatemia if phosphate intake is not adequate. In its more severe forms, hypophosphatemia can lead to anorexia, malaise, muscle weakness, and osteomalacia.

**Advantages:** In addition to the fast acting antacid ingredients, Aluminum Hydroxide and Magnesium Hydroxide, MAALOX® Antacid/Antigas contains the powerful antigas ingredient, simethicone, to provide concurrent fast relief from discomfort associated with gas.

### How Supplied:
**Maalox® Cooling Mint** Suspension is available in plastic bottles of 5 oz. (148 mL), 12 oz. (355 mL) and 26 oz. (769 mL)

**Maalox® Smooth Cherry** Suspension is available in plastic bottles of 12 oz. (355 mL)
*Shown in Product Identification Guide, page 515*

---

## Quick Dissolve MAALOX® Regular Strength Antacid.
### Calcium Carbonate Chewable Tablets
### Assorted, Lemon and Wild Berry flavors. Quick Dissolving Tablets

### Drug Facts:
**MAALOX® Regular Strength**

| Active Ingredient: (in each tablet) | Purpose: |
|---|---|
| Calcium carbonate 600 mg | Antacid |

**Uses:** For the relief of
- acid indigestion
- heartburn
- sour stomach
- upset stomach associated with these symptoms

**Warnings:**
**Ask a doctor or pharmacist before use if you are:** presently taking a prescription drug. Antacids may interact with certain prescription drugs
**Stop use and ask a doctor** if symptoms last for more than 2 weeks.
**Keep out of reach of children.**

### Directions:
- Chew 1 to 2 tablets as symptoms occur or as directed by a physician
- do not take more than 12 tablets in a 24-hour period or use the maximum dosage for more than 2 weeks except under the advice and supervision of a physician

### Other Information:
- Phenylketonurics: Contains Phenylalanine, .5 mg per tablet
- store at controlled room temperature 20–25°C (68–77°F)
- keep tightly closed and dry
- Acid neutralizing capacity (per 2 tablets) is 21.6 mEq.

**Inactive Ingredients:** Aspartame, colloidal silicon dioxide, croscarmellose sodium, D&C Red #30 aluminum lake, D&C Yellow #10 aluminum lake, dextrose, FD&C Blue #1 aluminum lake, flavors, magnesium stearate, maltodextrin, mannitol, pregelatinized starch. May also contain: corn starch, sodium chloride.

### How Supplied:
Lemon — Plastic Bottles of 45 and 85 Tablets.
Wild Berry — Plastic Bottles of 45 Tablets.
Assorted — Plastic Bottles of 85 and 145 Tablets.
**Questions? call 1-800-452-0051** 24 hours a day, 7 days a week.
*Shown in Product Identification Guide, page 515*

---

## Quick Dissolve MAALOX® Max Maximum Strength
### Antacid/Antigas.
### Calcium Carbonate and Simethicone Chewable Tablets
### Assorted, Lemon and Wild Berry Flavors. Quick Dissolving Tablets

### Drug Facts:
**MAALOX® Max Maximum Strength**

| Active Ingredients: (in each tablet) | Purpose: |
|---|---|
| Calcium carbonate 1000 mg | Antacid |
| Simethicone 60 mg | Antigas |

**Uses:** For the relief of
- acid indigestion
- heartburn
- sour stomach
- upset stomach associated with these symptoms
- bloating and pressure commonly referred to as gas

**Warnings:**
**Allergy Alert:** contains FD&C Yellow #5 aluminum lake (tartrazine) as a color additive
**Ask a doctor or pharmacist before use if you are:** presently taking a prescription drug. Antacids may interact with certain prescription drugs.
**Stop use and ask a doctor if:** symptoms last for more than 2 weeks.
**Keep out of reach of children.**

### Directions:
- Chew 1 to 2 tablets as symptoms occur or as directed by a physician
- do not take more than 8 tablets in a 24-hour period or use the maximum dosage for more than 2 weeks except under the advice and supervision of a physician

### Other Information:
- store at controlled room temperature 20–25°C (68–77°F)
- keep tightly closed and dry
- Acid neutralizing capacity (per 2 tablets) is 34mEq.

**Inactive Ingredients:** acesulfame K, colloidal silicon dioxide, croscarmellose sodium, dextrose, FD&C Red #40 aluminum lake, FD&C Yellow #5 aluminum lake, FD&C Yellow #6 aluminum lake, flavors, magnesium stearate, maltodextrin, mannitol, pregelatinized starch.

### How Supplied:
Lemon — Plastic Bottles of 35 and 65 Tablets.
Wild Berry — Plastic Bottles of 35 and 65 Tablets.

Assorted — Plastic Bottles of 35, 65, 90 and 115 Tablets.

**Questions? call 1-800-452-0051** 24 hours a day, 7 days a week.

*Shown in Product Identification Guide, page 515*

---

## TAVIST® Allergy Antihistamine Tablets
**Nonprescription Drug**
**Clemastine Fumarate**

### Active ingredient:
**(in each tablet)**
Clemastine fumarate, USP 1.34 mg (equivalent to 1 mg clemastine) ........................ Antihistamine

**Uses:** Temporarily reduces these symptoms of the common cold, hay fever, and other respiratory allergies:
• runny nose
• itchy, watery eyes
• sneezing
• itching of the nose or throat

**Warnings:**
**Ask a doctor before use if you have:**
• a breathing problem such as emphysema or chronic bronchitis
• glaucoma
• trouble urinating due to an enlargement of the prostate gland

**Ask a doctor or pharmacist before use if you are** taking sedatives or tranquilizers

**When using this product**
• avoid alcoholic drinks
• drowsiness may occur
• alcohol, sedatives, and tranquilizers may increase drowsiness
• be careful when driving a motor vehicle or operating machinery
• excitability may occur, especially in children

**If pregnant or breast-feeding,** ask a health professional before use.

**Keep out of reach of children.** In case of overdose, get medical help or contact a poison control center right away.

**Directions**
• adults and children 12 years of age and older: take 1 tablet every 12 hours, not more than 2 tablets in 24 hours unless directed by a doctor
• children under 12 years of age: consult a doctor

**Other information:**
• sodium free
• store at controlled room temperature 20–25°C (68–77°F)

**Inactive Ingredients** lactose, povidone, starch, stearic acid, talc.

**How Supplied:** Packets of 8 and 16 Tablets
**Novartis Consumer Health, Inc.**
Parsippany, NJ 07054-0622

*Shown in Product Identification Guide, page 515*

---

## TAVIST® Allergy/Sinus/Headache
**Antihistamine/Nasal Decongestant/Pain Reliever/Fever Reducer Caplets***
***Capsule-shaped tablet**
Clemastine fumarate 0.335 mg (equivalent to 0.25 mg clemastine), pseudoephedrine HCl 30 mg tablets, and acetaminophen 500 mg

**Drug Facts:**

**Active ingredients**
**(in each tablet)** **Purpose:**
Acetaminophen 500 mg ... Pain reliever/fever reducer
Clemastine fumarate 0.335 mg (equivalent to 0.25 mg clemastine) ........................ Antihistamine
Pseudoephedrine HCl 30 mg ........ Nasal decongestant

**Uses:** Temporarily relieves these symptoms of hay fever or other upper respiratory allergies, and common cold: sinus congestion and pressure, nasal congestion, headaches, itchy watery eyes, sneezing, runny nose, itching of the nose or throat, minor aches and pains, fever

**Warnings:**
**Alcohol Warning:** If you consume 3 or more alcoholic drinks daily, ask your doctor whether you should take acetaminophen or other pain relievers/fever reducers. Acetaminophen may cause liver damage.
**Do not use** if you are now taking a prescription monoamine oxidase inhibitor [MAOI] (certain drugs for depression, psychiatric or emotional conditions, or Parkinson's disease), or for 2 weeks after stopping the MAOI drug. If you do not know if your prescription drug contains an MAOI, ask a doctor or pharmacist before taking this product.
**Ask a doctor before use if you have:** heart disease, high blood pressure, thyroid disease, diabetes, glaucoma, a breathing problem such as emphysema or chronic bronchitis, trouble urinating due to an enlarged prostate gland
**Ask a doctor or pharmacist before use if you are:**
• taking sedatives or tranquilizers
• under a doctor's care for any continuing medical condition
• taking other drugs on a regular basis
• using another product containing acetaminophen, clemastine fumarate or pseudoephedrine HCl
**When using this product • do not use more than directed:**
• drowsiness may occur
• avoid alcoholic drinks
• excitability may occur, especially in children
• alcohol, sedatives, and tranquilizers may increase drowsiness
• be careful when driving a motor vehicle or operating machinery
**Warnings:**
**Stop use and ask a doctor if**
• nervousness, dizziness or sleeplessness occurs
• symptoms continue or get worse
• a fever lasts for more than 3 days
• new or unexpected symptoms occur
• nasal congestion lasts for more than 7 days

**If pregnant or breast-feeding,** ask a health professional before use.
**Keep out of reach of children.** In case of overdose, get medical help or contact a poison control center right away. Prompt medical attention is critical for adults as well as children even if you do not notice any signs or symptoms.

**Directions:**
• adults and children 12 years of age and over: take 2 caplets every 6 hours as needed: not more than 8 caplets in 24 hours unless directed by a doctor
• children under 12 years of age: ask a doctor

**Other Information:**
• store at 20°–25°C (68°–77°F) • avoid excessive heat

**Inactive Ingredients:** Calcium sulfate, glyceryl behenate, maltodextrin, methylcellulose, methylparaben, polyethylene glycol, silicon dioxide, sodium lauryl sulfate, starch, titanium dioxide
**Questions** Call **1-800-452-0051** 24 hours a day, 7 days a week.

**How Supplied:** Available in 24 ct. and 48 ct. caplet packages.
**Novartis Consumer Health, Inc.**
**Parsippany, NJ 07054-0622** ©2001
*Shown in Product Identification Guide, page 515*

---

## THERAFLU® REGULAR STRENGTH
**Cold & Sore Throat Night Time Medicine**
**Cold & Cough Night Time Medicine**

**Description:** Each packet of TheraFlu Regular Strength **Cold & Sore Throat Night Time Medicine** contains: acetaminophen 650 mg, pseudoephedrine hydrochloride 60 mg, and chlorpheniramine maleate 4 mg. Each packet of TheraFlu Regular Strength **Cold & Cough Night Time Medicine** also contains dextromethorphan hydrobromide 20 mg.

**Inactive ingredients:** Acesulfame K, aspartame, citric acid, D&C Yellow 10, flavors, maltodextrin, silicon dioxide, sodium citrate, sucrose and tribasic calcium phosphate.

Each packet contains: sodium 19 mg Phenylketonurics: Contains Phenylalanine 11 mg (Cold & Sore Throat) and 13 mg (Cold & Cough) per adult dose

**Indications:** Temporarily relieves these symptoms: headache, minor aches and pains, fever, minor sore throat pain, nasal and sinus congestion, runny nose, itchy nose or throat, itchy, watery eyes and sneezing. TheraFlu Regular

*Continued on next page*

---

*Information on Novartis Consumer Health, Inc., products appearing on these pages is effective as of November 2001.*

## Theraflu—Cont.

Strength **Cold & Cough Night Time Medicine** also suppresses coughs due to minor throat and bronchial irritation.

**Warnings: Keep this and all drugs out of the reach of children.** In case of accidental overdose, seek professional assistance or contact a poison control center immediately. Prompt medical attention is critical for adults as well as children even if you do not notice any signs or symptoms.

**Do not exceed recommended dosage.** If nervousness, dizziness, or sleeplessness occur, discontinue use and consult a doctor. If symptoms do not improve within 7 days or are accompanied by fever, consult a doctor. May cause excitability especially in children. Do not take this product if you have heart disease, high blood pressure, thyroid disease, diabetes, glaucoma, a breathing problem such as emphysema or chronic bronchitis, or difficulty in urination due to enlargement of the prostate gland, unless directed by a doctor.

Do not take this product for pain for more than 10 days or for fever for more than 3 days unless directed by a doctor. If pain or fever persists or gets worse, if new symptoms occur, or if redness or swelling is present, consult a doctor because these could be signs of a serious condition. If sore throat is severe, persists for more than 2 days, is accompanied or followed by fever, headache, rash, nausea, or vomiting, consult a doctor promptly.

May cause marked drowsiness; alcohol, sedatives, and tranquilizers may increase the drowsiness effect. Avoid alcoholic beverages while taking this product. Do not take this product if you are taking sedatives or tranquilizers, without first consulting your doctor. Use caution when driving a motor vehicle or operating machinery.

A persistent cough may be a sign of a serious condition. If cough persists for more than 1 week, tends to recur, or is accompanied by a fever, rash, or persistent headache, consult a doctor. Do not take this product for persistent or chronic cough such as occurs with smoking, asthma, or emphysema, or if cough is accompanied by excessive phlegm (mucus) unless directed by a doctor.

As with any drug, if you are pregnant or nursing a baby, seek the advice of a health professional before using this product.

**Alcohol Warning:** If you consume 3 or more alcoholic drinks every day, ask your doctor whether you should take acetaminophen or other pain relievers/fever reducers. Acetaminophen may cause liver damage.

**Drug Interaction Precaution:** Do not use this product if you are now taking a prescription monoamine oxidase inhibitor [MAOI] (certain drugs for depression, psychiatric or emotional conditions,

or Parkinson's disease), or for 2 weeks after stopping the MAOI drug. If you are uncertain whether your prescription drug contains an MAOI, consult a health professional before taking this product.

**Directions:** Adults and children 12 years of age and over: dissolve contents of one packet in 6 oz. hot water; sip while hot. One packet every 4 to 6 hours; not to exceed 4 packets in 24 hours, or as directed by a doctor. Children under 12 years of age: consult a doctor. **Microwave heating instructions:** Add contents of packet and 6 oz. of cool water to a microwave-safe cup and stir briskly. Microwave on high $1\frac{1}{2}$ minutes or until hot. Do not boil water or overheat, and remember to stir liquid between reheatings. Sweeten to taste if desired.

**How Supplied:** TheraFlu Regular Strength **Cold & Sore Throat Night Time Medicine** powder in foil packets, 6 packets per carton. TheraFlu Regular Strength **Cold & Cough Night Time Medicine** powder in foil packets, 6 or 12 packets per carton.

---

## THERAFLU® MAXIMUM STRENGTH
### Flu & Sore Throat Night Time Hot Liquid Medicine

Each packet of Theraflu Maximum Strength **Flu & Sore Throat Night Time Hot Liquid Medicine** contains: acetaminophen 1000 mg, pseudoephedrine HCl 60 mg, chlorpheniramine maleate 4 mg.

**Inactive Ingredients:** Acesulfame K, aspartame, citric acid, D&C Yellow 10, FD&C Blue 1, FD&C Red 40, flavors, maltodextrin, silicon dioxide, sodium citrate, sucrose and tribasic calcium phosphate.

Each packet contains: sodium 12 mg Phenylketonurics: contains phenylalanine 22 mg per adult dose

**Indications:** Temporarily relieves these symptoms: headache, minor aches and pains, itchy nose or throat, itchy watery eyes, fever, minor sore throat pain, nasal and sinus congestion, runny nose and sneezing.

**Warnings: Keep this and all drugs out of the reach of children.** In case of accidental overdose, seek professional assistance or contact a poison control center immediately. Prompt medical attention is critical for adults as well as children even if you do not notice any signs or symptoms.

**Do not exceed recommended dosage.** If nervousness, dizziness, or sleeplessness occur, discontinue use and consult a doctor. If symptoms do not improve within 7 days or are accompanied by fever, consult a doctor. May cause excitability, especially in children. Do not take this product if you have heart disease, high blood pressure, thyroid disease, diabetes, glaucoma, a breathing problem such as emphysema or chronic

bronchitis, or difficulty in urination due to enlargement of the prostate gland, unless directed by a doctor.

Do not take this product for pain for more than 10 days or for fever for more than 3 days unless directed by a doctor. If pain or fever persists or gets worse, if new symptoms occur, or if redness or swelling is present, consult a doctor because these could be signs of a serious condition. If sore throat is severe, persists for more than 2 days, is accompanied or followed by fever, headache, rash, nausea, or vomiting, consult a doctor promptly.

May cause drowsiness; alcohol, sedatives and tranquilizers may increase the drowsiness effect. Avoid alcoholic beverages while taking this product. Do not take this product if you are taking sedatives or tranquilizers without first consulting your doctor. Use caution when driving a motor vehicle or operating machinery.

As with any drug, if you are pregnant or nursing a baby, seek the advice of a health professional before using this product.

**Alcohol Warning:** If you consume 3 or more alcoholic drinks every day ask your doctor whether you should take acetaminophen or other pain relievers/fever reducers. Acetaminophen may cause liver damage.

**Drug Interaction Precaution:** Do not use this product if you are now taking a prescription monoamine oxidase inhibitor [MAOI] (certain drugs for depression, psychiatric or emotional conditions, or Parkinson's Disease), or for 2 weeks after stopping the MAOI drug. If you are uncertain whether your prescription drug contains an MAOI, consult a health professional before taking this product.

**Directions:** Adults and children 12 years of age and over: dissolve one packet in 6 oz. of hot water; sip while hot. One packet every 6 hours, not to exceed 4 packets in 24 hours, or as directed by a doctor. Children under 12 years of age: consult a doctor. **Microwave Heating Instructions:** Add contents of packet and 6 oz. of cool water to a microwave-safe cup and stir briskly. Microwave on high $1\frac{1}{2}$ minutes or until hot. Do not boil water or overheat, and remember to stir liquid between reheatings. Sweeten to taste if desired.

**How Supplied:** Theraflu Maximum Strength **Flu & Sore Throat Night Time Hot Liquid Medicine** powder in foil packets, 6 packets per carton.

---

## THERAFLU® MAXIMUM STRENGTH
### Flu & Congestion Non-Drowsy Hot Liquid Medicine

**Description:** Each packet of TheraFlu Maximum Strength **Flu & Congestion Non-Drowsy Hot Liquid Medicine**

contains: acetaminophen 1000 mg, guaifenesin 400 mg, pseudoephedrine HCl 60 mg, dextromethorphan HBr 30 mg.

**Inactive Ingredients:** Acesulfame K, aspartame, calcium phosphate, citric acid, D&C yellow 10, FD&C Red 40, flavors, maltodextrin, silicon dioxide, sodium citrate, sucrose.

Each packet contains: sodium 15 mg Phenylketonurics: contains phenylalanine 24 mg per adult dose

**Indications:** Temporarily relieves these symptoms: headache, minor aches and pains, chest congestion, fever, minor sore throat pain, nasal and sinus congestion. TheraFlu Maximum Strength **Flu & Congestion Non-Drowsy Hot Liquid Medicine** also suppresses coughs due to minor throat and bronchial irritation.

**Warnings: Keep this and all drugs out of the reach of children.** In case of overdose, get medical help or contact a poison control center immediately. Prompt medical attention is critical for adults as well as for children even if you do not notice any signs or symptoms. As with any drug, if you are pregnant or nursing a baby, seek the advice of a health professional before using this product.

**Do not exceed recommended dosage.** If nervousness, dizziness, or sleeplessness occur, discontinue use and consult a doctor. Do not take this product if you have heart disease, high blood pressure, thyroid disease, diabetes, or difficulty in urination due to enlargement of the prostate gland.

If symptoms do not improve within 7 days or are accompanied by fever, consult a doctor. Do not take this product for pain for more than 10 days. A persistent cough may be a sign of a serious condition. If cough persists for more than 7 days, tends to recur, or is accompanied by fever, rash or persistent headache, fever that lasts for more than 3 days, or if new symptoms occur consult a doctor. Do not take this product: 1) cough is accompanied by excessive phlegm (mucus), 2) for persistent or chronic cough such as occurs with smoking, asthma, emphysema or chronic bronchitis, 3) if sore throat persists for more than 2 days, is accompanied or followed by fever, headache, rash, nausea, or vomiting, unless directed by a doctor.

**Alcohol Warning:** If you consume 3 or more alcoholic drinks every day, ask your doctor whether you should take acetaminophen or other pain relievers/fever reducers. Acetaminophen may cause liver damage.

**Drug Interaction Precaution:** Do not use this product if you are now taking a prescription monoamine oxidase inhibitor (MAOI) (certain drugs for depression, psychiatric or emotional conditions, or Parkinson's disease), or for 2 weeks after stopping the MAOI drug. If you are uncertain whether your prescription drug contains an MAOI, consult a health professional before taking this product.

**Directions:** Adults and children 12 years of age and over: dissolve contents of one packet in 6 oz. hot water; sip while hot. One packet every 6 hours, not to exceed 4 packets in 24 hours, or as directed by a doctor. Children under 12 years of age: consult a doctor.

**Microwave heating instructions:** Add contents of one packet and 6 oz. of cool water to a microwave-safe cup and stir briskly. Microwave on high 1 1/2 minutes or until hot. Do not boil water or overheat, and remember to stir liquid between reheatings.

Sweeten to taste if desired.

**How Supplied:** TheraFlu Maximum Strength **Flu & Congestion Non-Drowsy Hot Liquid Medicine** is available in 6 foil packets per carton.

---

**THERAFLU® MAXIMUM STRENGTH**
**Flu & Cough Night Time Hot Liquid Medicine**

**Active Ingredients:** Each packet of TheraFlu Maximum Strength **Flu & Cough Night Time Hot Liquid Medicine** contains: acetaminophen 1,000 mg, pseudoephedrine HCl 60 mg, dextromethorphan HBr 30 mg, chlorpheniramine maleate 4 mg.

**Inactive Ingredients:** Acesulfame K, aspartame, citric acid, FD&C Blue 1, FD&C Red 40, flavors, maltodextrin, silicon dioxide, sodium citrate, sucrose, tribasic calcium phosphate.

Each packet contains: sodium 14 mg Phenylketonurics: Contains phenylalanine 27 mg per adult dose

**Indications:** Temporarily relieves these symptoms: headache, minor aches and pains, itchy nose or throat, itchy, watery eyes, fever, minor sore throat pain, nasal and sinus congestion, runny nose and sneezing. TheraFlu Maximum Strength **Flu & Cough Night Time Hot Liquid Medicine** also suppresses coughs due to minor throat and bronchial irritation.

**Warnings: Keep this and all drugs out of the reach of children.** In case of accidental overdose, seek professional assistance or contact a poison control center immediately. Prompt medical attention is critical for adults as well as for children even if you do not notice any signs or symptoms.

**Do not exceed recommended dosage.** If nervousness, dizziness, or sleeplessness occur, discontinue use and consult a doctor. If symptoms do not improve within 7 days or are accompanied by fever, consult a doctor. May cause excitability, especially in children. Do not take this product if you have heart disease, high blood pressure, thyroid disease, diabetes, glaucoma, a breathing

problem such as emphysema or chronic bronchitis, or difficulty in urination due to enlargement of the prostate gland, unless directed by a doctor.

A persistent cough may be a sign of a serious condition. If cough persists for more than 1 week, tends to recur, or is accompanied by fever, rash, or persistent headache, consult a doctor. Do not take this product for persistent or chronic cough such as occurs with smoking, asthma, emphysema, or if cough is accompanied by excessive phlegm (mucus) unless directed by a doctor.

Do not take this product for pain for more than 10 days or for fever for more than 3 days unless directed by a doctor. If pain or fever persists or gets worse, if new symptoms occur, or if redness or swelling is present, consult a doctor because these could be signs of a serious condition. If sore throat is severe, persists for more than 2 days, is accompanied or followed by fever, headache, rash, nausea, or vomiting, consult a doctor promptly.

May cause marked drowsiness; alcohol, sedatives, and tranquilizers may increase the drowsiness effect. Avoid alcoholic beverages while taking this product. Do not take this product if you are taking sedatives or tranquilizers, without first consulting your doctor. Use caution when driving a motor vehicle or operating machinery.

As with any drug, if you are pregnant or nursing a baby, seek the advice of a health professional before using this product.

**Alcohol Warning:** If you consume 3 or more alcoholic drinks every day, ask your doctor whether you should take acetaminophen or other pain relievers/fever reducers. Acetaminophen may cause liver damage.

**Drug interaction Precaution:** Do not use this product if you are now taking a prescription monoamine oxide inhibitor [MAOI] (certain drugs for depression, psychiatric or emotional conditions, or Parkinson's disease), or for 2 weeks after stopping the MAOI drug. If you are uncertain whether your prescription drug contains an MAOI, consult a health professional before taking this product.

**Directions:** Adults and children 12 years of age and over: dissolve contents of one packet in 6 oz. hot water; sip while hot. One packet every 6 hours, not to exceed 4 packets in 24 hours, or as directed by a doctor. Children under 12 years of age: consult a doctor.

**Microwave heating instructions:** Add contents of one packet and 6 oz. of cool water to a microwave-safe cup and

*Continued on next page*

*Information on Novartis Consumer Health, Inc., products appearing on these pages is effective as of November 2001.*

## Theraflu Flu/Cough—Cont.

stir briskly. Microwave on high 1½ minutes or until hot. Do not boil water or overheat, and remember to stir liquid between reheatings.

Sweeten to taste if desired.

**How Supplied:** TheraFlu Maximum Strength **Flu & Cough Night Time Hot Liquid Medicine** is available in 6 foil packets per carton.

---

### THERAFLU® MAXIMUM STRENGTH
**Severe Cold & Congestion Night Time Hot Liquid Medicine and Caplets**

**Description:** Each packet of TheraFlu **Maximum Strength Severe Cold & Congestion Night Time Hot Liquid Medicine** contains: acetaminophen 1000 mg, dextromethorphan HBr 30 mg, pseudoephedrine HCl 60 mg, and chlorpheniramine maleate 4 mg.

**Inactive Ingredients:** Acesulfame K, aspartame, citric acid, D&C Yellow 10, flavors, maltodextrin, silicon dioxide, sodium citrate, sucrose, and tribasic calcium phosphate.

Each packet contains: Sodium 19 mg. Phenylketonurics: Contains Phenylalanine 17 mg per adult dose

TheraFlu **Maximum Strength Severe Cold & Congestion Night Time Caplets:** each caplet contains acetaminophen 500 mg, pseudoephedrine HCl 30 mg, dextromethorphan HBr 15 mg, and chlorpheniramine maleate 2 mg.

**Inactive Ingredients:** colloidal silicon dioxide, croscarmellose sodium, D&C Yellow 10 aluminum lake, FD&C Blue 1 aluminum lake, FD&C Yellow 6 aluminum lake, gelatin, hydroxypropyl cellulose, hydroxypropyl methylcellulose, lactose, magnesium stearate, methylparaben, polydextrose, polyethylene glycol, pregelatinized starch, titanium dioxide and triacetin.

Each caplet contains: sodium 6 mg

**Indications:** TheraFlu Hot Liquid and Caplets provide temporary relief of these symptoms: headache, minor aches and pains, itchy nose or throat, itchy watery eyes, fever, minor sore throat pain, nasal and sinus congestion, runny nose, sneezing, and coughs due to minor throat and bronchial irritation.

**Warnings: Keep this and all drugs out of the reach of children.** In case of accidental overdose, seek professional assistance or contact a poison control center immediately. Prompt medical attention is critical for adults as well as children even if you do not notice any signs or symptoms.

**Do not exceed recommended dosage.** If nervousness, dizziness, or sleeplessness occur, discontinue use and consult a doctor. If symptoms do not improve within 7 days or are accompanied by fe-

ver, consult a doctor. May cause excitability, especially in children. Do not take this product if you have heart disease, high blood pressure, thyroid disease, diabetes, glaucoma, a breathing problem such as emphysema or chronic bronchitis, or difficulty in urination due to enlargement of the prostate gland, unless directed by a doctor. A persistent cough may be a sign of a serious condition. If cough persists for more than 1 week, tends to recur, or is accompanied by a fever, rash, or persistent headache, consult a doctor. Do not take this product for persistent or chronic cough such as occurs with smoking, asthma, or emphysema, or if cough is accompanied by excessive phlegm (mucus) unless directed by a doctor.

Do not take this product for pain for more than 10 days or for fever for more than 3 days unless directed by a doctor. If pain or fever persists or gets worse, if new symptoms occur, or if redness or swelling is present, consult a doctor because these could be signs of a serious condition. If sore throat is severe, persists for more than 2 days, is accompanied or followed by fever, headache, rash, nausea, or vomiting, consult a doctor promptly.

May cause marked drowsiness; alcohol, sedatives, and tranquilizers may increase the drowsiness effect. Avoid alcoholic beverages while taking this product. Do not take this product if you are taking sedatives or tranquilizers, without first consulting your doctor. Use caution when driving a motor vehicle or operating machinery.

As with any drug, if you are pregnant or nursing a baby, seek the advice of a health professional before using this product.

**Alcohol Warning:** If you consume 3 or more alcoholic drinks every day ask your doctor whether you should take acetaminophen or other pain relievers/fever reducers. Acetaminophen may cause liver damage.

**Drug Interaction Precaution:** Do not use this product if you are now taking a prescription monoamine oxidase inhibitor [MAOI] (certain drugs for depression, psychiatric or emotional conditions, or Parkinson's disease), or for 2 weeks after stopping the MAOI drug. If you are uncertain whether your prescription drug contains an MAOI, consult a health professional before taking this product.

**Directions:** TheraFlu® **Maximum Strength Severe Cold & Congestion Night Time Hot Liquid Medicine:** Adults and children 12 years of age and over: dissolve contents of one packet in 6 oz. cup of hot water; sip while hot. Take every 6 hours, not to exceed 4 packets in 24 hours, or as directed by a doctor. Children under 12 years of age: consult a doctor. **Microwave Heating Instructions:** Add contents of one packet and 6 oz. of cool water to a microwave-safe cup and stir briskly. Microwave on high 1½ minutes or until hot. Do not boil water or

overheat, and remember to stir liquid between reheatings. Sweeten to taste if desired.

**TheraFlu Maximum Strength Severe Cold & Congestion Night Time** Caplets: Adults and children 12 years of age and over: two caplets every 6 hours, not to exceed 8 caplets in 24 hours or as directed by a doctor. Children under 12 years of age: consult a doctor.

**How Supplied:** TheraFlu Maximum Strength **Severe Cold & Congestion Night Time Hot Liquid Medicine** powder in foil packets, 6 or 12 packets per carton. TheraFlu Maximum Strength **Severe Cold & Congestion Night Time** Caplets in blister packs of 12's and 24's.

*Shown in Product Identification Guide, page 515*

---

### THERAFLU® MAXIMUM STRENGTH
**Severe Cold & Congestion Non-Drowsy Hot Liquid Medicine and Caplets**

**Description:** Each packet of TheraFlu Maximum Strength **Severe Cold & Congestion Non-Drowsy Hot Liquid Medicine** contains: acetaminophen 1000 mg, pseudoephedrine HCl 60 mg, dextromethorphan HBr 30 mg.

**Inactive Ingredients:** acesulfame K, aspartame, citric acid, D&C Yellow 10, flavors, maltodextrin, silicon dioxide, sodium citrate, sucrose, and tribasic calcium phosphate.

Each packet contains: sodium 19 mg Phenylketonurics: Contains Phenylalanine 17 mg per adult dose

Each TheraFlu Maximum Strength **Severe Cold & Congestion Non-Drowsy Caplet** contains: Acetaminophen 500 mg, pseudoephedrine HCl 30 mg, dextromethorphan HBr 15 mg.

**Inactive ingredients:** Colloidal silicon dioxide, croscarmellose sodium, D&C Yellow 10 aluminum lake, FD&C Red 40, FD&C Yellow 6 aluminum lake, gelatin, hydroxypropyl cellulose, hydroxypropyl methylcellulose, lactose, magnesium stearate, methylparaben, polydextrose, polyethylene glycol, pregelatinized starch, titanium dioxide and triacetin.

Each caplet contains: sodium 6 mg

**Indications:** Temporarily relieves these symptoms: headache, minor aches and pains, fever, minor sore throat pain, nasal and sinus congestion. TheraFlu Maximum Strength **Severe Cold & Congestion Non-Drowsy Medicine** also suppresses cough due to minor throat and bronchial irritation.

**Warnings: Keep this and all drugs out of the reach of children.** In case of accidental overdose, seek professional assistance or contact a poison control center immediately. Prompt medical attention is critical for adults as well as children even if you do not notice any signs or symptoms.

**Do not exceed recommended dosage.** If nervousness, dizziness, or sleeplessness occur, discontinue use and consult a doctor. If symptoms do not improve within 7 days or are accompanied by fever, consult a doctor. Do not take this product if you have heart disease, high blood pressure, thyroid disease, diabetes, or difficulty in urination due to enlargement of the prostate gland unless directed by a physician.

A persistent cough may be a sign of a serious condition. If cough persists for more than 1 week, tends to recur, or is accompanied by a fever, rash, or persistent headache, consult a doctor. Do not take this product for persistent or chronic cough such as occurs with smoking, asthma, or emphysema, or if cough is accompanied by excessive phlegm (mucus) unless directed by a doctor.

Do not take this product for pain for more than 10 days or for fever for more than 3 days unless directed by a doctor. If pain or fever persists or gets worse, if new symptoms occur, or if redness or swelling is present, consult a doctor, because these could be signs of a serious condition. If sore throat is severe, persists for more than 2 days, is accompanied or followed by fever, headache, rash, nausea, or vomiting, consult a doctor promptly.

As with any drug, if you are pregnant or nursing a baby, seek the advice of a health professional before using this product.

**Alcohol Warning:** If you consume 3 or more alcoholic drinks every day ask your doctor whether you should take acetaminophen or other pain relievers/fever reducers. Acetaminophen may cause liver damage.

**Drug Interaction Precaution:** Do not take this product if you are now taking a prescription monoamine oxidase inhibitor [MAOI] (certain drugs for depression, psychiatric or emotional conditions, or Parkinson's disease), or for 2 weeks after stopping the MAOI drug. If you are uncertain whether your prescription drug contains an MAOI, consult a health professional before taking this product.

**Directions: TheraFlu® Maximum Strength Severe Cold & Congestion Non-Drowsy Hot Liquid Medicine:** Adults and children 12 years of age and over: dissolve one packet in 6 oz. cup of hot water; sip while hot. Take every 6 hours, not to exceed 4 packets in 24 hours, or as directed by a doctor. Children under 12 years of age: consult a doctor. Microwave Heating Instructions: Add contents of one packet and 6 oz. of cool water to a microwave-safe cup and stir briskly. Microwave on high 1 1/2 minutes or until hot. Do not boil or overheat, and remember to stir liquid between reheatings. Sweeten to taste if desired.

TheraFlu **Maximum Strength Severe Cold & Congestion Non-Drowsy Caplet:**

Adults and Children 12 years of age and over: two caplets every 6 hours, not to exceed eight caplets in 24 hours or as directed by a doctor. Children under 12 years of age: Consult a doctor.

**How Supplied:** TheraFlu Maximum Strength **Severe Cold & Congestion Non-Drowsy Hot Liquid Medicine** powder in foil packets, 6 packets per carton. TheraFlu Maximum Strength **Severe Cold & Congestion Non-Drowsy gelatin coated caplets** in blister packs of 12 and 24.

---

## TRIAMINIC® Allergy Congestion
Nasal Decongestant-Orange Flavor

### Drug Facts

**Active ingredient**
**(in each 5 mL, 1 teaspoon)**
Pseudoephedrine HCl, USP,
15 mg ........................ Nasal decongestant

**Uses** temporarily relieves these symptoms:
• hay fever or other upper respiratory allergies • nasal and sinus congestion

**Warnings**
**Do not use** in a child who is taking a prescription monoamine oxidase inhibitor (MAOI) (certain drugs for depression, psychiatric or emotional conditions, or Parkinson's disease), or for 2 weeks after stopping the MAOI drug. If you do not know if the child's prescription drug contains an MAOI, ask a doctor or pharmacist before giving this product.
**Ask a doctor before use if the child has**
• heart disease • high blood pressure
• thyroid disease • diabetes
**When using this product**
• do not use more than directed
**Stop use and ask a doctor if**
• nervousness, dizziness, or sleeplessness occurs • symptoms do not improve within 7 days or occur with a fever. These could be signs of a serious condition.
**Keep out of reach of children.** In case of overdose, get medical help or contact a poison control center right away.

**Dosage and Administration** • take every 4 to 6 hours; not more than 4 doses in 24 hours or as directed by a doctor

| Age | Weight | Dose |
|---|---|---|
| 4 months to under 1 year[1] | 12 to 17 lb | ¼ tsp (1.25 mL) |
| 1 to under 2 years[1] | 18 to 23 lb | ½ tsp (2.5 mL) |
| 2 to under 6 years | 24 to 47 lb | 1 tsp (5 mL) |
| 6 to under 12 years | 48 to 95 lb | 2 tsp (10 mL) |
| 12 years to adult | 96+ lb | 4 tsp (20 mL) |

[1]The dosage for children under 2 years should be determined by the physician

on the basis of the patient's weight, physical condition or other appropriate considerations. Dosages are provided as guidelines.
**Other Information:**
• each teaspoon contains: **sodium 1 mg**
• contains no aspirin • store at controlled room temperature 20–25°C (68–77°F).
**Inactive Ingredients:** Benzoic acid, edetate disodium, flavors, purified water, sodium hydroxide, sorbitol, sucrose

**How Supplied:** Bottle of 4 fl. oz. (118 mL)
*Questions:* call **1-800-452-0051**
For more information about Triaminic® visit our website at www.triaminic.com
Novartis Consumer Health, Inc.
Parsippany, NJ 07054-0622 ©2002
*Shown in Product Identification Guide, page 516*

---

## TRIAMINIC® Chest Congestion
Expectorant, Nasal Decongestant
Citrus Flavor

### Drug Facts:

**Active ingredients:**
**(in each 5 mL, 1 teaspoon)**
Guaifenesin,
USP, 50 mg ........................ Expectorant
Pseudoephedrine HCl,
USP, 15 mg .............. Nasal decongestant

**Uses** temporarily relieves these symptoms:
• chest congestion by loosening phlegm (mucus) to help clear bronchial passageways • nasal and sinus congestion

**Warnings:**
**Do not use** in a child who is taking a prescription monoamine oxidase inhibitor (MAOI) (certain drugs for depression, psychiatric or emotional conditions, or Parkinson's disease), or for 2 weeks after stopping the MAOI drug. If you do not know if the child's prescription drug contains an MAOI, ask a doctor or pharmacist before giving this product.
**Ask a doctor before use if the child has**
• heart disease • high blood pressure
• thyroid disease • diabetes • glaucoma
• cough that occurs with too much phlegm (mucus) • chronic cough that lasts or a breathing problem such as asthma or chronic bronchitis
**When using this product**
• do not use more than directed
**Stop use and ask a doctor if**
• nervousness, dizziness, or sleeplessness occur • symptoms do not improve within 7 days or occur with a fever

*Continued on next page*

*Information on Novartis Consumer Health, Inc., products appearing on these pages is effective as of November 2001.*

        

## Triaminic Chest—Cont.

• cough persists for more than 7 days, comes back, or occurs with a fever, rash, or persistent headache. These could be signs of a serious condition.

**Keep out of reach of children.** In case of overdose, get medical help or contact a poison control center right away.

### Dosage and Administration
take every 4 to 6 hours; not more than 4 doses in 24 hours or as directed by a doctor

| Age | Weight | Dose |
|---|---|---|
| 4 months to under 1 year[1] | 12 to 17 lb | ¼ tsp (1.25 mL) |
| 1 to under 2 years[1] | 18 to 23 lb | ½ tsp (2.5 mL) |
| 2 to under 6 years | 24 to 47 lb | 1 tsp (5 mL) |
| 6 to under 12 years | 48 to 95 lb | 2 tsp (10 mL) |
| 12 years to adult | 96+ lb | 4 tsp (20 mL) |

[1]The dosage for children under 2 years should be determined by the physician on the basis of the patient's weight, physical condition or other appropriate considerations. Dosages are provided as guidelines.

### Other Information
• each teaspoon contains: **sodium 2 mg** • contains no aspirin • store at controlled room temperature 20–25°C (68–77°F)

**Inactive Ingredients:** Benzoic acid, D&C Yellow 10, edetate disodium, FD&C Yellow 6, flavors, glycerin, polyethylene glycol, propylene glycol, purified water, sorbitol, sucrose

**How Supplied:** Bottles of 4 fl. oz. (118 mL) and 8 fl. oz. (236 mL)
*Questions:* call **1-800-452-0051**
For more information about Triaminic® visit our website at www.triaminic.com
**Novartis Consumer Health, Inc.**
Parsippany, NJ 07054-0622 ©2002
*Shown in Product Identification Guide, page 516*

---

**TRIAMINIC® Cold & Allergy**
Antihistamine, Nasal Decongestant-Orange Flavor
**TRIAMINIC® Cold & Cough**
Antihistamine, Cough Suppressant, Nasal Decongestant-Cherry Flavor
**TRIAMINIC® Flu, Cough & Fever**
Antihistamine, Cough Suppressant, Fever Reducer/Pain Reliever, Nasal Decongestant-Bubble Gum Flavor
**TRIAMINIC® Cold & Night Time Cough**
Antihistamine, Cough Suppressant, Nasal Decongestant-Grape Flavor

## Drug Facts
### Active ingredients
**(in each 5 mL, 1 teaspoon)**
**TRIAMINIC® Cold & Allergy**
Orange Flavor
Chlorpheniramine maleate, USP, 1 mg .......................... Antihistamine
Pseudoephedrine HCl, USP, 15 mg .............. Nasal decongestant
**TRIAMINIC® Cold & Cough**
Cherry Flavor
Chlorpheniramine maleate, USP, 1 mg .......................... Antihistamine
Dextromethorphan HBr, USP, 5 mg ................. Cough suppressant
Pseudoephedrine HCl, USP, 15 mg .............. Nasal decongestant
**TRIAMINIC® Flu, Cough & Fever**
Bubble Gum Flavor
Acetaminophen, USP, 160 mg ............ Fever reducer/Pain reliever
Chlorpheniramine maleate, USP, 1 mg .......................... Antihistamine
Dextromethorphan HBr, USP, 7.5 mg ............. Cough suppressant
Pseudoephedrine HCl, USP, 15 mg .............. Nasal decongestant
**TRIAMINIC® Cold & Night Time Cough**
Grape Flavor
Chlorpheniramine maleate, USP, 1 mg .......................... Antihistamine
Dextromethorphan HBr, USP, 7.5 mg ............. Cough suppressant
Pseudoephedrine HCl, USP, 15 mg .............. Nasal decongestant

**Uses** temporarily relieves these symptoms:
**TRIAMINIC® Cold & Allergy**
Antihistamine, Nasal Decongestant-Orange Flavor
• itchy, watery eyes • runny nose • itchy nose or throat • sneezing • nasal and sinus congestion

**TRIAMINIC® Cold & Cough**
Antihistamine, Cough Suppressant, Nasal Decongestant-Cherry Flavor
• cough due to minor throat and bronchial irritation • runny nose • nasal and sinus congestion • sneezing • itchy nose or throat • itchy, watery eyes

**TRIAMINIC® Flu, Cough & Fever**
Antihistamine, Cough Suppressant, Fever Reducer/Pain Reliever, Nasal Decongestant-Bubble Gum Flavor
• fever • minor aches and pains • headache and sore throat • cough due to minor throat and bronchial irritation • nasal and sinus congestion • sneezing • itchy nose or throat • itchy, watery eyes

**TRIAMINIC® Cold & Night Time Cough**
Antihistamine, Cough Suppressant, Nasal Decongestant-Grape Flavor
• cough due to minor throat and bronchial irritation • runny nose • nasal and sinus congestion • sneezing • itchy nose or throat • itchy, watery eyes

### Warnings:
**Do not use** in a child who is taking a prescription monoamine oxidase inhibitor (MAOI) (certain drugs for depression, psychiatric or emotional conditions, or Parkinson's disease), or for 2 weeks after

stopping the MAOI drug. If you do not know if the child's prescription drug contains an MAOI, ask a doctor or pharmacist before giving this product.
**Specific to Flu, Cough & Fever:** together with another product containing acetaminophen
**Specific to Cold & Night Time Cough:** if a child is on a sodium-restricted diet unless directed by a doctor
**Ask a doctor before use if the child has**
• heart disease • high blood pressure • thyroid disease • diabetes • glaucoma • cough that occurs with too much phlegm (mucus) (does not apply to Cold & Allergy) • a breathing problem such as asthma or chronic bronchitis • chronic cough that lasts (does not apply to Cold & Allergy).
**Ask a doctor or pharmacist before use if the child is** taking sedatives or tranquilizers.
**When using this product**
• do not use more than directed • excitability may occur, especially in children • marked drowsiness may occur (does not apply to Cold & Allergy) • sedatives and tranquilizers may increase drowsiness
**Stop use and ask a doctor if**
• nervousness, dizziness, or sleeplessness occur
• symptoms do not improve within 7 days or occur with a fever (does not apply to Flu, Cough, Fever)
• cough persists for more than 7 days, comes back, or occurs with fever, rash, or persistent headache (does not apply to Cold & Allergy)
**Specific to Flu, Cough & Fever:**
• symptoms do not improve within 5 days (pain) or 3 days (fever).
• sore throat persists for more than 2 days or occurs with headache, fever, rash, nausea or vomiting (does not apply to Cold & Allergy, Cold & Cough, Cold & Night Time Cough)
These could be signs of a serious condition.
**Keep out of reach of children.** In case of overdose, get medical help or contact a poison control center right away.
**Pertains only to Flu, Cough & Fever: Prompt medical attention is critical even if you do not notice any signs or symptoms.**

### Dosage and Administration[1]
**TRIAMINIC® Cold & Allergy**
Antihistamine, Nasal Decongestant-Orange Flavor (see Triaminic® Cold & Cough)

**TRIAMINIC® Cold & Cough**
Antihistamine, Cough Suppressant, Nasal Decongestant-Cherry Flavor
Take every 4 to 6 hours; not more than 4 doses in 24 hours or as directed by a doctor.

**TRIAMINIC® Flu, Cough & Fever**
Antihistamine, Cough Suppressant, Fever Reducer/Pain Reliever, Nasal Decongestant-Bubble Gum Flavor (see Triaminic® Cold & Night Time Cough)

**TRIAMINIC® Cold & Night Time Cough**
Antihistamine, Cough Suppressant, Nasal Decongestant-Grape Flavor

Take every 6 hours; not more than 4 doses in 24 hours or as directed by a doctor.

| Age | Weight | Dose |
|---|---|---|
| 4 months to under 1 year[2] | 12–17 lb | ¼ tsp (1.25 mL) |
| 1 to under 2 years[2] | 18–23 lb | ½ tsp (2.5 mL) |
| 2 to under 6 years[1] | 24–47 lb | 1 tsp (5 mL) |
| 6 to under 12 years | 48–95 lb | 2 tsp (10 mL) |
| 12 years to adult | 96+ lb | 4 tsp (20 mL) |

[1] As with any antihistamine-containing product, use of Triaminic® Formulas containing antihistamines in children under 6 years of age should be only under the advice and supervision of a physician.

[2] The dosage for children under 2 years should be determined by the physician on the basis of patients weight, physical condition or other appropriate considerations. Dosages are provided as guidelines. Antihistamines should not be given to neonates and are contraindicated in newborns.

### Other Information

**TRIAMINIC® Cold & Allergy**

Antihistamine, Nasal Decongestant-Orange Flavor
- each teaspoon contains: **sodium 2 mg**
- contains no aspirin
- store at controlled room temperature 20–25°C (68–77°F).

**TRIAMINIC® Cold & Cough**

Antihistamine, Cough Suppressant, Nasal Decongestant-Cherry Flavor
- each teaspoon contains: **sodium 10 mg**
- contains no aspirin
- store at controlled room temperature 20–25°C (68–77°F).

**TRIAMINIC® Flu, Cough & Fever**

Antihistamine, Cough Suppressant, Fever Reducer/Pain Reliever, Nasal Decongestant-Bubble Gum Flavor
- each teaspoon contains: **sodium 3 mg**
- contains no aspirin
- protect from light
- store at controlled room temperature 20–25°C (68–77°F).

**TRIAMINIC® Cold & Night Time Cough**

Antihistamine, Cough Suppressant, Nasal Decongestant-Grape Flavor
- each teaspoon contains: **sodium 22 mg**
- contains no aspirin
- store at controlled room temperature 20–25°C (68–77°F).

### Inactive Ingredients

**TRIAMINIC® Cold & Allergy**

Antihistamine, Nasal Decongestant-Orange Flavor

benzoic acid, edetate disodium, FD&C Yellow 6, flavors, purified water, sorbitol, sucrose

**TRIAMINIC® Cold & Cough**

Antihistamine, Cough Suppressant, Nasal Decongestant-Cherry Flavor

benzoic acid, FD&C Red 40, flavors, propylene glycol, purified water, sodium chloride, sorbitol, sucrose

**TRIAMINIC® Flu, Cough & Fever**

Antihistamine, Cough Suppressant, Fever Reducer/Pain Reliever, Nasal Decongestant-Bubble Gum Flavor

acesulfame K, benzoic acid, citric acid, D&C Red 33, dibasic potassium phosphate, disodium edetate, FD&C Red 40, flavors, glycerin, polyethylene glycol, potassium chloride, propylene glycol, purified water, sucrose, other ingredients

**TRIAMINIC® Cold & Night Time Cough**

Antihistamine, Cough Suppressant, Nasal Decongestant-Grape Flavor

benzoic acid, citric acid, D&C Red 33, dibasic sodium phosphate, FD&C Blue 1, flavors, propylene glycol, purified water, sorbitol, sucrose

### How Supplied:

**TRIAMINIC® Cold & Allergy**
**TRIAMINIC® Cold & Cough**
**TRIAMINIC® Cold & Night Time Cough**
Bottles of 4 fl. oz. (118 mL) and 8 fl.oz. (236 mL)
**TRIAMINIC® Flu, Cough & Fever**
Bottle of 4 fl. oz. (118 mL)
***Questions:*** call **1-800-452-0051**
**For more information about Triaminic® visit our website at www.triaminic.com**
**Novartis Consumer Health, Inc.**
Parsippany, NJ 07054-0622

*Shown in Product Identification Guide, page 516*

---

**TRIAMINIC® Cough**
**Cough Suppressant, Nasal Decongestant-Berry Flavor**

**TRIAMINIC® Cough & Congestion**
**Cough Suppressant, Nasal Decongestant-Orange Strawberry Flavor**

**TRIAMINIC® Cough & Sore Throat**
**Cough Suppressant, Nasal Decongestant, Pain Reliever-Fever Reducer-Grape Flavor**

### Drug Facts:

**Active ingredients**
**(in each 5 mL, 1 teaspoon)**
**TRIAMINIC® Cough**
Berry Flavor
Dextromethorphan HBr,
USP 5 mg ................. Cough suppressant
Pseudoephedrine, HCl,
USP, 15 mg .............. Nasal decongestant
**TRIAMINIC® Cough & Congestion**
Orange Strawberry Flavor
Dextromethorphan HBr,
USP, 7.5 mg ............ Cough suppressant
Pseudoephedrine, HCl,
USP, 15 mg .............. Nasal decongestant
**TRIAMINIC® Cough & Sore Throat**
Grape Flavor
Acetaminophen,
USP, 160 mg ..... Fever reducer, Pain reliever
Pseudoephedrine HCl,
USP, 15 mg .............. Nasal decongestant
Dextromethorphan HBr,
USP, 7.5 mg ............ Cough suppressant

**Uses:** Temporarily relieves these symptoms:
**TRIAMINIC® Cough**
Cough Suppressant, Nasal Decongestant-Berry Flavor (see Cough & Congestion)
**TRIAMINIC® Cough & Congestion**
Cough Suppressant, Nasal Decongestant-Orange Strawberry Flavor
- cough due to minor throat and bronchial irritation • nasal and sinus congestion
**TRIAMINIC® Cough & Sore Throat**
Cough Suppressant, Nasal Decongestant, Pain Reliever-Fever Reducer-Grape Flavor
- sore throat pain • minor aches and pains • cough due to minor throat and bronchial irritation • fever • nasal and sinus congestion

### Warnings

**Do not use** in a child who is taking a prescription monoamine oxidase inhibitor (MAOI) (certain drugs for depression, psychiatric or emotional conditions, or Parkinson's disease), or for 2 weeks after stopping the MAOI drug. If you do not know if the child's prescription drug contains an MAOI, ask a doctor or pharmacist before giving this product.
**Specific to Cough & Sore Throat:** together with another product containing acetaminophen
**Specific to Cough:** if child is on a sodium-restricted diet unless directed by a doctor
**Ask a doctor before use if the child has**
- heart disease • high blood pressure • thyroid disease • diabetes • glaucoma • cough that occurs with too much phlegm (mucus) • chronic cough that lasts or a breathing problem such as asthma or chronic bronchitis
**Ask a doctor or pharmacist before use if the child is** taking sedatives or tranquilizers.
**When using this product**
- do not use more than directed
**Stop use and ask a doctor if**
- nervousness, dizziness, or sleeplessness occurs • symptoms do not improve within 7 days or occur with a fever • cough persists for more than 7 days, comes back, or occurs with fever, rash, or persistent headache. These could be signs of a serious condition.
**Specific to Cough & Sore Throat:**
- sore throat persists for more than 2 days, or occurs with headache, fever, rash, nausea, or vomiting. These could be signs of a serious condition. • symptoms do not improve for 5 days (pain) or 3 days (fever)
**Keep out of reach of children.** In case of overdose, get medical help or contact a

*Continued on next page*

---

*Information on Novartis Consumer Health, Inc., products appearing on these pages is effective as of November 2001.*

## Triaminic Cough—Cont.

poison control center right away. (Not applicable to: Cough and Cough & Congestion). Prompt medical attention is critical even if you do not notice any signs or symptoms.

### Dosage and Administration
**Triaminic® Cough**
Cough Suppressant, Nasal Decongestant-Berry Flavor
Take every 4 to 6 hours; not more than 4 doses in 24 hours or as directed by a doctor.
**Triaminic® Cough & Congestion**
Cough Suppressant, Nasal Decongestant-Orange Strawberry Flavor
**Triaminic® Cough & Sore Throat**
Cough Suppressant, Nasal Decongestant, Pain Reliever-Fever Reducer-Grape Flavor
Take every 6 hours; not more than 4 doses in 24 hours or as directed by a doctor.

| Age | Weight | Dose |
|---|---|---|
| 4 mos. to under 1 yr[1] | 12–17 lb | ¼ tsp (1.25 mL) |
| 1 to under 2 years[1] | 18–23 lb | ½ tsp (2.5 mL) |
| 2 to under 6 years | 24–47 lb | 1 tsp (5 mL) |
| 6 to under 12 years | 48–95 lb | 2 tsp (10 mL) |
| 12 years to adult | 96 + lb | 4 tsp (20 mL) |

[1]The dosage for children under 2 years should be determined by the physician on the basis of patients weight, physical condition or other appropriate considerations. Dosages are provided as guidelines.

### Other Information
**TRIAMINIC® Cough**
Cough Suppressant, Nasal Decongestant-Berry Flavor
• each teaspoon contains: **sodium 20 mg**
• contains no aspirin • store at controlled room temperature 20–25°C (68–77°F)

### TRIAMINIC® Cough & Congestion
Cough Suppressant, Nasal Decongestant-Orange Strawberry Flavor
• each teaspoon contains: **sodium 7 mg**
• contains no aspirin • store at controlled room temperature 20–25°C (68–77°F)

### TRIAMINIC® Cough & Sore Throat
Cough Suppressant, Nasal Decongestant, Pain Reliever-Fever Reducer-Grape Flavor
• each teaspoon contains: **sodium 11 mg**
• contains no aspirin • store at controlled room temperature 20–25°C (68–77°F)

### Inactive Ingredients
**TRIAMINIC® Cough**
Cough Suppressant, Nasal Decongestant-Berry Flavor

benzoic acid, FD&C Blue 1, FD&C Red 40, flavors, propylene glycol, purified water, sodium chloride, sorbitol, sucrose

### TRIAMINIC® Cough & Congestion
Cough Suppressant, Nasal Decongestant-Orange Strawberry Flavor
benzoic acid, citric acid, dibasic sodium phosphate, edetate disodium, flavors, propylene glycol, purified water, sorbitol, sucrose

### TRIAMINIC® Cough & Sore Throat
Cough Suppressant, Nasal Decongestant, Pain Reliever-Fever-Reducer-Grape Flavor
benzoic acid, D&C Red 33, dibasic sodium phosphate, edetate disodium, FD&C Blue 1, FD&C Red 40, flavors, glycerin, polyethylene glycol, propylene glycol, purified water, sucrose, tartaric acid

### How Supplied:
**Triaminic® Cough**
**Triaminic® Cough & Congestion**
Bottles of 4 fl. oz. (118 mL)
**Triaminic® Cough & Sore Throat**
Bottles of 4 fl. oz. (118 mL) and 8 fl. oz (236 mL)
*Questions:* call **1-800-452-0051**
For more information about Triaminic® visit our website at www.triaminic.com
Novartis Consumer Health, Inc.
Parsippany, NJ 07054-0622 ©2002
*Shown in Product Identification Guide, page 516*

---

**TRIAMINIC® Softchews® Allergy Congestion—Orange Flavor**
Pseudoephedrine HCl—Nasal Decongestant
**TRIAMINIC® Softchews® Allergy Runny Nose & Congestion—Orange Flavor**
Antihistamine—Nasal Decongestant
**TRIAMINIC® Softchews® Allergy Sinus & Headache—Fruit Punch Flavor**
Pain Reliever—Nasal Decongestant

### Drug Facts:

**Active Ingredients** (in each tablet)
**TRIAMINIC® Softchews® Allergy Congestion**
Orange Flavor
Pseudoephedrine HCl, USP,
15 mg ........................ Nasal decongestant
**TRIAMINIC® Softchews® Allergy Runny Nose & Congestion**
Orange Flavor
Chlorpheniramine maleate, USP,
1 mg ...................... Antihistamine
Pseudoephedrine HCl, USP,
15 mg ........................ Nasal decongestant
**TRIAMINIC® Softchews® Allergy Sinus & Headache**
Fruit Punch Flavor
Acetaminophen, USP,
160 mg ...................... Pain reliever
Pseudoephedrine HCl, USP,
15 mg ........................ Nasal decongestant

**Uses:** Temporarily relieves these symptoms:

**TRIAMINIC® Softchews® Allergy Congestion**
Nasal Decongestant—Orange Flavor
• hay fever or other upper respiratory allergies
• nasal and sinus congestion
**TRIAMINIC® Softchews® Allergy Runny Nose & Congestion**
Antihistamine—Nasal Decongestant
Orange Flavor
• nasal and sinus congestion
• runny nose
• sneezing
• itchy nose or throat
• itchy, watery eyes
**TRIAMINIC® Softchews® Allergy Sinus & Headache**
Pain Reliever—Nasal Decongestant
Fruit Punch Flavor
• minor aches and pains
• headache
• nasal and sinus congestion
• hay fever or other upper respiratory allergies

### Warnings
**Do not use** in a child who is taking a prescription monoamine oxidase inhibitor (MAOI) (certain drugs for depression, psychiatric or emotional conditions, or Parkinson's disease), or for 2 weeks after stopping the MAOI drug. If you do not know if the child's prescription drug contains an MAOI, ask a doctor or pharmacist before giving this product.
**Specific to Sinus & Headache: Do not use** together with another product containing acetaminophen.
**Ask a doctor before use if the child has**
• heart disease • high blood pressure • thyroid disease • diabetes
**Specific to Runny Nose & Congestion:**
• glaucoma • a breathing problem such as chronic bronchitis
**Ask a doctor or pharmacist before use** if the child is taking sedatives or tranquilizers. (Not applicable to: Allergy Congestion or Allergy Sinus & Headache)
**When using this product**
• do not use more than directed
**Specific to Runny Nose & Congestion:**
• drowsiness may occur • sedatives and tranquilizers may increase drowsiness • excitability may occur, especially in children
**Stop use and ask a doctor if**
• nervousness, dizziness, or sleeplessness occur. These could be signs of a serious condition.
**Specific to Allergy Congestion:** symptoms do not improve within 7 days or occur with a fever. These could be signs of a serious condition.
**Specific to Runny Nose & Congestion:** symptoms do not improve within 7 days, or occur with fever, rash, or persistent headache.
**Specific to Sinus & Headache:** symptoms do not improve for 5 days (pain) or 3 days (fever), symptoms do not improve within 7 days or occur with a fever. These could be signs of a serious condition.

**Keep out of reach of children.** In case of overdose, get medical help or contact a poison control center right away. Prompt medical attention is critical even if you do not notice any signs or symptoms. (Not applicable to: Allergy Congestion and Runny Nose & Congestion.)

### Directions
- Let Softchews® tablet dissolve in mouth or chew Softchews® tablet before swallowing, whichever is preferred

**Specific to Congestion and Sinus & Headache:**
- take every 4 to 6 hours; not more than 4 doses in 24 hours or as directed by a doctor

| Age | Dose |
| --- | --- |
| children 6 to under 12 years of age | 2 tablets every 4 to 6 hours |
| children 2 to under 6 years of age | 1 tablet every 4 to 6 hours |
| children under 2 years of age | ask a doctor |

**Specific to Runny Nose & Congestion:**
- take every 4 to 6 hours; not more than 4 doses in 24 hours or as directed by a doctor

| Age | Dose |
| --- | --- |
| children 6 to under 12 years of age | 2 tablets every 4 to 6 hours |
| children under 6 years of age | ask a doctor |

### Other Information
**Specific to Allergy Congestion:**
- each Softchews® tablet contains: **sodium 5 mg**
- Phenylketonurics: Contains **Phenylalanine, 17.6 mg** per Softchews® tablet

**Specific to Runny Nose & Congestion:**
- each Softchews® tablet contains: **sodium 5 mg**
- Phenylketonurics: Contains **Phenylalanine, 17.6 mg** per Softchews® tablet

**Specific to Sinus & Headache:**
- each Softchews® tablet contains: **sodium 8 mg**
- Phenylketonurics: Contains **Phenylalanine, 11.2 mg** per Softchews® tablet
- contains no aspirin
- store at controlled room temperature 20–25°C (68–77°F)

### Inactive Ingredients
**TRIAMINIC Softchews Allergy Congestion**
Nasal Decongestant—Orange Flavor
aspartame, citric acid, crospovidone, ethylcellulose, FD&C Yellow 6 aluminum lake, flavors, fractionated coconut oil, hydroxypropyl methylcellulose, magnesium stearate, mannitol, microcrystalline cellulose, oleic acid, polyethylene glycol, sodium bicarbonate, sodium chloride, sorbitol, starch, sucrose, triethyl citrate

**TRIAMINIC Softchews Allergy Runny Nose & Congestion**
Antihistamine—Nasal Decongestant
Orange Flavor
aspartame, carnauba wax, citric acid, crospovidone, ethylcellulose, FD&C Yellow 6 aluminum lake, flavors, fractionated coconut oil, hydroxypropyl methylcellulose, magnesium stearate, mannitol, microcrystalline cellulose, mono- and di-glycerides, oleic acid, polyethylene glycol, silicon dioxide, sodium bicarbonate, sodium chloride, sorbitol, starch, sucrose, triethyl citrate.

**TRIAMINIC Softchews Allergy Sinus & Headache**
Pain Reliever—Nasal Decongestant
Fruit Punch Flavor
alpha-tocopherol, aspartame, citric acid, crospovidone, D&C Red 27, ethylcellulose, FD&C Blue 1, FD&C Red 40, flavors, fractionated coconut oil, hydroxypropyl methylcellulose, magnesium stearate, mannitol, microcrystalline cellulose, oleic acid, polyethylene glycol, sodium bicarbonate, sodium chloride, sorbitol, starch, sucrose, triethyl citrate

**How Supplied:** 18 Softchews® Tablets
***Questions?*** call **1-800-452-0051** 24 hours a day, 7 days a week.
For more information about Triaminic® visit our website at www.triaminic.com
*Shown in Product Identification Guide, page 516*

---

### TRIAMINIC® Softchews®
### Cold & Allergy
**Antihistamine, Nasal Decongestant-Orange Flavor**

### TRIAMINIC® Softchews®
### Cold & Cough
**Antihistamine, Cough Suppressant, Nasal Decongestant-Cherry Flavor**

**Drug Facts:**
**Active ingredients (in each tablet)**
**TRIAMINIC® Softchews® Cold & Allergy**-Orange Flavor
Chlorpheniramine maleate, USP,
1 mg ................................. Antihistamine
Pseudoephedrine, HCl, USP,
15 mg ........................ Nasal decongestant
**TRIAMINIC® Softchews® Cold & Cough**-Cherry Flavor
Pseudoephedrine HCl, USP,
15 mg ........................ Nasal decongestant
Dextromethorphan HBr, USP,
5 mg .......................... Cough suppressant
Chlorpheniramine maleate, USP,
1 mg ..................................... Antihistamine

**Uses** Temporarily relieves these symptoms:
**TRIAMINIC® Softchews® Cold & Allergy**
Antihistamine, Nasal Decongestant-Orange Flavor
- nasal and sinus congestion • runny nose • sneezing • itchy nose or throat • itchy, watery eyes

**TRIAMINIC® Softchews® Cold & Cough**
Antihistamine, Cough Suppressant, Nasal Decongestant-Cherry Flavor
- cough due to minor throat and bronchial irritation • runny nose • nasal and sinus congestion • sneezing • itchy nose or throat • itchy, watery eyes

**Warnings:**
**Do not use** in a child who is taking a prescription monoamine oxidase inhibitor (MAOI) (certain drugs for depression, psychiatric or emotional conditions, or Parkinson's disease), or for 2 weeks after stopping the MAOI drug. If you do not know if the child's prescription drug contains an MAOI, ask a doctor or pharmacist before giving this product.

**Ask a doctor before use if the child has**
- heart disease • high blood pressure • thyroid disease • diabetes • glaucoma • a breathing problem such as asthma or chronic bronchitis

**Specific to Cold & Cough:** cough that occurs with too much phlegm (mucus) or chronic cough that lasts.

**Ask a doctor or pharmacist before use** if the child is taking sedatives or tranquilizers.

**When using this product**
- do not use more than directed
- marked drowsiness may occur (only applies to Softchews Cold and Cough)
- sedatives and tranquilizers may increase drowsiness • excitability may occur, especially in children

**Stop use and ask a doctor if**
- nervousness, dizziness, or sleeplessness occurs • cough persists for more than 7 days (not applicable to: Cold & Allergy) • symptoms do not improve within 7 days, or occur with fever, rash, or persistent headache. These could be signs of a serious condition.

**Keep out of reach of children.** In case of overdose, get medical help or contact a poison control center right away.

**Dosage and Administration[1]:**
- Let Softchews® tablet dissolve in mouth or chew Softchews® tablet before swallowing, whichever is preferred
- take every 4 to 6 hours; not more than 4 doses in 24 hours or as directed by a doctor

| Age | Weight | Dose |
| --- | --- | --- |
| 2 to under 6 years[1] | 24 to 47 lb | 1 tablet |
| 6 to under 12 years | 48 to 95 lb | 2 tablets |
| 12 years to adult | 96 + lb | 4 tablets |

[1] As with any antihistamine-containing product, use of Triaminic® Formulas

*Continued on next page*

---

*Information on Novartis Consumer Health, Inc., products appearing on these pages is effective as of November 2001.*

## Triaminic Softchews Cold—Cont.

containing antihistamines in children under 6 years of age should be only under the advice and supervision of a physician.

**Other Information:**
• each Softchews® tablet contains: **sodium 5 mg** • contains no aspirin • store at controlled room temperature 20–25°C (68–77°F)

**Triaminic® Softchews® Cold & Allergy**
Antihistamine, Nasal Decongestant-Orange Flavor • Phenylketonurics: Contains: **Phenylalanine, 17.6 mg** per Softchews® tablet

**Triaminic® Softchews® Cold & Cough**
Antihistamine, Cough Suppressant, Nasal Decongestant-Cherry Flavor • Phenylketonurics: Contains: **Phenylalanine, 17.7 mg** per Softchews® tablet

**Inactive Ingredients:**
**TRIAMINIC® Softchews® Cold & Allergy**
Antihistamine, Nasal Decongestant-Orange Flavor
aspartame, carnauba wax, citric acid, crospovidone, ethylcellulose, FD&C Yellow 6 aluminum lake, flavors, fractionated coconut oil, hydroxypropyl methylcellulose, magnesium stearate, mannitol, microcrystalline cellulose, mono- and di-glycerides, oleic acid, polyethylene glycol, silicon dioxide, sodium bicarbonate, sodium chloride, sorbitol, starch, sucrose, triethyl citrate

**TRIAMINIC® Softchews® Cold & Cough**
Antihistamine, Cough Suppressant, Nasal Decongestant-Cherry Flavor
aspartame, carnauba wax, citric acid, crospovidone, D&C Red 27 aluminum lake, D&C Red 30 aluminum lake, ethylcellulose, FD&C Blue 2 aluminum lake, flavors, hydroxypropyl methylcellulose, magnesium stearate, mannitol, microcrystalline cellulose, mono- and di-glycerides, povidone, silicone dioxide, sodium bicarbonate, sucrose

**How Supplied:** 18 Softchews® Tablets.
*Questions:* call **1-800-452-0051**
**For more information about Triaminic® visit our website at www.triaminic.com
Novartis Consumer Health, Inc.**
Parsippany, NJ 07054-0622 ©2002
*Shown in Product Identification Guide, page 516*

---

**TRIAMINIC® Softchews® Cough**
Cough Suppressant-Strawberry Flavor
**TRIAMINIC® Softchews® Cough & Sore Throat**
Cough Suppressant, Nasal Decongestant, Pain Reliever-Fever Reducer-Grape Flavor

**Drug Facts:**
**Active Ingredient:** (in each tablet)
**TRIAMINIC® Softchews® Cough**
Strawberry Flavor
Dextromethorphan HBr, USP,
7.5 mg ............ Cough suppressant

**TRIAMINIC® Softchews® Cough & Sore Throat**
Grape Flavor
Acetaminophen, USP,
160 mg ...... Fever reducer, Pain reliever
Pseudoephedrine HCl, USP,
15 mg ........................ Nasal decongestant
Dextromethorphan HBr, USP,
5 mg ........................... Cough suppressant

**Uses:** Temporarily relieves these symptoms:
**TRIAMINIC® Softchews® Cough**
Cough Suppressant-Strawberry Flavor
• cough due to minor throat and bronchial irritation associated with the common cold
**TRIAMINIC® Softchews® Cough & Sore Throat**
Cough Suppressant, Nasal Decongestant, Pain Reliever-Fever Reducer-Grape Flavor
• fever • minor aches and pains
• headache and sore throat • cough due to minor throat and bronchial irritation
• nasal and sinus congestion

**Warnings:**
**Do not use** in a child who is taking a prescription monoamine oxidase inhibitor (MAOI) (certain drugs for depression, psychiatric or emotional conditions, or Parkinson's disease), or for 2 weeks after stopping the MAOI drug. If you do not know if the child's prescription drug contains an MAOI, ask a doctor or pharmacist before giving this product.
**Specific to Cough & Sore Throat:** other products containing acetaminophen
**Ask a doctor before use if the child has**
• a breathing problem such as chronic bronchitis or asthma • heart disease
• high blood pressure • thyroid disease
• diabetes • glaucoma
**Specific to Cough & Sore Throat:** cough that occurs with too much phlegm or chronic cough that lasts
**Ask a doctor or pharmacist before use** if the child is taking sedatives or tranquilizers
**When using this product**
• do not use more than directed
**Stop use and ask a doctor if**
**Specific to Cough:** • cough persists for more than 7 days, comes back, or occurs with a fever, rash, or persistent headache. These could be signs of a serious condition.
**Specific to Cough & Sore Throat:** • nervousness, dizziness, or sleeplessness occur • symptoms do not improve for 5 days (pain) or 3 days (fever) • cough persists for more than 7 days, comes back or occurs with fever, rash, or headache • sore throat persists for more than 2 days, or occurs with persistent headache, fever, rash, nausea or vomiting. These could be signs of a serious condition.
**Keep out of reach of children** In case of overdose, get medical help or contact a poison control center right away.

**Dosage and Administration**
Let *Softchews®* tablet dissolve in mouth or chew *Softchews®* tablet before swallowing, whichever is preferred.

**TRIAMINIC® Softchews® Cough**
Strawberry Flavor • take every 6 to 8 hours • not more than 4 doses in 24 hours
**TRIAMINIC® Softchews® Cough & Sore Throat**-Grape Flavor • take every 4 to 6 hours • not more than 4 doses in 24 hours.

| Age | Weight | Dose |
|---|---|---|
| 2 to under 6 years | 24 to 47 lb | 1 tablet |
| 6 to under 12 years | 48–97 lb | 2 tablets |
| 12 years to adult | 96+ lb | 4 tablets |

**Other Information**
• contains no aspirin • store at controlled room temperature 20°–25°C (68°–77°F)

**TRIAMINIC® Softchews® Cough**
Cough Suppressant-Strawberry Flavor
• each Softchews® tablet contains: **sodium 5 mg** • Phenylketonurics: Contains **Phenylalanine 22.5 mg** per tablet

**TRIAMINIC® Softchews® Cough & Sore Throat**
Cough Suppressant, Nasal Decongestant, Pain Reliever-Fever Reducer-Grape Flavor
• each Softchews® tablet contains **sodium 8 mg**
• Phenylketonurics: Contains **Phenylalanine, 28.1 mg** per tablet

**Inactive Ingredients:**
**TRIAMINIC® Softchews® Cough**
Cough Suppressant-Strawberry Flavor
aspartame, citric acid, crospovidone, ethylcellulose, FD&C Red 40 aluminum lake, flavors, magnesium stearate, mannitol, microcrystalline cellulose, povidone, silicon dioxide, sodium bicarbonate

**TRIAMINIC® Softchews® Cough & Sore Throat**
Cough Suppressant, Nasal Decongestant, Pain Reliever-Fever Reducer-Grape Flavor
aspartame, citric acid, crospovidone, D&C Red 27 aluminum lake, ethylcellulose, FD&C Blue 1 aluminum lake, flavors, magnesium stearate, mannitol, microcrystalline cellulose, povidone, silicon dioxide, sodium bicarbonate

**How Supplied:** 18 Softchews® Tablets
*Questions:* call **1-800-452-0051**
**For more information about Triaminic® visit our website at www.triaminic.com
Novartis Consumer Health, Inc.**
Parsippany, NJ 07054-0622 ©2002
*Shown in Product Identification Guide, page 516*

**TRIAMINIC® Vapor Patch
-Mentholated Cherry Scent
Cough Suppressant**

**TRIAMINIC® Vapor Patch
-Menthol Scent
Cough Suppressant**

**Drug Facts:**
**Active ingredients (in each patch)**
Camphor 4.7% ......... Cough suppressant
Menthol 2.6% .......... Cough suppressant

**Uses:** Temporarily relieves these symptoms:
• cough due to a cold • cough due to minor throat and bronchial irritation • cough to help you sleep

**Warnings:**
**For external use only**
**Flammable: Keep away from fire or flame**
**Do not use**
• near an open flame • by adding to hot water • in a microwave oven • in a container in which water is being heated
**Ask a doctor before use if the child has**
• cough that occurs with too much phlegm (mucus) • a persistent or chronic cough such as occurs with asthma
**When using this product**
• do not use more than directed • do not take by mouth or place in nostrils • do not apply to eyes, wounds, or damaged skin
**Stop use and ask a doctor if**
• a cough persists for more than 7 days, comes back, or occurs with fever, rash, or persistent headache. These could be signs of a serious condition • too much skin irritation occurs or gets worse
**Keep out of reach of children.** If swallowed, get medical help or contact a poison control center right away.

**Dosage and Administration**
Children 2 to under 12 years of age:
• Remove plastic backing • Apply to the throat or chest • Clothing should be left loose about the throat and chest to help the vapors rise to reach the nose and mouth • More than one patch may be used • Applications may be repeated up to three times daily or as directed by a doctor • May use with other cough suppressant products
Children under 2 years of age: Ask a doctor

**Other Information:**
• store at controlled room temperature 20–25°C (68–77°F) • protect from excessive heat

**Inactive Ingredients:**
**TRIAMINIC® Vapor Patch
-Mentholated Cherry Scent Cough Suppressant**
acrylic ester copolymer, aloe vera gel, eucalyptus oil, glycerin, karaya, propylene glycol, purified water, wild cherry fragrance

**TRIAMINIC® Vapor Patch
-Menthol Scent Cough Suppressant**
acrylic ester, copolymer, aloe vera gel, eucalyptus oil, glycerin, karaya, purified water, spirits of turpentine

**How Supplied:** Packet of 6 patches, ointment on a breathable cloth patch.
*Questions:* call **1-800-452-0051**
For more information about Triaminic® visit our website at www.triaminic.com
Novartis Consumer Health, Inc.,
Parsippany, NJ 07054-0622
©2002
*Shown in Product Identification Guide, page 516*

---

## Pfizer Consumer Group, Pfizer Inc.

**201 TABOR ROAD
MORRIS PLAINS, NJ 07950**

**Direct Inquiries to:**
1-(800) 223-0182

**For Consumer Product Information Call:**
1-(800) 524-2854 – Celestial Seasonings Soothers (only)
1-(800) 223-0182

**CELESTIAL SEASONINGS®
SOOTHERS® Herbal Throat Drops**

**Active Ingredients:** Menthol and Pectin.

**Inactive Ingredients:** *HARVEST CHERRY®*—Ascorbic Acid (Vitamin C); Cherry and Elderberry Juices; Citric Acid; Corn Syrup; Natural Flavoring; Oils of Angelica Root, Anise Star, Ginger, Lemon Grass, Sage and White Thyme; Sodium Ascorbate and Sucrose. *HONEY-LEMON CHAMOMILE*—Ascorbic Acid (Vitamin C); Chamomile Flower Extract; Citric Acid; Corn Syrup; Honey; Lemon Juice; Natural Flavoring; Oils of Angelica Root, Anise Star, Ginger, Lemon Grass, Sage and White Thyme; Sodium Ascorbate; Sucrose and Tea Extract. *SUNSHINE CITRUS™*—Ascorbic Acid (Vitamin C); Beta Carotene; Citric Acid; Corn Syrup; Natural Flavoring; Oils of Angelica Root, Anise Star, Ginger, Lemon Grass, Sage and White Thyme; Orange Juice; Sodium Ascorbate, and Sucrose.

**Indications:** For temporary relief of occasional minor irritation, pain, sore mouth and sore throat. Provides temporary protection of irritated areas in sore mouth and sore throat.

**Warnings:** If sore throat is severe, persists for more than 2 days, is accompanied or followed by fever, headache, rash, nausea, or vomiting, consult a doctor promptly. If sore mouth symptoms do not improve in 7 days, see your dentist or doctor promptly. KEEP THIS AND ALL DRUGS OUT OF THE REACH OF CHILDREN.

**Dosage and Administration:** Adults and children 5 years and over: Dissolve 2 drops (one at a time) slowly in the mouth. May be repeated every 2 hours as needed or as directed by a dentist or doctor. Children under 5 years: Consult a dentist or doctor.

**How Supplied:** Celestial Seasonings Soothers Throat Drops are available in bags of 24 drops. They are available in three flavors: Harvest Cherry, Honey-Lemon Chamomile, Sunshine Citrus.
*Shown in Product Identification Guide, page 516*

---

**HALLS® MENTHO–LYPTUS®
Cough Suppressant Drops**
[*Hols* ]

**Active Ingredient:** *MENTHO-LYPTUS®:* Menthol 7 mg per drop. *CHERRY:* Menthol 7.6 mg per drop. *HONEY-LEMON:* Menthol 8.6 mg per drop. *ICE BLUE PEPPERMINT:* Menthol 12 mg per drop. *SPEARMINT:* Menthol 6 mg per drop. *STRAWBERRY:* Menthol 3.5 mg per drop.

**Inactive Ingredients:** *MENTHO-LYPTUS®:* Eucalyptus Oil, Flavoring, Glucose Syrup and Sucrose. *CHERRY:* Blue 2, Eucalyptus Oil, Flavoring, Glucose Syrup, Red 40 and Sucrose. *HONEY-LEMON:* Beta Carotene, Eucalyptus Oil, Flavoring, Glucose Syrup and Sucrose. *ICE BLUE PEPPERMINT:* Blue 1, Eucalyptus Oil, Flavoring, Glucose Syrup and Sucrose. *SPEARMINT:* Beta Carotene, Blue 1, Eucalyptus Oil, Flavoring, Glucose Syrup and Sucrose. *STRAWBERRY:* Eucalyptus Oil, Flavoring, Glucose Syrup, Red 40 and Sucrose.

**Indications:** For temporary relief of minor throat irritation and coughs due to colds or inhaled irritants.

**Warnings:** A persistent cough may be a sign of a serious condition. If cough persists for more than 1 week, tends to recur, or is accompanied by fever, rash or persistent headache, consult a doctor. Do not take this product for persistent or chronic cough such as occurs with smoking, asthma, or emphysema, or if cough is accompanied by excessive phlegm (mucus) unless directed by a doctor. If sore throat is severe, persists for more than 2 days, is accompanied or followed by fever, headache, rash, swelling, nausea, or vomiting, consult a doctor promptly. KEEP THIS AND ALL DRUGS OUT OF THE REACH OF CHILDREN.

**Dosage and Administration:** *MENTHO-LYPTUS®, CHERRY, HONEY LEMON, ICE BLUE PEPPERMINT* and *SPEARMINT:* Adults and children 5 years and over: dissolve 1 drop slowly in

*Continued on next page*

## Halls Mentho-Lyptus—Cont.

mouth. Repeat every hour as needed or as directed by a doctor. Children under 5 years: consult a doctor.
*STRAWBERRY:* Adults and children 5 years and over: for sore throat dissolve 1 or 2 drops (one at a time) slowly in the mouth, for cough dissolve 2 drops (one at a time) slowly in the mouth. Repeat every hour as needed or as directed by a doctor. Children under 5 years: consult a doctor.

**How Supplied:** Halls® *Mentho-Lyptus®* Cough Suppressant Drops are available in single sticks of 9 drops each and in bags of 30. They are available in six flavors: *Regular Mentho-Lyptus®, Cherry, Honey-Lemon, Ice Blue Peppermint, Spearmint* and *Strawberry.* Regular Mentho-Lyptus®, Cherry and Honey-Lemon flavors are also available in bags of 80 drops. *Mentho-Lyptus®* and *Cherry* are also available in bags of 200 drops.
*Shown in Product Identification Guide, page 516*

---

## HALLS® PLUS
### Cough Suppressant/Throat Drops
[Hols ]

**Active Ingredients:** Each drop contains Menthol 10 mg and Pectin.

**Inactive Ingredients:** MENTHO-LYPTUS®: Carrageenan, Eucalyptus Oil, Flavoring, Glucose Syrup, Glycerin and Sucrose. CHERRY: Blue 2, Carrageenan, Eucalyptus Oil, Flavoring, Glucose Syrup, Glycerin, Red 40 and Sucrose. HONEY-LEMON: Beta Carotene, Carrageenan, Eucalyptus Oil, Flavoring, Glucose Syrup, Glycerin, Honey and Sucrose.

**Indications:** For temporary relief of minor throat irritation and coughs due to colds or inhaled irritants. Provides temporary protection of irritated areas in sore throat.

**Warnings:** A persistent cough may be a sign of a serious condition. If cough persists for more than 1 week, tends to recur, or is accompanied by fever, rash, or persistent headache, consult a doctor. Do not take this product for persistent or chronic cough such as occurs with smoking, asthma, or emphysema, or if cough is accompanied by excessive phlegm (mucous) unless directed by a doctor. If sore throat is severe, persists for more than 2 days, is accompanied or followed by fever, headache, rash, swelling, nausea, or vomiting, consult a doctor promptly. KEEP THIS AND ALL DRUGS OUT OF THE REACH OF CHILDREN.

**Dosage and Administration:** Adults and children 5 years and over: dissolve 1 drop slowly in the mouth. Repeat every hour as needed or as directed by a doctor. Children under 5 years: consult a doctor.

**How Supplied:** Halls® Plus Cough Suppressant / Throat Drops are available in single sticks of 10 drops each and in bags of 25 drops. They are available in three flavors: Regular Mentho-Lyptus®, Cherry and Honey-Lemon.
*Shown in Product Identification Guide, page 516*

---

## HALLS® SUGAR FREE
## HALLS® SUGAR FREE SQUARES
## MENTHO-LYPTUS®
### Cough Suppressant Drops
[Hols ]

**Active Ingredient:** Halls® Sugar Free: BLACK CHERRY and CITRUS BLEND: Menthol 5 mg per drop. MOUNTAIN MENTHOL: Menthol 5.8 mg per drop.
Halls® Sugar Free Squares: BLACK CHERRY: Menthol 5.8 mg per drop. MOUNTAIN MENTHOL: Menthol 6.8 mg per drop.

**Inactive Ingredients:** BLACK CHERRY: Acesulfame Potassium, Aspartame, Blue 1, Citric Acid, Eucalyptus Oil, Flavoring, Isomalt and Red 40. **Phenylketonurics: Contains 2 mg Phenylalanine Per Drop.** CITRUS BLEND: Acesulfame Potassium, Aspartame, Citric Acid, Eucalyptus Oil, Flavoring, Isomalt and Yellow 5 (Tartrazine). **Phenylketonurics: Contains 2 mg Phenylalanine Per Drop.** MOUNTAIN MENTHOL: Acesulfame Potassium, Aspartame, Eucalyptus Oil, Flavoring and Isomalt. **Phenylketonurics: Contains 2 mg Phenylalanine Per Drop.**

**Indications:** For temporary relief of minor throat irritation and coughs due to colds or inhaled irritants.

**Warnings:** A persistent cough may be a sign of a serious condition. If cough persists for more than 1 week, tends to recur, or is accompanied by fever, rash, or persistent headache, consult a doctor. Do not take this product for persistent or chronic cough such as occurs with smoking, asthma, or emphysema, or if cough is accompanied by excessive phlegm (mucus) unless directed by a doctor. If sore throat is severe, persists for more than 2 days, is accompanied or followed by fever, headache, rash, swelling, nausea, or vomiting, consult a doctor promptly. KEEP THIS AND ALL DRUGS OUT OF THE REACH OF CHILDREN.

**Dosage and Administration:** Adults and children 5 years and over: dissolve 1 drop slowly in mouth. Repeat every hour as needed or as directed by a doctor. Children under 5 years: consult a doctor.

**Additional Information:**
Halls® Sugar Free:
Exchange Information*:
1 Drop = Free Exchange
10 Drops = 1 Fruit
*The dietary exchanges are based on the *Exchange Lists for Meal Planning,* Copy-

right ©1989 by the American Diabetes Association, Inc. and the American Dietetic Association.

Excess consumption may have a laxative effect.

**How Supplied:** Halls® Sugar Free: Halls® Sugar Free Mentho-Lyptus® Cough Suppressant Drops are available in bags of 25 drops. They are available in three flavors: Black Cherry, Citrus Blend and Mountain Menthol. Halls® Sugar Free Squares: Halls® Sugar Free Squares Mentho-Lyptus® Cough Suppressant Drops are available in single sticks of 9 drops each. They are available in two flavors: Black Cherry and Mountain Menthol.
*Shown in Product Identification Guide, page 516*

---

## HALLS DEFENSE™ Vitamin C
## Supplement Drops
[Hols]

**Ingredients:** *ASSORTED CITRUS FLAVORS:* Sugar, Glucose Syrup, Sodium Ascorbate, Citric Acid, Natural Flavoring, Ascorbic Acid, Color Added and Red 40. *STRAWBERRY:* Sugar, Glucose Syrup, Sodium Ascorbate, Citric Acid, Ascorbic Acid, Natural and Artificial Flavoring, Color Added.

**Description:** Halls Defense™ Vitamin C Supplement Drops are delicious way to get 100% of the Daily Value of Vitamin C. Each drop provides 60 mg of Vitamin C (100% of the Daily Value).

**Indications:** Dietary Supplementation.

**How Supplied:** Halls Defense™ Vitamin C Supplement Drops are available in a Citrus Assortment (lemon, sweet grapefruit, orange) with all natural flavors and Strawberry in sticks of 9 drops each and in bags of 30 drops. Citrus assortment is also available in bags of 80 drops.
*Shown in Product Identification Guide, page 516*

---

## TRIDENT FOR KIDS™
### Sugarless Gum with Recaldent™
[Tri-dent for kids]

**Ingredients:** *BERRY BUBBLE GUM:* Sorbitol, Gum Base, Mannitol, Glycerin, Artificial and Natural Flavoring, Xylitol, Calcium Casein Peptone-Calcium Phosphate (Lactose-Free Milk Derivative)**, Soy Lecithin, Acetylated Monoglycerides, Sucralose, Red 40 Lake and Blue 2 Lake. **Contains a Milk-Based Ingredient.**

RECALDENT™**: A patented ingredient derived from casein, a bovine phosphoprotein found in milk. RECALDENT™ is a trademark of Bonlac Bioscience PTY Ltd.

**Description:** Trident For Kids™ is a dental care gum that remineralizes tooth enamel by safely delivering calcium and phosphate directly to teeth. In addition to strengthening teeth, chewing Trident for Kids™ may reduce the risk of tooth decay.

**Directions:** Trident For Kids™ chewed after meals provides an ideal way to deliver the benefits of Recaldent™, to help remove food particles that may adhere to teeth, and to help minimize plaque acids.

**How Supplied:** Trident For Kids™ with Recaldent™ is available in Berry Bubble Gum Flavor in an 8-stick pack.

*Shown in Product Identification Guide, page 516*

---

## TRIDENT WHITE™
[*Tri-dent White*]
**Sugarless Gum with Recaldent™**

**Ingredients:** *PEPPERMINT*: Sorbitol, Gum Base, Maltitol, Mannitol, Artificial and Natural Flavoring; Less Than 2% of: Acacia, Acesulfame Potassium, Aspartame, BHT (To Maintain Freshness), Calcium Casein Peptone-Calcium Phosphate (Lactose-Free Milk Derivative)**, Candelilla Wax, Sodium Stearate and Titanium Dioxide (Color).
**Contains a Milk Derived Ingredient.**
**Phenylketonurics:     Contains Phenylalanine.**
*WINTERGREEN:* Sorbitol, Gum Base, Maltitol, Mannitol, Artificial and Natural Flavoring; Less Than 2% of: Acacia, Acesulfame Potassium, Aspartame, BHT (To Maintain Freshness), Calcium Casein Peptone-Calcium Phosphate (Lactose-Free Milk Derivative)**, Candelilla Wax, Glycerin, Sodium Stearate, Soy Lecithin and Titanium Dioxide (Color).
**Contains a Milk Derived Ingredient.**
**Phenylketonurics:     Contains Phenylalanine.**
RECALDENT™**: A patented ingredient derived from casein, a bovine phosphoprotein found in milk. RECALDENT is a trademark of Bonlac Bioscience International PTY LTD.

**Description:** Trident White™ is a whitening gum that uses proprietary surfactant technology to help break up and gently remove stains from teeth. In addition to whitening teeth, chewing Trident White™ remineralizes tooth enamel by delivering calcium and phosphate beneath the tooth's surface.

**Directions:** When used as a part of a daily oral care regimen, Trident White helps gently remove stains caused by common beverages and food items consumed every day.

**How Supplied:** Trident White™ is available in Peppermint and Wintergreen flavors in a 12-pellet blister foil.

*Shown in Product Identification Guide, page 517*

---

## Pfizer Consumer Healthcare, Pfizer Inc.
**201 TABOR ROAD**
**MORRIS PLAINS, NJ 07950**

**Address Questions & Comments to:**
Consumer Affairs, Pfizer CHC
182 Tabor Road
Morris Plains, NJ 07950

**For Medical Emergencies/Information Contact:**
1-(800)-223-0182
1-(800)-732-7529 (BenGay, Bonine, Cortizone, Desitin Unisom, Visine, and Wart-Off products)
1-(800)-378-1783 (e.p.t.)
1-(800)-337-7266 (e.p.t.-Spanish)

---

## ACTIFED® Cold & Allergy Tablets
[*ăk 'tuh-fĕd* ]

**Drug Facts:**

**Active Ingredients:**
| (in each tablet) | Purposes: |
| --- | --- |
| Pseudoephedrine HCl 60 mg ............. | Nasal decongestant |
| Triprolidine HCl 2.5 mg ...................... | Antihistamine |

**Uses:**
* temporarily relieves these symptoms of hay fever or other upper respiratory allergies:
  * runny nose
  * sneezing
  * itchy, watery eyes
  * itching of the nose or throat
* temporarily relieves nasal congestion due to the common cold

**Warnings:**
**Do not use** if you are now taking a prescription monoamine oxidase inhibitor (MAOI) (certain drugs for depression, psychiatric, or emotional conditions, or Parkinson's disease), or for 2 weeks after stopping the MAOI drug. If you do not know if your prescription drug contains an MAOI, ask a doctor or pharmacist before taking this product.
**Ask a doctor before use if you have:**
* heart disease
* glaucoma
* thyroid disease
* diabetes
* high blood pressure
* trouble urinating due to an enlarged prostate gland
* a breathing problem such as emphysema or chronic bronchitis
**Ask a doctor or pharmacist before use if you are** taking sedatives or tranquilizers
**When using this product:**
* **do not use more than directed**
* drowsiness may occur
* avoid alcoholic drinks
* alcohol, sedatives, and tranquilizers may increase drowsiness
* be careful when driving a motor vehicle or operating machinery
* excitability may occur, especially in children
**Stop use and ask a doctor if:**
* you get nervous, dizzy, or sleepless

---

* symptoms do not improve within 7 days or are accompanied by fever
**If pregnant or breast-feeding,** ask a health professional before use.
**Keep out of reach of children.** In case of overdose, get medical help or contact a Poison Control Center right away.

**Directions:**
* take every 4 to 6 hours
* do not take more than 4 doses in 24 hours

| adults and children 12 years of age and over | 1 tablet |
| --- | --- |
| children 6 to under 12 years of age | ½ tablet |
| children under 6 years of age | ask a doctor |

**Other Information:**
* store at 59° to 77°F in a dry place
* protect from light

**Inactive Ingredients:** Corn starch, flavor, hydroxypropyl methylcellulose, lactose, magnesium stearate, polyethylene glycol, potato starch, povidone, sucrose, and titanium dioxide

**Questions?** call **1-800-223-0182,** Monday to Friday, 9 AM – 5 PM EST

**How Supplied:** Boxes of 12 and 24 tablets.

*Shown in Product Identification Guide, page 517*

---

## ACTIFED® Cold & Sinus MS Caplets (also available in Tablets)
**Maximum Strength**
[*ak 'tuh-fed*]

**Drug Facts:**

**Active Ingredients:**
| (in each caplet)† | Purposes: |
| --- | --- |
| Acetaminophen 500 mg ......... | Pain reliever/fever reducer |
| Chlorpheniramine maleate 2 mg .................... | Antihistamine |
| Pseudoephedrine HCl 30 mg ............... | Nasal decongestant |

†Dissolution differs from USP specification

**Uses:**
* temporarily relieves sinus congestion and pressure
* temporarily relieves these symptoms of hay fever:

*Continued on next page*

---

*This product information was prepared in November 2001. On these and other Pfizer Consumer Healthcare Products, detailed information may be obtained by addressing Pfizer Consumer Healthcare, Pfizer, Inc., Morris Plains, NJ 07950*

## Actifed Cold & Sinus—Cont.

- itchy, watery eyes
- sneezing
- itching of the nose or throat
- runny nose
- temporarily relieves these symptoms due to the common cold:
  - nasal congestion
  - headache
  - minor aches and pains
  - fever

### Warnings:
**Alcohol warning:** If you consume 3 or more alcoholic drinks every day, ask your doctor whether you should take acetaminophen or other pain relievers/fever reducers. Acetaminophen may cause liver damage.

**Do not use:**
- with any other product containing acetaminophen
- if you are now taking a prescription monoamine oxidase inhibitor (MAOI) (certain drugs for depression, psychiatric, or emotional conditions, or Parkinson's disease), or for 2 weeks after stopping the MAOI drug. If you do not know if your prescription drug contains an MAOI, ask a doctor or pharmacist before taking this product.

**Ask a doctor before use if you have:**
- heart disease
- glaucoma
- diabetes
- thyroid disease
- high blood pressure
- trouble urinating due to an enlarged prostate gland
- a breathing problem such as emphysema or chronic bronchitis

**Ask a doctor or pharmacist before use if you are** taking sedatives or tranquilizers

**When using this product:**
- **do not use more than directed**
- drowsiness may occur
- excitability may occur, especially in children
- avoid alcoholic drinks
- alcohol, sedatives, and tranquilizers may increase drowsiness
- be careful when driving a motor vehicle or operating machinery

**Stop use and ask a doctor if:**
- you get nervous, dizzy, or sleepless
- new symptoms occur
- symptoms do not improve
- you need to use more than 10 days
- fever occurs and lasts more than 3 days
- redness or swelling is present

**If pregnant or breast-feeding,** ask a health professional before use.

**Keep out of reach of children.** In case of overdose, get medical help or contact a Poison Control Center right away. Quick medical attention is critical for adults as well as for children even if you do not notice any signs or symptoms.

### Directions:
- adults and children 12 years of age and over: 2 caplets
- take every 6 hours while symptoms persist
- do not take more than 8 caplets in 24 hours, or as directed by a doctor
- children under 12 years of age: ask a doctor

### Other Information:
- store at 59° to 77°F in a dry place

**Inactive Ingredients:** Calcium stearate, croscarmellose sodium, crospovidone, D&C yellow no. 10 aluminum lake, FD&C yellow no. 6 aluminum lake, hydroxypropyl methylcellulose, microcrystalline cellulose, polyethylene glycol, polysorbate 80, povidone, pregelatinized starch, stearic acid, and titanium dioxide

**Questions?** call **1-800-223-0182**, Monday to Friday, 9AM – 5PM EST

**How Supplied:** Boxes of 20
*Shown in Product Identification Guide, page 517*

---

## ANUSOL®
### Hemorrhoidal Ointment
[ă′nū-sōl″]

**Active Ingredient:** Pramoxine HCl 1%, Zinc Oxide 12.5%, and Mineral Oil. Also contains: Benzyl Benzoate, Calcium Phosphate Dibasic, Cocoa Butter, Glyceryl Monooleate, Glyceryl Monostearate, Kaolin, Peruvian Balsam and Polyethylene Wax.

**Actions:** Anusol Ointment helps to relieve burning, itching and discomfort arising from irritated anorectal tissues. Pramoxine Hydrochloride in Anusol Ointment is a rapidly acting local anesthetic for the skin and mucous membranes in the lower portion of the anal canal. Pramoxine HCl is chemically distinct from procaine, cocaine, and dibucaine. Surface analgesia lasts for several hours.

**Indications:** Temporarily relieves the pain, soreness, burning and itching associated with hemorrhoids and anorectal disorders while temporarily forming a protective coating over inflamed tissues to help prevent the drying of tissues. Anusol Ointment is to be applied externally or in the lower portion of the anal canal (The enclosed dispensing cap is designed to control dispersion of the ointment to the affected area in the lower portion of the anal canal only.)

**Warnings:** If condition worsens or does not improve within 7 days, consult a physician. Certain persons can develop allergic reactions to ingredients in this product. If the symptom being treated does not subside or if redness, irritation, swelling, pain or other symptoms develop or increase, discontinue use and consult a physician promptly. Do not exceed the recommended daily dosage unless directed by a physician. Do not put this product into the rectum by using fingers or any mechanical device or applicator. KEEP THIS AND ALL DRUGS OUT OF THE REACH OF CHILDREN. In case of accidental ingestion seek professional assistance or contact a Poison Control Center immediately.

**Directions:** Adults: When practical, cleanse the affected area with mild soap and warm water and rinse thoroughly. Gently dry by patting with

toilet tissue or a soft cloth before application of this product. Apply externally to the affected up to 5 times daily. To use dispensing cap, attach it to tube, lubricate well, then gently insert part way into the anal canal. Squeeze tube to deliver medication. Thoroughly cleanse dispensing cap after use. Children under 12 years of age: Consult a physician.

**How Supplied:**—1-oz (28.3g) tubes with plastic applicator. Store at room temperature (59° to 77°F).
*Shown in Product Identification Guide, page 517*

---

## ANUSOL®
### Hemorrhoidal Suppositories
[ă′nū-sōl″]

**Drug Facts:**

**Active Ingredient**
**(in each suppository)**        **Purpose:**
Topical starch 51% ........... Hemorrhoidal suppository

**Uses:**
- temporarily relieves these symptoms associated with hemorrhoids and other anorectal disorders:
  - itching
  - burning
  - discomfort
- temporarily forms a protective coating over inflamed tissues to help protect drying of tissue

**Warnings:**
**When using this product:**
- do not use more than directed

**Stop use and ask a doctor if**
- rectal bleeding occurs
- condition worsens or does not improve within 7 days

**If pregnant or breast-feeding,** ask a health professional before use.

**Keep out of reach of children.** If swallowed, get medical help or contact a Poison Control Center right away.

**Directions:**
- remove wrapper before inserting into rectum
- adults: insert one (1) suppository rectally up to six times daily or after each bowel movement by following these steps:
  - when practical, clean the affected area with mild soap and warm water and rinse thoroughly
  - gently dry by patting or blotting with toilet tissue or a soft cloth before application
  - remove one suppository from wrapper and insert suppository into the rectum
- children under 12 years of age: ask a doctor
- Directions for opening Suppository Wrapper:
  - Detach (1) one suppository from the strip of suppositories.
  - Remove wrapper before inserting into the rectum as follows: Hold suppository upright (with words "pull apart" at top) and carefully separate

foil by inserting tip of fingernail at foil split.

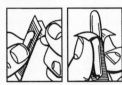

- Peel foil slowly and evenly down both sides, exposing suppository.
- Avoid excessive handling of suppository which is designed to melt at body temperature. If suppository seems soft, hold in foil wrapper under cold water for 2 or 3 minutes.

**Other Information:** • store at 59° to 77°F to avoid melting

**Inactive Ingredients:** Benzyl alcohol, hydrogenated vegetable oil, and tocopheryl acetate

**Questions?** Call toll-free **1-800-223-0182**, Monday to Friday 9 AM–5 PM EST

**How Supplied:** In boxes of 12 or 24 in silver foil strips. Store at 59–77°F to avoid melting.
*Shown in Product Identification Guide, page 517*

---

### ANUSOL HC-1 Hydrocortisone Anti-Itch
[ă′nū-sōl″]

**Active Ingredient:** Hydrocortisone Acetate (equivalent to 1% Hydrocortisone). Also contains: Diazolidinyl Urea, Methylparaben, Microcrystalline Wax, Mineral Oil, Propylene Gylcol, Propylparaben, Sorbitan Sesquioleate and White Petrolatum.

**Indications:** For temporary relief of itching associated with minor skin irritations, rashes and for external anal itching. Other uses of this product should be only under the advice and supervision of a physician.

**Warnings:** For external use only. Avoid contact with the eyes. If condition worsens, or if symptoms persist for more than 7 days or clear up and occur again within a few days, stop use of this product and do not begin use of any other hydrocortisone product unless you have consulted a physician. Do not exceed the recommended daily dosage unless directed by a physician. In case of bleeding, consult a physician promptly. Do not put this product into the rectum by using fingers or any mechanical device or applicator. Do not use for treatment of diaper rash. Consult a physician. KEEP THIS AND ALL DRUGS OUT OF THE REACH OF CHILDREN. In case of accidental ingestion, seek professional assistance or contact a Poison Control Center immediately.

**Directions:** Adults: When practical, cleanse the affected area with mild soap and warm water and rinse thoroughly. Gently dry by patting or blotting with toilet tissue or soft cloth before application of this product. Apply to affected area not more than 3 to 4 times daily. Children under 12 years: consult a physician.

**How Supplied:** 0.7oz (19.8g) tube. Store at 59° to 77°F.
*Shown in Product Identification Guide, page 517*

---

### BENADRYL® Allergy Kapseals® Capsules (also available in Ultratab™ Tablets)
[bĕ ′nă-drĭl ]

**Drug Facts:**

**Active Ingredient:**      **Purpose:**
(in each capsule)
Diphenhydramine HCl
25 mg ............................. Antihistamine

**Uses:**
- temporarily relieves these symptoms due to hay fever or other upper respiratory allergies:
  - runny nose
  - sneezing
  - itchy, watery eyes
  - itching of the nose or throat
- temporarily relieves these symptoms due to the common cold:
  - runny nose
  - sneezing

**Warnings:**
**Do not use** with any other product containing diphenhydramine, including one applied topically

**Ask a doctor before use if you have:**
- glaucoma
- trouble urinating due to an enlarged prostate gland
- a breathing problem such as emphysema or chronic bronchitis

**Ask a doctor or pharmacist before use if you are** taking sedatives or tranquilizers

**When using this product:**
- marked drowsiness may occur
- avoid alcoholic drinks
- alcohol, sedatives, and tranquilizers may increase drowsiness
- be careful when driving a motor vehicle or operating machinery
- excitability may occur, especially in children

**If pregnant or breast-feeding,** ask a health professional before use.

**Keep out of reach of children.** In case of overdose, get medical help or contact a Poison Control Center right away.

**Directions:**
- take every 4 to 6 hours
- do not take more than 6 doses in 24 hours

| adults and children 12 years of age and over | 25 mg to 50 mg (1 to 2 capsules) |
|---|---|
| children 6 to under 12 years of age | 12.5 mg** to 25 mg (1 capsule) |
| children under 6 years of age | ask a doctor |

**12.5 mg dosage strength is not available in this package. Do not attempt to break capsules.

**Other Information:**
- store at 59° to 77°F in a dry place
- protect from light

**Inactive Ingredients** D&C red no. 28, FD&C blue no. 1, FD&C red no. 3, FD&C red no. 40, gelatin, glyceryl monooleate, lactose, magnesium stearate, and titanium dioxide. Printed with black edible ink.

**Questions?** call **1-800-524-2624** (English/Spanish), weekdays, 9 AM–5 PM EST

**How Supplied:** Benadryl tablets are supplied in boxes of 24 and 48, bottle of 100; capsules are supplied in boxes of 24 and 48.
*Shown in Product Identification Guide, page 517*

---

### BENADRYL® Dye-Free Allergy Liqui-Gels® Softgels
[bĕ ′nă-drĭl ]

**Drug Facts:**

**Active Ingredient:**
(in each softgel)      **Purpose:**
Diphenhydramine
HCl 25 mg ..................... Antihistamine

**Uses:**
- temporarily relieves these symptoms due to hay fever or other upper respiratory allergies:
  - runny nose
  - sneezing
  - itchy, watery eyes
  - itching of the nose or throat
- temporarily relieves these symptoms due to the common cold:
  - runny nose
  - sneezing

**Warnings:**
**Do not use** with any other product containing diphenhydramine, including one applied topically

**Ask a doctor before use if you have:**
- glaucoma
- trouble urinating due to an enlarged prostate gland
- a breathing problem such as emphysema or chronic bronchitis

**Ask a doctor or pharmacist before use if you are** taking sedatives or tranquilizers

**When using this product:**
- marked drowsiness may occur
- avoid alcoholic drinks
- alcohol, sedatives, and tranquilizers may increase drowsiness
- be careful when driving a motor vehicle or operating machinery
- excitability may occur, especially in children

**If pregnant or breast-feeding,** ask a health professional before use.

*Continued on next page*

---

*This product information was prepared in November 2001. On these and other Pfizer Consumer Healthcare Products, detailed information may be obtained by addressing Pfizer Consumer Healthcare, Pfizer, Inc., Morris Plains, NJ 07950*

## Benadryl Allergy—Cont.

**Keep out of reach of children.** In case of overdose, get medical help or contact a Poison Control Center right away.

**Directions:**
- take every 4 to 6 hours
- do not take more than 6 doses in 24 hours

| adults and children 12 years of age and over | 25 mg to 50 mg (1 to 2 softgels) |
| children 6 to under 12 years of age | 12.5 mg** to 25 mg (1 softgel) |
| children under 6 years of age | ask a doctor |

**\*\*12.5 mg dosage strength is not available in this package. Do not attempt to break softgels.

**Other Information:**
- store at 59° to 77°F in a dry place
- protect from heat, humidity, and light

**Inactive Ingredients:** Gelatin, glycerin, polyethylene glycol 400, and sorbitol. Softgels are imprinted with edible dye-free ink.

**Questions?** call **1-800-524-2624** (English/Spanish), weekdays, 9 AM–5 PM EST

**How Supplied:** Benadryl® Dye-Free Allergy Liqui-Gels® Softgels are supplied in boxes of 24.
Liqui-Gels is a registered trademark of R.P. Scherer Corporation.
*Shown in Product Identification Guide, page 517*

---

## BENADRYL® ALLERGY & COLD CAPLETS
[bĕ 'nă-drĭl ]
**Capsule shaped tablets**

**Drug Facts:**

**Active Ingredients:**
**(in each caplet)**                  **Purposes:**
Acetaminophen
  500 mg ...... Pain reliever/fever reducer
Diphenhydramine HCl
  12.5 mg ............................ Antihistamine
Pseudoephedrine HCl
  30 mg ...................... Nasal decongestant

**Uses:**
- temporarily relieves these symptoms of hay fever and the common cold:
  - runny nose
  - nasal congestion
  - headache
  - fever
  - sore throat
  - muscular aches
  - sneezing
  - minor aches and pains
- temporarily relieves these additional symptoms of hay fever:
  - itching of the nose or throat
  - itchy, watery eyes

**Warnings:**
**Alcohol warning:** If you consume 3 or more alcoholic drinks every day, ask your doctor whether you should take acetaminophen or other pain relievers/fever reducers. Acetaminophen may cause liver damage.
**Do not use:**
- with any other product containing acetaminophen
- if you are now taking a prescription monoamine oxidase inhibitor (MAOI) (certain drugs for depression, psychiatric, or emotional conditions, or Parkinson's disease), or for 2 weeks after stopping the MAOI drug. If you do not know if your prescription drug contains an MAOI, ask a doctor or pharmacist before taking this product.
- with any other product containing diphenhydramine, including one applied topically.
**Ask a doctor before use if you have:**
- heart disease
- glaucoma
- thyroid disease
- diabetes
- high blood pressure
- trouble urinating due to an enlarged prostate gland
- a breathing problem such as emphysema or chronic bronchitis
**Ask a doctor or pharmacist before use if you are** taking sedatives or tranquilizers
**When using this product:**
- **do not use more than directed**
- marked drowsiness may occur
- excitability may occur, especially in children
- avoid alcoholic drinks
- alcohol, sedatives, and tranquilizers may increase drowsiness
- be careful when driving a motor vehicle or operating machinery
**Stop use and ask a doctor if:**
- new symptoms occur
- sore throat is severe
- you get nervous, dizzy, or sleepless
- symptoms do not get better
- you need to use more than 10 days
- redness or swelling is present
- fever occurs and lasts more than 3 days
- sore throat lasts for more than 2 days, is accompanied or followed by fever, headache, rash, swelling, nausea, or vomiting
**If pregnant or breast-feeding,** ask a health professional before use.
**Keep out of reach of children.** In case of overdose, get medical help or contact a Poison Control Center right away. Quick medical attention is critical for adults as well as for children even if you do not notice any signs or symptoms.

**Directions:**
- adults and children 12 years of age and over: 2 caplets
- children under 12 years of age: ask a doctor
- take every 6 hours while symptoms persist
- do not take more than 8 caplets in 24 hours or as directed by a doctor

**Other Information**
- store at 59° to 77°F in a dry place
**Inactive Ingredients:** Corn starch, croscarmellose sodium, hydroxypropyl cellulose, hydroxypropyl methylcellulose, microcrystalline cellulose, polyethylene glycol, pregelatinized starch, sodium starch glycolate, stearic acid, titanium dioxide, and zinc stearate

***Questions?*** call **1-800-524-2624** (English/Spanish), weekdays, 9 AM - 5 PM EST

**How Supplied:** Benadryl® Allergy & Cold tablets are supplied in boxes of 24 caplets.
*Shown in Product Identification Guide, page 517*

---

## BENADRYL®
## Allergy & Sinus Tablets
## (Formerly Benadryl Allergy/ Congestion)
[bĕ 'nă-drĭl ]

**Drug Facts:**

**Active Ingredients:**
**(in each tablet)**                  **Purposes:**
Diphenhydramine HCl
  25 mg ................................. Antihistamine
Pseudoephedrine HCl
  60 mg ...................... Nasal decongestant

**Uses:**
- temporarily relieves these symptoms due to hay fever or other upper respiratory allergies:
  - runny nose
  - sneezing
  - itchy, watery eyes
  - nasal congestion
  - itching of the nose or throat
- temporarily relieves these symptoms due to the common cold:
  - runny nose
  - sneezing
  - nasal congestion

**Warnings:**
**Do not use**
- if you are now taking a prescription monoamine oxidase inhibitor (MAOI) (certain drugs for depression, psychiatric, or emotional conditions, or Parkinson's disease), or for 2 weeks after stopping the MAOI drug. If you do not know if your prescription drug contains an MAOI, ask a doctor or pharmacist before taking this product.
- with any other product containing diphenhydramine, including one applied topically.
**Ask a doctor before use if you have:**
- heart disease
- glaucoma
- thyroid disease
- diabetes
- high blood pressure
- trouble urinating due to an enlarged prostate gland
- a breathing problem such as emphysema or chronic bronchitis
**Ask a doctor or pharmacist before use if you are** taking sedatives or tranquilizers
**When using this product:**
- **do not use more than directed**
- marked drowsiness may occur
- avoid alcoholic drinks
- alcohol, sedatives, and tranquilizers may increase drowsiness
- be careful when driving a motor vehicle or operating machinery
- excitability may occur, especially in children

**Stop use and ask a doctor if:**
- you get nervous, dizzy, or sleepless
- symptoms do not improve within 7 days or are accompanied by fever

**If pregnant or breast-feeding,** ask a health professional before use.

**Keep out of reach of children.** In case of overdose, get medical help or contact a Poison Control Center right away.

**Directions:**
- adults and children 12 years of age and over: one (1) tablet
- take every 4 to 6 hours
- do not take more than 4 tablets in 24 hours
- children under 12 years of age: ask a doctor

**Other Information:**
- protect from light
- store at 59° to 77°F in a dry place

**Inactive Ingredients:** Croscarmellose sodium, dibasic calcium phosphate dihydrate, FD&C blue no. 1 aluminum lake, hydroxypropyl methylcellulose, microcrystalline cellulose, polyethylene glycol, polysorbate 80, pregelatinized starch, stearic acid, titanium dioxide and zinc stearate. Printed with edible black ink.

**Questions?** call **1-800-524-2624** (English/Spanish), weekdays, 9 AM – 5 PM EST

**How Supplied:** Benadryl Allergy & Sinus Tablets are supplied in boxes of 24.
*Shown in Product Identification Guide, page 517*

---

**BENADRYL® Allergy & Sinus Headache Caplets***
**(also available in Gelcaps)**
[bĕ 'nă-drĭl ]
*Capsule shaped tablets

**Description:** BENADRYL ALLERGY & SINUS HEADACHE is specially formulated to provide effective relief of your upper respiratory allergy symptoms complicated by sinus and headache problems. It combines the strength of BENADRYL to relieve your runny nose, sneezing, itchy, water eyes, itchy nose or throat, with a maximum strength NASAL DECONGESTANT to relieve nasal and sinus congestion, and a maximum strength non-aspirin PAIN RELIEVER to relieve sinus pain and headache.

**Drug Facts:**

**Active Ingredients:**
**(in each caplet)**                **Purposes:**
Acetaminophen 500 mg .... Pain reliever
Diphenhydramine HCl
  12.5 mg ........................... Antihistamine
Pseudoephedrine HCl
  30 mg ...................... Nasal decongestant

**Uses:**
- temporarily relieves these symptoms of hay fever and the common cold:
  - runny nose
  - sneezing
  - headache
  - minor aches and pains
  - nasal congestion
- temporarily relieves these additional symptoms of hay fever:
  - itching of the nose or throat
  - itchy, watery eyes

**Warnings:**
**Alcohol warning:** If you consume 3 or more alcoholic drinks every day, ask your doctor whether you should take acetaminophen or other pain relievers/fever reducers. Acetaminophen may cause liver damage.
**Do not use:**
- with any other product containing acetaminophen
- if you are now taking a prescription monoamine oxidase inhibitor (MAOI) (certain drugs for depression, psychiatric, or emotional conditions, or Parkinson's disease), or for 2 weeks after stopping the MAOI drug. If you do not know if your prescription drug contains an MAOI, ask a doctor or pharmacist before taking this product.
- with any other product containing diphenhydramine, including one applied topically.

**Ask a doctor before use if you have:**
- heart disease
- glaucoma
- thyroid disease
- diabetes
- high blood pressure
- trouble urinating due to an enlarged prostate gland
- a breathing problem such as emphysema or chronic bronchitis

**Ask a doctor or pharmacist before use if you are** taking sedatives or tranquilizers
**When using this product:**
- **do not use more than directed**
- marked drowsiness may occur
- excitability may occur, especially in children
- avoid alcoholic drinks
- alcohol, sedatives, and tranquilizers may increase drowsiness
- be careful when driving a motor vehicle or operating machinery

**Stop use and ask a doctor if:**
- you get nervous, dizzy, or sleepless
- new symptoms occur
- symptoms do not get better
- you need to use more than 10 days
- fever occurs and lasts more than 3 days

**If pregnant or breast-feeding,** ask a health professional before use.
**Keep out of reach of children.** In case of overdose, get medical help or contact a Poison Control Center right away. Quick medical attention is critical for adults as well as for children even if you do not notice any signs or symptoms.

**Directions:**
- take every 6 hours while symptoms persist
- do not take more than 8 caplets in 24 hours or as directed by a doctor
- adults and children 12 years of age and over: 2 caplets
- children under 12 years of age: ask a doctor

**Other Information**
- store at 59° to 77°F in a dry place
**Inactive Ingredients:** Croscarmellose sodium, D&C yellow no. 10 aluminum lake, FD&C blue no. 1 aluminum lake, FD&C yellow no. 6 aluminum lake, hydroxypropyl cellulose, hydroxypropyl methylcellulose, microcrystalline cellulose, polyethylene glycol, polysorbate 80,

pregelatinized starch, sodium starch glycolate, stearic acid, titanium dioxide, and zinc stearate

**Questions?** call **1-800-524-2624** (English/Spanish), weekdays, 9 AM - 5 PM EST

**How Supplied:** Benadryl Allergy & Sinus Headache is available in boxes of 24 and 48 caplets, and box of 24, 48 and 72 gelcaps.
*Shown in Product Identification Guide, page 517*

---

**BENADRYL MAXIMUM STRENGTH SEVERE ALLERGY† & SINUS HEADACHE CAPLETS***
[be' na drĭll]
* **Capsule shaped tablets**
† **Upper Respiratory Allergies Only**

**Benadryl Severe Allergy & Sinus Headache** is specially formulated to provide effective relief of your upper respiratory allergy symptoms complicated by sinus and headache problems. It combines the maximum strength of BENADRYL to relieve your runny nose, sneezing, itchy, watery eyes, itchy nose or throat, with a maximum strength NASAL DECONGESTANT to relieve nasal and sinus congestion, and a maximum strength non-aspirin PAIN RELIEVER to relieve sinus pain and headache.

**Drug Facts:**

**Active Ingredients:**
**(in each caplet)**                **Purposes:**
Acetaminophen
  500 mg ................................ Pain reliever
Diphenhydramine
  HCl 25 mg ....................... Antihistamine
Pseudoephedrine
  HCl 30 mg ............. Nasal decongestant

**Uses:**
- temporarily relieves these symptoms of hay fever and the common cold:
  - runny nose
  - headache
  - sneezing
  - minor aches and pains
  - nasal congestion
- temporarily relieves these additional symptoms of hay fever:
  - itching of the nose or throat
  - itchy, watery eyes

**Warnings:**
**Alcohol warning:** If you consume 3 or more alcoholic drinks every day, ask your doctor whether you should take acetaminophen or other pain relievers/fever reducers. Acetaminophen may cause liver damage.

*Continued on next page*

---

*This product information was prepared in November 2001. On these and other Pfizer Consumer Healthcare Products, detailed information may be obtained by addressing Pfizer Consumer Healthcare, Pfizer, Inc., Morris Plains, NJ 07950*

## Benadryl Severe Allergy—Cont.

**Do not use:**
- with any other product containing acetaminophen
- if you are now taking a prescription monoamine oxidase inhibitor (MAOI) (certain drugs for depression, psychiatric, or emotional conditions, or Parkinson's disease), or for 2 weeks after stopping the MAOI drug. If you do not know if your prescription drug contains an MAOI, ask a doctor or pharmacist before taking this product.
- with any other product containing diphenhydramine, including one applied topically.

**Ask a doctor before use if you have:**
- heart disease
- glaucoma
- thyroid disease
- diabetes
- high blood pressure
- trouble urinating due to an enlarged prostate gland
- a breathing problem such as emphysema or chronic bronchitis

**Ask a doctor or pharmacist before use if you are** taking sedatives or tranquilizers

**When using this product:**
- do not use more than directed
- marked drowsiness may occur
- excitability may occur, especially in children
- avoid alcoholic drinks
- alcohol, sedatives, and tranquilizers may increase drowsiness
- be careful when driving a motor vehicle or operating machinery

**Stop use and ask a doctor if:**
- you get nervous, dizzy, or sleepless
- new symptoms occur
- symptoms do not get better
- you need to use more than 10 days
- fever occurs and lasts more than 3 days

**If pregnant or breast-feeding,** ask a health professional before use.

**Keep out of reach of children.** In case of overdose, get medical help or contact a Poison Control Center right away. Quick medical attention is critical for adults as well as for children even if you do not notice any signs or symptoms.

**Directions:**
- take every 6 hours while symptoms persist
- do not take more than 8 caplets in 24 hours or as directed by a doctor
- adults and children 12 years of age and over: 2 caplets
- children under 12 years of age: ask a doctor

**Other Information:**
- store at 59° to 77°F in a dry place

**Inactive Ingredients:** Carnauba wax, crospovidone, FD&C blue no. 1 aluminum lake, hydroxypropyl methylcellulose, magnesium stearate, microcrystalline cellulose, polyethylene glycol, polysorbate 80, povidone, pregelatinized starch, sodium starch glycolate, stearic acid, and titanium dioxide

**Questions?** call **1-800-524-2624** (English/Spanish), weekdays, 9 AM – 5 PM EST

**How Supplied:** Available in 20 Caplets (capsule-shaped tablets).
*Shown in Product Identification Guide, page 517*

---

## BENADRYL® ALLERGY & SINUS FASTMELT™
### Dissolving Tablets
[bĕ′nădrĭl]

**Drug Facts:**

**Active Ingredients:**
(in each tablet)                 **Purposes:**
Diphenhydramine citrate
  19 mg* ............................. Antihistamine
Pseudoephedrine
  HCl 30 mg ............ Nasal decongestant

*equivalent to 12.5 mg of diphenhydramine HCl

**Uses:**
- temporarily relieves these symptoms of hay fever or the common cold:
  - runny nose
  - sneezing
  - nasal congestion
- temporarily relieves these additional symptoms of hay fever:
  - itching of the nose or throat
  - itchy, watery eyes

**Warnings:**
**Do not use:**
- if you are now taking a prescription monoamine oxidase inhibitor (MAOI) (certain drugs for depression, psychiatric, or emotional conditions, or Parkinson's disease), or for 2 weeks after stopping the MAOI drug. If you do not know if your prescription drug contains an MAOI, ask a doctor or pharmacist before taking this product.
- with any other product containing diphenhydramine, including one applied topically.

**Ask a doctor before use if you have:**
- heart disease
- high blood pressure
- thyroid disease
- diabetes
- glaucoma
- trouble urinating due to an enlarged prostate gland
- a breathing problem such as emphysema or chronic bronchitis

**Ask a doctor or pharmacist before use if you are** taking sedatives or tranquilizers

**When using this product:**
- do not use more than directed
- marked drowsiness may occur
- excitability may occur, especially in children
- avoid alcoholic drinks
- alcohol, sedatives, and tranquilizers may increase drowsiness
- be careful when driving a motor vehicle or operating machinery

**Stop use and ask a doctor if:**
- you get nervous, dizzy, or sleepless
- symptoms do not improve within 7 days or are accompanied by fever

**If pregnant or breast-feeding,** ask a health professional before use.

**Keep out of reach of children.** In case of overdose, get medical help or contact a Poison Control Center right away.

**Directions:**
- adults and children 12 years of age and over: 2 tablets

- place in mouth and allow to dissolve
- take every 4 to 6 hours
- do not take more than 8 tablets in 24 hours, or as directed by a doctor

**Other Information:**
- **phenylketonurics:** contains phenylalanine 4.6 mg per tablet
- store at 59° to 77°F in a dry place

**Inactive Ingredients:** Aspartame, citric acid, D&C red no. 7 calcium lake, ethylcellulose, flavor, lactitol, magnesium stearate, mannitol, and stearic acid

**Questions?** call **1-800-524-2624** (English/Spanish), weekdays, 9 AM – 5 PM EST

**How Supplied:** Available in 20 count dissolving tablets.
*Shown in Product Identification Guide, page 517*

---

## Children's BENADRYL® Allergy Liquid Medication
[bĕ ′nă-drĭl ]

**Drug Facts:**

**Active Ingredient:**          **Purpose:**
(in each 5 mL)
Diphenhydramine
  HCl 12.5 mg .................. Antihistamine

**Uses:**
- temporarily relieves these symptoms due to hay fever or other upper respiratory allergies:
  - runny nose
  - sneezing
  - itchy, watery eyes
  - itching of the nose or throat
- temporarily relieves these symptoms due to the common cold:
  - runny nose
  - sneezing

**Warnings:**
**Do not use** with any other product containing diphenhydramine, including one applied topically.

**Ask a doctor before use if you have:**
- glaucoma
- trouble urinating due to an enlarged prostate gland
- a breathing problem such as emphysema or chronic bronchitis

**Ask a doctor or pharmacist before use if you are** taking sedatives or tranquilizers

**When using this product:**
- marked drowsiness may occur
- avoid alcoholic drinks
- alcohol, sedatives, and tranquilizers may increase drowsiness
- be careful when driving a motor vehicle or operating machinery
- excitability may occur, especially in children

**If pregnant or breast-feeding,** ask a health professional before use.

**Keep out of reach of children.** In case of overdose, get medical help or contact a Poison Control Center right away.

**Directions:**
- take every 4 to 6 hours
- do not take more than 6 doses in 24 hours

| children under 6 years of age | ask a doctor |
|---|---|
| children 6 to under 12 years of age | 1 to 2 teaspoonfuls (12.5 mg to 25 mg) |
| adults and children 12 years of age and over | 2 to 4 teaspoonfuls (25 mg to 50 mg) |

**Other Information:**
• store at 59° to 77°F

**Inactive Ingredients:** Citric acid, D&C red no. 33, FD&C red no. 40, flavors, glycerin, poloxamer 407, purified water, sodium benzoate, sodium chloride, sodium citrate, and sugar

**Questions?** call **1-800-524-2624** (English/Spanish), weekdays, 9 AM–5 PM EST

**How Supplied:** Children's Benadryl Allergy Liquid Medication is supplied in 4 and 8 fluid ounce bottles.

*Shown in Product Identification Guide, page 517*

## Children's BENADRYL® Dye-Free Allergy Liquid Medication
[bĕ 'nă-drĭl ]
**Bubble Gum Flavor**

**Drug Facts:**

**Active Ingredient:**
**(in each 5 mL)**                    **Purpose:**
Diphenhydramine
HCl 12.5 mg ...................... Antihistamine

**Uses:**
• temporarily relieves these symptoms due to hay fever or other upper respiratory allergies:
  • runny nose
  • sneezing
  • itchy, watery eyes
  • itching of the nose or throat
• temporarily relieves these symptoms due to the common cold:
  • runny nose
  • sneezing

**Warnings:**
**Do not use** with any other product containing diphenhydramine, including one applied topically.
**Ask a doctor before use if you have**
• glaucoma
• trouble urinating due to an enlarged prostate gland
• a breathing problem such as emphysema or chronic bronchitis
**Ask a doctor or pharmacist before use if you are** taking sedatives or tranquilizers
**When using this product:**
• marked drowsiness may occur
• avoid alcoholic drinks
• alcohol, sedatives, and tranquilizers may increase drowsiness
• be careful when driving a motor vehicle or operating machinery
• excitability may occur, especially in children
**If pregnant or breast-feeding,** ask a health professional before use.

**Keep out of reach of children.** In case of overdose, get medical help or contact a Poison Control Center right away.

**Directions:**
• take every 4 to 6 hours
• do not take more than 6 doses in 24 hours

| children under 6 years of age | ask a doctor |
|---|---|
| children 6 to under 12 years of age | 1 to 2 teaspoonfuls (12.5 mg to 25 mg) |
| adults and children 12 years of age and over | 2 to 4 teaspoonfuls (25 mg to 50 mg) |

**Other Information**
• store at 59° to 77°F

**Inactive Ingredients:** Carboxymethylcellulose sodium, citric acid, flavor, glycerin, purified water, saccharin sodium, sodium benzoate, sodium citrate, and sorbitol solution

**Questions?** call **1-800-524-2624** (English/Spanish), weekdays, 9 AM – 5 PM EST

**How Supplied:** Children's Benadryl Dye-Free Allergy Liquid Medication is supplied in 4 fl. oz. bottles.

*Shown in Product Identification Guide, page 517*

---

## Children's BENADRYL® Allergy & Sinus Liquid Medication (Formerly Children's Allergy/ Congestion)
[bĕ 'nă-drĭl ]

**Drug Facts:**

**Active Ingredients:**
**(in each 5 mL)\***                    **Purposes:**
Diphenhydramine
  HCl 12.5 mg .................... Antihistamine
Pseudoephedrine
  HCl 30 mg ............ Nasal decongestant

*\*5 mL = one teaspoonful*

**Uses:**
• temporarily relieves these symptoms due to hay fever or other upper respiratory allergies:
  • runny nose
  • sneezing
  • itchy, watery eyes
  • nasal congestion
  • itching of the nose or throat
• temporarily relieves these symptoms due to the common cold:
  • runny nose
  • sneezing
  • nasal congestion

**Warnings:**
**Do not use**
• if you are now taking a prescription monoamine oxidase inhibitor (MAOI) (certain drugs for depression, psychiatric, or emotional conditions, or Parkinson's disease), or for 2 weeks after stopping the MAOI drug. If you do not know if your prescription drug contains an MAOI, ask a doctor or pharmacist before taking this product.
• with any other product containing diphenhydramine, including one applied topically

**Ask a doctor before use if you have:**
• heart disease
• glaucoma
• thyroid disease
• diabetes
• high blood pressure
• trouble urinating due to an enlarged prostate gland
• a breathing problem such as emphysema or chronic bronchitis
**Ask a doctor or pharmacist before use if you are** taking sedatives or tranquilizers
**When using this product:**
• **do not use more than directed**
• marked drowsiness may occur
• avoid alcoholic drinks
• alcohol, sedatives, and tranquilizers may increase drowsiness
• be careful when driving a motor vehicle or operating machinery
• excitability may occur, especially in children
**Stop use and ask a doctor if:**
• you get nervous, dizzy, or sleepless
• symptoms do not improve within 7 days or are accompanied by fever
**If pregnant or breast-feeding,** ask a health professional before use.
**Keep out of reach of children.** In case of overdose, get medical help or contact a Poison Control Center right away.

**Directions:**
• take every 4 to 6 hours
• do not take more than 4 doses in 24 hours

| children under 6 years of age | ask a doctor |
|---|---|
| children 6 to under 12 years of age | 1 teaspoonful |
| adults and children 12 years of age and over | 2 teaspoonfuls |

**Other Information:**
• store at 59° to 77°F

**Inactive Ingredients:** Citric acid, FD&C blue no. 1, FD&C red no. 40, flavors, glycerin, poloxamer 407, polysorbate 20, purified water, saccharin sodium, sodium benzoate, sodium chloride, sodium citrate, and sorbitol solution

**Questions?** call **1-800-524-2624** (English/Spanish), weekdays, 9 AM – 5 PM EST

*Continued on next page*

*This product information was prepared in November 2001. On these and other Pfizer Consumer Healthcare Products, detailed information may be obtained by addressing Pfizer Consumer Healthcare, Pfizer, Inc., Morris Plains, NJ 07950*

## Benadryl Allergy/Sinus —Cont.

**How Supplied:** Benadryl Allergy & Sinus Liquid Medication is supplied in 4 fl. oz. bottles.

*Shown in Product Identification Guide, page 518*

## CHILDREN'S BENADRYL® ALLERGY CHEWABLES
[bĕ 'nă-drĭl ]

**Drug Facts:**

**Active Ingredient:**
**(in each tablet)** **Purpose:**
Diphenhydramine HCl
12.5 mg ........................... Antihistamine

**Uses:**
- temporarily relieves these symptoms due to hay fever or other upper respiratory allergies:
  - runny nose
  - sneezing
  - itchy, watery eyes
  - itching of the nose or throat
- temporarily relieves these symptoms due to the common cold:
  - runny nose
  - sneezing

**Warnings:**
**Do not use** with any other product containing diphenhydramine, including one applied topically.
**Ask a doctor before use if you have:**
- glaucoma
- trouble urinating due to an enlarged prostate gland
- a breathing problem such as emphysema or chronic bronchitis
**Ask a doctor or pharmacist before use if you are** taking sedatives or tranquilizers
**When using this product:**
- marked drowsiness may occur
- avoid alcoholic drinks
- alcohol, sedatives, and tranquilizers may increase drowsiness
- be careful when driving a motor vehicle or operating machinery
- excitability may occur, especially in children
**If pregnant or breast-feeding,** ask a health professional before use.
**Keep out of reach of children.** In case of overdose, get medical help or contact a Poison Control Center right away.

**Directions:**
- chew tablets thoroughly before swallowing
- take every 4 to 6 hours
- do not take more than 6 doses in 24 hours

| children under 6 years of age | ask a doctor |
|---|---|
| children 6 to under 12 years of age | 1 to 2 tablets (12.5 mg to 25 mg) |
| adults and children 12 years of age and over | 2 to 4 tablets (25 mg to 50 mg) |

**Other Information:**
- **phenylketonurics:** contains phenylalanine 4.2 mg per tablet

- store at 59° to 77°F in a dry place
- protect from heat, humidity, and light

**Inactive Ingredients:** Aspartame, dextrates, D&C red no. 27 aluminum lake, FD&C blue no. 1 aluminum lake, flavors, magnesium stearate, magnesium trisilicate, and tartaric acid

**Questions?** call **1-800-524-2624** (English/Spanish), weekdays, 9 AM – 5 PM EST

**How Supplied:** Children's Benadryl® Allergy Chewables are supplied in boxes of 24 tablets.

*Shown in Product Identification Guide, page 518*

## CHILDREN'S BENADRYL® ALLERGY/COLD FASTMELT™
Dissolving Tablets
[bĕ 'nă-drĭl]

**Drug Facts:**

**Active Ingredients:** **Purposes:**
**(in each tablet)**
Diphenhydramine citrate
19 mg* ................. Antihistamine/cough suppressant
Pseudoephedrine HCl
30 mg ...................... Nasal decongestant

*equivalent to 12.5 mg of diphenhydramine HCl

**Uses:**
- temporarily relieves these symptoms of hay fever or the common cold:
  - runny nose
  - sneezing
  - nasal congestion
  - cough
- temporarily relieves these additional symptoms of hay fever:
  - itching of the nose or throat
  - itchy, watery eyes

**Warnings:**
**Do not use**
- if you are now taking a prescription monoamine oxidase inhibitor (MAOI) (certain drugs for depression, psychiatric, or emotional conditions, or Parkinson's disease), or for 2 weeks after stopping the MAOI drug. If you do not know if your prescription drug contains an MAOI, ask a doctor or pharmacist before taking this product.
- with any other product containing diphenhydramine, including one applied topically.
**Ask a doctor before use if you have:**
- heart disease
- high blood pressure
- thyroid disease
- trouble urinating due to an enlarged prostate gland
- diabetes
- cough accompanied by excessive phlegm (mucus)
- glaucoma
- a breathing problem such as emphysema or chronic bronchitis
- persistent or chronic cough such as occurs with smoking, asthma, or emphysema
**Ask a doctor or pharmacist before use if you are** taking sedatives or tranquilizers
**When using this product:**
- **do not use more than directed**

- marked drowsiness may occur
- excitability may occur, especially in children
- avoid alcoholic drinks
- alcohol, sedatives, and tranquilizers may increase drowsiness
- be careful when driving a motor vehicle or operating machinery
**Stop use and ask a doctor if:**
- you get nervous, dizzy, or sleepless
- symptoms do not improve within 7 days or are accompanied by fever
- cough persists for more than 1 week, tends to recur, or is accompanied by fever, rash, or persistent headache. These could be signs of a serious condition.
**If pregnant or breast-feeding,** ask a health professional before use.
**Keep out of reach of children.** In case of overdose, get medical help or contact a Poison Control Center right away.

**Directions:**
- place in mouth and allow to dissolve
- take every 4 hours

| adults and children 12 years of age and over | 2 tablets; do not take more than 8 tablets in 24 hours or as directed by a doctor |
|---|---|
| children 6 to under 12 years of age | 1 tablet; do not take more than 4 tablets in 24 hours or as directed by a doctor |
| children under 6 years of age | ask a doctor |

**Other Information:**
- **phenylketonurics:** contains phenylalanine 4.6 mg per tablet
- store at 59° to 77°F in a dry place

**Inactive Ingredients:** Aspartame, citric acid, D&C red no. 7 calcium lake, ethylcellulose, flavor, lactitol, magnesium stearate, mannitol, and stearic acid

**Questions?** call **1-800-524-2624** (English/Spanish), weekdays, 9 AM - 5 PM EST

**How Supplied:** Cherry Flavor: Available in 20 dissolving tablets.

*Shown in Product Identification Guide, page 518*

## BENAMIST™
**From the Makers of Benadryl®**
**Without Drowsiness**
**Allergy Prevention Nasal Spray**
**Does not contain an antihistamine**

**Drug Facts:**

**Active ingredient:** **Purpose:**
**(per spray)**
Cromolyn sodium
5.2 mg ..... Nasal allergy symptom controller

**Uses:** To prevent and relieve nasal symptoms of hay fever and other nasal allergies:

- runny/itchy nose
- sneezing
- allergic stuffy nose

**Warnings:**
**Do not use**
- if you are allergic to any of the ingredients

**Ask a doctor before use if you have:**
- fever
- discolored nasal discharge
- sinus pain
- wheezing

**When using this product:**
- it may take several days of use to notice an effect. Your best effect may not be seen for 1 to 2 weeks.
- brief stinging or sneezing may occur right after use
- do not use it to treat sinus infection, asthma, or cold symptoms
- do not share this bottle with anyone else as this may spread germs

**Stop use and ask a doctor if:**
- shortness of breath, wheezing, or chest tightness occurs
- hives or swelling of the mouth or throat occurs
- your symptoms worsen
- you have new symptoms
- your symptoms do not begin to improve within two weeks
- you need to use for more than 12 weeks

**If pregnant or breast-feeding,** ask a health professional before use.

**Keep out of reach of children.** If swallowed, get medical help or contact a Poison Control Center right away.

**Directions:**
- see package insert on how to use pump
- parent or care provider must supervise the use of this product by young children
- adults and children 2 years and older:
  - spray once into each nostril. Repeat 3–4 times a day (every 4–6 hours). If needed, may be used up to 6 times a day.
  - use every day while in contact with the cause of your allergies (pollen, molds, pets, and dust)
  - to **prevent** nasal allergy symptoms, use before contact with the cause of your allergies. For best results, start using up to one week before contact.
  - if desired, you can use this product with other medicines, including other allergy medicines.
- children under 2 years: Do not use unless directed by a doctor

**Other Information:**
- store between 20°–25°C (68°–77°F)
- keep away from light
- keep carton and package insert. They contain important instructions.

**Inactive Ingredients:** Benzalkonium chloride, edetate disodium, purified water

**Questions?**
Call **1-800-524-2624**
(English/Spanish),
weekdays, 9 AM–5 PM EST
Before using any medication read all label directions. Keep carton and package insert. They contain important information.

BenaMist Nasal Spray is convenient and easy to administer using the metered spray pump. See package insert for spray pump directions.

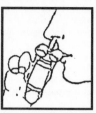

**What Makes the Active Ingredient in BenaMist Allergy Prevention Unique?**
**Nasal Allergy Symptom Prevention**
BenaMist can prevent nasal allergy symptoms when used before exposure to the cause of your nasal allergies, and will build protection against future symptoms as long as you continue to use BenaMist as directed.
**Effective Relief**
BenaMist provides original prescription-strength relief of nasal allergy symptoms, including congestion, sneezing and runny or itchy nose.
**Works only in your nose**
BenaMist is a nasal spray that works only in your nose—where nasal allergens attack. It helps to stop the cells in your nose from reacting to pollen, pet dander, and other allergens, so you don't experience nasal allergy symptoms.
**Safe**
- No drowsiness
- No jitters
- No "rebound" nasal congestion
- Safe to use with other medicines, including other allergy medicines
- Non habit forming
- Safe to use throughout your allergy season
- Good for year-round allergies
- Safe for children as young as two years old

**How Supplied:** Available in .44 and .88 fl. oz. Nasal Spray.
00750701C1                        VC104016
                                  02-0361-03
*Shown in Product Identification Guide, page 518*

---

**BENADRYL® Itch Relief Stick Extra Strength**
**Topical Analgesic/Skin Protectant**
[bĕ 'nă-drĭl ]

**Active    Ingredients:** Diphenhydramine Hydrochloride 2%, Zinc Acetate 0.1%.

**Inactive Ingredients:** Alcohol 73.5% v/v, Glycerin, Povidone, Purified Water and Tromethamine.

**Indications:** For the temporary relief of itching and pain associated with insect bites, minor skin irritations and rashes due to poison ivy, poison oak, or poison sumac. Dries the oozing and weeping of poison ivy, poison oak and poison sumac.

**Warnings:** FOR EXTERNAL USE ONLY. Do not use on chicken pox, measles, blisters, or on extensive areas of skin, except as directed by a physician. Avoid contact with the eyes. If condition worsens, or does not improve within 7 days or if symptoms persist for more than 7 days or clear up and occur again within a few days, discontinue use of this product and consult a physician. Do not use on children under 6 years of age without consulting a physician. **Do not use any other drugs containing diphenhydramine while using this product.** KEEP THIS AND ALL DRUGS OUT OF THE REACH OF CHILDREN. In case of accidental ingestion, seek professional assistance or contact a Poison Control Center immediately. **Flammable.** Keep away from fire or flame.

**Directions:** Adults and children 6 years of age and older: Apply to the affected area not more than 3 to 4 times daily. Children under 6 years of age: Consult a physician.

**How Supplied:** Benadryl® Itch Relief Stick is available in a .47 fl. oz (14 mL) dauber.
*Shown in Product Identification Guide, page 518*

---

**BENADRYL® Itch Stopping Cream Original Strength & Extra Strength**
[bĕ 'nă-drĭl ]

**Active Ingredients:**
Original Strength:  Diphenhydramine Hydrochloride 1% and Zinc Acetate 0.1%.
Extra Strength:  Diphenhydramine Hydrochloride 2% and Zinc Acetate 0.1%.

**Inactive Ingredients:** Cetyl Alcohol, Diazolidinyl Urea, Methylparaben, Polyethylene Glycol Monostearate 1000, Propylene Glycol, Propylparaben and Purified Water.

**Indications:** For the temporary relief of itching and pain associated with insect bites, minor skin irritations and rashes due to poison ivy, poison oak or poison sumac. Dries the oozing and weeping of poison ivy, poison oak and poison sumac.

**Actions:** Benadryl  Itch  Stopping Cream:
- Stops your itch at the source by blocking the histamine that causes itch.
- Provides local anesthetic itch and pain relief in a greaseless vanishing cream.
- Blocks the histamine hydrocortisone can't.

*Continued on next page*

---

*This product information was prepared in November 2001. On these and other Pfizer Consumer Healthcare Products, detailed information may be obtained by addressing Pfizer Consumer Healthcare, Pfizer, Inc., Morris Plains, NJ 07950*

## Benadryl Itch Cream—Cont.

Original Strength:
- Contains 1% diphenhydramine hydrochloride - for itch relief that is appropriate for the whole family to use (ages 2 and up).

Extra Strength:
- Contains the maximum amount of diphenhydramine hydrochloride - for times when you need extra strength itch relief (ages 12 and up).

**Warnings:** FOR EXTERNAL USE ONLY.

Original Strength: Do not use on chicken pox, measles, blisters or on extensive areas of skin, except as directed by a physician. Avoid contact with the eyes. If condition worsens, or does not improve within 7 days or if symptoms persist for more than 7 days or clear up and occur again within a few days, discontinue use of this product and consult a physician. Do not use on children under 2 years of age without consulting a physician. **Do not use any other drugs containing diphenhydramine while using this product.** KEEP THIS AND ALL DRUGS OUT OF THE REACH OF CHILDREN. In case of accidental ingestion, seek professional assistance or contact a Poison Control Center immediately.

Extra Strength: Do not use on chicken pox, measles, blisters or on extensive areas of skin, except as directed by a physician. Avoid contact with the eyes. If condition worsens, or does not improve within 7 days or if symptoms persist for more than 7 days or clear up and occur again within a few days, discontinue use of this product and consult a physician. Do not use on children under 12 years of age without consulting a physician. **Do not use any other drugs containing diphenhydramine while using this product.** KEEP THIS AND ALL DRUGS OUT OF THE REACH OF CHILDREN. In case of accidental ingestion, seek professional assistance or contact a Poison Control Center immediately.

**Directions:** Original Strength: Adults and children 2 years of age and older: Apply to affected area not more than 3 to 4 times daily. Children under 2 years of age: Consult a physician. Extra Strength: Adults and children 12 years of age and older: Apply to affected area not more than 3 to 4 times daily. Children under 12 years of age: Consult a physician.

**How Supplied:** Benadryl Itch Stopping Cream is available in 1 oz (28.3 g) Original Strength and 1 oz (28.3 g) Extra Strength tubes.

*Shown in Product Identification Guide, page 518*

---

## BENADRYL® Itch Stopping Gel
## Original Strength & Extra Strength
[bĕ 'nă-drĭl ]

**Active Ingredients:**
Original Strength: Diphenhydramine Hydrochloride 1%.

Extra Strength: Diphenhydramine Hydrochloride 2%.

**Inactive Ingredients:** SD Alcohol 38B, Camphor, Citric Acid, Diazolidinyl Urea, Glycerin, Hydroxypropyl Methylcellulose, Methylparaben, Propylene Glycol, Propylparaben, Purified Water, and Sodium Citrate.

**Indications:** For the temporary relief of itching and pain associated with insect bites, minor skin irritations and rashes due to poison ivy, poison oak or poison sumac.

**Actions**: Original Strength: Benadryl Original Strength Gel stops your itch at the source by blocking the histamine that causes itch. It contains 1% diphenhydramine hydrochloride for itch relief appropriate for the whole family to use (ages 6 and up). It provides local anesthetic itch and pain relief. Benadryl Itch Stopping Gel blocks the histamine hydrocortisone can't!

Extra Strength: Benadryl Extra Strength Gel stops your itch at the source by blocking the histamine that causes itch. It contains the maximum amount of diphenhydramine hydrochloride for times when you need extra stength itch relief. It provides local anesthetic itch and pain relief (ages 12 and up). Benadryl Itch Stopping Gel blocks the histamine hydrocortisione can't!

**Warnings:** FOR EXTERNAL USE ONLY.

Do not use on chicken pox, measles, blisters or on extensive areas of skin, except as directed by a physician. Avoid contact with the eyes. If condition worsens, or if symptoms persist for more than 7 days or clear up and occur again within a few days, discontinue use of this product and consult a physician. **Do not use any other drugs containing diphenhydramine while using this product.** KEEP THIS AND ALL DRUGS OUT OF THE REACH OF CHILDREN. In case of accidental ingestion, seek professional assistance or contact a Poison Control Center immediately.

**Directions:** Original Strength: Shake well. Adults and children 6 years of age and older: Apply to affected area not more than 3 to 4 times daily. Children under 6 years of age: Consult a physician.

Extra Strength: Shake well. Adults and children 12 years of age and older: Apply to affected area not more than 3 to 4 times daily. Children under 12 years of age: Consult a physician.

**How Supplied:** Benadryl Itch Stopping Gel is supplied in 4 fl. oz. (118mL) bottles in both Original and Extra.

---

## BENADRYL® Itch Stopping Spray
## Original Strength & Extra Strength
[bĕ 'nă-drĭl ]

**Active Ingredients:**
Original Strength: Diphenhydramine Hydrochloride 1% and Zinc Acetate 0.1%.

Extra Strength: Diphenhydramine Hydrochloride 2% and Zinc Acetate 0.1%.

**Inactive Ingredients:** Alcohol up to 73.6% v/v, Glycerin, Povidone, Purified Water and Tromethamine.

**Indications:** For the temporary relief of itching and pain associated with insect bites, minor skin irritations and rashes due to poison ivy, poison oak or poison sumac. Dries the oozing and weeping of poison ivy, poison oak and poison sumac.

**Warnings:** FOR EXTERNAL USE ONLY.

Original Strength: Do not use on chicken pox, measles, blisters or on extensive areas of skin, except as directed by a physician. Avoid contact with the eyes. If condition worsens or does not improve within 7 days, or if symptoms persist for more than 7 days or clear up and occur again within a few days, discontinue use of this product and consult a physician. Do not use on children under 2 years of age without consulting a physician. **Do not use any other drugs containing diphenhydramine while using this product.** KEEP THIS AND ALL DRUGS OUT OF THE REACH OF CHILDREN. In case of accidental ingestion, seek professional assistance or contact a Poison Control Center immediately. **Flammable**. Keep away from fire or flame.

Extra Strength: Do not use on chicken pox, measles, blisters or on extensive areas of skin, except as directed by a physician. Avoid contact with the eyes. If condition worsens or does not improve within 7 days, or if symptoms persist for more than 7 days or clear up and occur again within a few days, discontinue use of this product and consult a physician. Do not use on children under 12 years of age without consulting a physician. **Do not use any other drugs containing diphenhydramine while using this product.** KEEP THIS AND ALL DRUGS OUT OF THE REACH OF CHILDREN. In case of accidental ingestion, seek professional assistance or contact a Poison Control Center immediately. Flammable. Keep away from fire or flame.

**Directions:** Original Strength: Adults and children 2 years of age and older: Apply to affected area not more than 3 to 4 times daily. Children under 2 years of age: Consult a physician. Extra Strength: Adults and children 12 years of age and older: Apply to affected area not more than 3 to 4 times daily. Children under 12 years of age: Consult a physician.

**How Supplied:** Benadryl Itch Stopping Spray Original and Extra Strength is available in a 2 fl. oz. (59mL) pump spray bottle.

*Shown in Product Identification Guide, page 518*

## BENGAY® External Analgesic Products

**Description:** BENGAY products contain menthol in an alcohol base gel, combinations of methyl salicylate and menthol in cream and ointment bases, as well as a combination of methyl salicylate, menthol and camphor in a non-greasy cream base; all suitable for topical application.

In addition to the Original Formula Pain Relieving Ointment (methyl salicylate, 18.3%; menthol, 16%), BENGAY is offered as BENGAY Greaseless Pain Relieving Cream (methyl salicylate, 15%; menthol, 10%), an Arthritis Formula NonGreasy Pain Relieving Cream (methyl salicylate, 30%; menthol, 8%), an Ultra Strength NonGreasy Pain Relieving Cream (methyl salicylate 30%; menthol 10%; camphor 4%), Vanishing Scent NonGreasy Pain Relieving Gel (2.5% menthol), and S.P.A. (Site Penetrating Action) Pain Relieving Cream (10% menthol) with a fresh scent.

**Action and Uses:** Methyl salicylate, menthol and camphor are external analgesics which stimulate sensory receptors of warmth and/or cold. This produces a counter-irritant response which provides temporary relief of minor aches and pains of muscles and joints associated with simple backache, arthritis, strains and sprains.

Several double-blind clinical studies of BENGAY products containing menthol-methyl salicylate have shown the effectiveness of this combination in counteracting minor pain of skeletal muscle stress and arthritis.

Three studies involving a total of 102 normal subjects in which muscle soreness was experimentally induced showed statistically significant beneficial results from use of the active product vs. placebo for lowered Muscle Action Potential (spasms), greater rise in threshold of muscular pain and greater reduction in perceived muscular pain. Six clinical studies of a total of 207 subjects suffering from minor pain due to osteoarthritis and rheumatoid arthritis showed the active product to give statistically significant beneficial results vs. placebo for greater relief of perceived pain, increased range of motion of the affected joints and increased digital dexterity. In two studies designed to measure the effect of topically applied BENGAY vs. placebo on muscular endurance, discomfort, onset of exercise pain and fatigue, 30 subjects performed a submaximal three-hour run and another 30 subjects performed a maximal treadmill run. BENGAY was found to significantly decrease the discomfort during the submaximal and maximal runs, and increase the time before onset of fatigue during the maximal run.

Applied before workouts, BENGAY relaxes tight muscles and increases circulation to make exercising more comfortable, longer.

To help reduce muscle ache and soreness after exercise, BENGAY can be applied and allowed to work before taking a shower.

**Directions:** Apply to affected area not more than 3 to 4 times daily.

**Warnings:** For external use only. Use only as directed. Do not use with a heating pad. Keep away from children to avoid accidental ingestion. Do not swallow. If swallowed, get medical help or contact a Poison Control Center immediately. Do not bandage tightly. Keep away from eyes, mucous membranes, broken or irritated skin. If skin redness or excessive irritation develops, pain lasts for more than 10 days, or with arthritis-like conditions in children under 12, do not use and call a physician.

*Shown in Product Identification Guide, page 518*

---

## BENYLIN® Adult Formula Cough Suppressant
[bĕ '-nă-lĭn ]

### Drug Facts:

**Active Ingredient:**          **Purpose:**
**(in each 5 mL)\***
Dextromethorphan
  HBr 15 mg ............................ Antitussive

*5 mL = one teaspoonful

### Use:
• temporarily relieves cough due to minor throat and bronchial irritation due to the common cold

### Warnings:
**Do not use** if you are now taking a prescription monoamine oxidase inhibitor (MAOI) (certain drugs for depression, psychiatric, or emotional conditions, or Parkinson's disease), or for 2 weeks after stopping the MAOI drug. If you do not know if your prescription drug contains an MAOI, ask a doctor or pharmacist before taking this product.
**Ask a doctor before use if you have:**
• cough accompanied by excessive phlegm (mucus)
• persistent or chronic cough such as occurs with smoking, asthma, or emphysema
**Stop use and ask a doctor if:**
• cough persists for more than 1 week, tends to recur, or is accompanied by fever, rash, or persistent headache. These could be signs of a serious condition.
**If pregnant or breast-feeding,** ask a health professional before use.
**Keep out of reach of children.** In case of overdose, get medical help or contact a Poison Control Center right away.

### Directions:
• take every 6 to 8 hours
• do not take more than 4 doses in 24 hours

| | |
|---|---|
| adults and children 12 years of age and over | two (2) teaspoonfuls |
| children 6 to under 12 years of age | one (1) teaspoonful |
| children 2 to under 6 years of age | one-half (1/2) teaspoonful |
| children under 2 years of age | ask a doctor |

### Other Information:
• store at 59° to 77°F

**Inactive Ingredients:** Caramel, citric acid, D&C red no. 33, FD&C red no. 40, flavors, glycerin, poloxamer 407, polysorbate 20, purified water, saccharin sodium, sodium benzoate, sodium carboxymethyl cellulose, sodium citrate, and sorbitol solution

**Questions?** Call **1-800-223-0182**, Monday to Friday, 9 AM–5 PM EST

**How Supplied:** Benylin Adult Formula is supplied in 4 fl. oz. (118 mL) bottles.
*Shown in Product Identification Guide, page 518*

---

## BENYLIN® Expectorant Cough Suppressant/Expectorant
[bĕ '-nă-lĭn ]

### Drug Facts:

**Active Ingredients:**
**(in each 5 mL)\***          **Purpose:**
Dextromethorphan HBr
  5 mg ........................................ Antitussive
Guaifenesin 100 mg ............. Expectorant

* 5 ml = one teaspoonful

### Uses:
• temporarily relieves cough due to minor throat and bronchial irritation due to the common cold
• helps loosen phlegm (mucus) and thin bronchial secretions to make coughs more productive

### Warnings:
**Do not use** if you are now taking a prescription monoamine oxidase inhibitor (MAOI) (certain drugs for depression, psychiatric or emotional conditions, or Parkinson's disease), or for 2 weeks after stopping the MAOI drug. If you do not know if your prescription drug contains an MAOI, ask a doctor or pharmacist before taking this product.
**Ask a doctor before use if you have:**
• cough accompanied by excessive phlegm (mucus)

***Continued on next page***

*This product information was prepared in November 2001. On these and other Pfizer Consumer Healthcare Products, detailed information may be obtained by addressing Pfizer Consumer Healthcare, Pfizer, Inc., Morris Plains, NJ 07950*

## Benylin Expectorant—Cont.

- persistent or chronic cough such as occurs with smoking, asthma, chronic bronchitis, or emphysema

**Stop use and ask a doctor if:**
- cough persists for more than 1 week, tends to recur, or is accompanied by a fever, rash, or persistent headache. These could be signs of a serious condition.

**If pregnant or breast-feeding**, ask a health professional before use.

**Keep out of reach of children**. In case of overdose, get medical help or contact a Poison Control Center right away.

**Directions:**
- take every 4 hours
- do not take more than 6 doses in 24 hours

| | |
|---|---|
| adults and children 12 years of age and over | four (4) teaspoonfuls |
| children 6 to under 12 years of age | two (2) teaspoonfuls |
| children 2 to under 6 years of age | one (1) teaspoonful |
| children under 2 years of age | ask a doctor |

**Other Information:**
- store at 59° to 77°F

**Inactive Ingredients:** Caramel, citric acid, D&C red no. 33, edetate disodium, FD&C red no. 40, flavors, poloxamer 407, polyethylene glycol, propyl gallate, propylene glycol, purified water, saccharin sodium, sodium benzoate, sodium chloride, sodium citrate, and sorbitol solution

**Questions?** Call **1-800-223-0182**, Monday to Friday, 9 AM – 5 PM EST

**How Supplied:** Benylin Expectorant is available in 4 fl. oz. (118 mL) bottles.

*Shown in Product Identification Guide, page 518*

---

## BENYLIN® Pediatric Cough Suppressant

[bĕ '-nă-lĭn ]

### Drug Facts:

**Active Ingredient:**
(in each 5 mL)*               **Purpose:**
Dextromethorphan HBr
   7.5 mg ..................................... Antitussive

* 5 ml = one teaspoonful

**Uses:**
- temporarily relieves cough due to minor throat and bronchial irritation due to the common cold

**Warnings:**
**Do not use** if you are now taking a prescription monoamine oxidase inhibitor (MAOI) (certain drugs for depression, psychiatric or emotional conditions, or Parkinson's disease), or for 2 weeks after stopping the MAOI drug. If you do not

know if your prescription drug contains an MAOI, ask a doctor or pharmacist before taking this product.

**Ask a doctor before use if you have:**
- cough accompanied by excessive phlegm (mucus)
- persistent or chronic cough such as occurs with smoking, asthma, or emphysema

**Stop use and ask a doctor if:**
- cough persists for more than 1 week, tends to recur, or is accompanied by fever, rash, or persistent headache. These could be signs of a serious condition.

**If pregnant or breast-feeding,** ask a health professional before use.

**Keep out of reach of children.** In case of overdose, get medical help or contact a Poison Control Center right away.

**Directions:**
- take every 6 to 8 hours
- do not take more than 4 doses in 24 hours

| | |
|---|---|
| children under 2 years of age | ask a doctor |
| children 2 to under 6 years of age | one (1) teaspoonful |
| children 6 to under 12 years of age | two (2) teaspoonfuls |
| adults and children 12 years of age and over | four (4) teaspoonfuls |

**Other Information:**
- store at 59° to 77°F

**Inactive Ingredients:** Citric acid, FD&C blue no. 1, FD&C red no. 40, flavors, glycerin, poloxamer 407, polysorbate 20, purified water, saccharin sodium, sodium benzoate, sodium carboxymethyl cellulose, sodium citrate, and sorbitol solution

**Questions?** Call **1-800-223-0182**, Monday to Friday, 9 AM – 5 PM EST

**How Supplied:** Benylin Pediatric is supplied in 4 fl. oz. (118 mL) bottles.

*Shown in Product Identification Guide, page 518*

---

## BONINE®
## (Meclizine hydrochloride)
## Chewable Tablets

**Action:** BONINE® (meclizine) is an $H_1$ histamine receptor blocker of the piperazine side chain group. It exhibits its action by an effect on the Central Nervous System (CNS), possibly by its ability to block muscarinic receptors in the brain.

**Indications:** For the prevention and treatment of nausea, vomiting, or dizziness associated with motion sickness.

**Warnings:** Do not take this product, unless directed by a doctor, if you have a breathing problem such as emphysema or chronic bronchitis, or if you have glaucoma or difficulty in urination due to enlargement of the prostate gland. Do not give to children under 12 years of age un-

less directed by a doctor. May cause drowsiness; alcohol, sedatives, and tranquilizers may increase the drowsiness effect. Avoid alcoholic beverages while taking this product. Do not take this product if you are taking sedatives or tranquilizers without first consulting your doctor. Use caution when driving a motor vehicle or operating machinery. Do not exceed recommended dosage. Keep this and all drugs out of the reach of children. In case of accidental overdose, seek professional assistance or contact a Poison Control Center immediately. As with any drug, if you are pregnant or nursing a baby, seek the advise of a health professional before using this product.

**Directions:** BONINE® should be taken one hour before travel starts. Adults and children 12 years of age and over: oral dosage is 1 to 2 tablets once daily, or as directed by a doctor.

**How Supplied:** BONINE® (meclizine HCl) is available in convenient packets of 8 and 16 chewable tablets of 25 mg. meclizine HCl.

**Inactive Ingredients:** FD&C Red #40, Lactose, Magnesium Stearate, Purified Siliceous Earth, Raspberry Flavor, Saccharin Sodium, Starch, Talc.

*Shown in Product Identification Guide, page 518*

---

## CALADRYL® Lotion
## CALADRYL® Clear™ Lotion

[că 'lă drĭl " ]

**Active Ingredients:** Caladryl Lotion: Calamine 8%, and Pramoxine Hydrochloride 1%.
Caladryl Clear Lotion: Pramoxine Hydrochloride 1% and Zinc Acetate 0.1%.

**Inactive Ingredients:** Caladryl Lotion: Alcohol USP, Camphor, Diazolidinyl Urea, Fragrance, Hydroxypropyl Methylcellulose, Methylparaben, Oil of Lavender, Oil of Rosemary, Polysorbate 80, Propylene Glycol, Propylparaben, Purified Water and Xanthan Gum.
Caladryl Clear Lotion: Alcohol USP, Camphor, Citric Acid, Diazolidinyl Urea, Fragrance, Glycerin, Hydroxypropyl Methylcellulose, Methylparaben, Oil of Lavender, Oil of Rosemary, Polysorbate 40, Propylene Glycol, Propylparaben, Purified Water and Sodium Citrate.

**Indications:** For the temporary relief of itching and pain associated with rashes due to poison ivy, poison oak or poison sumac, insect bites and minor skin irritations. Dries the oozing and weeping of poison ivy, poison oak and poison sumac.

**Warnings:** FOR EXTERNAL USE ONLY. Avoid contact with the eyes. If condition worsens or does not improve within 7 days, or if symptoms persist for more than 7 days or clear up and occur again within a few days, discontinue use of this product and consult a physician.

KEEP THIS AND ALL DRUGS OUT OF THE REACH OF CHILDREN. In case of accidental ingestion, seek professional assistance or contact a Poison Control Center immediately.

Do not use on children under 2 years of age without consulting a physician.

**Directions:** SHAKE WELL Before application, wash affected area of skin. Adults and children 2 years of age and older: Apply to affected area not more than 3 to 4 times daily. Children under 2 years of age: Consult a physician.

**How Supplied:** Caladryl Clear Lotion—6 fl. oz. (177 mL) bottles Caladryl Lotion—6 fl. oz. (177 mL) bottles

*Shown in Product Identification Guide, page 518*

----

## CORTIZONE•5®
### Creme and Ointment
## CORTIZONE FOR KIDS™
### Creme Anti-itch
(0.5% hydrocortisone)

**Description:** CORTIZONE•5® creme (with aloe) and ointment are topical anti-itch preparations.

**Active Ingredient:** Hydrocortisone 0.5%.

**Inactive Ingredients:** Creme: Aloe Barbadensis Gel, Aluminum Sulfate, Calcium Acetate, Cetearyl Alcohol, Glycerin, Light Mineral Oil, Maltodextrin, Methylparaben, Potato Dextrin, Propylparaben, Purified Water, Sodium Cetearyl Sulfate, Sodium Lauryl Sulfate, White Petrolatum, White Wax.
Ointment: Aloe Barbadensis Extract, White Petrolatum.

**Indications:** CORTIZONE•5® is recommended for the temporary relief of itching associated with minor skin irritations, inflammation and rashes due to: eczema, insect bites, poison ivy, oak, sumac, soaps, detergents, cosmetics, jewelry, seborrheic dermatitis, psoriasis, external anal and genital itching. Other uses of this product should be only under the advice and supervision of a doctor.

**Warnings:** For external use only. Avoid contact with the eyes. If condition worsens, or if symptoms persist for more than 7 days or clear up and occur again within a few days, stop use of this product and do not begin use of any other hydrocortisone product unless you have consulted a doctor. Do not use in genital area if you have a vaginal discharge, consult a doctor. Do not use for the treatment of diaper rash or for the treatment of chicken pox, consult a doctor.
**Warnings For External Anal Itching Users:** Do not exceed the recommended daily dosage unless directed by a doctor. In case of bleeding, consult a doctor promptly. Do not put this product into the rectum by using fingers or any mechanical device or applicator.

Keep this and all drugs out of the reach of children. In case of accidental ingestion, seek professional assistance or contact a poison control center immediately.

**Dosage and Administration:** Adults and children 2 years of age and older: Apply to affected area not more than 3 to 4 times daily. Children under 2 years of age: Do not use, consult a doctor.
**Directions For External Anal Itching Users:** Adults: When practical, cleanse the affected area with mild soap and warm water and rinse thoroughly. Gently dry by patting or blotting with toilet tissue or a soft cloth before application of this product. Children under 12 years of age: Consult a doctor.

**How to Store:** Store at controlled room temperature 15°–30°C (59°–86°F).

**How Supplied:** CORTIZONE•5® creme: 1 oz. and 2 oz. tubes. CORTIZONE•5® ointment: 1 oz. tube. CORTIZONE for KIDS™ creme: 1 oz. tubes.

*Shown in Product Identification Guide, page 518*

----

## CORTIZONE•10®
### Creme and Ointment
## CORTIZONE•10®
### Quick Shot Spray

**Description:** CORTIZONE•10® creme (with aloe), ointment and Quick Shot Spray are topical anti-itch preparations and are the maximum strength available without a prescription.

**Active Ingredient:** Hydrocortisone 1%.

**Inactive Ingredients:** Creme: Aloe Barbadensis Gel, Aluminum Sulfate, Calcium Acetate, Cetearyl Alcohol, Glycerin, Light Mineral Oil, Maltodextrin, Methylparaben, Potato Dextrin, Propylparaben, Purified Water, Sodium Cetearyl Sulfate, Sodium Lauryl Sulfate, White Petrolatum, White Wax.
Ointment: White Petrolatum.
Quick Shot Spray: Benzyl Alcohol, Propylene Glycol, Purified Water, SD Alcohol 40-2 (60% v/v).

**Indications:** Cortizone•10® is recommended for the temporary relief of itching associated with minor skin irritations, inflammation and rashes due to: eczema, insect bites, poison ivy, oak, sumac, soaps, detergents, cosmetics, jewelry, seborrheic dermatitis, psoriasis, external anal and genital itching. Other uses of this product should be only under the advice and supervision of a doctor.

**Warnings:** For external use only. Avoid contact with the eyes. If condition worsens, or if symptoms persist for more than 7 days or clear up and occur again within a few days, stop use of this product and do not begin use of any other hydrocortisone product unless you have consulted a doctor. Do not use in genital area if you have a vaginal discharge, consult a doctor. Do not use for the treatment of dia-

per rash, consult a doctor. CORTIZONE•10® Creme and Ointment only:
**Warnings For External Anal Itching Users:** Do not exceed the recommended daily dosage unless directed by a doctor. In case of bleeding, consult a doctor promptly. Do not put this product into the rectum by using fingers or any mechanical device or applicator.
Keep this and all drugs out of the reach of children. In case of accidental ingestion, seek professional assistance or contact a poison control center immediately.

**Dosage and Administration:** Adults and children 2 years of age and older: Apply to affected area not more than 3 to 4 times daily. Children under 2 years of age: Do not use, consult a doctor.
CORTIZONE•10® Creme and Ointment Only:

**Directions For External Anal Itching Users:** Adults: When practical, cleanse the affected area with mild soap and warm water. Rinse thoroughly. Gently dry by patting or blotting with toilet tissue or a soft cloth before application of this product. Children under 12 years of age: Consult a doctor.

**How to Store:** Store at controlled room temperature 15°–30°C (59°–86°F).
Quick Shot Spray only:
Flammable—Keep away from fire or flame.

**How Supplied:** CORTIZONE•10® creme: .5 oz, 1 oz. and 2 oz. tubes. CORTIZONE•10® ointment: 1 oz. and 2 oz. tubes.
CORTIZONE•10® Quick Shot Spray: 1.5 oz. pump bottle.
*Shown in Product Identification Guide, page 519*

----

## CORTIZONE•10® Plus
### Creme

**Description:** CORTIZONE•10® Plus creme is a topical anti-itch preparation containing 10 moisturizers.

**Active Ingredient:** Hydrocortisone 1%.

**Inactive Ingredients:** Aloe Barbadensis Gel, Aluminum Sulfate, Calcium Acetate, Cetearyl Alcohol, Cetyl Alcohol, Corn Oil, Glycerin, Isopropyl Palmitate, Light Mineral Oil, Maltodextrin, Methylparaben, Potato Dextrin, Propylene Glycol, Propylparaben, Purified Wa-

*Continued on next page*

*This product information was prepared in November 2001. On these and other Pfizer Consumer Healthcare Products, detailed information may be obtained by addressing Pfizer Consumer Healthcare, Pfizer, Inc., Morris Plains, NJ 07950*

## Cortizone•10 Plus—Cont.

ter, Sodium Cetearyl Sulfate, Sodium Lauryl Sulfate, Vitamin A Palmitate, Vitamin D, Vitamin E, White Petrolatum, White Wax.

**Indications:** CORTIZONE•10® Plus is recommended for the temporary relief of itching associated with minor skin irritations, inflammation and rashes due to: eczema, insect bites, poison ivy, oak, sumac, soaps, detergents, cosmetics, jewelry, seborrheic dermatitis, psoriasis, external anal and genital itching. Other uses of this product should be only under the advice and supervision of a doctor.

**Warnings:** For external use only. Avoid contact with the eyes. If condition worsens, or if symptoms persist for more than 7 days or clear up and occur again within a few days, stop use of this product and do not begin use of any other hydrocortisone product unless you have consulted a doctor. Do not use in genital area if you have a vaginal discharge, consult a doctor. Do not use for the treatment of diaper rash consult a doctor.

**Warnings For External Anal Itching Users:** Do not exceed the recommended daily dosage unless directed by a doctor. In case of bleeding, consult a doctor promptly. Do not put this product into the rectum by using fingers or any mechanical device or applicator.

Keep this and all drugs out of the reach of children. In case of accidental ingestion, seek professional assistance or contact a poison control center immediately.

**Dosage and Administration:** Adults and children 2 years of age and older: Apply to affected area not more than 3 to 4 times daily. Children under 2 years of age: Do not use, consult a doctor.

**Directions For External Anal Itching Users:** Adults: When practical, cleanse the affected area with mild soap and warm water and rinse thoroughly. Gently dry by patting or blotting with toilet tissue or a soft cloth before application of this product. Children under 12 years of age: Consult a doctor.

**How to Store:** Store at controlled room temperature 15°–30°C (59°–86°F).

**How Supplied:** CORTIZONE•10® Plus creme: 1 oz and 2 oz. tubes.

*Shown in Product Identification Guide, page 519*

---

## DESITIN® CORNSTARCH BABY POWDER
**(with Zinc Oxide)**

**Description:** Desitin Cornstarch Baby Powder combines zinc oxide (10%) with topical starch (cornstarch) for topical application. Also contains: fragrance and tribasic calcium phosphate.

**Actions and Uses:** Desitin Cornstarch Baby Powder with zinc oxide and topical starch (cornstarch) is designed to protect from wetness, help prevent and treat diaper rash, and other minor skin irritations. It offers all the benefits of a talc-free, absorbent cornstarch powder, but with the addition of zinc oxide, the same protective ingredient found in Desitin Ointment. Cornstarch also prevents friction. Zinc oxide provides an additional physical barrier by forming a protective coating over the skin or mucous membranes which serves to reduce further effects of irritants on affected areas.

**Directions:** Change wet and soiled diapers promptly, cleanse the diaper area, and allow to dry.

Apply powder close to the body away from child's face. Carefully shake the powder into the diaper or into the hand and apply to diaper area. Apply liberally as often as necessary with each diaper change, especially at bedtime, or anytime when exposure to wet diapers may be prolonged. Use liberally in all body creases, and whenever chafing, prickly heat or other minor skin irritations occur.

**Warning:** For external use only. Do not use on broken skin. Avoid contact with eyes. Keep powder away from child's face to avoid inhalation. If diaper rash worsens or does not improve within 7 days, consult a doctor.

**How Supplied:** Desitin Cornstarch Baby Powder with Zinc Oxide is available in 14 ounce (397g) containers with sifter-top caps.

*Shown in Product Identification Guide, page 519*

---

## DESITIN® CREAMY WITH ALOE and VITAMIN E
**Zinc Oxide Diaper Rash Ointment**

**Drug Facts:**

**Active Ingredient:**       **Purpose:**
Zinc oxide 10% .... Diaper rash ointment

**Uses:**
• helps treat and prevent diaper rash
• protects chafed skin due to diaper rash and helps seal out wetness

**Warnings:**
**For external use only**
**When using this product**
• avoid contact with the eyes
**Stop use and ask a doctor if:**
• condition worsens or does not improve within 7 days
**Keep out of reach of children.** If swallowed, get medical help or contact a Poison Control Center right away.

**Directions:**
• change wet and soiled diapers promptly
• cleanse the diaper area
• allow to dry
• apply ointment liberally as often as necessary, with each diaper change, especially at bedtime or anytime when exposure to wet diapers may be prolonged

**Other Information:**
• store at between 15° and 30°C (59° to 86°F)

**Inactive Ingredients:** aloe barbadensis gel, cyclomethicone, dimethicone, fragrance, methylparaben, microcrystalline wax, mineral oil, propylparaben, purified water, sodium borate, sorbitan sesquioleate, vitamin E, white petrolatum, and white wax

**Questions?** Call **1-800-723-7529,** Monday to Friday, 9 AM–5 PM EST

**How Supplied:** Desitin Creamy with Aloe and Vitamin E is available in 2 oz. (57g) and 4 oz. (113g) tubes.

*Shown in Product Identification Guide, page 519*

---

## DESITIN® OINTMENT

**Description:** Desitin Ointment combines Zinc Oxide (40%) with Cod Liver Oil in a petrolatum-lanolin base suitable for topical application. Also contains: BHA, fragrance, methylparaben, talc and water.

**Actions and Uses:** Desitin Ointment helps treat and prevent diaper rash. Desitin also protects chafed skin due to diaper rash and helps seal out wetness. In addition to healing diaper rash, Desitin is excellent first aid to treat and protect minor burns, cuts, scrapes, sunburn, and skin irritations. Use for superficial non-infected wounds and burns only.

Relief and protection is afforded by Zinc Oxide in a unique hypoallergenic formula. This ingredient together with cod liver oil and the petrolatum-lanolin base provide a physical barrier by forming a protective coating over skin or mucous membranes which serves to reduce further effects of irritants on the affected area and relieves burning, pain or itch produced by them.

Several studies have shown the effectiveness of Desitin Ointment in the relief and prevention of diaper rash.

Two clinical studies involving 90 infants demonstrated the effectiveness of Desitin Ointment in curing diaper rash. The diaper rash area was treated with Desitin Ointment at each diaper change for a period of 24 hours, while the untreated site served as controls. A significant reduction was noted in the severity and area of diaper dermatitis on the treated area.

Ninety-seven (97) babies participated in a 12-week study to show that Desitin Ointment helps prevent diaper rash. Approximately half of the infants (49) were treated with Desitin Ointment on a regular daily basis. The other half (48) received the ointment as necessary to treat any diaper rash which occurred. The incidence as well as the severity of diaper rash was significantly less among the babies using the ointment on a regular daily basis.

In a comparative study of the efficacy of Desitin Ointment vs. a baby powder, forty-five (45) babies were observed for a total of eight (8) weeks. Results support the conclusion that Desitin Ointment is a better prophylactic against diaper rash than the baby powder.

In another study, Desitin was found to be dramatically more effective in reducing the severity of medically diagnosed diaper rash than a commercially available diaper rash product in which only anhydrous lanolin and petrolatum were listed as ingredients. Fifty (50) infants participated in the study, half of whom were treated with Desitin and half with the other product. In the group (25) treated with Desitin, seventeen (17) infants showed significant improvement within 10 hours which increased to twenty-three improved infants within 24 hours. Of the group (25) treated with the other product, only three showed improvement at ten hours with a total of four improved within twenty-four hours. These results are statistically valid to conclude that Desitin Ointment reduces severity of diaper rash within ten hours.

Several other studies show that Desitin Ointment helps relieve other skin disorders, such as contact dermatitis.

**Directions:** To treat and prevent diaper rash, change wet and soiled diapers promptly, cleanse the diaper area and allow to dry. Apply Desitin Ointment liberally as often as necessary, with each diaper change, especially at bedtime or anytime when exposure to wet diapers may be prolonged.

**Treatment:** If diaper rash is present, or at the first sign of redness, minor skin irritation or chafing, simply apply Desitin Ointment three or four times daily as needed. In superficial noninfected surface wounds and minor burns, apply a thin layer of Desitin Ointment, using a gauze dressing, if necessary. For external use only.

**Warnings:** For external use only. Avoid contact with eyes. If condition worsens or does not improve within 7 days, consult your doctor. Keep this and all drugs out of the reach of children. In case of accidental ingestion, seek professional assistance or contact a poison control center immediately. Store between 15° and 30°C (59° and 86°F).

**How Supplied:** Desitin Ointment is available in 1 ounce (28g), 2 ounce (57g), and 4 ounce (114g) tubes, and 9 ounce (255g) and 1 lb. (454g) jars.

*Shown in Product Identification Guide, page 519*

---

## e.p.t® PREGNANCY TEST
### Over 99% Accurate in Laboratory Tests

**PLEASE READ INSTRUCTIONS CAREFULLY:**
[See figure at top of page]
**How to use:** Remove the **e.p.t.** test stick from its foil packet just prior to use. Remove the purple cap to expose the absorbent tip. Hold the test stick by its thumb grip. Point the absorbent tip

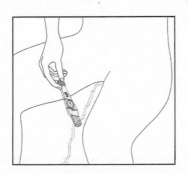

Cap    Absorbent Tip    Sealed Splashguard    Thumb Grip

ept

Round Window    Square Window

downward. Place the absorbent tip in the urine flow for just 5 seconds, or dip the absorbent tip into a clean container of urine for just 5 seconds.

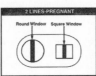

Place the test stick on a flat surface with the windows facing up for at least 3 minutes. (If you wish, replace the cap to cover the absorbent tip.) You may notice a light pink color moving across the windows.

**Important: To avoid affecting the test result, wait at least 3 minutes before lifting the stick.**

**How to Read the Results:**
Wait 3 minutes to read the result. A line will appear in the square window showing the test is complete. Be sure to read the result before 20 minutes have passed.

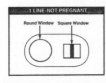

**2 LINES-PREGNANT**
Round Window    Square Window

Two distinct parallel lines, one in each window, indicate that you are **pregnant.** The lines can be different shades of pink. Please see your doctor to discuss your pregnancy and the next steps. Early prenatal care is important to ensure the health of you and your baby.

**1 LINE-NOT PREGNANT**
Round Window    Square Window

One line in the square window but none in the round window indicates that you are **not pregnant.** If your period does not start within a week, repeat the test. If you still get a negative result and your period has not started, please see your doctor.

**Important:  If no line appears in the square window, the test result is invalid. Do not read the result. Call**

toll-free number 1-800-378-1783 (1-800-EPT-1STEP).

**Questions?** Call toll-free 1-800-378-1783 Registered nurses available 8:30 am - 5:00 pm EST weekdays, consumer specialists available until 8:00 pm, and recorded help available 24 hours, (including weekends).

**Questions and Answers about e.p.t.®**
**When can I use e.p.t?**
**e.p.t** can be used any time of day as soon as you miss your period and any day thereafter.

**How does e.p.t work?**
**e.p.t** detects hCG (human Chorionic Gonadotropin), a hormone present in urine only during pregnancy. **e.p.t** can detect hCG in your urine as early as the first day your period is late.

**What if the lines in the round and square windows are different shades of pink?** As long as 2 parallel lines appear, one in each window, the result is positive, even if the two lines are different shades of pink.

**What if I think the test result is incorrect?** Following the instructions carefully should yield an accurate reading. If you think the result is incorrect, or if it is difficult to detect a line in the round window, repeat the test after 2–3 days with a new **e.p.t** stick.

**Are there any factors that can affect the test result?** Yes. Certain drugs which contain hCG or are used in combination with hCG (such as Humegon™, Pregnyl, Profasi, Pergonal, APL) and rare medical conditions. If you repeat the test and continue to get an unexpected result, contact your doctor.

Using **e.p.t** within 8 weeks of giving birth or having a miscarriage may cause a false positive result. The test may detect hCG still in your system from a previous pregnancy. You should ask your doctor for help in interpreting the result of your **e.p.t** test if you have recently been pregnant.

*Continued on next page*

---

*This product information was prepared in November 2001. On these and other Pfizer Consumer Healthcare Products, detailed information may be obtained by addressing Pfizer Consumer Healthcare, Pfizer, Inc., Morris Plains, NJ 07950*

## E.P.T. Pregnancy Test—Cont.

Factors which should <u>not</u> affect the test result include alcohol, analgesics (pain killers), antibiotics, birth control pills or hormone therapies containing clomiphene citrate (Clomid or Serophen). Store at room temperature 15°–30°C (59°–86°F). FOR IN-VITRO DIAGNOSTIC USE. (NOT FOR INTERNAL USE.) KEEP OUT OF THE REACH OF CHILDREN.
**Please call our toll-free number 1-800-378-1783 with any questions about using e.p.t.**

*Shown in Product Identification Guide, page 519*

---

## LISTERINE® Antiseptic
[lĭs 'tərēn ]

**Active Ingredients:** Thymol 0.064%, Eucalyptol 0.092%, Methyl Salicylate 0.060% and Menthol 0.042%.

**Inactive Ingredients:** Water, Alcohol 26.9%, Benzoic Acid, Poloxamer 407, Sodium Benzoate and Caramel.

**Indications:** Use Listerine twice daily to help:
• Prevent & Reduce Plaque
• Prevent & Reduce Gingivitis
• Fight Bad Breath
• Kill Germs Between Teeth

**Actions:** Listerine® Antiseptic has been shown to help prevent and reduce supragingival plaque accumulation and gingivitis when used in a conscientiously applied program of oral hygiene and regular professional care. Its effect on periodontitis has not been determined. Listerine is the only leading nonprescription mouthrinse that has received the American Dental Association's Council on Scientific Affairs Seal of Acceptance for helping to prevent and reduce plaque above the gumline and gingivitis.

**Directions:** Rinse full strength for 30 seconds with 20 ml ($^2/_3$ fl. ounce or 4 teaspoonfuls) morning and night. If bad breath persists, see your dentist.

**Warnings:** Do not administer to children under twelve years of age. **Keep this and all drugs out of the reach of children.** Do not swallow. In case of accidental ingestion, seek professional assistance or contact a poison control center immediately.
Cold weather may cloud Listerine. Its antiseptic properties are not affected. Store at 59° to 77°F.

**How Supplied:** Listerine® Antiseptic is supplied in 250 ml, 500 ml, 1.0 liter and 1.5 liter bottles, as well as 3 fl. oz. bottles. It is also available to professionals in 3 fl. oz. bottles and in gallons.

*Shown in Product Identification Guide, page 519*

---

## COOL MINT LISTERINE® ANTISEPTIC
[lĭs 'tərēn ]

**Active Ingredients:** Thymol 0.064%, Eucalyptol 0.092%, Methyl Salicylate 0.060% and Menthol 0.042%.

**Inactive Ingredients:** Water, Alcohol 21.6%, Sorbitol Solution, Flavoring, Poloxamer 407, Benzoic Acid, Sodium Saccharin, Sodium Benzoate and FD&C Green No. 3.

**Indications:** To help prevent and reduce plaque and gingivitis/For bad breath. Use Cool Mint Listerine Antiseptic twice Daily to help:
• Prevent & Reduce Plaque
• Prevent & Reduce Gingivitis
• Fight Bad Breath
• Kills Germs Between teeth.

**Actions:** Cool Mint Listerine® Antiseptic has been shown to help prevent and reduce supragingival plaque accumulation and gingivitis when used in a conscientiously applied program of oral hygiene and regular professional care. Its effect on periodontitis has not been determined. Listerine is the only leading nonprescription mouthrinse that has received the American Dental Association's Council on Scientific Affairs Seal of Acceptance for helping to prevent and reduce plaque above the gumline and gingivitis.

**Directions:** Rinse full strength for 30 seconds with 20 ml ($^2/_3$ fl. ounce or 4 teaspoonfuls) morning and night. If bad breath persists, see your dentist.

**Warnings:** Do not administer to children under twelve years of age. **Keep this and all drugs out of the reach of children.** Do not swallow. In case of accidental ingestion, seek professional assistance or contact a poison control center immediately. Cold weather may cloud Cool Mint Listerine. Its Antiseptic properties are not affected. Store at 59° to 77°F.

**How Supplied:** Cool Mint Listerine® Antiseptic is supplied in 250 ml, 500 ml, 1.0 liter and 1.5 liter bottles, as well as 3 and 58 fl. oz. bottles. It is also available to professionals in 3 fl. oz. bottles and in gallon bottles.

*Shown in Product Identification Guide, page 519*

---

## FRESHBURST LISTERINE® ANTISEPTIC
[lĭs 'tərēn ]

**Active Ingredients:** Thymol 0.064%, Eucalyptol 0.092%, Methyl Salicylate 0.060% and Menthol 0.042%.

**Inactive Ingredients:** Water, Alcohol 21.6%, Sorbitol Solution, Flavoring, Poloxamer 407, Benzoic Acid, Sodium Saccharin, Sodium Benzoate, D&C Yellow No. 10 and FD&C Green No. 3.

**Indications:** To help prevent and reduce plaque and gingivitis/For bad breath. Use FreshBurst Listerine Antiseptic Twice Daily to help:
• Prevent & Reduce Plaque
• Prevent & Reduce Gingivitis
• Fight Bad Breath
• Kill Germs Between Teeth

**Actions:** FreshBurst Listerine® Antiseptic has been shown to help prevent and reduce supragingival plaque accumulation and gingivitis when used in a conscientiously applied program of oral hygiene and regular professional care. Its effect on periodontitis has not been determined. Listerine is the only leading nonprescription mouthrinse that has received the American Dental Association's Council on Scientific Affairs Seal of Acceptance for helping to prevent and reduce plaque above the gumline and gingivitis.

**Directions:** Rinse full strength for 30 seconds with 20 ml ($^2/_3$ fl. ounce or 4 spoonfuls) morning and night. If bad breath persists, see your dentist.

**Warnings:** Do not administer to children under twelve years of age. **Keep this and all drugs out of the reach of children.** Do not swallow. In case of accidental ingestion, seek professional assistance or contact a poison control center immediately. Cold weather may cloud FreshBurst Listerine. Its antiseptic properties are not affected. Store at 59° to 77°F.

**How Supplied:** FreshBurst Listerine® antiseptic is supplied in 250 ml, 500 ml, 1.0 liter and 1.5 liter bottles, as well as 3 fl. oz. bottles. It is also available to professionals in 3 fl. oz. bottles and in gallon bottles.

*Shown in Product Identification Guide, page 519*

---

## TARTAR CONTROL LISTERINE® Antiseptic
[lys'tərĕn]

**Active Ingredients:** Thymol 0.064%, Eucalyptol 0.092%, Methyl Salicylate 0.060%, and Menthol 0.042.%.

**Inactive Ingredients:** Water, Alcohol (21.6%), Sorbitol Solution, Flavoring, Poloxamer 407, Sodium Saccharin, Benzoic Acid, Zinc Chloride, Sodium Benzoate, and FD&C Blue # 1.

**Indications:** To help prevent and reduce plaque and gingivitis, prevent tartar buildup, and fight bad breath. Use Tartar Control Listerine Antiseptic twice daily to help:
• Prevent & Fight Tartar Build-up
• Prevent & Reduce Plaque
• Prevent & Reduce Gingivitis
• Fight Bad Breath
• Kill Germs Between Teeth

**Actions:** Tartar Control Listerine® Antiseptic has been shown to help prevent and reduce supragingival plaque accumulation and gingivitis when used in a conscientiously applied program of oral hygiene and regular professional care. It has also been shown to help reduce the formation of tartar above the gumline. Its effect on periodontitis has not been determined. Listerine is the only leading nonprescription mouthrinse that has received the American Dental Association's Council on Scientific Affairs Seal of Acceptance for helping to prevent and reduce plaque above the gumline and gingivitis.

**Directions:** Rinse full strength for 30 seconds with 20ml (2/3 fluid ounce or 4 teaspoonfuls) morning and night. If bad breath persists, see your dentist.

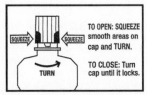

**Warnings:** Do not administer to children under twelve years of age. **KEEP THIS AND ALL DRUGS OUT OF THE REACH OF CHILDREN.** Do not swallow. Incase of accidental overdose, seek professional assistance or contact a Poison Control Center immediately. **Cold weather may cloud Tartar Control Listerine. Its antiseptic properties are not affected.**
Store at 59° to 77°F.

**How Supplied:** Tartar Control. Listerine® Antiseptic is suppled in 250 ml, 500 ml, 1.0 litter and 1.5 litter bottles, as well as 3 fl. oz. bottles.
*Shown in Product Identification Guide, page 519*

## LISTERMINT®
### Alcohol-Free Mouthwash
[lĭs 'tər mĭnt ]

**Ingredient:** Water, Glycerin, Poloxamer 335, PEG 600, Flavors, Sodium Lauryl Sulfate, Sodium Benzoate, Sodium Saccharin, Benzoic Acid, Zinc Chloride, D&C Yellow No. 10, FD&C Green No. 3.

**Indications:** Freshens breath; contains no fluoride.

**Directions:** Rinse with 30 ml (1 fl. oz.) for 30 seconds to freshen breath in the morning and after meals as needed.

**Warnings:** Do not swallow. Keep out of reach of children.

**How Supplied:** Listermint® is supplied to consumers in a 32 fl. oz. bottle and is available to professionals in 3 fl. oz. bottles and in gallons.
*Shown in Product Identification Guide, page 519*

## LUBRIDERM® Advanced Therapy
### Creamy Lotion
[lū brĭ dĕrm ]

**Ingredients:** Water, Cetyl Alcohol, Glycerin, Mineral Oil, Cyclomethicone,

Propylene Glycol Dicaprylate/Dicaprate, PEG-40 Stearate, Isopropyl Isostearate, Emulsifying Wax, Lecithin, Carbomer 940, Diazolidinyl Urea, Titanium Dioxide, Sodium Benzoate, BHT, Tri(PPG-3 Myristyl Ether) Citrate, Disodium EDTA, Retinyl Palmitate, Tocopheryl Acetate, Sodium Pyruvate, Iodopropynyl Butylcarbamate, Fragrance, Sodium Hydroxide, Xanthan Gum.

**Uses:** Lubriderm Advanced Therapy's nourishing, rich and creamy formula helps heal extra-dry skin. Its unique combination of nutrient-enriched moisturizers penetrate dry skin leaving you with soft, smooth and comfortable skin. This non-greasy feeling lotion absorbs quickly and is non-comedogenic.

**Directions:** Smooth Lubriderm on hands and body every day.
For external use only.

**How Supplied:** Available in 6, 10, 16, and 19.6 fl. oz. plastic bottles and a 3.3 fl. oz. tube.
*Shown in Product Identification Guide, page 519*

## LUBRIDERM® Daily UV Lotion
### w/Sunscreen
[lū brĭ dĕrm]

**Active Ingredients:** Octyl Methoxycinnamate 7.5%, Octyl Salicylate 4%, Oxybenzone 3%. **Inactive Ingredients:** Purified Water, C12-15 Alkyl Benzoate, Cetearyl Alcohol (and) Ceteareth-20, Cetyl Alcohol, Glyceryl Monostearate, Propylene Glycol, Petrolatum, Diazolidinyl Urea, Triethanolamine, Disodium EDTA, Xanthan Gum, Acrylates/C10-30 Alkyl Acrylate Crosspolymer, Tocopheryl Acetate, Iodopropynyl Butylcarbamate, Fragrance, Carbomer.

**Actions and Uses:** Lubriderm Daily UV Lotion's unique formula combines light, daily moisturization with dermatologist-recommended SPF 15 sun protection. This non-greasy feeling lotion moisturizes dry skin and helps protect against the damaging rays of the sun.

**Directions:** Apply liberally as often as necessary. Children under 6 months of age: consult a doctor.

**Warnings:** For external use only. Avoid contact with the eyes. If contact occurs, rinse eyes thoroughly with water. Discontinue use if signs of irritation or rash appear. If irritation or rash persists, consult a doctor. Keep out of reach of children. In case of accidental ingestion, seek professional assistance or contact a Poison Control Center immediately.
Store between 59°–77°F.

**How Supplied:** Available in 6, 10, 16 fl. oz plastic bottles and a 3.3 fl. oz. tube.
*Shown in Product Identification Guide, page 519*

## LUBRIDERM®
### Seriously Sensitive® Lotion
[lū brĭ dĕrm ]

**Ingredients:** Water, Butylene Glycol, Mineral Oil, Petrolatum, Glycerin, Cetyl Alcohol, Propylene Glycol Dicaprylate/ Dicaprate, PEG-40 Stearate, C11-13 Isoparaffin, Glyceryl Stearate, Tri (PPG-3 Myristyl Ether) Citrate, Emulsifying Wax, Dimethicone, DMDM Hydantoin, Methylparaben, Carbomer 940, Ethylparaben, Propylparaben, Titanium Dioxide, Disodium EDTA, Sodium Hydroxide, Butylparaben, Xanthan Gum.

**Uses:** Lubriderm Seriously Sensitive Lotion's unique combination of emollients provides sensitive dry skin with the moisture it needs while helping to create a protective layer. It is non-comedogenic, 100% lanolin free, fragrance free, and dye free so its appropriate for skin that is sensitive to these ingredients. It is nongreasy feeling and absorbs quickly.

**Directions:** Smooth on hands and body everyday. Particularly effective when used after showering or bathing. For external use only.

**How Supplied:** Available in 1, 6, 10, and 16 fl. oz. plastic bottles and 3.3 fl. oz. tube.
*Shown in Product Identification Guide, page 519*

## LUBRIDERM®
### Skin Firming Body Lotion
[lū brĭ dĕrm]

**Ingredients:** Water, isostearic acid, stearic acid, steareth-21, sodium lactate, PPG 12/SMDI copolymer, lactic acid, steareth-2, magnesium aluminum silicate, cetyl alcohol, imidurea, fragrance, potassium sorbate, xanthan gum.

**Uses:** Lubriderm Skin Firming Body Lotion, with its unique dual action formula of Alpha Hydroxy Acid and moisturizers, will improve the firmness and appearance of your skin. This advanced non-greasy feeling lotion has been shown in a clinical study to help increase skin firmness in just 8 weeks, leaving improved skin texture and healthy-looking skin.

**Directions:** Apply liberally twice daily. Gently massage lotion all over body. Rub in a circular motion to stimulate circula-

*Continued on next page*

*This product information was prepared in November 2001. On these and other Pfizer Consumer Healthcare Products, detailed information may be obtained by addressing Pfizer Consumer Healthcare, Pfizer, Inc., Morris Plains, NJ 07950*

## Lubriderm Firming—Cont.

tion and promote firming in problem areas like legs, thighs and arms. Daily use of sun protection (such as Lubriderm Daily UV) is advisable when using this product.

**How Supplied:** Available in 10 fl. oz. plastic bottles.

*Shown in Product Identification Guide, page 519*

---

## LUBRIDERM®
### Skin Therapy Moisturizing Lotion
[lū brĭ dĕrm ]

**Ingredients: Scented**—Water, Mineral Oil, Petrolatum, Sorbitol Solution, Stearic Acid, Lanolin, Lanolin Alcohol, Cetyl Alcohol, Glyceryl Stearate/PEG-100 Stearate, Triethanolamine, Dimethicone, Propylene Glycol, Microcrystalline Wax, Tri(PPG-3 Myristyl Ether) Citrate, Disodium EDTA, Methylparaben, Ethylparaben, Propylparaben, Fragrance, Xanthan Gum, Butylparaben, Methyldibromo Glutaronitrile.
**Fragrance Free**—Contains Water, Mineral Oil, Petrolatum, Sorbitol Solution, Stearic Acid, Lanolin, Lanolin Alcohol, Cetyl Alcohol, Glyceryl Stearate/PEG-100 Stearate, Triethanolamine, Dimethicone, Propylene Glycol, Microcrystalline Wax, Tri(PPG-3 Myristyl Ether) Citrate, Disodium EDTA, Methylparaben, Ethylparaben, Propylparaben, Xanthan Gum, Butylparaben, Methyldibromo Glutaronitrile.

**Uses:** Lubriderm provides the essential moisturizing elements that contribute to healthy skin. Its unique combination of emollients penetrate dry skin to effectively moisturize without leaving a greasy feel. Lubriderm helps heal and protect skin from dryness, absorbs rapidly for a clean, natural feel and is noncomedogenic so it won't clog pores.

**Directions:** Smooth on hands and body every day. Particularly effective when used after showering or bathing. For external use only.

**How Supplied:**
**Scented:** Available in 6, 10, 16 and 19.6 oz. plastic bottles.
**Fragrance Free:** Available in 6, 10 and 16 fl. oz. plastic bottles and 3.3 fl. oz. tube.

*Shown in Product Identification Guide, page 519*

---

## NEOSPORIN® Ointment
[nē 'uh-spō 'rŭn ]

**Each Gram Contains:** Polymyxin B Sulfate 5,000 units, Bacitracin Zinc 400 units and Neomycin 3.5 mg. Also contains a base of Cocoa Butter*, Cottonseed Oil*, Olive Oil*, Sodium Pyruvate*, Tocopheryl Acetate* and White Petrolatum.

*U.S. Patent # 5,652,274

**Indications:** First aid to help prevent infection in minor cuts, scrapes, and burns.

**Directions:** Clean the affected area. Apply a small amount of this product (an amount equal to the surface area of the tip of a finger) on the area 1 to 3 times daily. May be covered with a sterile bandage.

**Warnings:** For external use only. Do not use in the eyes or apply over large areas of the body. In case of deep or puncture wounds, animal bites, or serious burns, consult a physician. Stop use and consult a physician if the condition persists or gets worse, or if a rash or other allergic reaction develops. Do not use if you are allergic to any of the ingredients. Do not use longer than 1 week unless directed by a physician. KEEP THIS AND ALL DRUGS OUT OF THE REACH OF CHILDREN. In case of accidental ingestion, seek professional assistance or contact a Poison Control Center immediately.

**How Supplied:** Tubes, 1/2 oz (14.2 g) (with applicator tip), 1 oz (28.3 g), 1/32 oz (0.9 g) foil packets packed 10 per box (Neo To Go™) or 144 per box. Store at 59° to 77°F.

*Shown in Product Identification Guide, page 519*

---

## NEOSPORIN® + PAIN RELIEF MAXIMUM STRENGTH Cream
[nē "uh-spō 'rŭn ]

**Each Gram Contains:** Polymyxin B Sulfate 10,000 units, Neomycin 3.5 mg, and Pramoxine Hydrochloride 10 mg. Also contains: Emulsifying Wax, Methylparaben 0.25% (added as a preservative), Mineral Oil, Poloxamer 188, Propylene Glycol, Purified Water, and White Petrolatum.

**Indications:** First aid to help prevent infection and provide temporary relief of pain or discomfort in minor cuts, scrapes, and burns.

**Directions:** Adults and children 2 years of age and older: Clean the affected area. Apply a small amount of this product (an amount equal to the surface area of the tip of a finger) on the area 1 to 3 times daily. May be covered with a sterile bandage. Children under 2 years of age: Consult a physician.

**Warnings:** For external use only. Do not use in the eyes or apply over large areas of the body. In case of deep or puncture wounds, animal bites, or serious burns, consult a physician. Stop use and consult a physician if the condition persists or gets worse, or if symptoms persist for more than 1 week or clear up and occur again within a few days, or if a rash or other allergic reaction develops. Do not use if you are allergic to any of the ingredients. Do not use longer than 1

week unless directed by a physician. KEEP THIS AND ALL DRUGS OUT OF THE REACH OF CHILDREN. In case of accidental ingestion, seek professional assistance or contact a Poison Control Center immediately.

**How Supplied:** 1/2 oz (14.2 g) (with applicator tip) tubes. Store at 59° to 77°F.

*Shown in Product Identification Guide, page 520*

---

## NEOSPORIN® + PAIN RELIEF MAXIMUM STRENGTH Ointment
[nē "uh-spō 'rŭn ]

**Each Gram Contains:** Polymyxin B Sulfate 10,000 units, Bacitracin Zinc 500 units, Neomycin 3.5 mg, and Pramoxine Hydrochloride 10 mg, in a custom blend of White Petrolatum.

**Indications:** First aid to help prevent infection and provide temporary relief of pain or discomfort in minor cuts, scrapes, and burns.

**Directions:** Adults and children 2 years of age and older: Clean the affected area. Apply a small amount of this product (an amount equal to the surface area of the tip of a finger) on the area 1 to 3 times daily. May be covered with a sterile bandage. Children under 2 years of age: Consult a physician.

**Warnings:** For external use only. Do not use in the eyes or apply over large areas of the body. In case of deep or puncture wounds, animal bites, or serious burns, consult a physician. Stop use and consult a physician if the condition persists or gets worse, or if symptoms persist for more than 1 week or clear up and occur again within a few days, or if a rash or other allergic reaction develops. Do not use if you are allergic to any of the ingredients. Do not use longer than 1 week unless directed by a physician. KEEP THIS AND ALL DRUGS OUT OF THE REACH OF CHILDREN. In case of accidental ingestion, seek professional assistance or contact a Poison Control Center immediately.

**How Supplied:** 1/2 oz (14.2 g) (with applicator tip) and 1 oz (28.3 g) tubes. Store at 59° to 77°F.

*Shown in Product Identification Guide, page 520*

---

## NIX® Creme Rinse
### Permethrin
### Lice Treatment
[nĭks ]

**Each Fluid Ounce Contains:** Active Ingredient: permethrin 280 mg (1%). Also contains: balsam canada, cetyl alcohol, citric acid, FD&C Yellow No. 6, fragrance, hydrolyzed animal protein, hydroxyethylcellulose, polyoxyethylene 10 cetyl ether, propylene glycol, stearalkonium chloride, water, isopropyl alcohol 5.6 g (20%), methylparaben 56 mg (0.2%), and propylparaben 22 mg (0.08%).

**Product Benefits:** Nix Creme Rinse kills lice and their unhatched eggs with usually only one application. Nix protects against head lice reinfestation for 14 days. The creme rinse formula leaves hair manageable and easy to comb.

**Indications:** For the treatment of head lice.

**Directions for Use:** Nix Creme Rinse should be used after hair has been washed with your regular shampoo, rinsed with water and towel dried. A sufficient amount should be applied to saturate hair and scalp (especially behind the ears and on the nape of the neck). Leave on hair for 10 minutes but no longer. Rinse with water. A single application is usually sufficient. If live lice are observed seven days or more after the first application of this product, a second treatment should be given. For proper head lice management, remove nits with the nit comb provided.

Head lice live on the scalp and lay small white eggs (nits) on the hair shaft close to the scalp. The nits are most easily found on the nape of the neck or behind the ears. All personal headgear, scarfs, coats, and bed linen should be disinfected by machine washing in hot water and drying, using the hot cycle of a dryer for at least 20 minutes. Personal articles of clothing or bedding that cannot be washed may be dry-cleaned, sealed in a plastic bag for a period of about 2 weeks, or sprayed with a product specifically designed for this purpose. Personal combs and brushes may be disinfected by soaking in hot water (above 130°F) for 5 to 10 minutes. Thorough vacuuming of rooms inhabited by infected patients is recommended.

Shake well before using.

**Warnings:** For external use only. Keep out of eyes when rinsing hair. Adults and children: Close eyes and do not open eyes until product is rinsed out. If product gets into the eyes, immediately flush with water. Do not use near the eyes or permit contact with mucous membranes, such as inside the nose, mouth, or vagina, as irritation may occur. Children: Also protect children's eyes with a washcloth, towel, or other suitable material or method. This product should not be used on children less than 2 months of age. Itching, redness, or swelling of the scalp may occur. If skin irritation persists or infection is present or develops, discontinue use and consult a doctor. Consult a doctor if infestation of eyebrows or eyelashes occurs. This product may cause breathing difficulty or an asthmatic episode in susceptible persons. As with any drug, if you are pregnant or nursing a baby, seek the advice of a health professional before using this product. Keep this and all drugs out of the reach of chil-

dren. In case of accidental ingestion, seek professional assistance or contact a Poison Control Center immediately.

**Professional Labeling:**
**Indications:** For the treatment of head lice. For prophylactic use during head lice epidemics.

**Warnings:** For external use only. Keep out of eyes when rinsing hair. Adults and children: Close eyes and do not open eyes until product is rinsed out. If product gets into the eyes, immediately flush with water. Do not use near the eyes or permit contact with mucous membranes, such as inside the nose, mouth, or vagina, as irritation may occur. Children: Also protect children's eyes with a washcloth, towel, or other suitable material or method. This product should not be used on pediatric patients less than 2 months of age. Itching, redness, or swelling of the scalp may occur. If skin irritation persists or infection is present or develops, discontinue use and consult a doctor. Consult a doctor if infestation of eyebrows or eyelashes occurs. This product may cause breathing difficulty or an asthmatic episode in susceptible persons. As with any drug, if you are pregnant or nursing a baby, seek the advice of a health professional before using this product. Keep this and all drugs out of the reach of children. In case of accidental ingestion, seek professional assistance or contact a Poison Control Center immediately.

**Dosage and Administration**
*Treatment*
Nix Creme Rinse should be used after hair has been washed with patient's regular shampoo, rinsed with water and towel dried. A sufficient amount should be applied to saturate hair and scalp (especially behind the ears and on the nape of the neck). Leave on hair for 10 minutes but no longer. Rinse with water. A single application is usually sufficient. If live lice are observed seven days or more after the first application of this product, a second treatment should be given. For proper head lice management, remove nits with the nit comb provided.

Head lice live on the scalp and lay small white eggs (nits) on the hair shaft close to the scalp. The nits are most easily found on the neck or behind the ears. All personal headgear, scarfs, coats, and bed linen should be disinfected by machine washing in hot water and drying, using the hot cycle of a dryer for a least 20 minutes. Personal articles of clothing or bedding that cannot be washed may be dry-cleaned, sealed in a plastic bag for a period of about 2 weeks, or sprayed with a product specifically designed for this purpose. Personal combs and brushes may be disinfected by soaking in hot water (above 130°F) for 5 to 10 minutes. Thorough vacuuming of rooms inhabited by infected patients is recommended.

*Prophylaxis*
Prophylactic use of Nix Creme Rinse is only recommended for individuals ex-

posed to head lice epidemics in which at least 20% of the population at an institution are infested and for immediate household members of infested individuals. Casual use is strongly discouraged. The method of application of Nix Creme Rinse for prophylaxis is identical to that described above for treatment of a lice infestation except nit removal is not required.

*Directions for Use*
One application of Nix Creme Rinse has been shown to protect greater than 95% of patients against reinfestation for at least two weeks. In epidemic settings, a second prophylactic application is recommended two weeks after the first because the life cycle of a head louse is approximately four weeks.

**How Supplied:** Bottles of 2 fl. oz. (59 mL) with nit removal comb and Family Pack of 2 bottles, 2 fl. oz. (59 mL) each, with two nit removal combs. Store at 15° to 25°C (59° to 77°F).

*Shown in Product Identification Guide, page 520*

---

## NIX® LICE CONTROL SPRAY
**For Bedding and Furniture**

**NOT FOR USE IN HUMANS**

**Directions for Use:** It is a violation of Federal law to use this product in a manner inconsistent with its labeling.

**FOR USE IN NON-FOOD AREA OF HOMES**

**Indoor Application:** Surface Spraying: To kill lice, spray in an inconspicuous area to test for possible staining or discoloration. Inspect again after drying, then proceed to spray entire area to be treated. Spray from a distance of 8 to 10 inches. Treat only those garments and parts of bedding, including mattresses and furniture that cannot be either laundered or dry cleaned. Allow all treated articles to dry thoroughly before use.

Do not use in food/feed areas of food/feed handling establishments, restaurants or other areas where food/feed is commercially prepared or processed. Do not use in serving areas while food is exposed or facility is in operation. Serving areas are areas where prepared foods are served such as dining rooms, but excluding areas where foods may be prepared or held.

*Continued on next page*

---

*This product information was prepared in November 2001. On these and other Pfizer Consumer Healthcare Products, detailed information may be obtained by addressing Pfizer Consumer Healthcare, Pfizer, Inc., Morris Plains, NJ 07950*

## Nix Spray—Cont.

In the home, cover all food handling surfaces, cover or remove all food and cooking utensils or wash thoroughly after treatment.

Do not apply to classrooms while in use. Not for use in Federally Inspected Meat and Poultry Plants.

**Storage and Disposal:** Do not contaminate water, food or feed by storing or disposal.

**Pesticide Storage and Spill Procedures:** Keep from freezing. Store upright at room temperature. Avoid exposure to extreme temperatures. In case of spill or leakage, soak up with an absorbent material such as sand, sawdust, earth, fuller's earth, etc. Dispose of with chemical waste.

**Pesticide Disposal:** Pesticide or rinse water that cannot be used according to label instructions must be disposed of at or by an approved waste disposal facility.

**Container Disposal:** Do not reuse empty container. Wrap container and put in trash collection.

## READ ENTIRE LABEL BEFORE EACH USE.

> Observe all precautionary statements and follow directions for use carefully.

**Environmental Hazards:** This product is extremely toxic to fish and aquatic organisms. Do not apply directly to any body of water. Do not contaminate water when disposing of equipment washwater. This pesticide is toxic to honey bees and other beneficial pollinators exposed to an application. Do not apply when bees are actively visiting blooming plants (vegetables, flowers, fruit/ornamental trees) Do not allow this product to come in direct contact with bee hives at any time.

**QUESTIONS OR COMMENTS:**
Call Toll Free 1-888-542-3546
*Shown in Product Identification Guide, page 520*

## POLYSPORIN® Ointment
[pŏl 'ē-spō 'rŭn ]

**Each Gram Contains:** Polymyxin B Sulfate 10,000 units and Bacitracin Zinc 500 units in a special White Petrolatum Base.

**Indications:** First aid to help prevent infection in minor cuts, scrapes, and burns.

**Directions:** Clean the affected area. Apply a small amount of this product (an amount equal to the surface area of the tip of a finger) on the area 1 to 3 times daily. May be covered with a sterile bandage.

**Warnings:** For external use only. Do not use in the eyes or apply over large areas of the body. In case of deep or puncture wounds, animal bites, or serious burns, consult a physician. Stop use and consult a physician if the condition persists or gets worse, or if a rash or other allergic reaction develops. Do not use if you are allergic to any of the ingredients. Do not use longer than 1 week unless directed by a physician. KEEP THIS AND ALL DRUGS OUT OF THE REACH OF CHILDREN. In case of accidental ingestion, seek professional assistance or contact a Poison Control Center immediately

**How Supplied:** Tubes, ¹/₂ oz (14.2 g) with applicator tip, 1 oz (28.3 g); ¹/₃₂ oz (0.9 g) foil packets packed in cartons of 144.
Store at 59° to 77°F.
*Shown in Product Identification Guide, page 520*

## POLYSPORIN® Powder
[pŏl 'ē-spō 'rŭn ]

**Each Gram Contains:** Polymyxin B Sulfate 10,000 units and Bacitracin Zinc 500 units in a Lactose Base.

**Indications:** First aid to help prevent infection in minor cuts, scrapes, and burns.

**Directions:** Clean the affected area. Apply a light dusting of the powder on the area 1 to 3 times daily. May be covered with a sterile bandage.

**Warnings:** For external use only. Do not use in the eyes or apply over large areas of the body. In case of deep or puncture wounds, animal bites, or serious burns, consult a physician. Stop use and consult a physician if the condition persists or gets worse, or if a rash or other allergic reaction develops. Do not use if you are allergic to any of the ingredients. Do not use longer than 1 week unless directed by a physician. KEEP THIS AND ALL DRUGS OUT OF THE REACH OF CHILDREN. In case of accidental ingestion, seek professional assistance or contact a Poison Control Center immediately.

**How Supplied:** 0.35 oz (10 g) shaker-vial.
Store at 15° to 25°C (59° to 77°F). Do not store under refrigeration.
*Shown in Product Identification Guide, page 520*

## ROLAIDS® Antacid Tablets
Original Peppermint, Spearmint, and Cherry

**Active Ingredients:** Calcium Carbonate 550 mg and Magnesium Hydroxide 110 mg per tablet.

**Inactive Ingredients:** *Peppermint and Spearmint Flavors:* Dextrose, Flavoring, Magnesium Stearate, Polyethylene Glycol, Pregelatinized Starch and Sucrose.

*Cherry Flavor:* Dextrose, Flavoring, Magnesium Stearate, Polyethylene Glycol, Pregelatinized Starch, D&C Red No. 27 Aluminum Lake, and Sucrose.

**Indications:** For the relief of heartburn, sour stomach or acid indigestion and upset stomach due to these symptoms.

**Actions:** Rolaids® provides rapid neutralization of stomach acid. Each tablet has an acid-neutralizing capacity of 14.7 mEq and the ability to maintain the pH of stomach contents at 3.5 or greater for a significant period of time.

**Warnings:** Do not take more than 12 tablets in a 24 hour period or use the maximum dosage of this product for more than 2 weeks except under the advice and supervision of a physician. KEEP THIS AND ALL DRUGS OUT OF THE REACH OF CHILDREN.

**Drug Interaction Precaution:** Antacids may interact with certain prescription drugs. If you are presently taking a prescription drug, do not take this product without checking with your physician or other health professional.

**Dosage and Administration:** Chew 2 to 4 tablets as symptoms occur. Repeat hourly if symptoms return, or as directed by a physician.

**How Supplied:** Rolaids® is available in 12-tablet rolls, 3-packs containing three 12-tablet rolls and in bottles containing 150 or 300 tablets.
*Shown in Product Identification Guide, page 520*

## EXTRA STRENGTH ROLAIDS®
Antacid Tablets
Freshmint and Fruit Flavors

**Active Ingredients:** Calcium Carbonate 675 mg and Magnesium Hydroxide 135 mg per tablet.

**Inactive Ingredients:** *Freshmint Flavor:* Dextrose, Flavoring, Magnesium Stearate, Polyethylene Glycol, Pregelatinized Starch and Sucrose.

*Fruit Flavor:* Dextrose, Flavoring, Magnesium Stearate, Polyethylene Glycol, Pregelatinized Starch, Sucrose and FD & C Yellow No. 5 Aluminum Lake (tartrazine).

**Indications:** For the relief of heartburn, sour stomach or acid indigestion and upset stomach due to these symptoms.

**Actions:** Extra Strength Rolaids® provides rapid neutralization of stomach acid. Each tablet has an acid-neutralizing capacity of 18.2 mEq and the ability to maintain the pH of stomach contents at 3.5 or greater for a significant period of time.

**Warnings:** Do not take more than 10 tablets in a 24 hour period or use the maximum dosage of this product for more than 2 weeks except under the advice of and supervision of a physician. KEEP THIS AND ALL DRUGS OUT OF THE REACH OF CHILDREN.

**Drug Interaction Precaution:** Antacids may interact with certain prescription drugs. If you are presently taking a prescription drug, do not take this product without checking with your physician or other health professional.

**Dosage and Administration:** Chew 2 to 4 tablets as symptoms occur. Repeat hourly if symptoms return, or as directed by a physician.

**How Supplied:** Extra Strength Rolaids® is available in 10-tablet rolls, 3-packs containing three 10-tablet rolls and in bottle containing 100 and 250 tablets.

*Shown in Product Identification Guide, page 520*

---

## SINUTAB® Non-Drying Liquid Caps
[sîn 'ū tăb ]

### Drug Facts:

**Active Ingredients:**          **Purposes:**
**(in each liquid cap)**
Guaifenesin
  200 mg ................................ Expectorant
Pseudoephedrine
  HCl 30 mg ........... Nasal decongestant

### Uses:
- temporarily relieves nasal congestion associated with sinusitis
- helps loosen phlegm (mucus) and thin bronchial secretions to drain bronchial passageways of bothersome mucus and make coughs more productive

### Warnings:
**Do not use** if you are now taking a prescription monoamine oxidase inhibitor (MAOI) (certain drugs for depression, psychiatric, or emotional conditions, or Parkinson's disease), or for 2 weeks after stopping the MAOI drug. If you do not know if your prescription drug contains an MAOI, ask a doctor or pharmacist before taking this product.

**Ask a doctor before use if you have:**
- heart disease
- high blood pressure
- thyroid disease
- diabetes
- trouble urinating due to an enlarged prostate gland
- persistent or chronic cough such as occurs with smoking, asthma, chronic bronchitis, or emphysema
- cough occurs with too much phlegm (mucus)

**When using this product:**
- **do not use more than directed**

**Stop use and ask a doctor if:**
- you get nervous, dizzy, or sleepless
- symptoms do not improve within 7 days or are accompanied by fever
- cough persists for more than 1 week, tends to recur, or is accompanied by a fever, rash, or persistent headache. These could be signs of a serious condition.

**If pregnant or breast-feeding,** ask a health professional before use.

**Keep out of reach of children.** In case of overdose, get medical help or contact a Poison Control Center right away.

### Directions:
- adults and children 12 years of age and over: 2 liquid caps
- children under 12 years of age: ask a doctor
- take every 4 hours
- do not take more than 8 liquid caps in 24 hours

### Other Information:
- store at 59° to 77° F
- protect from heat, humidity, and light

**Inactive Ingredients:** FD&C blue no. 1, gelatin, glycerin, polyethylene glycol 400, povidone, propylene glycol, and sorbitol. Printed with edible white ink.

**Questions?** Call **1-800-223-0182,** Monday to Friday, 9 AM–5 PM EST

**How Supplied:** Sinutab® Non-Drying supplied in a box of 24 liquid caps.

*Shown in Product Identification Guide, page 520*

---

## SINUTAB® Sinus Allergy Medication, Maximum Strength Formula, Caplets
[sîn 'ū tăb ]

### Drug Facts:

**Active Ingredients:**
**(in each caplet)**[+]          **Purposes:**
Acetaminophen 500 mg .... Pain reliever
Chlorpheniramine maleate
  2 mg ........................ Antihistamine
Pseudoephedrine HCl
  30 mg ...................... Nasal decongestant

---

[+]Dissolution differs from USP specification.

**Uses:** Temporarily relieves these symptoms of hay fever or other upper respiratory allergies:
- runny nose
- sneezing
- itchy, watery eyes
- itching of the nose or throat
- headache
- minor aches and pains
- nasal congestion

### Warnings:
**Alcohol warning:** If you consume 3 or more alcoholic drinks every day, ask your doctor whether you should take acetaminophen or other pain relievers/fever reducers. Acetaminophen may cause liver damage.

**Do not use:**
- with any other product containing acetaminophen
- if you are now taking a prescription monoamine oxidase inhibitor (MAOI) (certain drugs for depression, psychiatric, or emotional conditions, or Parkinson's disease), or for 2 weeks after stopping the MAOI drug. If you do not know if your prescription drug contains an MAOI, ask a doctor or pharmacist before taking this product.

**Ask a doctor before use if you have:**
- glaucoma

- high blood pressure
- heart disease
- thyroid disease
- diabetes
- trouble urinating due to an enlarged prostate gland
- a breathing problem such as emphysema or chronic bronchitis

**Ask a doctor or pharmacist before use if you are** taking sedatives or tranquilizers

**When using this product:**
- **do not use more than directed**
- drowsiness may occur
- excitability may occur, especially in children
- avoid alcoholic drinks
- alcohol, sedatives, and tranquilizers may increase drowsiness
- be careful when driving a motor vehicle or operating machinery

**Stop use and ask a doctor if:**
- you get nervous, dizzy, or sleepless
- new symptoms occur
- symptoms do not get better
- you need to use more than 10 days
- fever occurs and lasts more than 3 days

**If pregnant or breast-feeding,** ask a health professional before use.

**Keep out of reach of children.** In case of overdose, get medical help or contact a Poison Control Center right away. Quick medical attention is critical for adults as well as for children even if you do not notice any signs or symptoms.

### Directions:
- adults and children 12 years of age and over: 2 caplets
- children under 12 years of age: ask a doctor
- take every 6 hours while symptoms persist
- do not take more than 8 caplets in 24 hours or as directed by a doctor

### Other Information:
- store at 59° to 77°F in a dry place

**Inactive Ingredients:** Calcium stearate, croscarmellose sodium, crospovidone, D&C yellow no. 10 aluminum lake, FD&C yellow no. 6 aluminum lake, hydroxypropyl methylcellulose, microcrystalline cellulose, polyethylene glycol, polysorbate 80, povidone, pregelatinized starch, stearic acid, and titanium dioxide

**Questions?** call **1-800-223-0182,** Monday to Friday, 9 AM – 5 PM EST

**How Supplied:** Sinutab® Sinus Allergy Medication, Maximum Strength Formula Caplets are supplied in child-resistant blister packs in boxes of 24 tablets or caplets.

*Shown in Product Identification Guide, page 520*

*Continued on next page*

---

*This product information was prepared in November 2001. On these and other Pfizer Consumer Healthcare Products, detailed information may be obtained by addressing Pfizer Consumer Healthcare, Pfizer, Inc., Morris Plains, NJ 07950*

## SINUTAB® Sinus Medication, Maximum Strength Without Drowsiness Formula, Caplets (also available in Tablets)
[sĭn 'ū tăb ]

**Drug Facts:**

**Active Ingredients:**
(in each caplet)                    **Purposes:**
Acetaminophen 500 mg ... Pain reliever
Pseudoephedrine
   HCl 30 mg ............ Nasal decongestant

**Uses:**
• temporarily relieves nasal congestion associated with sinusitis
• temporarily relieves headache, minor aches, and pains

**Warnings:**
**Alcohol warning:** If you consume 3 or more alcoholic drinks every day, ask your doctor whether you should take acetaminophen or other pain relievers/fever reducers. Acetaminophen may cause liver damage.
**Do not use:**
• with any other product containing acetaminophen
• if you are now taking a prescription monoamine oxidase inhibitor (MAOI) (certain drugs for depression, psychiatric, or emotional conditions, or Parkinson's disease), or for 2 weeks after stopping the MAOI drug. If you do not know if your prescription drug contains an MAOI, ask a doctor or pharmacist before taking this product.
**Ask a doctor before use if you have:**
• heart disease
• high blood pressure
• thyroid disease
• diabetes
• trouble urinating due to an enlarged prostate gland
**When using this product:**
• do not use more than directed
**Stop use and ask a doctor if:**
• you get nervous, dizzy, or sleepless
• new symptoms occur
• symptoms do not get better
• you need to use more than 10 days
• fever occurs and lasts more than 3 days
**If pregnant or breast-feeding,** ask a health professional before use.
**Keep out of reach of children.** In case of overdose, get medical help or contact a Poison Control Center right away. Quick medical attention is critical for adults as well as for children even if you do not notice any signs or symptoms.

**Directions:**
• adults and children 12 years of age and over: 2 caplets
• children under 12 years of age: ask a doctor
• take every 6 hours while symptoms persist
• do not take more than 8 caplets in 24 hours or as directed by a doctor

**Other Information:**
• store at 59° to 77°F in a dry place
**Inactive Ingredients:** Calcium stearate, croscarmellose sodium, crospovidone, FD&C yellow no. 6 aluminum lake, hydroxypropyl methylcellulose, microcrystalline cellulose, polyethylene glycol, polysorbate 80, povidone, pregelatinized starch, stearic acid, and titanium dioxide

**Questions?** call **1-800-223-0182,** Monday to Friday, 9 AM – 5 PM EST
**How Supplied:** Sinutab® Sinus Medication, Maximum Strength Without Drowsiness Formula, Caplets and Tablets are supplied in child-resistant blister packs in boxes of 24 tablets or caplets.
*Shown in Product Identification Guide, page 520*

---

## SUDAFED® 12 Hour Long-Acting Nasal Decongestant Non-Drowsy MS Tablets
[sū 'duh-fĕd ]
*Capsule-shaped Tablets

**Drug Facts:**

**Active Ingredient:**
(in each tablet)                    **Purpose:**
Pseudoephedrine
   HCl 120 mg ........... Nasal decongestant

**Uses:**
• temporarily relieves nasal congestion due to the common cold, hay fever or other upper respiratory allergies, and nasal congestion associated with sinusitis
• temporarily relieves sinus congestion and pressure

**Warnings:**
**Do not use** if you are now taking a prescription monoamine oxidase inhibitor (MAOI) (certain drugs for depression, psychiatric, or emotional conditions, or Parkinson's disease), or for 2 weeks after stopping the MAOI drug. If you do not know if your prescription drug contains an MAOI, ask a doctor or pharmacist before taking this product.
**Ask a doctor before use if you have:**
• heart disease
• high blood pressure
• thyroid disease
• diabetes
• trouble urinating due to an enlarged prostate gland
**When using this product:**
• do not use more than directed
**Stop use and ask a doctor if:**
• you get nervous, dizzy, or sleepless
• symptoms do not improve within 7 days or are accompanied by fever
**If pregnant or breast-feeding,** ask a health professional before use.
**Keep out of reach of children.** In case of overdose, get medical help or contact a Poison Control Center right away.

**Directions:**
• adults and children 12 years of age and over: one tablet every 12 hours not to exceed two tablets in 24 hours
• children under 12 years of age: use of product not recommended

**Other Information:**
• store at 59° to 77°F in a dry place
• protect from light
**Inactive Ingredients:** hydroxypropyl methylcellulose, magnesium stearate, microcrystalline cellulose, polyethylene glycol, povidone, and titanium dioxide. May also contain: candelilla wax or carnauba wax. Printed with edible blue ink.

**Questions?** call **1-800-524-2624** (English/Spanish), weekdays, 9 AM–5 PM EST
**How Supplied:** Boxes of 10 and 20.
*Shown in Product Identification Guide, page 521*

---

## SUDAFED® 24 Hour Tablets Non-Drowsy
[sū 'duh-fĕd]

**Drug Facts:**

**Active Ingredient:**
(in each tablet)                    **Purpose:**
Pseudoephedrine
   HCl 240 mg ........... Nasal decongestant

**Uses:**
• temporarily relieves nasal congestion due to the common cold, hay fever or other upper respiratory allergies, and nasal congestion associated with sinusitis
• reduces swelling of nasal passages
• relieves sinus pressure

**Warnings:**
**Do not use** if you are now taking a prescription monoamine oxidase inhibitor (MAOI) (certain drugs for depression, psychiatric, or emotional conditions, or Parkinson's disease), or for 2 weeks after stopping the MAOI drug. If you do not know if your prescription drug contains an MAOI, ask a doctor or pharmacist before taking this product.
**Ask a doctor before use if you have:**
• heart disease
• high blood pressure
• thyroid disease
• trouble urinating due to an enlarged prostate gland
• diabetes
• had obstruction or narrowing of the bowel. Rarely, tablets of this kind may cause bowel obstruction (blockage), usually in people with severe narrowing of the bowel (esophagus, stomach or intestine).
**When using this product:**
• do not use more than directed
**Stop use and ask a doctor if:**
• you get nervous, dizzy, or sleepless
• symptoms do not improve within 7 days or are accompanied by fever
• you experience persistent abdominal pain or vomiting
**If pregnant or breast-feeding,** ask a health professional before use.
**Keep out of reach of children.** In case of overdose, get medical help or contact a Poison Control Center right away.

**Directions:**
• adults and children 12 years of age and over: **swallow one** whole tablet with fluid every 24 hours
• **do not exceed one tablet in 24 hours**
• **do not divide, crush, chew or dissolve the tablet**
• the tablet does not completely dissolve and may be seen in the stool (this is normal)
• not for use in children under 12 years of age

**Other Information:**
• store at 59° to 77°F in a dry place

**Inactive Ingredients:** Cellulose, cellulose acetate, hydroxypropyl cellulose, hydroxypropyl methylcellulose, magnesium stearate, polyethylene glycol, polysorbate 80, povidone, sodium chloride, and titanium dioxide

**Questions?** call **1-800-524-2624** (English/Spanish), weekdays, 9 AM – 5 PM EST

**How Supplied:** Box of 5 tablets and 10 tablets. **BLISTER PACKAGED FOR YOUR PROTECTION. DO NOT USE IF INDIVIDUAL SEALS ARE BROKEN.**

*Shown in Product Identification Guide, page 521*

---

## SUDAFED® Cold & Cough Liquid Caps
[sū 'duh-fĕd ]

**Drug Facts:**

**Active Ingredients:** Purposes:
**(in each liquid cap)**
Acetaminophen
  250 mg ..... Pain reliever/fever reducer
Dextromethorphan
  HBr 10 mg ............. Cough suppressant
Guaifenesin 100 mg ............ Expectorant
Pseudoephedrine HCl
  30 mg ...................... Nasal decongestant

**Uses:**
* temporarily relieves these symptoms due to the common cold:
  * nasal congestion
  * headache
  * minor aches and pains
  * muscular aches
  * fever
  * sore throat
  * cough
* helps loosen phlegm (mucus) and thin bronchial secretions to drain bronchial tubes and make coughs more productive

**Warnings:**
**Alcohol warning:** If you consume 3 or more alcoholic drinks every day, ask your doctor whether you should take acetaminophen or other pain relievers/fever reducers. Acetaminophen may cause liver damage.
**Do not use:**
* with any other product containing acetaminophen
* if you are now taking a prescription monoamine oxidase inhibitor (MAOI) (certain drugs for depression, psychiatric, or emotional conditions, or Parkinson's disease), or for 2 weeks after stopping the MAOI drug. If you do not know if your prescription drug contains an MAOI, ask a doctor or pharmacist before taking this product.
**Ask a doctor before use if you have:**
* heart disease
* thyroid disease
* diabetes
* high blood pressure
* trouble urinating due to an enlarged prostate gland
* cough accompanied by excessive phlegm (mucus)

* persistent or chronic cough such as occurs with smoking, asthma, chronic bronchitis, or emphysema
**When using this product:**
* **do not use more than directed**
**Stop use and ask a doctor if:**
* new symptoms occur
* redness or swelling is present
* symptoms do not improve
* sore throat is severe
* you get nervous, dizzy, or sleepless
* sore throat lasts for more than 2 days, is accompanied or followed by fever, headache, rash, swelling, nausea, or vomiting
* you need to use more than 10 days
* cough persists for more than 7 days, tends to recur, or is accompanied by rash, persistent headache, fever that lasts more than 3 days. These could be signs of a serious condition.
**If pregnant or breast-feeding,** ask a health professional before use.
**Keep out of reach of children.** In case of overdose, get medical help or contact a Poison Control Center right away. Quick medical attention is critical for adults as well as for children even if you do not notice any signs or symptoms.

**Directions:**
* adults and children 12 years of age and over: 2 liquid caps
* take every 4 hours while symptoms persist
* do not take more than 8 liquid caps in 24 hours, or as directed by a doctor
* children under 12 years of age: ask a doctor

**Other Information:**
* store at 59° to 77°F in a dry place

**Inactive Ingredients:** D&C yellow no. 10, FD&C red no. 40, gelatin, glycerin, polyethylene glycol 400, povidone, propylene glycol, purified water, and sorbitol. Printed with edible white ink.

**Questions?** call **1-800-524-2624** (English/Spanish), weekdays, 9 AM – 5 PM EST

**How Supplied:** Boxes of 10 and 20.
*Shown in Product Identification Guide, page 520*

---

## SUDAFED® Non-Drowsy MS Nasal Decongestant 30-mg Tablets
[sū 'duh-fĕd ]

**Drug Facts:**

**Active Ingredient:**
**(in each tablet)** Purpose:
Pseudoephedrine HCl
  30 mg ...................... Nasal decongestant

**Uses:**
* temporarily relieves nasal congestion due to the common cold, hay fever or other upper respiratory allergies, and nasal congestion associated with sinusitis
* temporarily relieves sinus congestion and pressure

**Warnings:**
**Do not use** if you are now taking a prescription monoamine oxidase inhibitor (MAOI) (certain drugs for depression, psychiatric, or emotional conditions, or Parkinson's disease), or for 2 weeks after stopping the MAOI drug. If you do not know if your prescription drug contains an MAOI, ask a doctor or pharmacist before taking this product.

**Ask a doctor before use if you have:**
* heart disease
* high blood pressure
* thyroid disease
* diabetes
* trouble urinating due to an enlarged prostate gland
**When using this product:**
* **do not use more than directed**
**Stop use and ask a doctor if:**
* you get nervous, dizzy, or sleepless
* symptoms do not improve within 7 days or are accompanied by fever
**If pregnant or breast-feeding,** ask a health professional before use.
**Keep out of reach of children.** In case of overdose, get medical help or contact a Poison Control Center right away.

**Directions:**
* take every 4 to 6 hours
* do not take more than 4 doses in 24 hours

| | |
|---|---|
| adults and children 12 years of age and over | 2 tablets |
| children 6 to under 12 years of age | 1 tablet |
| children under 6 years of age | ask a doctor |

**Other Information:**
* store at 59° to 77°F in a dry place

**Inactive Ingredients:** Acacia, candelilla wax, corn starch, FD&C red no. 40 aluminum lake, FD&C yellow no. 6 aluminum lake, hydroxypropyl methylcellulose, lactose, magnesium stearate, pharmaceutical glaze, poloxamer 407, polyethylene glycol, polyethylene oxide, polysorbate 60, povidone, sodium benzoate, sodium lauryl sulfate, stearic acid, sucrose, and titanium dioxide. Printed with edible black ink.

**Questions?** call **1-800-524-2624** (English/Spanish), weekdays, 9 AM – 5 PM EST

**How Supplied:** Boxes of 24, 48 and 96.
*Shown in Product Identification Guide, page 520*

*Continued on next page*

*This product information was prepared in November 2001. On these and other Pfizer Consumer Healthcare Products, detailed information may be obtained by addressing Pfizer Consumer Healthcare, Pfizer, Inc., Morris Plains, NJ 07950*

## SUDAFED® NON-DRYING, NON-DROWSY MS LIQUID CAPS
[sū 'duh-fĕd ]

**Drug Facts:**

**Active Ingredients:**     **Purposes:**
**(in each liquid cap)**
Guaifenesin 200 mg ............ Expectorant
Pseudoephedrine
  HCl 30 mg ............. Nasal decongestant

**Uses:**
- temporarily relieves nasal congestion associated with sinusitis
- promotes nasal and/or sinus drainage
- temporarily relieves sinus congestion and pressure
- helps loosen phlegm (mucus) and thin bronchial secretions to rid the bronchial passageways of bothersome mucus and make coughs more productive

**Warnings:**
**Do not use** if you are now taking a prescription monoamine oxidase inhibitor (MAOI) (certain drugs for depression, psychiatric, or emotional conditions, or Parkinson's disease), or for 2 weeks after stopping the MAOI drug. If you do not know if your prescription drug contains an MAOI, ask a doctor or pharmacist before taking this product.
**Ask a doctor before use if you have:**
- heart disease
- high blood pressure
- thyroid disease
- diabetes
- trouble urinating due to an enlarged prostate gland
- cough that occurs with too much phlegm (mucus)
- persistent or chronic cough such as occurs with smoking, asthma, chronic bronchitis, or emphysema
**When using this product:**
- **do not use more than directed**
**Stop use and ask a doctor if:**
- you get nervous, dizzy, or sleepless
- symptoms do not improve within 7 days or are accompanied by fever
- cough persists for more than 1 week, tends to recur, or is accompanied by a fever, rash, or persistent headache. These could be signs of a serious condition.
**If pregnant or breast-feeding**, ask a health professional before use.
**Keep out of reach of children.** In case of overdose, get medical help or contact a Poison Control Center right away.

**Directions:**
- adults and children 12 years of age and over: swallow 2 liquid caps
- take every 4 hours
- do not exceed 8 liquid caps in 24 hours
- children under 12 years of age: ask a doctor

**Other Information:**
- store at 59° to 77°F
- protect from heat, humidity, and light

**Inactive Ingredients:** FD&C blue no. 1, gelatin, glycerin, polyethylene glycol 400, povidone, propylene glycol, and sorbitol. Printed with edible white ink.

**Questions?** call **1-800-524-2624** (English/Spanish), weekdays, 9 AM - 5 PM EST

**How Supplied:** Sudafed Non-Drying Sinus is supplied in boxes of 24 liquid caps.

*Shown in Product Identification Guide, page 520*

## SUDAFED® Severe Cold Caplets
(Formerly Sudafed Severe Cold Formula)
[sū 'duh-fĕd]

**Drug Facts:**

**Active Ingredients:**     **Purpose:**
**(in each caplet)**
Acetaminophen
  500 mg ...... Pain reliever/fever reducer
Dextromethorphan HBr
  15 mg .................................... Antitussive
Pseudoephedrine HCl
  30 mg ..................... Nasal decongestant

**Uses:**
- temporarily relieves these symptoms due to the common cold:
  - nasal congestion
  - headache
  - minor aches and pains
  - muscular aches
  - cough
  - sore throat
  - fever

**Warnings:**
**Alcohol warning:** If you consume 3 or more alcoholic drinks every day, ask your doctor whether you should take acetaminophen or other pain relievers/fever reducers. Acetaminophen may cause liver damage.
**Do not use:**
- with any other product containing acetaminophen
- if you are now taking a prescription monoamine oxidase inhibitor (MAOI) (certain drugs for depression, psychiatric, or emotional conditions, or Parkinson's disease), or for 2 weeks after stopping the MAOI drug. If you do not know if your prescription drug contains an MAOI, ask a doctor or pharmacist before taking this product.
**Ask a doctor before use if you have:**
- heart disease
- thyroid disease
- diabetes
- high blood pressure
- trouble urinating due to an enlarged prostate gland
- cough accompanied by excessive phlegm (mucus)
- persistent or chronic cough as occurs with smoking, asthma, or emphysema
**When using this product:**
- **do not use more than directed**
**Stop use and ask a doctor if:**
- new symptoms occur
- sore throat is severe
- you get nervous, dizzy, or sleepless
- symptoms do not get better
- you need to use more than 10 days
- redness or swelling is present
- fever gets worse or lasts more than 3 days
- cough persists for more than 7 days, tends to recur, or is accompanied by rash, or persistent headache. These could be signs of a serious condition.
- sore throat lasts for more than 2 days, is accompanied or followed by fever, headache, rash, swelling, nausea, or vomiting
**If pregnant or breast-feeding**, ask a health professional before use.
**Keep out of reach of children.** In case of overdose, get medical help or contact a Poison Control Center right away. Quick medical attention is critical for adults as

well as for children even if you do not notice any signs or symptoms.

**Directions:**
- adults and children 12 years of age and over: 2 caplets
- children under 12 years of age: ask a doctor
- take every 6 hours while symptoms persist
- do not take more than 8 caplets in 24 hours or as directed by a doctor

**Other Information:**
- store at 59° to 77°F in a dry place

**Inactive Ingredients:** Carnauba wax, crospovidone, hydroxypropyl methylcellulose, magnesium stearate, microcrystalline cellulose, polyethylene glycol, polyethylene oxide, povidone, pregelatinized starch, stearic acid, and titanium dioxide

**Questions?** call toll free **1-800-524-2624,** Monday to Friday, 9 AM – 5 PM EST

**How Supplied:** Boxes of 12 and 24 caplets; boxes of 12 tablets.
*Shown in Product Identification Guide, page 521*

## SUDAFED® Sinus & Allergy Tablets
(Formerly Cold & Allergy)
[sū 'duh-fĕd ]

**Drug Facts:**

**Active Ingredients:**     **Purposes:**
**(in each tablet)**
Chlorpheniramine maleate
  4 mg ............................... Antihistamine
Pseudoephedrine HCl
  60 mg .................... Nasal decongestant

**Uses:**
- temporarily relieves these symptoms due to hay fever (allergic rhinitis) or other upper respiratory allergies:
  - runny nose
  - sneezing
  - itchy, watery eyes
  - nasal congestion
  - itching of the nose or throat
- temporarily relieves these symptoms due to the common cold:
  - runny nose
  - sneezing
  - nasal congestion

**Warnings:**
**Do not use** if you are now taking a prescription monoamine oxidase inhibitor (MAOI) (certain drugs for depression, psychiatric, or emotional conditions, or Parkinson's disease), or for 2 weeks after stopping the MAOI drug. If you do not know if your prescription drug contains an MAOI, ask a doctor or pharmacist before taking this product.
**Ask a doctor before use if you have:**
- high blood pressure
- thyroid disease
- heart disease
- glaucoma
- diabetes
- trouble urinating due to an enlarged prostate gland
- a breathing problem such as emphysema or chronic bronchitis
**Ask a doctor or pharmacist before use if you are** taking sedatives or tranquilizers
**When using this product:**
- **do not use more than directed**
- drowsiness may occur

- excitability may occur, especially in children
- avoid alcoholic drinks
- alcohol, sedatives, and tranquilizers may increase drowsiness
- be careful when driving a motor vehicle or operating machinery

**Stop use and ask a doctor if:**
- you get nervous, dizzy, or sleepless
- symptoms do not improve within 7 days or are accompanied by fever

**If pregnant or breast-feeding**, ask a health professional before use.

**Keep out of reach of children.** In case of overdose, get medical help or contact a Poison Control Center right away.

**Directions:**
- take every 4 to 6 hours
- do not take more than 4 doses in 24 hours

| adults and children 12 years of age and over | 1 tablet |
| --- | --- |
| children 6 to under 12 years of age | ½ tablet |
| children under 6 years of age | ask a doctor |

**Other Information:**
- store at 59° to 77°F in a dry place

**Inactive Ingredients:** Lactose, magnesium stearate, potato starch, and povidone

**Questions?** call **1-800-524-2624** (English/Spanish), weekdays, 9 AM–5 PM EST

**How Supplied:** Boxes of 24 tablets.
*Shown in Product Identification Guide, page 520*

---

## SUDAFED® SINUS & COLD
### (Formerly Cold & Sinus)
### Liquid Caps
[sū 'duh-fed]

**Drug Facts:**

**Active Ingredients:**
**(in each liquid cap)**      **Purposes:**
Acetaminophen
   325 mg .... Pain reliever/fever reducer
Pseudoephedrine HCl
   30 mg ................... Nasal decongestant

**Uses:**
- temporarily relieves these symptoms due to the common cold:
  - nasal congestion
  - headache
  - minor aches and pains
  - muscular aches
  - sore throat
  - fever
  - temporarily restores freer breathing through the nose
  - temporarily relieves sinus congestion and pressure

**Warnings:**
**Alcohol warning:** If you consume 3 or more alcoholic drinks every day, ask your doctor whether you should take acetaminophen or other pain relievers/fever reducers. Acetaminophen may cause liver damage.

**Do not use:**
- with any other product containing acetaminophen
- if you are now taking a prescription monoamine oxidase inhibitor (MAOI) (certain drugs for depression, psychiatric, or emotional conditions, or Parkinson's disease), or for 2 weeks after stopping the MAOI drug. If you do not know if your prescription drug contains an MAOI, ask a doctor or pharmacist before taking this product.

**Ask a doctor before use if you have:**
- heart disease
- thyroid disease
- diabetes
- high blood pressure
- trouble urinating due to an enlarged prostate gland

**When using this product:**
- do not use more than directed

**Stop use and ask a doctor if:**
- redness or swelling is present
- you get nervous, dizzy, or sleepless
- new symptoms occur
- you need to use more than 10 days
- symptoms do not improve
- fever gets worse or lasts more than 3 days
- sore throat is severe
- sore throat lasts for more than 2 days, is accompanied or followed by fever, headache, rash, swelling, nausea, or vomiting

**If pregnant or breast-feeding,** ask a health professional before use.

**Keep out of reach of children.** In case of overdose, get medical help or contact a Poison Control Center right away. Quick medical attention is critical for adults as well as for children even if you do not notice any signs or symptoms.

**Directions:**
- adults and children 12 years of age and over: 2 liquid caps
- take every 4 to 6 hours while symptoms persist
- do not take more than 8 liquid caps in 24 hours, or as directed by a doctor
- children under 12 years of age: ask a doctor

**Other Information:**
- store at 59° to 77°F
- protect from heat, humidity, and light

**Inactive Ingredients:** FD&C blue no. 1, FD&C red no. 40, gelatin, glycerin, polyethylene glycol, povidone, sodium acetate, and sorbitol. Printed with edible white ink.

**Questions?** call **1-800-524-2624** (English/Spanish), weekdays, 9 AM – 5 PM EST

**How Supplied:** Boxes of 10 and 20 liquid caps.
*Shown in Product Identification Guide, page 520*

---

## SUDAFED® Sinus Headache Caplets and Tablets
[sū 'duh-fĕd ]

**Drug Facts:**

**Active Ingredients:**
**(in each caplet)**      **Purposes:**
Acetaminophen 500 mg .... Pain reliever
Pseudoephedrine
   HCl 30 mg ........... Nasal decongestant

**Uses:**
- temporarily relieves nasal congestion associated with sinusitis
- temporarily relieves headache, minor aches, and pains

**Warnings:**
**Alcohol warning:** If you consume 3 or more alcoholic drinks every day, ask your doctor whether you should take acetaminophen or other pain relievers/fever reducers. Acetaminophen may cause liver damage.

**Do not use:**
- with any other product containing acetaminophen
- if you are now taking a prescription monoamine oxidase inhibitor (MAOI) (certain drugs for depression, psychiatric, or emotional conditions, or Parkinson's disease), or for 2 weeks after stopping the MAOI drug. If you do not know if your prescription drug contains an MAOI, ask a doctor or pharmacist before taking this product.

**Ask a doctor before use if you have:**
- heart disease
- thyroid disease
- diabetes
- high blood pressure
- trouble urinating due to an enlarged prostate gland

**When using this product:**
- do not use more than directed

**Stop use and ask a doctor if:**
- you get nervous, dizzy, or sleepless
- new symptoms occur
- symptoms do not get better
- you need to use more than 10 days
- fever occurs and lasts for more than 3 days

**If pregnant or breast-feeding,** ask a health professional before use.

**Keep out of reach of children.** In case of overdose, get medical help or contact a Poison Control Center right away. Quick medical attention is critical for adults as well as for children even if you do not notice any signs or symptoms.

**Directions:**
- children under 12 years of age: ask a doctor
- adults and children 12 years of age and over: 2 caplets every 6 hours while symptoms persist
- do not take more than 8 caplets in 24 hours or as directed by a doctor

**Other Information:**
- store at 59° to 77°F in a dry place

**Inactive Ingredients:** crospovidone, FD&C yellow no. 6 aluminum lake, hydroxypropyl methylcellulose, microcrystalline cellulose, polyethylene glycol, polysorbate 80, povidone, pregelatinized starch, stearic acid and titanium dioxide may also contain: calcium stearate, carnauba wax, croscarmellose sodium and magnesium stearate.

*Continued on next page*

---

*This product information was prepared in November 2001. On these and other Pfizer Consumer Healthcare Products, detailed information may be obtained by addressing Pfizer Consumer Healthcare, Pfizer, Inc., Morris Plains, NJ 07950*

## Sudafed Sinus—Cont.

**Questions?** call **1-800-524-2624** (English/Spanish), weekdays, 9 AM–5 PM EST

**How Supplied:** Boxes of 24 and 48 caplets; boxes of 24 tablets.

*Shown in Product Identification Guide, page 521*

## SUDAFED® SINUS NIGHTTIME
[sū' duh-fĕd]

### Drug Facts:

**Active Ingredients:**
**(in each tablet)**          **Purposes:**
Pseudoephedrine HCl
 60 mg ..................... Nasal decongestant
Triprolidine HCl
 2.5 mg ............................ Antihistamine

### Uses:
• temporarily relieves these symptoms of hay fever or other upper respiratory allergies:
  • runny nose
  • sneezing
  • nasal and sinus congestion
  • itchy, watery eyes
  • itching of the nose or throat
• temporarily relieves nasal and sinus congestion due to the common cold or associated with sinusitis

### Warnings:
**Do not use** if you are now taking a prescription monoamine oxidase inhibitor (MAOI) (certain drugs for depression, psychiatric, or emotional conditions, or Parkinson's disease), or for 2 weeks after stopping the MAOI drug. If you do not know if your prescription drug contains an MAOI, ask a doctor or pharmacist before taking this product.

**Ask a doctor before use if you have:**
• high blood pressure
• heart disease
• thyroid disease
• diabetes
• glaucoma
• trouble urinating due to an enlarged prostate gland
• a breathing problem such as emphysema or chronic bronchitis

**Ask a doctor or pharmacist before use if you are** taking sedatives or tranquilizers

**When using this product**
• **do not use more than directed**
• drowsiness may occur
• avoid alcoholic drinks
• alcohol, sedatives, and tranquilizers may increase drowsiness
• be careful when driving a motor vehicle or operating machinery
• excitability may occur, especially in children

**Stop use and ask a doctor if**
• you get nervous, dizzy, or sleepless
• symptoms do not improve within 7 days or are accompanied by fever

**If pregnant or breast-feeding,** ask a health professional before use.

**Keep out of reach of children.** In case of overdose, get medical help or contact a Poison Control Center right away.

### Directions:
• take every 4 to 6 hours
• do not take more than 4 doses in 24 hours

| | |
|---|---|
| adults and children 12 years of age and over | 1 tablet |
| children 6 to under 12 years of age | 1/2 tablet |
| children under 6 years of age | ask a doctor |

### Other Information:
• store at 59° to 77°F in a dry place
• protect from light

**Inactive Ingredients:** Flavor, hydroxypropyl methylcellulose, lactose, magnesium stearate, polyethylene glycol, potato starch, povidone, sucrose, and titanium dioxide

**Questions?** call **1-800-524-2624** (English/Spanish), weekdays, 9 AM–5 PM EST

**How Supplied:** Boxes of 12 tablets.

*Shown in Product Identification Guide, page 521*

## SUDAFED® Sinus Nighttime Plus Pain Relief
[sū'duh - fĕd]

### Drug Facts:

**Active Ingredients:**
**(in each caplet)**          **Purposes:**
Acetaminophen
 500 mg .............................. Pain reliever
Diphenhydramine HCl
 25 mg ............................. Antihistamine
Pseudoephedrine HCl
 30 mg .................... Nasal decongestant

### Uses:
• temporarily relieves these symptoms of hay fever, the common cold or other upper respiratory allergies:
  • runny nose
  • sneezing
  • nasal and sinus congestion
  • headache
  • minor aches and pains
• temporarily relieves these additional symptoms of hay fever or other upper respiratory allergies:
  • itching of the nose or throat
  • itchy, watery eyes
• temporarily relieves nasal and sinus congestion associated with sinusitis

### Warnings:
**Alcohol warning:** If you consume 3 or more alcoholic drinks every day, ask your doctor whether you should take acetaminophen or other pain relievers/fever reducers. Acetaminophen may cause liver damage.

**Do not use:**
• with any other product containing acetaminophen
• if you are now taking a prescription monoamine oxidase inhibitor (MAOI) (certain drugs for depression, psychiatric, or emotional conditions, or Parkinson's disease), or for 2 weeks after stopping the MAOI drug. If you do not know if your prescription drug contains an MAOI, ask a doctor or pharmacist before taking this product.
• with any other product containing diphenhydramine, including one applied topically

**Ask a doctor before use if you have:**
• heart disease
• glaucoma
• thyroid disease
• diabetes
• high blood pressure
• trouble urinating due to an enlarged prostate gland
• a breathing problem such as emphysema or chronic bronchitis

**Ask a doctor or pharmacist before use if you are** taking sedatives or tranquilizers

**When using this product:**
• **do not use more than directed**
• marked drowsiness may occur
• avoid alcoholic drinks
• alcohol, sedatives, and tranquilizers may increase drowsiness
• excitability may occur, especially in children
• be careful when driving a motor vehicle or operating machinery

**Stop use and ask a doctor if:**
• you get nervous, dizzy, or sleepless
• new symptoms occur
• fever occurs and lasts more than 3 days
• symptoms do not get better
• you need to use more than 10 days

**If pregnant or breast-feeding,** ask a health professional before use.

**Keep out of reach of children.** In case of overdose, get medical help or contact a Poison Control Center right away. Quick medical attention is critical for adults as well as for children even if you do not notice any signs or symptoms.

### Directions:
• take every 6 hours while symptoms persist
• do not take more than 8 caplets in 24 hours or as directed by a doctor
• adults and children 12 years of age and over: 2 caplets
• children under 12 years of age: ask a doctor

### Other Information:
• store at 59° to 77°F in a dry place

**Inactive Ingredients:** Carnauba wax, crospovidone, FD&C blue no. 1 aluminum lake, hydroxypropyl methylcellulose, magnesium stearate, microcrystalline cellulose, polyethylene glycol, polysorbate 80, povidone, pregelatinized starch, sodium starch glycolate, stearic acid, and titanium dioxide

**Questions?** call **1-800-524-2624** (English/Spanish), weekdays, 9 AM – 5 PM EST

**How Supplied:** Boxes of 20 caplets. Capsule shaped tablets.

*Shown in Product Identification Guide, page 521*

## CHILDREN'S SUDAFED®
**Cold & Cough Non-Drowsy Liquid**
[sū 'duh-fĕd]

### Drug Facts:

**Active Ingredients:**          **Purposes:**
**(in each 5 mL*)**
Dextromethorphan HBr
 5 mg ....................................... Antitussive

Pseudoephedrine HCl
15 mg ..................... Nasal decongestant

---

*5 mL = one teaspoonful

**Uses:**
- temporarily relieves nasal congestion due to the common cold
- temporarily quiets cough due to minor throat and bronchial irritation occurring with a cold or inhaled irritants

**Warnings:**
**Do not use** if you are now taking a prescription monoamine oxidase inhibitor (MAOI) (certain drugs for depression, psychiatric, or emotional conditions, or Parkinson's disease), or for 2 weeks after stopping the MAOI drug. If you do not know if your prescription drug contains an MAOI, ask a doctor or pharmacist before taking this product.
**Ask a doctor before use if you have:**
- heart disease
- thyroid disease
- diabetes
- high blood pressure
- trouble urinating due to an enlarged prostate gland
- cough accompanied by excessive phlegm (mucus)
- persistent or chronic cough such as occurs with smoking, asthma, or emphysema
**When using this product:**
- **do not use more than directed**
**Stop use and ask a doctor if:**
- you get nervous, dizzy, or sleepless
- symptoms do not improve within 7 days or are accompanied by fever
- cough persists for more than 1 week, tends to recur, or is accompanied by fever, rash, or persistent headache. These could be signs of a serious condition.
**If pregnant or breast-feeding,** ask a health professional before use.
**Keep out of reach of children.** In case of overdose, get medical help or contact a Poison Control Center right away.

**Directions:**
- take every 4 hours
- do not take more than 4 doses in 24 hours, or as directed by a doctor

| children under 2 years of age | ask a doctor |
|---|---|
| children 2 to under 6 years of age | one (1) teaspoonful |
| children 6 to under 12 years of age | two (2) teaspoonfuls |
| adults and children 12 years of age and over | four (4) teaspoonfuls |

**Other Information:**
- store at 59° to 77°F

**Inactive Ingredients:** Carboxymethylcellulose sodium, citric acid, D&C red no. 33, FD&C red no. 40, flavors, glycerin, poloxamer 407, polyethylene glycol 1450, purified water, saccharin sodium, sodium benzoate, sodium chloride, sodium citrate, and sorbitol solution

**Questions?** call **1-800-524-2624** (English/Spanish), weekdays, 9 AM–5 PM EST

**How Supplied:** Sudafed Children's Cold and Cough Non-Drowsy Liquid is supplied in 4 fl. oz. bottles.
*Shown in Product Identification Guide, page 521*

---

## CHILDREN'S SUDAFED®
**Nasal Decongestant Chewables**
[sū ' duh-fĕd ]

**Drug Facts:**

**Active Ingredient:**
**(in each tablet)**      **Purpose:**
Pseudoephedrine HCl
15 mg ..................... Nasal decongestant

**Uses:**
- temporarily relieves nasal congestion due to the common cold, hay fever or other upper respiratory allergies, and nasal congestion associated with sinusitis
- temporarily relieves sinus congestion and pressure
- promotes nasal and/or sinus drainage

**Warnings:**
**Do not use** if you are now taking a prescription monoamine oxidase inhibitor (MAOI) (certain drugs for depression, psychiatric, or emotional conditions, or Parkinson's disease), or for 2 weeks after stopping the MAOI drug. If you do not know if your prescription drug contains an MAOI, ask a doctor or pharmacist before taking this product.
**Ask a doctor before use if you have:**
- heart disease
- high blood pressure
- thyroid disease
- diabetes
- trouble urinating due to an enlarged prostate gland
**When using this product:**
- **do not use more than directed**
**Stop use and ask a doctor if:**
- you get nervous, dizzy, or sleepless
- symptoms do not improve within 7 days or are accompanied by fever
**If pregnant or breast-feeding,** ask a health professional before use.
**Keep out of reach of children.** In case of overdose, get medical help or contact a Poison Control Center right away.

**Directions:**
- take every 4 to 6 hours
- do not take more than 4 doses in 24 hours

| children under 2 years of age | ask a doctor |
|---|---|
| children 2 to under 6 years of age | one (1) chewable tablet |
| children 6 to under 12 years of age | two (2) chewable tablets |
| adults and children 12 years of age and over | four (4) chewable tablets |

**Other Information:**
- **phenylketonurics:** contains phenylalanine 0.78 mg per tablet
- store at 59° to 77°F in a dry place
- protect from light

**Inactive Ingredients:** Ascorbic acid, aspartame, carnauba wax, citric acid, crospovidone, FD&C yellow no. 6 aluminum lake, flavors, hydroxypropyl methylcellulose, magnesium stearate, mannitol, microcrystalline cellulose, sodium chloride, and tartaric acid

**Questions?** call **1-800-524-2624** (English/Spanish), weekdays, 9 AM – 5 PM EST

**How Supplied:** Box of 24 chewable tablets.
*Shown in Product Identification Guide, page 521*

---

## SUDAFED®
**CHILDREN'S NASAL DECONGESTANT LIQUID MEDICATION**
[sū 'duh-fĕd ]

**Drug Facts:**

**Active Ingredient:**
**(in each 5 mL*)**      **Purpose:**
Pseudoephedrine HCl
15 mg ..................... Nasal decongestant

---

*5 mL = one teaspoonful

**Uses:**
- temporarily relieves nasal congestion due to the common cold, hay fever or other upper respiratory allergies, and nasal congestion associated with sinusitis
- temporarily relieves sinus congestion and pressure
- promotes nasal and/or sinus drainage

**Warnings:**
**Do not use** if you are now taking a prescription monoamine oxidase inhibitor (MAOI) (certain drugs for depression, psychiatric, or emotional conditions, or Parkinson's disease), or for 2 weeks after stopping the MAOI drug. If you do not know if your prescription drug contains an MAOI, ask a doctor or pharmacist before taking this product.
**Ask a doctor before use if you have:**
- heart disease
- high blood pressure
- thyroid disease
- diabetes
- trouble urinating due to an enlarged prostate gland
**When using this product:**
- **do not use more than directed**
**Stop use and ask a doctor if:**
- you get nervous, dizzy, or sleepless
- symptoms do not improve within 7 days or are accompanied by fever

*Continued on next page*

---

***This product information was prepared in November 2001. On these and other Pfizer Consumer Healthcare Products, detailed information may be obtained by addressing Pfizer Consumer Healthcare, Pfizer, Inc., Morris Plains, NJ 07950***

## Sudafed Children's Nasal—Cont.

**If pregnant or breast-feeding,** ask a health professional before use.

**Keep out of reach of children.** In case of overdose, get medical help or contact a Poison Control Center right away.

### Directions:
- take every 4 to 6 hours
- do not take more than 4 doses in 24 hours

| children under 2 years of age | ask a doctor |
|---|---|
| children 2 to under 6 years of age | one (1) teaspoonful |
| children 6 to under 12 years of age | two (2) teaspoonfuls |
| adults and children 12 years of age and over | four (4) teaspoonfuls |

### Other Information:
- store at 59° to 77°F

**Inactive Ingredients:** Citric acid, edetate disodium, FD&C red no. 40, FD&C blue no. 1, flavors, glycerin, poloxamer 407, polyethylene glycol 1450, povidone K-90, purified water, saccharin sodium, sodium benzoate, sodium citrate, and sorbitol solution

**Questions?** Call **1-800-524-2624** (English/Spanish), weekdays, 9 AM – 5 PM EST

**How Supplied:** Sudafed Children's Nasal Decongestant is supplied in 4 fl. oz. bottles

*Shown in Product Identification Guide, page 521*

---

## TUCKS®
### Pre-moistened Hemorrhoidal/Vaginal Pads
[tŭks ]

**Active Ingredients:** Soft pads are pre-moistened with a solution containing Witch Hazel 50%.

**Inactive Ingredients:** Water, Glycerin, Alcohol, Propylene Glycol, Sodium Citrate, Diazolidinyl Urea, Citric Acid, Methylparaben, Propylparaben.

**Indications:** For the temporary relief of external itching, burning and irritation associated with hemorrhoids.

### Other Uses:
Hygienic Wipe: TUCKS Pads are effective for everyday personal hygienic use on outer rectal and vaginal areas. Used in place of toilet tissue, TUCKS Pads gently and thoroughly remove irritation-causing matter. They are especially handy during menstrual periods.
Vaginal Care: Gentle, soft TUCKS Pads can be used daily to freshen and cleanse.
Moist Compress: For additional relief, TUCKS Pads can be folded and used as a compress on inflamed tissue. TUCKS Pads are particularly helpful in relieving discomfort following childbirth, rectal or vaginal surgery.
Baby Care: TUCKS Pads are recommended as a final cleansing step at diaper changing time.

**Directions:** For external use only. *As a hemorrhoidal treatment* —Adults: When practical, cleanse the affected area with mild soap and warm water and rinse thoroughly. Gently dry by patting or blotting with toilet tissue or soft cloth before application of this product. Gently apply to affected area by patting and then discard. Can be used up to six times daily or after each bowel movement. Children under 12 years of age: consult a physician. *As a hygienic wipe* —Use as a wipe instead of toilet tissue. *As a moist compress* —For soothing relief, fold pad and place in contact with irritated tissue. Leave in place for 5 to 15 minutes. Repeat as needed.

**Warnings:** If condition worsens or does not improve within 7 days, consult a physician. Do not exceed recommended daily dosage unless directed by a physician. In case of bleeding, consult a physician promptly. Do not put this product into the rectum by using fingers or any mechanical device or applicator. **KEEP THIS AND ALL DRUGS OUT OF THE REACH OF CHILDREN.** In case of accidental ingestion, seek professional assistance or contact a Poison Control Center immediately.
Store at 59° to 77°F.

**How Supplied:** Jars of 40 and 100 pads. Also available TUCKS® individual foil-wrapped towelettes.

*Shown in Product Identification Guide, page 521*

---

## MAXIMUM STRENGTH UNISOM SLEEPGELS®
### Nighttime Sleep Aid

**Description:** Maximum Strength Unisom SleepGels are liquid-filled, blue soft gelatin capsules.

**Active Ingredient:** Diphenhydramine Hydrochloride 50 mg.

**Inactive Ingredients:** FD&C Blue No. 1, Gelatin, Glycerin, Pharmaceutical Glaze, Polyethylene Glycol, Propylene Glycol, Purified Water, Sorbitol, Titanium Dioxide.

**Indications:** Helps to reduce difficulty falling asleep.

**Action:** Diphenhydramine Hydrochloride is an ethanolamine antihistamine with anticholinergic and sedative effects.

**Administration and Dosage:** Adults and children 12 years of age and over: Oral dosage is one softgel (50 mg) at bedtime if needed, or as directed by a doctor.

**Warnings:** Do not take this product, unless directed by a doctor, if you have a breathing problem such as emphysema or chronic bronchitis, or if you have glaucoma or difficulty in urination due to enlargement of the prostate gland. Do not take this product if pregnant or nursing a baby.
- Do not give to children under 12 years of age.
- If sleeplessness persists continuously for more than two weeks, consult your doctor. Insomnia may be a symptom of serious underlying medical illness.
- Avoid alcoholic beverages while taking this product. Do not take this product if you are taking sedatives or tranquilizers, without first consulting your doctor.
- **Do Not Use:** with any other product containing diphenhydramine, including one applied topically.
- Keep this and all drugs out of the reach of children.
- In case of accidental overdose, seek professional assistance or contact a poison control center immediately.

**Drug Interaction:** Monoamine oxidase (MAO) inhibitors prolong and intensify the anticholinergic effects of antihistamines. The CNS depressant effect is heightened by alcohol and other CNS depressant drugs.

**Symptoms of Oral Overdosage:** Antihistamine overdosage reactions may vary from central nervous system depression to stimulation.
Stimulation is particularly likely in children. Atropine-like signs and symptoms, such as dry mouth, fixed and dilated pupils, flushing, and gastrointestinal symptoms, may also occur.

**Attention:** Use only if softgel blister seals are unbroken.

**How Supplied:** Boxes of 16 liquid filled softgels in child resistant blisters and boxes of 8 with non-child resistant packaging. Also in a 32 count easy to open child resistant bottle.
Store between 15° and 30°C (59° and 86°F)

*Shown in Product Identification Guide, page 521*

---

## UNISOM® SleepTabs™
[yu 'na-som]
### Nighttime Sleep Aid
(doxylamine succinate)

## PRODUCT OVERVIEW

**Key Facts:** Unisom is an ethanolamine antihistamine (doxylamine) which characteristically shows a high incidence of sedation. It produces a reduced latency to end of wakefulness and early onset of sleep.

**Major Uses:** Unisom has been shown to be clinically effective as a sleep aid when 1 tablet is given 30 minutes before retiring.

**Safety Information:** Unisom is contraindicated in pregnancy and nursing mothers. It is also contraindicated in patients with asthma, glaucoma, and enlargement of the prostate. Caution should be used if taken when alcohol is being consumed. Caution is also indicated when taken concurrently with other medications due to the anticholinergic properties of antihistamines.

**Description:** Pale blue oval scored tablets containing 25 mg. of doxylamine succinate, 2-[α-(2-dimethylaminoethoxy)α-methylbenzyl]pyridine succinate.

**Inactive Ingredients:** Dibasic Calcium Phosphate, FD&C Blue #1 Aluminum Lake, Magnesium Stearate, Microcrystalline Cellulose, Sodium Starch Glycolate.

**Administration and Dosage:** One tablet 30 minutes before going to bed. Take once daily or as directed by a doctor. Not for children under 12 years of age.

**Warnings:** Do not take this product, unless directed by a doctor, if you have a breathing problem such as emphysema or chronic bronchitis, or if you have glaucoma or difficulty in urination due to enlargement of the prostate gland. Do not take this product if pregnant or nursing a baby.
- If sleeplessness persists continuously for more than two weeks, consult your doctor. Insomnia may be a symptom of a serious underlying medical illness.
- Do not take this product if presently taking any other drug, without consulting your doctor or pharmacist.
- Take this product with caution if alcohol is being consumed.
- For adults only. Do not give to children under 12 years of age.
- Keep this and all medications out of the reach of children. This product contains an antihistamine and will cause drowsiness. It should be used only at bedtime.

**Side Effects:** Occasional anticholinergic effects may be seen.

**Attention:** Use only if tablet blister seals are unbroken.

**How Supplied:** Boxes of 8, 32 and 48 tablets in child resistant packaging. Boxes of 16 tablets in non-child resistant packaging.
*Shown in Product Identification Guide, page 521*

## VISINE® ORIGINAL
### Redness Reliever Eye Drops

**Drug Facts:**

| Active Ingredient: | Purpose: |
|---|---|
| Tetrahydrozoline HCl 0.05% ......................... | Redness reliever |

**Use:**
- for the relief of redness of the eye due to minor eye irritations

**Warnings:**
**Ask a doctor before use if you have** narrow angle glaucoma
**When using this product:**
- pupils may become enlarged temporarily
- overuse may cause more eye redness
- remove contact lenses before using
- do not use if this solution changes color or becomes cloudy

- do not touch tip of container to any surface to avoid contamination
- replace cap after each use

**Stop use and ask a doctor if:**
- you feel eye pain
- changes in vision occur
- redness or irritation of the eye lasts
- condition worsens or lasts more than 72 hours

**If pregnant or breast-feeding,** ask a health professional before use.
**Keep out of reach of children.** If swallowed, get medical help or contact a Poison Control Center right away.

**Directions:**
- put 1 to 2 drops in the affected eye(s) up to 4 times daily
- children under 6 years of age: ask a doctor

**Other Information:**
- store at 15° to 30°C (59° to 86°F)

**Inactive Ingredients:** benzalkonium chloride, boric acid, edetate disodium, purified water, sodium borate, and sodium chloride

**Questions?** call **1-800-223-0182**, Monday to Friday, 9 AM – 5 PM EST

**Caution:** Do not use if Visine-imprinted neckband on bottle is broken or missing.

**How Supplied:** In 0.5 fl. oz. and 1.0 fl. oz. plastic dispenser bottle and 0.5 fl. oz. plastic bottle with dropper.
*Shown in Product Identification Guide, page 521*

---

## VISINE-A®
### ANTIHISTAMINE & REDNESS RELIEVER EYE DROPS

**Drug Facts:**

| Active Ingredients: | Purpose: |
|---|---|
| Naphazoline hydrochloride 0.025% ........................ | Redness reliever |
| Pheniramine maleate 0.3% ................................. | Antihistamine |

**Uses:** Temporarily relieves itchy, red eyes due to:
- pollen
- ragweed
- grass
- animal hair and dander

**Warnings:**
**Do not use**
- if you are sensitive to any ingredient in this product

**Ask a doctor before use if you have:**
- heart disease
- high blood pressure
- narrow angle glaucoma
- trouble urinating due to an enlarged prostate gland

**When using this product:**
- pupils may become enlarged temporarily
- do not touch tip of container to any surface to avoid contamination
- replace cap after each use
- remove contact lenses before using
- do not use if this solution changes color or becomes cloudy
- overuse may cause more eye redness

**Stop use and ask a doctor if:**
- you feel eye pain
- changes in vision occur
- redness or irritation of the eye lasts
- condition worsens or lasts more than 72 hours

**Keep out of reach of children.** If swallowed, get medical help or contact a Poison Control Center right away. Accidental swallowing by infants and children may lead to coma and marked reduction in body temperature.

**Directions:**
- adults and children 6 years of age and over: put 1 or 2 drops in the affected eye(s) up to 4 times a day
- for children under 6 years of age: consult a doctor

**Other Information:**
- some users may experience a brief tingling sensation
- store between 15° and 25°C (59° and 77°F)

**Inactive Ingredients:** boric acid and sodium borate buffer system preserved with benzalkonium chloride (0.01%) and edetate disodium (0.1%), sodium hydroxide and/or hydrochloric acid (to adjust pH), and purified water

**Questions?** call **1-800-223-0182**, Monday to Friday, 9 AM – 5 PM EST

**Caution:** Do not use if Visine imprinted neckband on bottle is broken or missing.

**How Supplied:** In 0.5 fl. oz. plastic dispenser bottle.
*Shown in Product Identification Guide, page 521*

---

## VISINE A.C.®
### Astringent/Redness Reliever Eye Drops

**Drug Facts:**

| Active Ingredients: | Purposes: |
|---|---|
| Tetrahydrozoline HCl 0.05% ............... | Redness reliever |
| Zinc sulfate 0.25% ................. | Astringent |

**Use:**
- for temporary relief of discomfort and redness of the eye due to minor eye irritations

**Warnings:**
**Ask a doctor before use if you have** narrow angle glaucoma
**When using this product:**
- pupils may become enlarged temporarily
- overuse may cause more eye redness
- remove contact lenses before using

*Continued on next page*

---

*This product information was prepared in November 2001. On these and other Pfizer Consumer Healthcare Products, detailed information may be obtained by addressing Pfizer Consumer Healthcare, Pfizer, Inc., Morris Plains, NJ 07950*

## Visine A.C.—Cont.

- do not use if this solution changes color or becomes cloudy
- do not touch tip of container to any surface to avoid contamination
- replace cap after each use

**Stop use and ask a doctor if:**
- you feel eye pain
- changes in vision occur
- redness or irritation of the eye lasts
- condition worsens or lasts more than 72 hours

**If pregnant or breast-feeding,** ask a health professional before use.

**Keep out of reach of children.** If swallowed, get medical help or contact a Poison Control Center right away.

**Directions:**
- put 1 to 2 drops in the affected eye(s) up to 4 times daily
- children under 6 years of age: ask a doctor

**Other information:**
- some users may experience a brief tingling sensation
- store at 15° to 30°C (59° to 86°F)

**Inactive Ingredients:** benzalkonium chloride, boric acid, edetate disodium, purified water, sodium chloride, and sodium citrate

**Questions?** call **1-800-223-0182,** Monday to Friday, 9 AM – 5 PM EST

**Caution:** Do not use if Visine-imprinted neckband on bottle is broken or missing.

**How Supplied:** In 0.5 fl. oz. and 1.0 fl. oz. plastic dispenser bottle.
*Shown in Product Identification Guide, page 521*

---

## ADVANCED RELIEF VISINE®
**Lubricant/Redness Reliever Eye Drops**

**Drug Facts:**

| Active Ingredients: | Purposes: |
| --- | --- |
| Dextran 70 0.1% | Lubricant |
| Polyethylene glycol 400 1% | Lubricant |
| Povidone 1% | Lubricant |
| Tetrahydrozoline HCl 0.05% | Redness reliever |

**Uses:**
- for the relief of redness of the eye due to minor eye irritations
- for use as a protectant against further irritation or to relieve dryness of the eye

**Warnings:**
**Ask a doctor before use if you have** narrow angle glaucoma
**When using this product:**
- pupils may become enlarged temporarily
- overuse may cause more eye redness
- remove contact lenses before using
- do not use if this solution changes color or becomes cloudy
- do not touch tip of container to any surface to avoid contamination
- replace cap after each use

**Stop use and ask a doctor if:**
- you feel eye pain
- changes in vision occur

- redness or irritation of the eye lasts
- condition worsens or lasts more than 72 hours

**If pregnant or breast-feeding,** ask a health professional before use.

**Keep out of reach of children.** If swallowed, get medical help or contact a Poison Control Center right away.

**Directions:**
- put 1 or 2 drops in the affected eye(s) up to 4 times daily
- children under 6 years of age: ask a doctor

**Other Information:**
- store at 15° to 30°C (59° to 86°F)

**Inactive Ingredients:** benzalkonium chloride, boric acid, edetate disodium, purified water, sodium borate, and sodium chloride

**Questions?** call **1-800-223-0182,** Monday to Friday, 9 AM – 5 PM EST

**Caution:** Do not use if Visine-imprinted neckband on bottle is broken or missing.

**How Supplied:** In 0.5 fl. oz. and 1.0 fl. oz. plastic dispenser bottle.
*Shown in Product Identification Guide, page 521*

---

## VISINE L.R.®
**Redness Reliever Eye Drops**

**Drug Facts:**

| Active Ingredient: | Purpose: |
| --- | --- |
| Oxymetazoline HCl 0.025% | Redness reliever |

**Use:**
- for the relief of redness of the eye due to minor eye irritations

**Warnings:**
**Ask a doctor before use if you have** narrow angle glaucoma
**When using this product:**
- overuse may cause more eye redness
- remove contact lenses before using
- do not use if this solution changes color or becomes cloudy
- do not touch tip of container to any surface to avoid contamination
- replace cap after each use

**Stop use and ask a doctor if:**
- you feel eye pain
- changes in vision occur
- redness or irritation of the eye lasts
- condition worsens or lasts more than 72 hours

**If pregnant or breast-feeding,** ask a health professional before use.

**Keep out of reach of children.** If swallowed, get medical help or contact a Poison Control Center right away.

**Directions:**
- adults and children 6 years of age and over: put 1 or 2 drops in the affected eye(s)
- this may be repeated as needed every 6 hours or as directed by a doctor
- children under 6 years of age: ask a doctor

**Other Information:**
- store at 15° to 30°C (59° to 86°F)

**Inactive Ingredients:** benzalkonium chloride, boric acid, edetate disodium, purified water, sodium borate, and sodium chloride

**Questions?** call **1-800-223-0182,** Monday to Friday, 9 AM – 5 PM EST

**Caution:** Do not use if Visine-imprinted neckband on bottle is broken or missing.

**How Supplied:** In 0.5 fl. oz. and 1.0 fl. oz. plastic dispenser bottle.
*Shown in Product Identification Guide, page 521*

---

## VISINE TEARS® (Multi-Dose)
**Lubricant Eye Drops**

**Drug Facts:**

| Active Ingredients: | Purpose: |
| --- | --- |
| Glycerin 0.2% | Lubricant |
| Hydroxypropyl methylcellulose 0.2% | Lubricant |
| Polyethylene glycol 400 1% | Lubricant |

**Uses:**
- for the temporary relief of burning and irritation due to dryness of the eye
- for protection against further irritation

**Warnings:**
**When using this product:**
- remove contact lenses before using
- do not use if this solution changes color or becomes cloudy
- do not touch tip of container to any surface to avoid contamination
- replace cap after each use

**Stop use and ask a doctor if:**
- you feel eye pain
- changes in vision occur
- redness or irritation of the eye lasts
- condition worsens or lasts more than 72 hours

**If pregnant or breast-feeding,** ask a health professional before use.

**Keep out of reach of children.** If swallowed, get medical help or contact a Poison Control Center right away.

**Directions:**
- put 1 or 2 drops in the affected eye(s) as needed
- children under 6 years of age: ask a doctor

**Other Information:**
- store at 15° to 30°C (59° to 86°F)

**Inactive Ingredients:** ascorbic acid, benzalkonium chloride, boric acid, dextrose, disodium phosphate, glycine, magnesium chloride, potassium chloride, purified water, sodium borate, sodium chloride, sodium citrate, and sodium lactate

**Questions?** call **1-800-223-0182,** Monday to Friday, 9 AM – 5 PM EST

**Caution:** Do not use if Visine-imprinted neckband on bottle is broken or missing.

**How Supplied:** In 0.5 fl. oz. and 1 fl. oz. plastic dispenser bottle.
*Shown in Product Identification Guide, page 521*

## VISINE TEARS®
### Preservative Free, Single-Use Containers
### Lubricant Eye Drops

**Drug Facts:**

| Active Ingredients: | Purpose: |
|---|---|
| Glycerin 0.2% ........................... | Lubricant |
| Hydroxypropyl methylcellulose 0.2% .......................................... | Lubricant |
| Polyethylene glycol 400 1% ... | Lubricant |

**Uses:**
- for the temporary relief of burning and irritation due to dryness of the eye
- for protection against further irritation

**Warnings:**
**When using this product**
- remove contact lenses before using
- do not use if this solution changes color or becomes cloudy
- do not touch tip of container to any surface to avoid contamination
- do not reuse; once opened, discard

**Stop use and ask a doctor if:**
- you feel eye pain
- changes in vision occur
- redness or irritation of the eye lasts
- condition worsens or lasts more than 72 hours

**If pregnant or breast-feeding,** ask a health professional before use.
**Keep out of reach of children.** If swallowed, get medical help or contact a Poison Control Center right away.

**Directions:**
- put 1 or 2 drops in the affected eye(s) as needed
- children under 6 years of age: ask a doctor

**Other Information:**
- store at 15° to 30°C (59° to 86°F)

**Inactive Ingredients:** ascorbic acid, dextrose, disodium phosphate, glycine, magnesium chloride, potassium chloride, purified water, sodium chloride, sodium citrate, sodium lactate, and sodium phosphate

**Questions?** call **1-800-223-0182**, Monday to Friday, 9 AM - 5 PM EST

**Caution:** Use only if unit dose container is intact.

**How Supplied:** 1 box contains 28 single-use containers, 0.01 fl. oz. (0.4 mL) each

*Shown in Product Identification Guide, page 521*

---

## MAXIMUM STRENGTH WART–OFF®
### SALICYLIC ACID • WART REMOVER
### Liquid

**Drug Facts:**

| Active Ingredient: | Purpose: |
|---|---|
| Salicylic acid 17% w/w .... | Wart remover |

**Uses:** For the removal of common warts and plantar warts on the bottom of the foot. The common wart is easily recognized by the rough "cauliflower-like" appearance of the surface. The plantar wart is recognized by its location only on the bottom of the foot, its tenderness, and the interruption of the footprint pattern.

**Warnings:**
**For external use only.**
**Extremely flammable:** Keep away from fire or flame
**Do not use:**
- on irritated skin, on any area that is infected or reddened, if you are a diabetic, or if you have poor blood circulation
- on moles, birthmarks, warts with hair growing from them, genital warts, or warts on the face or mucous membranes

**When using this product:**
- if product gets into the eye, flush with water for 15 minutes
- avoid inhaling vapors
- cap bottle tightly and store at room temperature away from heat

**Stop use and ask a doctor if**
- discomfort persists

**Keep out of reach of children.** If swallowed, get medical help or contact a Poison Control Center right away.

**Directions:**
- wash affected area
- dry area thoroughly
- apply one drop at a time with applicator to sufficiently cover each wart
- let dry
- repeat this procedure once or twice daily as needed (until wart is removed) for up to 12 weeks

**Other Information:**
- store at 15° to 30°C (59° to 86°F)

**Inactive Ingredients:**
Alcohol 26.3% w/w, *t*-butyl alcohol, denatonium benzoate, flexible collodion, and propylene glycol dipelargonate.

**Questions?** Call **1-800-723-7529**, Monday to Friday, 9 AM – 5 PM EST

**How Supplied:** 0.45 fluid ounce (13.3mL) bottle.

---

## ZANTAC® 75
### Ranitidine Tablets 75 mg
### Acid Reducer
[*zan ' tak*]

**Drug Facts:**

| Active Ingredient: (in each tablet) | Purpose: |
|---|---|
| Ranitidine 75 mg (as ranitidine hydrochloride 84 mg) ......... | Acid reducer |

**Uses:**
- relieves heartburn associated with acid indigestion and sour stomach
- prevents heartburn associated with acid indigestion and sour stomach brought on by certain foods and beverages

**Warnings:**
**Allergy alert:** Do not use if you are allergic to ranitidine or other acid reducers
**Do not use:**
- if you have trouble swallowing
- with other acid reducers

**Stop use and ask a doctor if:**
- stomach pain continues
- you need to take this product for more than 14 days

**If pregnant or breast-feeding,** ask a health professional before use.
**Keep out of reach of children.** In case of overdose, get medical help or contact a Poison Control Center right away.

**Directions:**
- adults and children 12 years and over:
  - to **relieve** symptoms, swallow 1 tablet with a glass of water
  - to **prevent** symptoms, swallow 1 tablet with a glass of water **30 to 60 minutes before** eating food or drinking beverages that cause heartburn
  - can be used up to twice daily (up to 2 tablets in 24 hours)
- children under 12 years: ask a doctor

**Other Information:**
- do not use if foil under bottle cap or individual blister unit is open or torn
- store at 20°–25°C (68°–77°F)
- avoid excessive heat or humidity
- this product is sodium and sugar free

**Inactive Ingredients:** Hydroxypropyl methylcellulose, magnesium stearate, microcrystalline cellulose, synthetic red iron oxide, titanium dioxide, triacetin

**Read the Label:** Read the directions, consumer information leaflet and warnings before use. Keep the carton. It contains important information.

**Questions?** call **1-800-223-0182**. Information is available 24 hours a day, 7 days a week.

**How Supplied:** Zantac 75 is available in convenient blister packs in boxes of 4, 10, 20 and 30 tablets, and in bottles of 60, 80 and 100 count.

Zantac is a registered trademark of the Glaxo Wellcome group of companies.
*Shown in Product Identification Guide, page 522*

---

## Pharmacia Consumer Healthcare
**PEAPACK, NJ 07977**

**For Medical and Pharmaceutical Information, Including Emergencies:**
(616) 833-8244
(800) 253-8600 ext. 3-8244

## CORTAID®
### Maximum Strength, Sensitive Skin and Intensive Therapy
### Cream and Ointment
### (hydrocortisone 1% and ¹/₂%)
### Anti-itch products

**Description:** CORTAID Maximum Strength contains the highest strength of hydrocortisone available without a prescription. CORTAID Sensitive Skin has been specially formulated with aloe and ¹/₂% hydrocortisone. CORTAID Intensive Therapy's special formula of 1% hydrocortisone is recommended for eczema and psoriasis sufferers. The vanishing action

*Continued on next page*

## Cortaid—Cont.

of CORTAID Cream makes it cosmetically acceptable when the skin itch or rash treated is on exposed parts of the body such as the hands or arms. CORTAID Ointment is best used where protection, lubrication, and soothing of dry and scaly lesions are required. The ointment is also recommended for treating itchy genital and anal areas.

**Active Ingredients:**
CORTAID Maximum Strength Cream: Hydrocortisone 1%
CORTAID Maximum Strength Ointment: Hydrocortisone acetate 1%
CORTAID Intensive Therapy Cream: Hydrocortisone 1%
CORTAID Sensitive Skin Cream: Hydrocortisone acetate $1/2$%

**Indications:** Use CORTAID for the temporary relief of itching associated with minor skin irritations, inflammation, and rashes due to eczema, psoriasis, seborrheic dermatitis, poison ivy, poison oak, or poison sumac, insect bites, soaps, detergents, cosmetics, jewelry, and for external feminine and anal itching. Other uses of this product should be only under the advice and supervision of a physician.

**Directions:** *Adults and children 2 years of age and older:* Apply to affected area not more than 3 to 4 times daily. *Children under 2 years of age:* Do not use, consult a physician. *Adults:* For external anal itching, when practical, cleanse the affected area with mild soap and warm water and rinse thoroughly by patting or blotting with an appropriate cleansing pad. Gently dry by patting or blotting with toilet tissue or a soft cloth before application of this product. *Children under 12 years of age:* For external anal itching, consult a physician.

**Warnings:** For external use only. Avoid contact with the eyes. If condition worsens, or if symptoms persist for more than 7 days or clear up and occur again within a few days, stop use of this product and do not begin use of any other hydrocortisone product unless you have consulted a physician. Do not use for the treatment of diaper rash. Consult a physician. For external feminine itching, do not use if you have a vaginal discharge. Consult a physician. For external anal itching, do not exceed the recommended daily dosage unless directed by a physician. In case of bleeding, consult a physician promptly. Do not put this product into the rectum by using fingers or any mechanical device or applicator.
**Keep this and all drugs out of the reach of children. In case of accidental ingestion, seek professional assistance or contact a Poison Control Center immediately.**

**Inactive Ingredients:**
**Maximum Strength Products:** *Maximum Strength Cream:* Aloe vera, benzyl alcohol, ceteareth-20, cetearyl alcohol, glycerin, isopropyl myristate, isostearyl neopentanoate, methylparaben, mixed fatty acid esters, polyoxyl 40 stearate, and purified water.
*Maximum Strength Ointment:* butylparaben, cholesterol, methylparaben, microcrystalline wax, mineral oil, and white petrolatum.
**Sensitive Skin Products:**
*Sensitive Skin Cream:* aloe vera, butylparaben, glyceryl stearate, methylparaben, mixed fatty acid esters, polyethylene glycol, stearamidoethyl diethylamine, and purified water.
**Intensive Therapy Products:**
*Intensive Therapy Cream:* cetyl alcohol, citric acid, glyceryl stearate, isopropyl myristate, methylparaben, polyoxyl 40 stearate, polysorbate 60, propylene glycol, propylparaben, purified water, sodium citrate, sorbic acid, sorbitan monostearate, stearyl alcohol and white wax.

**How Supplied:** Maximum Strength Cream: $1/2$ oz., 1 oz., and 2 oz. tubes
Maximum Strength Ointment: $1/2$ oz. and 1 oz. tubes
Sensitive Skin Cream: $1/2$ oz. tube
Intensive Therapy Cream: 2 oz. tube

---

## DRAMAMINE® Original Formula Tablets

## DRAMAMINE® Chewable Formula Tablets
**Antiemetic**

**Description:** DRAMAMINE Original Formula Tablets and DRAMAMINE Chewable Formula Tablets contain dimenhydrinate, which is the chlorotheophylline salt of the antihistaminic agent diphenhydramine.

**Active Ingredient:** Dimenhydrinate 50 mg per tablet.

**Indications:** For prevention and treatment of the symptoms associated with motion sickness including nausea, vomiting, and dizziness

**Directions:** To prevent motion sickness, the first dose should be taken ½ to 1 hour before starting activity. To prevent or treat motion sickness, use the following dosing.
Adults and children 12 years and over: 1 to 2 tablets every 4–6 hours; not more than 8 tablets in 24 hours, or as directed by a doctor
Children 6 to under 12 years: ½ to 1 tablet every 6–8 hours: not more than 3 tablets in 24 hours, or as directed by a doctor
Children 2 to under 6 years: ¼ to ½ tablet every 6–8 hours; not more than 1 ½ tablets in 24 hours, or as directed by a doctor

**Warnings:**
**Do not use** in children under 2 years of age unless directed by a doctor.

**Ask a doctor before use if you have**
• a breathing problem such as emphysema or chronic bronchitis • glaucoma • difficulty in urination due to enlargement of the prostate gland
**Ask a doctor or pharmacist before use if you are** taking sedatives or tranquilizers
**When using these products**
• marked drowsiness may occur • avoid alcoholic drinks • alcohol, sedatives, and tranquilizers may increase drowsiness • be careful when driving a motor vehicle or operating machinery
**If pregnant or breast-feeding,** ask a health professional before use.
**Keep out of reach of children.**
In case of overdose, get medical help or contact a Poison Control Center right away.

**Other Information:**
Chewable Formula Tablets: Phenylketonurics: contains **phenylalanine** 1.5 mg per tablet. Also contains FD&C yellow No. 5 (tartrazine) as a color additive

**Inactive Ingredients:** DRAMAMINE Original Formula Tablets: colloidal silicon dioxide, croscarmellose sodium, lactose, magnesium stearate, microcrystalline cellulose
DRAMAMINE Chewable Formula Tablets: aspartame, citric acid, FD&C yellow no. 5, FD&C yellow no. 6, flavor, magnesium stearate, methacrylic acid copolymer, sorbitol

**How Supplied:** Original Formula Tablets: scored, white tablets, available in 12 ct. vials, 36 ct. and 100 ct. packages
Chewable Formula Tablets: scored, orange tablets, available in 8 ct. and 24 ct. packages
Store at room temperature

---

## DRAMAMINE® Less Drowsy Formula Tablets
**Antiemetic**

**Description:** DRAMAMINE Less Drowsy Formula contains meclizine hydrochloride.
**Active Ingredient:** Meclizine hydrochloride 25 mg per tablet

**Indications:** for prevention and treatment of the symptoms associated with motion sickness including nausea, vomiting, and dizziness

**Directions:** To prevent motion sickness, the first dose should be taken 1 hour before starting activity. To prevent or treat motion sickness, use the following dosing.
Adults and children 12 years and over: 1 to 2 tablets once daily, or as directed by a doctor

**Warnings:**
**Do not use** in children under 12 years of age unless directed by a doctor.
**Ask a doctor before use if you have:**
• a breathing problem such as emphysema or chronic bronchitis • glaucoma • difficulty in urination due to enlargement of the prostate gland

**Ask a doctor or pharmacist before use if you are** taking sedatives or tranquilizers
**When using these products:**
• drowsiness may occur • avoid alcoholic drinks • alcohol, sedatives, and tranquilizers may increase drowsiness • be careful when driving a motor vehicle or operating machinery
**If pregnant or breast-feeding,** ask a health professional before use.
**Keep out of reach of children.**
In case of overdose, get medical help or contact a Poison Control Center right away.

**Inactive Ingredients:** Colloidal silicon dioxide, corn starch, D&C yellow no. 10 (aluminum lake), lactose, magnesium stearate, microcrystalline cellulose

**How Supplied:** Yellow tablets in 8 ct. vials
Store at controlled room temperature 20°–25°C (68°–77°F)

---

## EMETROL®
**(Phosphorated Carbohydrate Solution)**
**For the relief of nausea associated with upset stomach**

**Description:** EMETROL is an oral solution containing balanced amounts of dextrose (glucose) and levulose (fructose) and phosphoric acid with controlled hydrogen ion concentration. Available in original lemon-mint or cherry flavor. EMETROL quickly relieves nausea by local action on the wall of the hyperactive G.I. tract.

**Active Ingredients:** Each 5 mL teaspoonful contains dextrose (glucose), 1.87 g; levulose (fructose), 1.87 g; and phosphoric acid, 21.5 mg.

**Indications:** For the relief of nausea due to upset stomach from intestinal flu and food or drink indiscretions. For other conditions, take only as directed by your physician.

**Directions:**

**Usual Adult Dose:** One or two tablespoonfuls (1 tbsp equals 3 tsps). Repeat every 15 minutes until distress subsides.

**Usual Children's Dose (2 to 12 years):** One or two teaspoonfuls. Repeat dose every 15 minutes until distress subsides.

**Important:** For maximum effectiveness never dilute EMETROL or drink fluids of any kind immediately before or after taking a dose.

**Caution:** Not to be taken for more than one hour (5 doses) without consulting a physician. If nausea continues or recurs frequently, consult a physician promptly as it may be a sign of a serious condition.

**Warnings:** This product contains fructose and should not be taken by persons with hereditary fructose intolerance (HFI).

As with any drug, if you are pregnant or nursing a baby, seek the advice of a health professional before using this product.
**This product contains sugar and should not be taken by diabetics except under the advice and supervision of a physician.**
**Keep this and all medications out of the reach of children.**
**In case of accidental overdose, contact a Poison Control Center or physician immediately.**

**Inactive Ingredients:** glycerin, methylparaben, purified water; D&C Yellow No. 10 and natural lemon-mint flavor in lemon-mint Emetrol; FD&C Red No. 40 and artificial cherry flavor in cherry Emetrol.

**How Supplied:** Yellow, Lemon-Mint: Bottles of 4 & 8 fluid ounces.
Red, Cherry:
Bottles of 4 & 8 fluid ounces.

---

## NASALCROM® Nasal Spray
**Nasal Allergy Symptom Controller**

**Description:** NASALCROM Nasal Spray contains a liquid formulation of cromolyn sodium that stabilizes mast cells that release histamine. NASALCROM is neither an antihistamine nor a decongestant nor a corticosteroid. In addition to treating nasal allergy symptoms, it decreases the allergic reaction by reducing the release of histamine, the trigger of allergy symptoms, from mast cells. NASALCROM has no known drug interactions and is safe to use with medications including other allergy medications.
**Active Ingredient: (per spray)** Cromolyn sodium 5.2mg

**Indications:** To prevent and relieve nasal symptoms of hay fever and other nasal allergies:
• runny/itchy nose • sneezing • allergic stuffy nose

**Directions:**
• parent or care provider must supervise the use of this product by young children. Adults and children 2 years and older:
• spray once into each nostril. Repeat 3–4 times a day (every 4–6 hours). If needed, may be used up to 6 times a day.
• use every day while in contact with the cause of your allergies (pollen, molds, pets, and dust)
• to **prevent** nasal allergy symptoms, use before contact with the cause of your allergies. For best results, start using up to one week before contact.
• if desired, you can use this product with other medications, including other allergy medications.
• children under 2 years: Do not use unless directed by a doctor

**Warnings:**
**Do not use** • if you are allergic to any of the ingredients

**Ask a doctor before use if you have**
• fever • discolored nasal discharge • sinus pain • wheezing
**When using this product** • it may take several days of use to notice an effect. Your best effect may not be seen for 1 to 2 weeks • brief stinging or sneezing may occur right after use • do not use to treat sinus infection, asthma, or cold symptoms • do not share this bottle with anyone else as this may spread germs
**Stop use and ask a doctor if**
• shortness of breath, wheezing, or chest tightness occurs • hives or swelling of the mouth or throat occurs • your symptoms worsen • you have new symptoms • your symptoms do not begin to improve within two weeks • you need to use more than 12 weeks
**If pregnant or breast feeding** ask a health professional before use.
**Keep out of reach of children.** If swallowed, get medical help or contact a Poison Control Center right away.

**Inactive Ingredients:** benzalkonium chloride, edetate disodium, purified water

**How Supplied:** NASALCROM Nasal Spray is available in 13mL (100 metered sprays) and 26mL (200 metered sprays) sizes
Store between 20°–25°C (68°–77°F). Keep away from light.

---

**PEDIACARE® Multisymptom Cold Liquid**
**PEDIACARE® NightRest Cough-Cold Liquid**
**PEDIACARE® Cold & Allergy Liquid**
**PEDIACARE® Long-Acting Cough Plus Cold Liquid**
**PEDIACARE® Infants' Drops Decongestant**
**PEDIACARE® Infants' Drops Decongestant Plus Cough**

**Description:** PEDIACARE products are available in six different formulas, allowing you to select the ideal product to temporarily relieve your patient's symptoms. **PEDIACARE® Multisymptom Cold Liquid** contains an antihistamine, chlorpheniramine maleate, a nasal decongestant, pseudoephedrine HCl, and a cough suppressant, dextromethorphan hydrobromide, to provide temporary relief of nasal congestion, runny nose, sneezing and coughing due to the common cold, hay fever or other upper respiratory allergies. **PEDIACARE® NightRest Cough-Cold Liquid** contains a decongestant, pseudoephedrine hydrochloride, an antihistamine, chlorpheniramine maleate, and a cough suppressant, dextromethorphan hydrobromide, to provide temporary relief of coughs, nasal congestion, runny nose and sneezing due to the common cold hayfever or other upper respiratory allergies.

*Continued on next page*

## Pediacare—Cont.

**PEDIACARE® Cold & Allergy Liquid** contains a decongestant, pseudoephedrine hydrochloride and an antihistamine, chlorpheniramine maleate to provide temporary relief of nasal congestion, runny nose and sneezing due to the common cold, hayfever or other respiratory allergies. **PEDIACARE® Long-Acting Cough Plus Cold Liquid** contains a decongestant, pseudoephedrine hydrochloride and a cough suppressant, dextromethorphan hydrobromide to provide temporary relief of nasal congestion and coughing due to the common cold, hayfever or other respiratory allergies. **PEDIACARE® Infants' Drops Decongestant** contains a decongestant, pseudoephedrine hydrochloride, to provide temporary relief of nasal congestion due to the common cold, hay fever or other upper respiratory allergies. **PEDIACARE® Infants' Drops Decongestant Plus Cough** contains a decongestant, pseudoephedrine hydrochloride, and a cough suppressant, dextromethorphan hydrobromide to provide temporary relief of nasal congestion and coughing due to common cold, hay fever or other upper respiratory allergies.

**Active Ingredients:** Each 5 mL of **PEDIACARE® Multisymptom Cold Liquid** contains pseudoephedrine hydrochloride 15 mg, chlorpheniramine maleate 1 mg and dextromethorphan hydrobromide 5 mg. Each 0.8 mL oral dropper of **PEDIACARE® Infants' Drops Decongestant** contains pseudoephedrine hydrochloride 7.5 mg. Each 0.8 mL of **PEDIACARE® Infants' Drops Decongestant Plus Cough** contains pseudoephedrine hydrochloride 7.5 mg and dextromethorphan hydrobromide 2.5 mg. Each 5 mL of **PEDIACARE® NightRest Cough-Cold Liquid** contains pseudoephedrine hydrochloride 15 mg, chlorpheniramine maleate 1 mg and dextromethorphan hydrobromide 7.5 mg. Each 5mL of **PEDIACARE® Cold & Allergy Liquid** contains pseudoephedrine hydrochloride 15mg and chlorpheniramine maleate 1mg. Each 5mL of **PEDIACARE® Long-Acting Cough Plus Cold Liquid** contains pseudoephedrine hydrochloride 15mg and dextromethorphan hydrobromide 7.5mg. **PEDIACARE® Multisymptom Cold Liquid** and **NightRest Cough-Cold Liquid** are cherry flavored, alcohol free and red in color. **PEDIACARE® Cold & Allergy Liquid** is bubblegum flavored, alcohol free and pink in color. **PEDIACARE® Long-Acting Cough Plus Cold Liquid** is grape flavored, alcohol free and purple in color. **PEDIACARE® Infants' Drops Decongestant** is fruit flavored alcohol free and red in color. **PEDIACARE® Infants' Drops Decongestant Plus Cough** is cherry flavored, alcohol free and clear, non-staining in color.

**Professional Dosage:** A calibrated dosage cup is provided for accurate dosing of the **PEDIACARE** Liquid formulas. A calibrated oral dropper is provided for accurate dosing of **PEDIACARE® Infants' Drops**. All doses of **PEDIACARE® Multisymptom Cold, Cold & Allergy Liquid**, as well as **PEDIACARE® Infants' Drops** may be repeated every 4–6 hours, not to exceed 4 doses in 24 hours. **PEDIACARE® NightRest Liquid** and **Long-Acting Cough Plus Cold Liquid** may be repeated every 6–8 hrs, not to exceed 4 doses in 24 hours.
[See table below]

**Warnings: Keep this and all medication out of the reach of children.** In case of accidental overdosage, contact a physician or poison control center immediately.

The following information appears on the appropriate package labels:

**PEDIACARE® Multisymptom Cold Liquid, Night Rest Cough-Cold Liquid, Cold & Allergy Liquid:** Do not exceed recommended dosage. If nervousness, dizziness or sleeplessness occur, discontinue use and consult a doctor. If symptoms do not improve within 7 days or are accompanied by fever, consult a doctor. A persistent cough may be a sign of a serious condition. If cough persists for more than one week, tends to recur or is accompanied by fever, rash, or persistent headache, consult a doctor. Do not give this product for persistent or chronic cough such as occurs with asthma or if cough is accompanied by excessive phlegm (mucus) unless directed by a doctor. May cause excitability especially in children. May cause drowsiness. Sedatives and tranquilizers may increase the drowsiness effect. Do not give this product to children who are taking sedatives or tranquilizers without first consulting the child's doctor. Do not give this product to children who have a breathing problem such as chronic bronchitis, or who have glaucoma, heart disease, high blood pressure, thyroid disease or diabetes, without first consulting the child's doctor.

**PEDIACARE® Long-Acting Cough Plus Cold Liquid:** Do not exceed recommended dosage. If nervousness, dizziness, or sleeplessness occur, discontinue

| Age Group | 0–3 mos | 4–11 mos | 12–23 mos | 2–3 yrs | 4–5 yrs | 6–8 yrs | 9–10 yrs | 11 yrs | Dosage |
|---|---|---|---|---|---|---|---|---|---|
| Weight (lbs) | 6–11 lbs | 12–17 lbs | 18–23 lbs | 24–35 lbs | 36–47 lbs | 48–59 lbs | 60–71 lbs | 72–95 lbs | |
| PEDIACARE® Infants' Drops Decongestant* | ½ dropper (0.4 mL) | 1 dropper (0.8 mL) | 1½ droppers (1.2 mL) | 2 droppers (1.6 mL) | | | | | q4–6h |
| PEDIACARE® Infants' Drops Decongestant Plus Cough* | ½ dropper (0.4 mL) | 1 dropper (0.8 mL) | 1½ droppers (1.2 mL) | 2 droppers (1.6 mL) | | | | | q4–6h |
| PEDIACARE® Long-Acting Cough Plus Cold Liquid* | | | ½ tsp | 1 tsp | 1½ tsp | 2 tsp | 2½ tsp | 3 tsp | q6–8h |
| PEDIACARE® Multisymptom Cold Liquid** | | | | 1 tsp | 1½ tsp | 2 tsp | 2½ tsp | 3 tsp | q4–6h |
| PEDIACARE® NightRest Liquid** | | | | 1 tsp | 1½ tsp | 2 tsp | 2½ tsp | 3 tsp | q6–8h |
| PEDIACARE® Cold & Allergy Liquid** | | | | 1 tsp | 1½ tsp | 2 tsp | 2½ tsp | 3 tsp | q4–6h |

*Administer to children under 2 years only on the advice of a physician.
**Administer to children under 6 years only on the advice of a physician.

use and consult a doctor. If symptoms do not improve within 7 days or are accompanied by fever, consult a doctor. A persistent cough may be a sign of a serious condition. If cough persists for more than one week, tends to recur or is accompanied by fever, rash, or persistent headache, consult a doctor. Do not give this product for persistent or chronic cough such as occurs with asthma or if cough is accompanied by excessive phlegm (mucus) unless directed by a doctor. Do not give this product to a child who has heart disease, high blood pressure, thyroid disease or diabetes unless directed by a doctor. Take by mouth only.

**PEDIACARE® Infants' Drops Decongestant:** Do not exceed the recommended dosage. If nervousness, dizziness or sleeplessness occur discontinue use and consult a doctor. If symptoms do not improve within 7 days or are accompanied by fever, consult a physician. Do not give this product to a child who has heart disease, high blood pressure, thyroid disease or diabetes unless directed by a doctor. Take by mouth only. Not for nasal use.

**PEDIACARE® Infants' Drops Decongestant Plus Cough:** Do not exceed recommended dosage. If nervousness, dizziness, or sleeplessness occur, discontinue use and consult a doctor. If symptoms do not improve within 7 days or are accompanied by fever, consult a doctor. A persistent cough may be a sign of a serious condition. If cough persists for more than one week, tends to recur or is accompanied by fever, rash, or persistent headache, consult a doctor. Do not give this product for persistent or chronic cough such as occurs with asthma or if cough is accompanied by excessive phlegm (mucus) unless directed by a doctor. Do not give this product to a child who has heart disease, high blood pressure, thyroid disease or diabetes unless directed by a doctor. Take by mouth only. Not for nasal use.

**Drug Interaction Precaution:** Do not give this product to a child who is taking a prescription monoamine oxidase inhibitor (MAOI) (certain drugs for depression, psychiatric or emotional conditions), or for 2 weeks after stopping the MAOI drug. If you are uncertain whether your child's prescription drug contains an MAOI, consult a health professional before giving this product.

**Overdosage:** Acute dextromethorphan overdose usually does not result in serious signs and symptoms unless massive amounts have been ingested. Signs and symptoms of a substantial overdose may include nausea and vomiting, visual disturbances, CNS disturbances, and urinary retention. Symptoms from pseudoephedrine overdose consist most often of mild anxiety, tachycardia and/or mild hypertension. Symptoms usually appear within 4 to 8 hours of ingestion and are transient, usually requiring no treatment. Chlorpheniramine toxicity should be treated as you would an antihistamine/anticholinergic overdose and is likely to be present within a few hours after acute ingestion.

**Inactive Ingredients: PEDIACARE® Multisymptom Cold Liquid:** citric acid, corn syrup, FD&C red 40, flavors, glycerin, propylene glycol, purified water, sodium benzoate, sodium carboxymethylcellulose, sorbitol.
**PEDIACARE® NightRest Cough-Cold:** citric acid, corn syrup, FD&C red 40, flavors, glycerin, propylene glycol, purified water, sodium benzoate, sodium carboxymethylcellulose, sorbitol.
**PEDIACARE® Cold & Allergy Liquid:** citric acid, corn syrup, FD&C red #40, flavors, glycerin, propylene glycol, purified water, sodium benzoate, sodium carboxymethylcellulose, sorbitol.
**PEDIACARE® Long-Acting Cough Plus Cold Liquid:** citric acid, corn syrup, FD&C blue #1, FD&C red #40, flavors, glycerin, propylene glycol, purified water, sodium benzoate, sodium carboxymethylcellulose, sorbitol.
**PEDIACARE® Infants' Drops Decongestant:** benzoic acid, citric acid, FD&C red #40, flavors, glycerin, polyethylene glycol, propylene glycol, purified water, sodium benzoate, sorbitol, sucrose.
**PEDIACARE® Infants' Drops Decongestant Plus Cough:** citric acid, flavors, glycerin, purified water, sodium benzoate, sorbitol.

**How Supplied: PEDIACARE® Multisymptom Cold Liquid, NightRest Cough-Cold Liquid** (color red), **Cold & Allergy** (color pink), and **Long-Acting Cough Plus Cold** (color purple)-bottles of 4 fl. oz. (120 mL) with child-resistant safety cap and calibrated dosage cup. **PEDIACARE® Infants' Drops Decongestant** (color red) and **PEDIACARE® Infants' Drops Decongestant Plus Cough** (clear)—bottles of ¹/₂ fl. oz. (15 mL) with calibrated dropper.
Store bottled product in original outer carton until depleted.

---

## ROGAINE® FOR MEN EXTRA STRENGTH
**(5% Minoxidil Topical Solution) Hair Regrowth Treatment**

**Description:** ROGAINE For Men Extra Strength is a colorless solution for use only on the scalp to help regrow hair in men.

**Active Ingredient:** Minoxidil 5% w/v

**Indication:** Hair regrowth treatment for men

**Directions:** Apply 1 mL (twice a day, every day, directly onto the scalp) in the hair loss area. Using more or using more often will not improve results.

**Warnings:**
**For external use only**
**Flammable:** Keep away from fire or flame
**Do not use if:**
• you are a woman
• you have no family history of hair loss
• your hair loss is sudden and/or patchy
• you do not know the reason for your hair loss
• you are under 18 years of age
• your scalp is red, inflamed, infected, irritated, or painful

• you are using other medications on the scalp
**Ask a doctor before use if you have** heart disease
**When using this product:**
• do not apply on other parts of the body
• avoid contact with the eyes. In case of accidental contact, rinse eyes with large amounts of cool tap water.
• some people have experienced changes in hair color and/or texture
• it may take 2 to 4 months before you see results.
• the amount of hair regrowth is different for each person. This product will not work for all men.
**Stop use and ask a doctor if:**
• unwanted facial hair growth occurs
• chest pain, rapid heartbeat, faintness, or dizziness occurs
• sudden, unexplained weight gain occurs
• your hands or feet swell
• scalp irritation occurs, and continues or worsens
• you do not see hair regrowth in 4 months
**Not for use by women. May grow facial hair. May be harmful if used during pregnancy or breast-feeding.**
**Keep out of reach of children.** If swallowed, get medical help or contact a Poison Control Center right away.

**Inactive Ingredients:** Alcohol (30% v/v), propylene glycol (50% v/v), and purified water.

**How Supplied:** ROGAINE For Men Extra Strength is available in packs of one, three, or four 60 mL bottles. (One 60 mL bottle is a one-month supply.) Store at controlled room temperature 20° to 25°C (68° to 77°F).

---

## ROGAINE® For Women
**(2% Minoxidil Topical Solution) Hair Regrowth Treatment**

**Description:** ROGAINE is a colorless liquid medication for use on the scalp to help regrow hair.

**Active Ingredient:** Minoxidil 2% w/v

**Indication:** Hair regrowth treatment.

**Directions:** Apply one mL (twice a day, every day, directly onto the scalp) in the hair loss area. Using more or using more often will not improve results.

**Warnings:**
**For external use only**
**Flammable:** Keep away from fire or flame
**Do not use if**
• you have no family history of hair loss
• your hair loss is sudden and/or patchy
• hair loss is associated with childbirth
• you do not know the reason for your hair loss
• you are under 18 years of age
• your scalp is red, inflamed, infected, irritated, or painful
• you use other topical prescription products on the scalp
**Ask a doctor before use if you have heart disease**
**When using this product**
• do not apply on other parts of the body
• avoid contact with the eyes. In case of

*Continued on next page*

## Rogaine For Women—Cont.

accidental contact, rinse eyes with large amounts of cool tap water.
- some people have experienced changes in hair color and/or texture
- it takes time to regrow hair. You may need to use this product daily for at least 4 months before you see results.
- the amount of hair regrowth is different for each person. This product will not work for everyone

**Stop use and ask a doctor if**
- unwanted facial hair growth occurs
- chest pain, rapid heartbeat, faintness, or dizziness occurs
- sudden, unexplained weight gain occurs
- your hands or feet swell
- redness or irritation occurs
- you do not see hair regrowth in 8 months

**If pregnant or breast-feeding** ask a health professional before use.

**Keep out of reach of children.** If swallowed, get medical help or contact a Poison Control Center right away.

## Side Effects:

The most common side effects are itching and other skin irritations of the treated area of the scalp. If scalp irritation continues, stop use and see a doctor.

Although unwanted facial hair growth has been reported on the face and on other parts of the body, such reports have been infrequent. The unwanted hair growth may be caused by the transfer of ROGAINE to areas other than the scalp, or by absorption into the circulatory system of low levels of the active ingredient, or by a medical condition not related to the use of ROGAINE. If you experience unwanted hair growth, discontinue using ROGAINE and see your doctor for recommendations about appropriate treatment. After stopping use of ROGAINE, the unwanted hair, if caused by the use of ROGAINE, should go away over time.

**Inactive Ingredients:** Alcohol (60% v/v), propylene glycol (20% v/v), and purified water.

**How Supplied**: ROGAINE For Women is available in packs of one, three, or four 60 mL bottles. (One 60 mL bottle is a one-month supply.)
Store at Controlled Room Temperature 20° to 25°C (68° to 77°F).

---

## SURFAK® LIQUI-GELS®
**Stool Softener Laxative**

**Description:** SURFAK®, a stool softener, is indicated for the relief of occasional constipation. SURFAK is a convenient, once a day therapy, which provides gentle prevention and superior relief from the discomfort associated with passing stools related to trauma, lifestyle, or aging. It works gently by drawing water into the stool, making it softer and easier to pass. Regularity can be expected to return in 12 to 72 hours.

**Active Ingredients:** Each soft gelatin Liqui-Gel contains 240 mg docusate calcium.

**Indication:** Stool softener laxative

**Directions:** Adults and children 12 years of age and over: one Liqui-Gel by mouth daily for several days or until bowel movements are normal. For use in children under 12, consult a physician.

**Warnings:** Do not use laxative products when abdominal pain, nausea, or vomiting are present unless directed by a doctor. If you have noticed a sudden change in bowel habits that persists over a period of 2 weeks, consult a doctor before using a laxative. Laxative products should not be used for a period longer than 1 week unless directed by a doctor. Rectal bleeding or failure to have a bowel movement after use of a laxative may indicate a serious condition. Discontinue use and consult your doctor. Keep this and all drugs out of the reach of children. In case of accidental overdose, seek professional assistance or contact a Poison Control Center immediately. As with any drug, if you are pregnant or nursing a baby, seek the advice of a health professional before using this product.

**Drug Interaction Precaution:** Do not take this product if you are presently taking mineral oil, unless directed by a doctor.

**Inactive Ingredients:** Also contains corn oil, FD&C Blue #1 and Red #40, gelatin, glycerin, parabens, sorbitol, and other ingredients.

**How Supplied:** Red soft gelatin capsules in packages of 10, 30 and 100. LIQUI-GELS® is a registered trademark of RP Scherer Corp.

---

## The Procter & Gamble Company
**P. O. BOX 559**
**CINCINNATI, OH 45201**

**Direct Inquiries to:**
Consumer Relations
(800) 832–3064

---

## METAMUCIL® FIBER LAXATIVE
[met uh-mū sil]
**(psyllium husk)**
*Also see **Metamucil Dietary Fiber Supplement** in Dietary Supplement Section*

**Description:** Metamucil contains psyllium husk (from the plant *Plantago*

*ovata*), a bulk forming, natural therapeutic fiber for restoring and maintaining regularity when recommended by a physician. Metamucil contains no chemical stimulants and does not disrupt normal bowel function. Each dose contains approximately 3.4 grams of psyllium husk (or 2.4 grams of soluble fiber). Inactive ingredients, sodium, calcium, potassium, calories, carbohydrate, dietary fiber, and phenylalanine content are shown in the following table for all versions and flavors. Metamucil Smooth Texture Sugar-Free Regular Flavor contains no sugar and no artificial sweeteners; Metamucil Smooth Texture Sugar-Free Orange Flavor contains aspartame (phenylalanine content per dose is 25 mg). Metamucil powdered products are gluten-free. Metamucil Fiber Wafers contain gluten: Apple Crisp contains 0.7g/dose, Cinnamon Spice contains 0.5g/dose. Each two-wafer dose contains 5 grams of fat.

**Actions:** The active ingredient in Metamucil is psyllium husk, a natural fiber which promotes elimination due to its bulking effect in the colon. This bulking effect is due to both the water-holding capacity of undigested fiber and the increased bacterial mass following partial fiber digestion. These actions result in enlargement of the lumen of the colon, and softer stool, thereby decreasing intraluminal pressure and straining, and speeding colonic transit in constipated patients.

**Indications:** Metamucil is indicated for the treatment of occasional constipation, and when recommended by a physician, for chronic constipation and constipation associated with irritable bowel syndrome, diverticulosis, hemorrhoids, convalescence, senility and pregnancy. Pregnancy: Category B. If considering use of Metamucil as part of a cholesterol-lowering program, see **Metamucil Dietary Fiber Supplement** in Dietary Supplement Section.

**Drug Facts**

**Active Ingredient:**
(in each DOSE)                    **Purpose:**
Psyllium husk
 approximately 3.4 g ..... Fiber therapy
                                    for regularity

**Uses:**
- effective in treating occasional constipation and restoring regularity

**Warnings:**
**Choking:** Taking this product without adequate fluid may cause it to swell and block your throat or esophagus and may cause choking. Do not take this product if you have difficulty in swallowing. If

| Adults 12 yrs. & older | Powders: 1 dose in 8 oz of liquid. Wafers: 1 dose with 8 oz of liquid. Take at the first sign of irregularity; can be taken up to 3 times daily. Generally produces effect in 12 – 72 hours. |
| --- | --- |
| 6 – 11 yrs. | Powders: ½ adult dose in 8 oz of liquid. Wafers: 1 wafer with 8 oz of liquid. Can be taken up to 3 times daily |
| Under 6 yrs. | consult a doctor |

## Metamucil Fiber Laxative/Dietary Fiber Supplement

| Versions/Flavors | Ingredients (alphabetical order) | Sodium mg/ dose | Calcium mg/ dose | Potassium mg/ dose | Calories kcal/ dose | Total Carbohydrate g/dose | Dietary Fiber/ (Soluble) g/dose | Dosage (Weight in gms) | How Supplied |
|---|---|---|---|---|---|---|---|---|---|
| **Smooth Texture Orange** Flavor Metamucil Powder | Citric Acid, FD&C Yellow #6, Natural and Artificial Flavor, Psyllium Husk, Sucrose | 5 | 7 | 30 | 45 | 12 | 3 (2.4) | 1 rounded tablespoon ~12g | Canisters: Doses: 48, 72, 114; Cartons: 30 single-dose packets. |
| **Smooth Texture Sugar-Free Orange** Flavor Metamucil Powder | Aspartame, Citric Acid, FD&C Yellow #6, Maltodextrin, Natural and Artificial Flavor, Psyllium Husk | 5 | 7 | 30 | 20 | 5 | 3 (2.4) | 1 rounded teaspoon ~5.8g | Canisters: Doses: 30, 48, 72 114, 180; Cartons: 30 single-dose packets. |
| **Smooth Texture Sugar-Free Regular** Flavor Metamucil Powder | Citric Acid, Maltodextrin, Psyllium Husk | 4 | 7 | 30 | 20 | 5 | 3 (2.4) | 1 rounded teaspoon ~5.4g | Canisters: Doses: 48, 72 114. |
| **Original Texture Regular** Flavor Metamucil Powder | Psyllium Husk, Sucrose | 3 | 6 | 30 | 25 | 7 | 3 (2.4) | 1 rounded teaspoon ~7g | Canisters: Doses: 48, 72 114. |
| **Original Texture Orange** Flavor Metamucil Powder | Citric Acid, FD&C Yellow #6, Natural and Artificial Flavor, Psyllium Husk, Sucrose | 5 | 6 | 30 | 40 | 11 | 3 (2.4) | 1 rounded tablespoon ~11g | Canisters: Doses: 48,72 114. |
| ***Fiber Laxative*** | | | | | | | | | |
| ***Wafers*** | | | | | | | | | |
| **Apple Crisp** (1) Metamucil Wafers | | 20 | 14 | 60 | 120 | 17 | 6 | 2 wafers 24 g | Cartons: 12 doses |
| **Cinnamon Spice** (2) Metamucil Wafers | | 20 | 14 | 60 | 120 | 17 | 6 | 2 wafers 24 g | Cartons: 12 doses |

(1) ascorbic acid, brown sugar, cinnamon, corn oil, corn starch, fructose, lecithin, molasses, natural and artificial flavors, oat hull fiber, psyllium husk, sodium bicarbonate, sucrose, water, wheat flour
(2) ascorbic acid, cinnamon, corn oil, corn starch, fructose, lecithin, molasses, natural and artificial flavors, nutmeg, oat hull fiber, oats, psyllium husk, sodium bicarbonate, sucrose, water, wheat flour

you experience chest pain, vomiting, or difficulty in swallowing or breathing after taking this product, seek immediate medical attention.
**Ask a doctor before use if you have:**
• a sudden change in bowel habits persisting for 2 weeks
• abdominal pain, nausea or vomiting
**When using this product:**
• may cause allergic reaction in people sensitive to inhaled or ingested psyllium
**Stop use and ask a doctor if:**
• constipation lasts more than 7 days
• rectal bleeding occurs
These may be signs of a serious condition.
**Keep out of reach of children.** In case of overdose, get medical help or contact a Poison Control Center right away.

**Directions:** For Powders: Put one dose into an empty glass. Fill glass with at least 8 oz of water or your favorite beverage. Stir briskly and drink promptly. If mixture thickens, add more liquid and stir. Mix this product (child or adult dose) with at least 8 ounces (a full glass) of water or other fluid. For Wafers: Take this product (child or adult dose) with at least 8 ounces (a full glass) of liquid. Taking

these products without enough liquid may cause choking. See choking warning.
[See table at bottom of previous page]
Laxatives, including bulk fibers, may affect how well other medicines work. If you are taking a prescription medicine by mouth, take this product at least 2 hours before or 2 hours after the prescribed medicine. As your body adjusts to increased fiber intake, you may experience changes in bowel habits or minor bloating. **New Users:** Start with 1 dose per day; gradually increase to 3 doses per day as necessary.

**Other Information:**
• **Each product contains:** sodium (See table for amount/dose)
• **PHENYLKETONURICS:** Smooth Texture Sugar Free Orange product **contains phenylalanine** 25 mg per dose
• Each product contains a 100% natural, therapeutic fiber

**Inactive Ingredients:** See table
Notice to Health Care Professionals: To minimize the potential for allergic reaction, health care professionals who frequently dispense powdered psyllium products should avoid inhaling airborne

dust while dispensing these products. Handling and Dispensing: To minimize generating airborne dust, spoon product from the canister into a glass according to label directions.

**How Supplied:** Powder: canisters and cartons of single-dose packets. Wafers: cartons of single dose packets. (See table) [See table above]
***Questions?*** **1-800-983-4237**
*Shown in Product Identification Guide, page 522*

---

**PEPTO-BISMOL®**
**ORIGINAL LIQUID,**
**MAXIMUM STRENGTH LIQUID,**
**ORIGINAL AND CHERRY FLAVOR**
**CHEWABLE TABLETS**
**AND EASY-TO-SWALLOW CAPLETS**
**For upset stomach, indigestion, heartburn, nausea and diarrhea.**

Multi-symptom Pepto-Bismol® contains bismuth subsalicylate and is the only leading OTC stomach remedy clinically

*Continued on next page*

## Pepto-Bismol Original—Cont.

proven effective for both upper and lower GI symptoms. It has been clinically proven in double-blind placebo-controlled trials for relief of upset stomach symptoms and diarrhea.

**Active Ingredient: (per tablespoon/per tablet/per caplet)**
**Original Liquid/Tablets/Caplets**
Bismuth subsalicylate 262 mg
**Maximum Strength Liquid**
Bismuth subsalicylate 525 mg

**Inactive Ingredients:**
**[Original Liquid]** benzoic acid, flavor, magnesium aluminum silicate, methylcellulose, red 22, red 28, saccharin sodium, salicylic acid, sodium salicylate, sorbic acid, water
**[Maximum Strength Liquid]** benzoic acid, flavor, magnesium aluminum silicate, methylcellulose, red 22, red 28, saccharin sodium, salicylic acid, sodium salicylate, sorbic acid, water
**[Original Tablets]** calcium carbonate, flavor, magnesium stearate, mannitol, povidone, red 27 aluminum lake, saccharin sodium, talc
**[Cherry Tablets]** adipic acid, calcium carbonate, flavor, magnesium stearate, mannitol, povidone, red 27 aluminum lake, red 40 aluminum lake, saccharin sodium, talc
**[Caplets]** calcium carbonate, magnesium stearate, mannitol, microcrystalline cellulose, polysorbate 80, povidone, red 27 aluminum lake, silicon dioxide, sodium starch glycolate.

**Other Information:**
**Sodium Content**
Original Liquid – each Tbsp contains: sodium 6 mg • low sodium
Maximum Strength Liquid - each Tbsp contains: sodium 6 mg • low sodium
Chewable Tablets – each Original or Cherry Flavor Tablet contains: sodium less than 1 mg • very low sodium
Caplets – each Caplet contains: sodium 2 mg • low sodium
**Salicylate Content**
Original Liquid – each Tbsp contains: salicylate 130 mg
Maximum Strength Liquid – each Tbsp contains: salicylate 236 mg
Chewable Tablets – each tablet contains: [original] salicylate 102 mg
[cherry] salicylate 99 mg
Caplets – each caplet contains: salicylate 99 mg
**All Forms are sugar free.**

**Indications:**
• relieves upset stomach symptoms (i.e., indigestion, heartburn, nausea and fullness caused by over-indulgence in food and drink) without constipating; and,
• controls diarrhea (including Travelers' Diarrhea).

**Actions:** For upset stomach symptoms, the active ingredient is believed to work via a topical effect on the stomach mucosa. For diarrhea, it is believed to work by several mechanisms in the gastrointestinal tract, including: 1) normalizing fluid movement via an antisecretory mechanism, 2) binding bacterial toxins and 3) antimicrobial activity.

**Warnings:**
**Do not use**
• for children and teenagers who have or are recovering from chicken pox or flu. If nausea or vomiting occurs, ask a doctor because this could be an early sign of Reye Syndrome, a rare but serious illness.
• if you are allergic to salicylates including aspirin
**Ask a doctor if you are** taking medicines for
• anticoagulation (thinning the blood)
• diabetes • gout
**Stop use and ask a doctor if**
• taken with other salicylates such as aspirin and ringing in the ears occurs
• diarrhea occurs with a fever or lasts more than 2 days
• other symptoms last more than 2 weeks
**If pregnant or breast feeding,** ask a health professional before use.
**Keep out of reach of children.**

**Notes:** May cause a temporary and harmless darkening of the tongue or stool. Stool darkening should not be confused with melena.

While no lead is intentionally added to Pepto-Bismol, this product contains certain ingredients that are mined from the ground and thus contain small amounts of naturally occurring lead. For example, bismuth, contained in the active ingredient of Pepto-Bismol, is mined and therefore contains some naturally occurring lead. The small amounts of naturally occurring lead in Pepto-Bismol are low in comparison to average daily lead exposure; this is for the information of healthcare professionals. Pepto-Bismol is indicated for treatment of acute upset stomach symptoms and diarrhea. It is not intended for chronic use.

**Overdosage:** In case of overdose, patients are advised to contact a physician or Poison Control Center. Emesis induced by ipecac syrup is indicated in large ingestions provided ipecac can be administered within one hour of ingestion. Activated charcoal should be administered after gastric emptying. Patients should be evaluated for signs and symptoms of salicylate toxicity.

**Directions:**
**Pepto-Bismol® Original Liquid, Original & Cherry Flavor Chewable Tablets, and Caplets**

[Original Liquid]
• shake well before using
• for easy dosing, use dose cup
[Original Tablet, Cherry Tablets]
• chew or dissolve in mouth
[Caplets]
• swallow with water, do not chew

| AGE | DOSAGE |
|---|---|
| adults & children 12 yrs & older | 2 Tbsp. or 30 ml, 2 tablets or 2 caplets |
| children 9 to under 12 yrs | 1 Tbsp or 15 ml, 1 tablet or 1 caplet |
| children 6 to under 9 yrs | 2 tsp or 10 ml, 2/3 tablet or 2/3 caplet |
| children 3 to under 6 yrs | 1 tsp or 5 ml, 1/3 tablet or 1/3 caplet |
| children under 3 yrs | ask a doctor |

• repeat every ½ to 1 hour as needed
• not more than 8 doses in 24 hours

**Pepto-Bismol® Maximum Strength Liquid**
• shake well before using
• for easy dosing, use dose cup

| AGE | DOSAGE |
|---|---|
| adults & children 12 yrs & older | 2 Tbsp. or 30 ml |
| children 9 to under 12 yrs | 1 Tbsp or 15 ml |
| children 6 to under 9 yrs | 2 tsp or 10 ml |
| children 3 to under 6 yrs | 1 tsp or 5 ml |
| children under 3 yrs | ask a doctor |

• repeat every hour as needed
• not more than 4 doses in 24 hours

**How Supplied:** Pepto-Bismol® Original and Maximum Strength Liquids are pink. Pepto-Bismol® Original Liquid is available in: 4, 8, 12 and 16 fl oz bottles. Pepto-Bismol® Maximum Strength Liquid is available in: 4, 8 and 12 fl oz bottles. Pepto-Bismol® Original and Cherry Flavor Tablets are pink, round, chewable tablets imprinted with a debossed triangle and "Pepto-Bismol" on one side. Tablets are available in: boxes of 30 and 48. Pepto-Bismol® Caplets are pink and imprinted with "Pepto-Bismol" on one side. Caplets are available in bottles of 24 and 40.
• avoid excessive heat (over 104°F or 40°C)
• protect liquids from freezing
**Questions:** 1-800-717-3786
www.pepto-bismol.com

*Shown in Product Identification Guide, page 522*

## THERMACARE®

[thərm' ă-kār]
**Therapeutic Heat Wraps
with Air-Activated Heat Discs**

### Uses:
**Back Wrap:** Provides temporary relief of minor muscular back aches and pains associated with overexertion, strains and sprains.
**Neck to Arm Wrap:** Provides temporary relief of minor muscular and joint aches and pains associated with overexertion, strains, sprains and arthritis.
**Menstrual Patch:** Provides temporary relief of minor menstrual cramp pain.

### Warnings:
**Skin warning** This product has the potential to cause skin irritation or burns. Do <u>not</u> use ThermaCare in the same location for more than 8 hours in any 24 hour period.
**Ingestion warning** Each heat disc contains iron (∼2 grams) which can be harmful if ingested. If ingested, rinse mouth with water and call a Poison Control Center right away. If heat disc contents come in contact with your skin or eyes, rinse right away with water.
**Flammability warning** To avoid the risk of fire, do not microwave or attempt to reheat this product.

### Do not use:
- if the material covering the heat discs is damaged or torn
- with medicated lotions, creams or ointments
- on skin that is damaged or broken
- on areas of bruising or swelling that have occurred within 48 hours
- on people unable to remove the product on their own, including children and infants
- on areas of the body where heat cannot be felt
- if you are bedridden or prone to skin ulcers
- with other forms of therapeutic heat, including electric heating pads

### Ask a doctor before use if you:
- are pregnant
- have diabetes
- have poor blood circulation
- have rheumatoid arthritis

### When using this product:
- it is normal to experience slight skin redness after removing the wrap. If your skin is still red after a few hours, stop using ThermaCare until the redness goes away completely. To reduce the risk of prolonged redness in the future, we recommend you:
  (a) wear ThermaCare for a shorter period of time
  (b) wear looser clothing when using ThermaCare
  (c) wear ThermaCare over a thin layer of clothing instead of directly against your skin
- be careful and periodically check your skin:
  (a) if you know your skin is sensitive to heat
  (b) if you feel your tolerance to heat has decreased over the years
  (c) when lying down or leaning against the product
  (d) when wearing a tight fitting belt or waistband over the product
- if you know your skin is sensitive to heat, consider wearing ThermaCare during the day to gain experience with the level of heat before deciding to use ThermaCare during sleep

### Stop use and ask a doctor if:
- after 7 days of product use (4 days for menstrual product) the pain you are treating gets worse or remains unchanged. This could be a sign of a more serious condition
- you experience any discomfort, swelling, rash or other changes in your skin that persist where the wrap is worn

**Keep out of reach of children and pets.**

**Directions:** Open the pouch when ready to use. It may take up to 30 minutes for ThermaCare to reach its therapeutic temperature. For maximum effectiveness, we recommend you wear ThermaCare for the full 8 hours. For sustained and enhanced benefits, use ThermaCare for 2 or 3 consecutive days. Do not use for more than 8 hours in any 24 hour period <u>OR</u> for more than 7 days in a row (4 days in a row for menstrual product).

Position heat discs directly over pain area of low back.

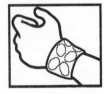

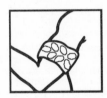

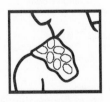

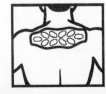

Peel away paper to reveal adhesive side. Place on muscle-pained area with adhesive side toward skin. Attach firmly.

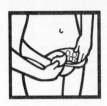

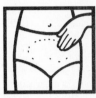

Position patch over pain area. Adhere adhesive side of patch to inside of panties.

### How Supplied:
**Back Wrap:** Available in trial size of 1 L/XL or in boxes of 2 S/M or L/XL wraps.
**Neck to Arm:** Available in boxes of 3 wraps.
**Menstrual:** Available in boxes of 3 patches.

*Shown in Product Identification Guide, page 522*

---

## VICKS® 44® COUGH RELIEF
**Dextromethorphan HBr/
Cough Suppressant
Alcohol 5%**

- Maximum Strength
- Non-Drowsy
- For Adults & Children

### Drug Facts:

### Active Ingredient:
| (per tablespoon, 15 ml) | Purpose: |
| --- | --- |
| Dextromethorphan HBr 30 mg ...................... | Cough suppressant |

**Uses:** Temporarily relieves
- cough due to minor throat and bronchial irritation associated with a cold

### Warnings:
**Do not use** if you are now taking a prescription monoamine oxidase inhibitor (MAOI) (certain drugs for depression, psychiatric or emotional conditions, or Parkinson's disease), or for 2 weeks after stopping the MAOI drug. If you do not know if your prescription drug contains an MAOI, ask a doctor or pharmacist before taking this product.

### Ask a doctor before use if you have:
- cough associated with excessive phlegm (mucus)
- persistent or chronic cough such as occurs with smoking, asthma, or emphysema

### Stop use and ask a doctor if:
- cough lasts more than 7 days, comes

*Continued on next page*

## Vicks 44—Cont.

back, or occurs with fever, rash, or headache that lasts. These could be signs of a serious condition.

**If pregnant or breast feeding,** ask a health professional before use.

**Keep out of reach of children.** In case of overdose, get medical help or contact a Poison Control Center right away.

**Directions:**
- use teaspoon (tsp), tablespoon (TBSP) or dose cup
  - Under 6 yrs. ...................... ask a doctor
  - 6–11 yrs. ..................... 1½ tsp or 7½ ml
  - 12 yrs. & older ........... 1 TBSP or 3 tsp or 15 ml
- Repeat every 6–8 hours, not to exceed 4 doses per 24 hours.

**Other Information:**
- store at room temperature
- **each tablespoon contains** sodium 31 mg

**Inactive Ingredients:** Alcohol, FD&C Blue 1, carboxymethylcellulose sodium, citric acid, flavor, high fructose corn syrup, polyethylene oxide, polyoxyl 40 stearate, propylene glycol, purified water, FD&C Red 40, saccharin sodium, sodium benzoate, sodium citrate.

**How Supplied:** Available in 4 FL OZ (118 ml) plastic bottle and ½ FL OZ (15 ml) pouch. A calibrated dose cup accompanies each bottle.

**TAMPER EVIDENT:** Do not use if imprinted shrinkband is missing or broken.

**Questions?** 1-800-342-6844

Dist. by Procter & Gamble, Cincinnati, OH 45202.

US Pat 5,458,879            42434792

*Shown in Product Identification Guide, page 522*

---

## VICKS® 44D®
### COUGH & HEAD CONGESTION RELIEF
**Cough Suppressant/ Nasal Decongestant**
Alcohol 5%
- Maximum Strength
- Non-Drowsy
- For Adults & Children

**Drug Facts:**

**Active Ingredients:**
**(per tablespoon, 15 ml)          Purpose:**
Dextromethorphan HBr
 30 mg .................... Cough suppressant
Pseudoephedrine HCl
 60 mg .................... Nasal decongestant

**Uses:** Temporarily relieves these cold symptoms
- cough
- nasal congestion

**Warnings:**
**Failure to follow these warnings could result in serious consequences.**

**Do not use** if you are now taking a prescription monoamine oxidase inhibitor (MAOI) (certain drugs for depression, psychiatric or emotional conditions, or Parkinson's disease), or for 2 weeks after stopping the MAOI drug. If you do not

know if your prescription drug contains an MAOI, ask a doctor or pharmacist before taking this product.

**Ask a doctor before use if you have:**
- heart disease
- asthma
- emphysema
- thyroid disease
- diabetes
- chronic bronchitis
- cough associated with smoking
- high blood pressure
- excessive phlegm (mucus)
- persistent or chronic cough
- trouble urinating due to enlarged prostate gland

**When using this product do not take more than directed.**

**Stop use and ask a doctor if:**
- symptoms do not get better within 7 days or are accompanied by fever.
- you get nervous, dizzy or sleepless
- cough lasts more than 7 days, comes back, or occurs with fever, rash, or headache that lasts.
  These could be signs of a serious condition.

**If pregnant or breast-feeding,** ask a health professional before use.

**Keep out of reach of children.** In case of overdose, get medical help or contact a Poison Control Center right away.

**Directions:**
- use teaspoon (tsp), tablespoon (TBSP) or dose cup
  - Under 6 yrs. ...................... ask a doctor
  - 6–11 yrs. .................. 1½ tsp or 7½ ml
  - 12 yrs. & older. ........... 1 TBSP or 3 tsp or 15 ml
- Repeat every 6 hours, not to exceed 4 doses per day.

**Other Information:**
- store at room temperature
- **each tablespoon contains** sodium 31 mg

**Inactive Ingredients:** Alcohol, FD&C Blue 1, carboxymethylcellulose sodium, citric acid, flavor, high fructose corn syrup, polyethylene oxide, polyoxyl 40 stearate, propylene glycol, purified water, FD&C Red 40, saccharin sodium, sodium benzoate, sodium citrate.

**How Supplied:** Available in 1 FL OZ (30 ml) 4 FL OZ (118 ml) and 8 FL OZ (236 ml) plastic bottles. A calibrated dose cup accompanies each bottle.

**TAMPER EVIDENT:** Do not use if imprinted shrinkband is missing or broken.

**Question?** 1-800-342-6844

Dist. by Procter & Gamble, Cincinnati OH 45202.

US Pat 5,458,879            42434796

*Shown in Product Identification Guide, page 522*

---

## VICKS® 44E®
### Cough & Chest Congestion Relief
**Cough Suppressant/Expectorant**
Alcohol 5%
- Non-Drowsy
- For Adults & Children

**Drug Facts:**

**Active Ingredients:**
**(per tablespoon, 15 ml)          Purpose:**
Dextromethorphan HBr
 20 mg ....................... Cough suppressant

Guaifenesin
 200 mg .................................. Expectorant

**Uses:**
- temporarily relieves cough due to the common cold
- helps loosen phlegm to rid the bronchial passageways of bothersome mucus

**Warnings:**
**Do not use**
- if you are on a sodium-restricted diet
- if you are now taking a prescription monoamine oxidase inhibitor (MAOI) (certain drugs for depression, psychiatric or emotional conditions, or Parkinson's disease), or for 2 weeks after stopping the MAOI drug. If you do not know if your prescription drug contains an MAOI, ask a doctor or pharmacist before taking this product.

**Ask a doctor before use if you have:**
- chronic bronchitis
- asthma
- persistent or chronic cough
- excessive phlegm (mucus)
- emphysema
- cough associated with smoking

**Stop use and ask a doctor if:**
- cough lasts more than 7 days, comes back, or occurs with fever, rash, or headache that lasts. These could be signs of a serious condition.

**If pregnant or breast-feeding,** ask a health professional before use.

**Keep out of reach of children.** In case of overdose, get medical help or contact a Poison Control Center right away.

**Directions:**
- use teaspoon (tsp), tablespoon (TBSP) or dose cup
  - Under 6 yrs. ................... ask a doctor
  - 6–11 yrs. ................ 1½ tsp or 7½ ml
  - 12 yrs. & older. . 1 TBSP or 3 tsp or 15 ml
- Repeat every 4 hours, not to exceed 6 doses per 24 hours.

**Other Information:**
- store at room temperature
- **each tablespoon contains** sodium 31 mg

**Inactive Ingredients:** Alcohol, FD&C Blue 1, carboxymethylcellulose sodium, citric acid, flavor, high fructose corn syrup, polyethylene oxide, polyoxyl 40 stearate, propylene glycol, purified water, FD&C Red 40, saccharin sodium, sodium benzoate, sodium citrate.

**How Supplied:** Available in 4 FL OZ (118 ml) and 8 FL OZ (236 ml) plastic bottles. A calibrated dose cup accompanies each bottle.

**TAMPER EVIDENT:** Do not use if imprinted shrinkband is missing or broken.

**Questions?** 1-800-342-6844

Dist. by Procter & Gamble, Cincinnati OH 45202.

US Pat 5,458,879            42434800

*Shown in Product Identification Guide, page 522*

## VICKS® 44M®
### COUGH, COLD & FLU RELIEF
**Cough Suppressant/Nasal Decongestant/Antihistamine/Pain Reliever–Fever Reducer**
**Alcohol 10%**

Maximum strength cough formula

**Drug Facts:**

**Active Ingredients:**
(per teaspoon, 5 ml)          **Purpose:**
Acetaminophen
  162.5 mg ... Pain reliever/fever reducer
Chlorpheniramine maleate
  1 mg .................................. Antihistamine
Dextromethorphan HBr
  7.5 mg ...................... Cough suppressant
Pseudoephedrine HCl
  15 mg ...................... Nasal decongestant

**Uses:** Temporarily relieves cough/cold/flu symptoms:
* cough
* sneezing
* headache
* muscular aches
* sore throat pain
* fever
* runny nose
* nasal congestion

**Warnings:**
**Failure to follow these warnings could result in serious consequences.**
**Alcohol warning** If you consume 3 or more alcoholic drinks every day, ask your doctor whether you should take acetaminophen or other pain relievers/fever reducers. Acetaminophen may cause liver damage.
**Sore throat warning** Severe or persistent sore throat or sore throat that occurs with high fever, headache, rash, nausea, and vomiting may be serious. Ask a doctor right away. Do not use more than 2 days or give to children under 12 years of age unless directed by a doctor.
**Do not use** if you are now taking a prescription monoamine oxidase inhibitor (MAOI) (certain drugs for depression, psychiatric or emotional conditions, or Parkinson's disease), or for 2 weeks after stopping the MAOI drug. If you do not know if your prescription drug contains an MAOI, ask a doctor or pharmacist before taking this product.
**Ask a doctor before use if you have:**
* heart disease
* asthma
* emphysema
* thyroid disease
* diabetes
* glaucoma
* high blood pressure
* excessive phlegm (mucus)
* breathing problems
* chronic bronchitis
* persistent or chronic cough
* cough associated with smoking
* trouble urinating due to enlarged prostate gland
**Ask a doctor or pharmacist before use if you are** taking sedatives or tranquilizers.
**When using this product:**
* **do not use more than directed**
* excitability may occur, especially in children
* drowsiness may occur
* avoid alcoholic drinks
* be careful when driving a motor vehicle or operating machinery
* do not use with other products containing acetaminophen
* alcohol, sedatives, and tranquilizers may increase drowsiness
**Stop use and ask a doctor if:**
* you get nervous, dizzy or sleepless
* fever gets worse or lasts more than 3 days
* new symptoms occur
* you need to use more than 7 days
* symptoms do not get better
* cough lasts more than 7 days, comes back, or occurs with fever, rash, or headache that lasts.
  These could be signs of a serious condition.
**If pregnant or breast-feeding,** ask a health professional before use.
**Keep out of reach of children.** In case of overdose, get medical help or contact a Poison Control Center right away. Quick medical attention is critical for adults as well as for children even if you do not notice any signs or symptoms.

**Directions:**
* children 12 and under: ask a doctor.
* 12 yrs. & older: take 4 teaspoons (tsp) or 20 ml (dose cup), repeat every 6 hours; no more than 4 doses per 24 hours.

**Other Information:**
* store at room temperature
* **each teaspoon contains** sodium 8 mg

**Inactive Ingredients:** Alcohol, FD&C Blue 1, carboxymethylcellulose sodium, citric acid, flavor, high fructose corn syrup, polyethylene glycol, polyethylene oxide, propylene glycol, purified water, FD&C Red 40, saccharin sodium, sodium citrate.

**How Supplied:** Available in 4 FL OZ (118 ml) and 8 FL OZ (236 ml) plastic bottles. A calibrated dose cup accompanies each bottle.
**TAMPER EVIDENT:** Do not use if imprinted shrinkband is missing or broken. Not recommended for children.
**Questions?** 1-800-342-6844
Dist. by Procter & Gamble, Cincinnati OH 45202.
US Pat 5,458,879          42434741
*Shown in Product Identification Guide, page 522*

---

## CHILDREN'S VICKS® NYQUIL®
### COLD/COUGH RELIEF
**Antihistamine/Nasal Decongestant/Cough Suppressant**

Children's NyQuil was specially formulated with three effective ingredients to relieve nighttime cough, nasal congestion, and runny nose so children can rest. Children's NyQuil® is alcohol free and analgesic free and has a pleasant cherry flavor.

**Drug Facts:**

**Active Ingredients:**          **Purpose:**
(per tablespoon, 15 ml)
Chlorpheniramine maleate
  2 mg .................................. Antihistamine
Dextromethorphan HBr
  15 mg ...................... Cough suppressant
Pseudoephedrine HCl
  30 mg ...................... Nasal decongestant

**Uses:** Temporarily relieves cold symptoms:
* cough
* sneezing
* runny nose
* nasal congestion

**Warnings:**
**Failure to follow these warnings could result in serious consequences.**
**Do not use**
* if you are on a sodium-restricted diet
* if you are now taking a prescription monoamine oxidase inhibitor (MAOI) (certain drugs for depression, psychiatric or emotional conditions, or Parkinson's disease), or for 2 weeks after stopping the MAOI durg. If you do not know if your prescription drug contains an MAOI, ask a doctor or pharmacist before taking this product.
**Ask a doctor before use if you have:**
* heart disease
* asthma
* emphysema
* thyroid disease
* diabetes
* glaucoma
* high blood pressure
* excessive phlegm (mucus)
* breathing problems
* chronic bronchitis
* persistent or chronic cough
* cough associated with smoking
* trouble urinating due to enlarged prostate gland
**Ask a doctor or pharmacist before use if you are** taking sedatives or tranquilizers.
**When using this product:**
* **do not use more than directed**
* excitability may occur, especially in children
* drowsiness may occur
* avoid alcoholic drinks
* be careful when driving a motor vehicle or operating machinery
* alcohol, sedatives, and tranquilizers may increase drowsiness
**Stop use and ask a doctor if:**
* you get nervous, dizzy or sleepless
* new symptoms occur
* you need to use more than 7 days
* symptoms do not get better within 7 days or accompanied by a fever
* cough lasts more than 7 days, comes back, or occurs with fever, rash, or headache that lasts.
  These could be signs of a serious condition.
**If pregnant or breast-feeding,** ask a health professional before use.
**Keep out of reach of children.** In case of overdose, get medical help or contact a Poison Control Center right away. Quick medical attention is critical for adults as well as for children even if you do not notice any signs or symptoms.

**Directions:**
* use tablespoon (TBSP) or dose cup
  under 6 yrs. ...................... ask a doctor
  6–11 yrs. ................... 1 TBSP or 15 ml
  12 yrs. & older ........ 2 TBSP or 30 ml

*Continued on next page*

## Vicks Children's Nyquil—Cont.

- Repeat every 6 hours, not to exceed 4 doses per 24 hours.

**Other Information:**
- store at room temperature
- **each tablespoon contains** sodium 70.5 mg

**Inactive Ingredients:** Citric acid, flavor, potassium sorbate, propylene glycol, purified water, FD&C Red 40, sodium citrate, sucrose.

**How Supplied:** Available in 4 FL OZ (115 ml) plastic bottles with child-resistant, tamper-evident cap and a calibrated medicine cup.
Questions? 1-800-362-1683
Exp. Date: See Bottom.          42434744
Dist. by Procter & Gamble, Cincinnati OH 45202.

*Shown in Product Identification Guide, page 522*

---

**VICKS® Cough Drops**
**Menthol Cough Suppressant/**
**Oral Anesthetic**
**Menthol and Cherry Flavors**

**CONSUMER INFORMATION:** Vicks Cough Drops provide fast and effective relief. Each drop contains effective medicine to suppress your impulse to cough as it dissolves into a soothing syrup to relieve your sore throat.

**Drug Facts:**

**Active Ingredients:**
Menthol:

| Active Ingredient: (per drop) | Purpose: |
|---|---|
| Menthol 3.3 mg ...... | Cough suppressant/ oral anesthetic |

Cherry:

| Active Ingredient: (per drop) | Purpose: |
|---|---|
| Menthol 1.7 mg ...... | Cough suppressant/ oral anesthetic |

**Uses:** Temporarily relieves:
- sore throat
- coughs due to colds or inhaled irritants

**Warnings:**
**Ask a doctor before use if you have:**
- cough associated with excessive phlegm (mucus)
- persistent or chronic cough such as those caused by asthma, emphysema, or smoking
- a severe sore throat accompanied by difficulty in breathing or that lasts more than 2 days
- a sore throat accompanied or followed by fever, headache, rash, swelling, nausea or vomiting

**Stop use and ask a doctor if:**
- you need to use more than 7 days
- cough lasts more than 7 days, comes back, or occurs with fever, rash, or headache that lasts. These could be the signs of a serious condition.

**If pregnant or breast-feeding,** ask a health professional before use.
**Keep out of reach of children.**

**Directions:**
- under 5 yrs.: ask a doctor (menthol)
- adults & children 5 yrs & older: allow 2 drops to dissolve slowly in mouth (cherry)
- adults & children 5 yrs & older: allow 3 drops to dissolve slowly in mouth
Cough: may be repeated every hour.
Sore Throat: may be repeated every 2 hours.

**Other Information:**
- store at room temperature

**Inactive Ingredients:**
Menthol: Ascorbic acid, caramel, corn syrup, eucalyptus oil, sucrose.
Cherry: Ascorbic acid, blue 1, citric acid, corn syrup, eucalyptus oil, flavor, FD&C Red 40, sucrose.

**How Supplied:** Vicks® Cough Drops are available in boxes of 20 triangular drops. Each red or green drop is debossed with "V."
Questions? 1-800-707-1709
Made in Mexico by Procter & Gamble Manufactura 5. de R.I. de C.V. Dist. by Procter & Gamble
Cincinnati OH 45202
50144381

---

**VICKS® DAYQUIL® LIQUID**
**VICKS® DAYQUIL® LIQUICAPS®**
**Multi-Symptom Cold/Flu Relief**
**Nasal Decongestant/**
**Pain Reliever/Cough**
**Suppressant/Fever Reducer**
**Non-drowsy**

**Drug Facts:**

**Active Ingredients:**

**LIQUID:**

| Active Ingredients: (per tablespoon, 15 ml) | Purpose: |
|---|---|
| Acetaminophen 325 mg ...... | Pain reliever/fever reducer |
| Dextromethorphan HBr 10 mg ...... | Cough suppressant |
| Pseudoephedrine HCl 30 mg ...... | Nasal decongestant |

**LIQUICAP®:**

| Active Ingredients: (per softgel) | Purpose: |
|---|---|
| Acetaminophen 250 mg ...... | Pain reliever/fever reducer |
| Dextromethorphan HBr 10 mg ...... | Cough suppressant |
| Pseudoephedrine HCl 30 mg ...... | Nasal decongestant |

**Uses:** Temporarily relieves common cold/flu symptoms:
- minor aches
- pains
- headache
- muscular aches
- sore throat pain
- fever
- nasal congestion
- cough

**Warnings:**
**Failure to follow these warnings could result in serious consequences.**

**Alcohol warning** If you consume 3 or more alcoholic drinks every day, ask your doctor whether you should take acetaminophen or other pain relievers/fever reducers. Acetaminophen may cause liver damage.
**Sore throat warning** If sore throat is severe, persists more than 2 days, is accompanied by fever, nausea, rash or vomiting, consult a doctor promptly.
LIQUID:   Do not use if you are on a sodium-restricted diet.
**Do not use** if you are now taking a prescription monoamine oxidase inhibitor (MAOI) (certain drugs for depression, psychiatric or emotional conditions, or Parkinson's disease), or for 2 weeks after stopping the MAOI drug. If you do not know if your prescription drug contains an MAOI, ask a doctor or pharmacist before taking this product.
**Ask a doctor before use if you have:**
- heart disease
- asthma
- emphysema
- thyroid disease
- diabetes
- cough associated with smoking
- high blood pressure
- excessive phlegm (mucus)
- breathing problems
- persistent or chronic cough
- trouble urinating due to enlarged prostate gland

**When using this product:**
- do not use more than directed
- do not use with other products containing acetaminophen
- avoid alcoholic drinks.

**Stop use and ask a doctor if:**
- you get nervous, dizzy or sleepless
- fever gets worse or lasts more than 3 days
- new symptoms occur
- symptoms do not get better within 7 days
- you need to use more than 7 days (adults) or 5 days (children)
- cough lasts more than 7 days (adults) or 5 days (chidren), comes back, or occurs with fever, rash, or headache that lasts. These could be the signs of a serious condition.

**If pregnant or breast-feeding,** ask a health professional before use.
**Keep out of reach of children.** In case of overdose, get medical help or contact a Poison Control Center right away. Quick medical attention is critical for adults as well as for children even if you do not notice any signs or symptoms.

**Directions:**
**LIQUID:**
- use teaspoon (tsp), tablespoon (TBSP) or dose cup
  under 6 yrs. ...................... ask a doctor
  6–11 yrs. ..... 1 TBSP or 3 tsp or 15 ml
  12 yrs. & older ........... 2 TBSP or 6 tsp or 30 ml
- Repeat every 4 hours, not to exceed 4 doses per 24 hours or use as directed by a doctor. If taking NyQuil® and DayQuil, limit total to 4 doses per 24 hours.
**LIQUICAP:**
  under 6 yrs. ...................... ask a doctor
  6–11 yrs. .............. 1 softgel with water

12 yrs. & older .. 2 softgels with water
- Repeat every 4 hours, not to exceed 4 doses per 24 hours or use as directed by a doctor. If taking NyQuil® and DayQuil, limit total to 4 doses per 24 hours.

**Other Information:**
**LIQUID:**
- store at room temperature
- **each tablespoon contains** sodium 70.5 mg
**LIQUICAP:**
- store at room temperature

**Inactive Ingredients:**
**LIQUID:** Citric acid, flavor, glycerin, polyethylene glycol, propylene glycol, purified water, saccharin sodium, sodium citrate, sucrose, FD&C Yellow 6.
**LIQUICAP:** Gelatin, glycerin, polyethylene glycol, povidone, propylene glycol, purified water, FD&C Red 40, sorbitol special, yellow 6.

**How Supplied:** Available in: **LIQUID** 6 FL OZ (177 ml) and 10 FL OZ (295 ml) plastic bottles with child-resistant, tamper-evident cap and a calibrated medicine cup.
**LIQUICAP:** in 2–count 12-count child-resistant packages and 20- and 36-count nonchild-resistant packages. Each softgel is imprinted: "DayQuil."
**LIQUID:**
**TAMPER EVIDENT:** Do not use if imprinted shrinkband is missing or broken.
**LIQUICAP:**
**TAMPER EVIDENT:** This package is safety sealed and child resistant. Use only if blisters are intact. If difficult to open, use scissors.
**Questions?** 1-800-251-3374
Made in Canada
Dist. by Procter & Gamble
Cincinnati OH 45202
42435018

*Shown in Product Identification Guide, page 522*

---

## VICKS® NYQUIL® COUGH
**Antihistamine**
**Cough Suppressant**
**All Night Cough Relief**
**Cherry Flavor**

alcohol 10%
**Drug Facts:**

**Active Ingredients:**　　　**Purpose:**
**(per tablespoon, 15 ml)**
Dextromethorphan HBr
　15 mg ..................... Cough suppressant
Doxylamine succinate
　6.25 mg .......................... Antihistamine

**Uses:**
Temporarily relieves cold symptoms
- cough
- runny nose and sneezing

**Warnings:**
**Do not use** if you are now taking a prescription monoamine oxidase inhibitor (MAOI) (certain drugs for depression, psychiatric or emotional conditions, or Parkinson's disease), or for 2 weeks after

stopping the MAOI drug. If you do not know if your prescription drug contains an MAOI, ask a doctor or pharmacist before taking this product.

**Ask a doctor before use if you have:**
- asthma
- emphysema
- breathing problems
- excessive phlegm (mucus)
- glaucoma
- chronic bronchitis
- persistent or chronic cough
- cough associated with smoking
- trouble urinating due to enlarged prostate gland

**Ask a doctor or pharmacist before use if you are:**
taking sedatives or tranquilizers.

**When using this product:**
- do not use more than directed
- marked drowsiness may occur
- avoid alcoholic drinks
- excitability may occur, especially in children
- be careful when driving a motor vehicle or operating machinery
- alcohol, sedatives, and tranquilizers may increase drowsiness

**Stop use and ask a doctor if:**
- cough lasts more than 7 days, comes back, or occurs with fever, rash, or headache that lasts.
These could be signs of a serious condition.

**If pregnant or breast-feeding,** ask a health professional before use.

**Keep out of reach of children.** In case of overdose, get medical help or contact a Poison Control Center right away.

**Directions:**
Use tablespoon (TBSP) or dose cup
Under 12 yrs. ........................ ask a doctor
12 yrs. & older ............. 2 TBSP or 30 ml
- Repeat every 6 hours, not to exceed 4 doses per day.
If taking NyQuil and DayQuil®, limit total to 4 doses per day.

**Other Information:**
- store at room temperature
- **each tablespoon contains** sodium 17.5 mg

**Inactive Ingredients:** Alcohol, blue 1, citric acid, flavor, high fructose corn syrup, polyethylene glycol, propylene glycol, purified water, red 40, saccharin sodium, sodium citrate.

**How Supplied:** Available in 1 FL OZ (30 ml) 6 FL OZ (177 ml), 10 FL OZ (295 ml) plastic bottles with child-resistant, tamper-evident cap and calibrated Medicine cup.

**TAMPER EVIDENT:** Do not use if imprinted shrinkband is missing or broken.

**Questions?** 1-800-362-1683
Dist. by Procter & Gamble,
Cincinnati OH 45202. 42437885

*Shown in Product Identification Guide, page 522*

## VICKS® NYQUIL® LIQUICAPS®
## VICKS® NYQUIL® LIQUID
**(Original and Cherry)**
**Multi-Symptom Cold/Flu Relief**
**Antihistamine/Cough**
**Suppressant/Pain Reliever/**
**Nasal Decongestant/**
**Fever Reducer**

Liquid (Original and Cherry)—alcohol 10%

**Drug Facts:**

**Active Ingredients:**
**LiquiCaps®:**
**Active Ingredients:**　　　　**Purpose:**
**(per softgel)**
Acetaminophen
　250 mg ...... Pain reliever/fever reducer
Dextromethorphan HBr
　10 mg ...................... Cough suppressant
Doxylamine succinate
　6.25 mg ........................... Antihistamine
Pseudoephedrine HCl
　30 mg ..................... Nasal decongestant
**Liquid (Original and Cherry):**
**Active Ingredients:**　　　　**Purpose:**
**(per tablespoon, 15 ml)**
Acetaminophen
　500 mg ...... Pain reliever/fever reducer
Dextromethorphan HBr
　15 mg ...................... Cough suppressant
Doxylamine succinate
　6.25 mg ........................... Antihistamine
Pseudoephedrine HCl
　30 mg ..................... Nasal decongestant

**Uses:**
**LiquiCaps®:**
Temporarily relieves these common cold/flu symptoms:
- minor aches and pains
- muscular aches
- fever
- headache
- nasal congestion
- runny nose and sneezing
- cough due to minor throat & bronchial irritation
**Liquid (Original and Cherry):**
Temporarily relieves these common cold/flu symptoms:
- minor aches and pains
- headache
- muscular aches
- sore throat
- fever
- runny nose and sneezing
- nasal congestion
- cough due to minor throat and bronchial irritation

**Warnings:**
**Failure to follow these warnings could result in serious consequences.**
**Alcohol warning** If you consume 3 or more alcoholic drinks every day, ask your doctor whether you should take acetaminophen or other pain relievers/fever reducers. Acetaminophen may cause liver damage.
**Sore throat warning** If sore throat is severe, persists more than 2 days, is accompanied or followed by fever, rash, nausea, or vomiting, consult a doctor promptly.

*Continued on next page*

## Vicks Nyquil—Cont.

**Do not use** if you are now taking a prescription monoamine oxidase inhibitor (MAOI) (certain drugs for depression, psychiatric or emotional conditions, or Parkinson's disease), or for 2 weeks after stopping the MAOI drug. If you do not know if your prescription drug contains an MAOI, ask a doctor or pharmacist before taking this product.

**Ask a doctor before use if you have:**
• heart disease
• asthma
• emphysema
• thyroid disease
• diabetes
• glaucoma
• high blood pressure
• excessive phlegm (mucus)
• breathing problems
• chronic bronchitis
• persistent or chronic cough
• cough associated with smoking
• trouble urinating due to enlarged prostate gland

**Ask a doctor or pharmacist before use if you are** taking sedatives or tranquilizers.

**When using this product**
• **do not use more than directed**
• excitability may occur, especially in children
• marked drowsiness may occur
• avoid alcoholic drinks
• do not use with other products containing acetaminophen
• be careful when driving a motor vehicle or operating machinery
• alcohol, sedatives, and tranquilizers may increase drowsiness

**Stop use and ask a doctor if:**
• symptoms do not get better within 7 days or are accompanied by fever.
• you get nervous, dizzy or sleepless
• fever gets worse or lasts more than 3 days
• new symptoms occur
• swelling or redness is present.
• cough lasts more than 7 days, comes back, or occurs with fever, rash, or headache that lasts. These could be signs of a serious condition.

**If pregnant or breast-feeding,** ask a health professional before use.

**Keep out of reach of children.** In case of overdose, get medical help or contact a Poison Control Center right away. Quick medical attention is critical for adults as well as for children even if you do not notice any signs or symptoms.

**Directions:**
**LiquiCaps®:**
• children under 12 yrs.: ask a doctor.
• 12 yrs. & older: swallow 2 softgels with water, repeat every 4 hours; no more than 4 doses per 24 hours. If taking NyQuil and DayQuil®, limit total to 4 doses per 24 hours.
**Liquid** (Original and cherry):
• children under 12 yrs.: ask a doctor.
• 12 yrs. & older: take 2 tablespoons (TBSP) or 30 ml (dose cup), repeat every 6 hours; no more than 4 doses per 24 hours. If taking NyQuil and DayQuil®, limit total to 4 doses per 24 hours.

**Other Information:**
**LiquiCaps®:**
• store at room temperature

**Liquid** (Original and Cherry):
• store at room temperature
• **each tablespoon contains** sodium 17 mg

**Inactive Ingredients:**
**LiquiCaps®:** FD&C Blue 1, gelatin, glycerin, polyethylene glycol, povidone, propylene glycol, purified water, sorbitol special, D&C Yellow 10.
**Liquid** (Original): Alcohol, citric acid, flavor, FD&C Green 3, high fructose corn syrup, polyethylene glycol, propylene glycol, purified water, saccharin sodium, sodium citrate, yellow 6, D&C Yellow 10.
**Liquid** (Cherry): Alcohol, FD&C Blue 1, citric acid, flavor, high fructose corn syrup, polyethylene glycol, propylene glycol, purified water, FD&C Red 40, saccharin sodium, sodium citrate.

**How Supplied:**
**LiquiCaps®:** Available in 2-count 12- and 36-count child-resistant blister packages and 20-count non-child resistant blister packages. Each softgel is imprinted: "NyQuil".
**Liquid:** Available in 1 FL OZ (30 ml) 6 and 10 FL OZ (177 ml and 295 ml, respectively) plastic bottles with child-resistant, tamper-evident cap and calibrated medicine cup.
**LiquiCaps®:**
**TAMPER EVIDENT:** This package is safety sealed and child resistant. Use only if blisters are intact. If difficult to open, use scissors.
**Liquid** (Original and cherry):
**TAMPER EVIDENT:** Do not use if imprinted shrinkband is missing or broken.
**Questions?** 1-800-362-1683
**Liqui Caps®:**
Made in Canada
Dist. by Procter & Gamble,
Cincinnati OH 45202.
©2001                                    42435017
**Liquid** (Original): Dist. by Procter & Gamble
Cincinnati OH 45202          42434786
**Liquid** (Cherry): Dist. by Procter & Gamble
Cincinnati OH 45202          42434789

*Shown in Product Identification Guide, page 522*

---

**PEDIATRIC VICKS® 44e®**
**Cough & Chest Congestion Relief**

• Non-drowsy
• Alcohol-free
• Aspirin-free

**Drug Facts:**

**Active Ingredients:**
| (per tablespoon, 15 ml) | Purpose: |
|---|---|
| Dextromethorphan HBr 10 mg | Cough suppressant |
| Guaifenesin 100mg | Expectorant |

**Uses:**
• temporarily relieves cough due to the common cold
• helps loosen phlegm to rid bronchial passageways of bothersome mucus

**Warnings:**
**Do not use**
• if you are on a sodium-restricted diet
• if you are now taking a prescription monoamine oxidase inhibitor (MAOI) (certain drugs for depression, psychiatric or emotional conditions, or Parkinson's disease), or for 2 weeks after stopping the MAOI drug. If you do not know if your prescription drug contains an MAOI, ask a doctor or pharmacist before taking this product.

**Ask a doctor before use if you have:**
• chronic bronchitis
• asthma
• emphysema
• excessive phlegm (mucus)
• breathing problems
• persistent or chronic cough
• cough associated with smoking
**Stop use and ask a doctor if:**
• cough lasts more than 7 days, comes back, or occurs with fever, rash, or headache that lasts. These could be signs of a serious condition.
**If pregnant or breast-feeding,** ask a health professional before use.
**Keep out of reach of children.** In case of overdose, get medical help or contact a Poison Control Center right away.

**Directions:**
• use tablespoon (TBSP) or dose cup
| Under 2 yrs. | ask a doctor |
| 2–5 yrs. | ½ TBSP or 7½ ml |
| 6–11 yrs. | 1 TBSP or 15 ml |
| 12 yrs.& older | 2 TBSP or 30 ml |
• Repeat every 4 hours, not to exceed 6 doses per 24 hours.

**Other Information:**
• store at room temperature
• **each tablespoon contains** sodium 30 mg

**Inactive Ingredients:** Carboxymethylcellulose sodium, citric acid, flavor, high fructose corn syrup, polyethylene oxide, polyoxyl 40 stearate, propylene glycol, purified water, FD&C Red 40, saccharin sodium, sodium benzoate, sodium citrate.

**How Supplied:** 4 FL OZ (118 ml) plastic bottles. A calibrated dose cup accompanies each bottle.
**TAMPER EVIDENT:** Do not use if imprinted shrinkband is missing or broken.
**Questions?** 1-800-342-6844
Dist. by Procter & Gamble, Cincinnati OH 45202.
US Pat 5,458,879                   42434802
*Shown in Product Identification Guide, page 522*

---

**PEDIATRIC VICKS® 44m®**
**Cough & Cold Relief**
**Cough Suppressant/Nasal Decongestant/Antihistamine**

• Alcohol-free
• Aspirin-free

**Drug Facts:**

**Active Ingredients:**
| (per tablespoon, 15 ml) | Purpose: |
|---|---|
| Chlorpheniramine maleate 2 mg | Antihistamine |
| Dextromethorphan HBr 15 mg | Cough suppressant |

Pseudoephedrine HCl
30 mg ...................... Nasal decongestant

**Uses:** Temporarily relieves cough/cold symptoms
- cough
- sneezing
- runny nose
- nasal congestion

**Warnings:**
**Failure to follow these warnings could result in serious consequences.**
**Do not use:**
- if you are on a sodium-restricted diet
- if you are now taking a prescription monoamine oxidase inhibitor (MAOI) (certain drugs for depression, psychiatric or emotional conditions, or Parkinson's disease), or for 2 weeks after stopping the MAOI drug. If you do not know if your prescription drug contains an MAOI, ask a doctor or pharmacist before taking this product.

**Ask a doctor before use if you have:**
- heart disease
- asthma
- emphysema
- thyroid disease
- diabetes
- glaucoma
- high blood pressure
- excessive phlegm (mucus)
- breathing problems
- chronic bronchitis
- persistent or chronic cough
- cough associated with smoking
- trouble urinating due to enlarge prostate gland

**Ask a doctor or pharmicist before use if you are** taking sedatives or tranquilizers.

**When using this product:**
- **do not use more than directed**
- excitability may occur, especially in children
- drowsiness may occur
- avoid alcoholic drinks
- be careful when driving a motor vehicle or operating machinery
- alcohol, sedatives, and tranquilizers may increase drowsiness

**Stop use and ask a doctor if:**
- fever gets worse or lasts more than 3 days
- you get nervous, dizzy or sleepless
- new symptoms occur
- symptoms do not get better within 7 days
- you need to use more than 7 days
- cough last more than 7 days, comes back, or occurs with fever, rash, or headache that lasts
  These could be signs of a serious condition.

**If pregnant or breast-feeding,** ask a health professional before use.

**Keep out of reach of children.** In case of overdose, get medical help or contact a Poison Control Center right away. Quick medical attention is critical for adults as well as for children, even if you do not notice any signs or symptoms.

**Directions:**
- use tablespoon (TBSP) or dose cup
  Under 6 yrs. ..................... ask a doctor
  6–11 yrs. ................... 1 TBSP or 15 ml
  12 yrs. & older ........ 2 TBSP or 30 ml
- Repeat every 6 hours, not to exceed 4 doses per 24 hours.

**Other Information:**
- store at room temperature
- **each tablespoon contains** sodium 30 mg

**Inactive Ingredients:** Carboxymethylcellulose sodium, citric acid, flavor, high fructose corn syrup, polyethylene oxide, polyoxyl 40 stearate, propylene glycol, purified water, FD&C Red 40, saccharin sodium, sodium benzoate, sodium citrate.

**How Supplied:** 4 FL OZ (118 ml) plastic bottles. A calibrated dose cup accompanies each bottle.

**TAMPER EVIDENT:** Do not use if imprinted shrinkband is missing or broken.
***Questions?*** 1-800-342-6844
Dist. by Procter & Gamble, Cincinnati OH 45202.
US Pat 5,458,879　　　　　42434743
*Shown in Product Identification Guide, page 522*

---

## VICKS® SINEX® [NASAL SPRAY]
[Ultra Fine Mist] for Sinus Relief
[sĭ 'něx ]
**Phenylephrine HCl Nasal Decongestant**

**Drug Facts:**

| **Active Ingredients:** | **Purpose:** |
| --- | --- |
| Phenylephrine HCl 0.5% .............. | Nasal decongestant |

**Uses:** Temporarily relieves sinus/nasal congestion due to
- colds
- hay fever
- upper respiratory allergies
- sinusitis

**Warnings:**
**Do not use**
- this container by more than one person; it may spread infection
- for more than 3 days

**Ask a doctor before use if you have:**
- heart disease
- thyroid disease
- diabetes
- high blood pressure
- trouble urinating due to enlarged prostate gland

**When using this product:**
- **do not exceed recommended dosage**
- temporary burning, stinging, sneezing, or increased nasal discharge may occur
- frequent or prolonged use may cause nasal congestion to recur or worsen

**Stop use and ask a doctor if:**
- symptoms persist for more than 3 days

**If pregnant or breast-feeding,** ask a health professional before use.

**Keep out of reach of children.** In case of accidental ingestion, get medical help or contact a poison control center right away.

**Directions:**
**Nasal Spray:**
- under 12 yrs. ask a doctor
- adults & children 12 yrs. & older: 2 or 3 sprays in each nostril without tilting your head, not more than every 4 hours.

**Ultra Fine Mist:** Remove protective cap. Before using for the first time, prime the

pump by firmly depressing its rim several times. Hold container with thumb at base and nozzle between first and second fingers. Without tilting your head, insert nozzle into nostril. Fully depress rim with a firm, even stroke and inhale deeply.
- under 12 yrs.: ask a doctor
- adults & children 12 yrs. & older: 2 or 3 sprays in each nostril, not more often than every 4 hours.

**Other Information:**
- store at room temperature

**Inactive Ingredients:** Benzalkonium chloride, camphor, chlorhexidine gluconate, citric acid, disodium EDTA, eucalyptol, menthol, purified water, tyloxapol

**How Supplied:** Available in 1/2 FL OZ (14.7 ml) plastic squeeze bottle and 1/2 FL OZ (14.7 ml) measured dose Ultra Fine mist pump. Note: This container is properly filled when approximately half full. Air space equal to one half of volume is necessary to propel the fine spray.

**TAMPER EVIDENT:**
Do not use if imprinted shrinkband is missing or broken.
**Questions?** 1-800-873-8276
Nasal Spray 42436771
Ultra Fine Mist 42436765
Dist. by Procter & Gamble
Cincinnati OH 45202

---

## VICKS® SINEX®
[sĭ 'něx ]
**12-HOUR [Nasal Spray]**
[Ultra Fine Mist] for Sinus Relief
**Oxymetazoline HCl**
**Nasal Decongestant**

**Drug Facts:**

| **Active Ingredients:** | **Purpose:** |
| --- | --- |
| Oxymetazoline HCl 0.05% ...................... | Nasal decongestant |

**Uses:** Temporarily relieves sinus/nasal congestion due to
- colds
- hay fever
- upper respiratory allergies
- sinusitis

**Warnings:**
**Do not use** • this container by more than one person; it may spread infection
• for more than 3 days

**Ask a doctor before use if you have:**
- heart disease
- thyroid disease
- diabetes
- high blood pressure
- trouble urinating due to enlarged prostate gland

**When using this product:**
- **do not exceed recommended dosage**
- temporary burning, stinging, sneezing, or increased nasal discharge may occur
- frequent or prolonged use may cause nasal congestion to recur or worsen

**Stop use and ask a doctor if:**
- symptoms persist for more than 3 days

**If pregnant or breast-feeding,** ask a health professional before use.

*Continued on next page*

## Vicks Sinex 12-Hour—Cont.

**Keep out of reach of children.** In case of accidental ingestion, get medical help or contact a poison control center right away.

### Directions:
**Nasal Spray:**
- under 6 yrs. ask a doctor
- adults & children 6 yrs. & older (with adult supervision): 2 or 3 sprays in each nostril without tilting your head, not more often than every 10 to 12 hours. Do not exceed 2 applications in any 24-hour period.

(Note: This container is properly filled when approximately half full. Air space equal to one half of volume is necessary to propel the fine spray).

**Ultra Fine Mist:** Remove protective cap. Before using for the first time, prime the pump by firmly depressing its rim several times. Hold container with thumb at base and nozzle between first and second fingers. Without tilting your head, insert nozzle into nostril. Fully depress rim with a firm, even stroke and inhale deeply.
- under 6 yrs.: ask a doctor
- adults & children 6 yrs. & older (with adult supervision): 2 or 3 sprays in each nostril, not more often than every 10 to 12 hours. Do not exceed 2 applications in any 24-hour period.

### Other Information:
- store at room temperature

**Inactive Ingredients:** Benzalkonium chloride, camphor, chlorhexidine gluconate, disodium EDTA, eucalyptol, menthol, potassium phosphate, purified water, sodium chloride, sodium phosphate, tyloxapol.

**How Supplied:** Available in ½ FL OZ (14.7 ml) plastic squeeze bottle and ½ FL OZ (14.7 ml) measured-dose Ultra Fine mist pump.
**TAMPER EVIDENT:** Do not use if imprinted shrinkband is missing or broken.
Nasal Spray 42436768
Ultra Fine Mist 42436763
*Questions?* 1-800-873-8276
Dist. by
Procter & Gamble,
Cincinnati OH 45202

---

## VICKS® VAPOR INHALER
### Levmetamfetamine/Nasal Decongestant

### Drug Facts:

| Active Ingredients: | Purpose: |
|---|---|
| (per inhaler) | |
| Levmetamfetamine | |
| 50 mg | Nasal decongestant |

**Uses:** Temporarily relieves nasal congestion due to:
- colds
- hay fever
- upper respiratory allergies
- sinusitis

### Warnings:
**Do not use**
- this container by more than one person; it may spread infection
- for more than 7 days

**Ask a doctor before use if you have:**
- heart disease
- thyroid disease
- diabetes
- high blood pressure
- trouble urinating due to enlarged prostate gland

**When using this product:**
- **do not exceed recommended dosage**
- temporary burning, stinging, sneezing, or increased nasal discharge may occur
- frequent or prolonged use may cause nasal congestion to recur or worsen

**Stop use and ask a doctor if:**
- symptoms persist

**If pregnant or breast-feeding,** ask a health professional before use.

**Keep out of reach of children.** If swallowed, get medical help or contact a poison control center right away.

### Directions:
The product delivers in each 800 ml air 0.04 to 0.15 mg of levmetamfetamine.
- under 6 yrs.: ask a doctor
- 6–11 yrs.: with adult supervision, 1 inhalation in each nostril not more often than every 2 hours.
- 12 yrs. & older: 2 inhalation in each nostril, not more often than every 2 hours.

### Other Information:
- store at room temperature
- keep inhaler tightly closed.
- This inhaler is effective for a minimum of 3 months after first use.

**Inactive Ingredients:** Bornyl acetate, camphor, lavender oil, menthol.

**How Supplied:** Available as a cylindrical plastic nasal inhaler.
Net weight: 0.007 OZ (198 mg).
**TAMPER EVIDENT:** Use only if imprinted wrap is intact.
*Questions?* 1-800-873-8276
Dist. by Procter & Gamble, Cincinnati OH 45202. ©2001 42438038

---

## VICKS® VAPORUB®
## VICKS® VAPORUB® CREAM
### (greaseless)
[vā 'pō-rub]
### Nasal Decongestant/Cough Suppressant/Topical Analgesic

### Drug Facts:

**Active Ingredients:**
**Vicks® VapoRub®:**

| Active Ingredients: | Purpose: |
|---|---|
| Camphor 4.8% | Cough suppressant, nasal decongestant & topical analgesic |
| Eucalyptus oil 1.2% | Cough suppressant & nasal decongestant |
| Menthol 2.6% | Cough suppressant, nasal decongestant & topical analgesic |

**Vicks® VapoRub® Cream:**

| Active Ingredients: | Purpose: |
|---|---|
| Camphor 5.2% | Cough suppressant, nasal decongestant & topical analgesic |
| Eucalyptus oil 1.2% | Cough suppressant & nasal decongestant |
| Menthol 2.8% | Cough suppressant, nasal decongestant & topical analgesic |

**Uses:** On chest & throat temporarily relieves
- cough
- nasal congestion due to the common cold

on aching muscles temporarily relieves
- minor aches & pains

### Warnings:
**Failure to follow these warnings could result in serious consequences.**
**For external use only; avoid contact with eyes.**
**Do not use:**
- by mouth
- with tight bandages
- in nostrils
- on wounds or damaged skin

**Ask a doctor before use if you have:**
- excessive phlegm (mucus)
- asthma
- emphysema
- persistent or chronic cough
- cough associated with smoking

**When using this product do not:**
- heat
- microwave
- use near an open flame
- add to hot water or any container where heating water. May cause splattering and result in burns.

**Stop use and ask a doctor if:**
- muscle aches/pains persist more than 7 days or come back
- cough lasts more than 7 days, comes back, or occurs with fever, rash, or headache that lasts.
  These could be signs of a serious condition.

**If pregnant or breast-feeding,** ask a health professional before use.

**Keep out of reach of children.** In case of accidental ingestion, get medical help or contact a Poison Control Center right away.

**Directions:** See important warnings under **"When using this product"**
- under 2 yrs.: ask a doctor
- adults and children 2 yrs. & older: Rub a thick layer on chest & throat or rub on sore aching muscles. If desired, cover with a soft cloth but keep clothing loose. Repeat up to three times per 24 hours.

### Other Information:
- store at room temperature

### Inactive Ingredients:
**Vicks® VapoRub®:** Cedarleaf oil, nutmeg oil, special petrolatum, thymol, turpentine oil

**Vicks® VapoRub® Cream:** Carbomer 954, cedarleaf oil, cetyl alcohol, cetyl palmitate, cyclomethicone copolyol, dimethicone copolyol, dimethicone, EDTA, glycerin, imidazolidinyl urea, isopropyl palmitate, methylparaben, nutmeg oil, peg-100 stearate, propylparaben, purified water, sodium hydroxide, stearic acid, stearyl alcohol, thymol, titanium dioxide, turpentine oil

### How Supplied:
**Vicks VapoRub®:** Available in 1.76 oz (50 g) 3.53 oz (100 g) and 6 oz (170 g) plastic jars 0.45 oz (12 g) tin.

**Vicks® VapoRub® Cream:** Available in 2 oz (60 g) tube ⅙ oz pouch.
**Questions? 1-800-873-8276**
www.vicks.com
Vicks® VapoRub® 50142932
Vicks® VapoRub® Cream 50117758
US Pat. 5,322,689
Made in Mexico by Procter & Gamble
Manufactura, S. de R.L. de C.V.
Dist. by Procter & Gamble,
Cincinnati OH 45202

---

## VICKS® VAPOSTEAM®

[vā ′pō ″stēm ]
**Liquid Medication for Hot Steam Vaporizers. Camphor/Cough Suppressant**

**Drug Facts:**

**Active Ingredient:**       **Purpose:**
Camphor 6.2% ......... Cough suppressant

**Uses:** Temporarily relieves cough associated with a cold.

**Warnings:**
**Failure to follow these warnings could result in serious consequences.**
**For external use only**
**Flammable** Keep away from fire or flame. Cap container tightly and store at room temperature away from heat.
**Ask a doctor before use if you have:**
• a persistent or chronic cough
• cough associated with smoking
• emphysema
• excessive phlegm (mucus)
• asthma
**When using this product do not**
• heat
• microwave
• use near an open flame
• take by mouth
• direct steam from the vaporizer too close to the face
• add to hot water or any container where heating water except when adding to cold water only in a hot steam vaporizer. May cause splattering and result in burns.
**Stop use and ask a doctor if:**
• cough lasts more than 7 days, comes back, or occurs with fever, rash, or headache that lasts.
These could be signs of a serious condition.
**Keep out of reach of children.** In case of eye exposure (flush eyes with water); or in case of accidental ingestion; seek medical help or contact a Poison Control Center right away.

**Directions:**
**see important warnings under "When using this product"**
• under 2 yrs.: ask a doctor
• adults & children 2 yrs. & older: use 1 tablespoon of solution for each quart of water or 1½ teaspoonsful of solution for each pint of water
• add solution directly to cold water only in a hot steam vaporizer
• follow manufacturer's directions for using vaporizer. Breathe in medicated vapors. May be repeated up to 3 times a day.

**Inactive Ingredients:** Alcohol 78%, cedarleaf oil, eucalyptus oil, laureth-7, menthol, nutmeg oil, poloxamer 124, silicone.

**How Supplied:** Available in 4 FL OZ (118 mL) and 8 FL OZ (235 mL) bottles.
**Questions? 1-800-873-8276**
Made in Mexico by Procter & Gamble
Manufactura S. de R.L. de C.V.
Dist. by Procter & Gamble
Cincinnati OH 45202
50144018

---

**EDUCATIONAL MATERIAL**

The Procter & Gamble Company offers to health care professionals a variety of journal reprints and patient education materials. For this information, please call **1-800-832-3064** or write:
Scientific Communications
The Procter & Gamble Company
P.O. Box 599
Cincinnati, OH 45201
Information is also available by visiting www.pg.com. Select the brand of interest from the *Product Help* section. Each brand site offers a *Contact Us* page in case of additional questions.

---

## Products on Demand

**1621 EAST FLAMINGO RD.**
**SUITE 15A**
**LAS VEGAS, NV 89119**
**www.vitara.com**
**(888) 806-0344**

**Direct Inquiries to:**
Shaina M. Toppo
(888) 806-0344
www.vitara.com

**Vitara™**
**Female Sexual Aid/Enhancer**

**Active Ingredients:** N-methylnicotinate, (FDA Monograph) Wild Yam Plant Extract (Discoreae)

**Inactive Ingredients:** Water, Propylene Glycol, Glycerin, Polyquaternium-37/Propylene Glycol Dicaprylate Dicaprate & PPG1 Trideceth-6, Sorbic Acid, Methyl & Propyl Paraben, Fragrance

**Description:** Several studies have shown that in excess of 40% of females suffer from some type of sexual dysfunction. Sexual dysfunction has been divided into four subclasses. Three of these four subclasses can be attributed to a decrease in blood flow to the female genitalia. In particular, the lack of blood flow to the clitoris makes reaching orgasm very difficult or impossible to attain. Vitara™ causes increased blood flow instanta-neously to the genitalia, which, with manual stimulation has shown to allow women to experience an orgasm. Also, the natural occurring estrogens and hormonal precursors found in the yams and DHEA increase vaginal moisture.

**Actions:** Used as directed, Vitara™ Female Sexual Enhancer causes immediate profound vasodialation to the female genitalia and with appropriate manipulation allows for female orgasm. Even in women who are diabetic, menopausal, or who take medication for high blood pressure, depression or anxiety. Also, women who have orgasms report greater intensity and frequency or orgasms. Vaginal mucosa also becomes more lubricated and women experience a very warm, "tingling" sensation wherever Vitara™ is applied.

**Warnings:** Vitara™ will cause vasodialation/dermal flush to any tissue.

**How Supplied:** Available in 1 Fl. oz Bottle.
*Shown in Product Identification Guide, page 522*

---

## The Purdue Frederick Company

**ONE STAMFORD FORUM**
**STAMFORD, CT 06901-3431**

**For Medical Information Contact:**
Medical Department
(888) 726–7535

**BETADINE® BRAND**
**First Aid Antibiotics**
**+ Moisturizer Ointment**

**Actions:** Topical broad-spectrum antibiotics polymyxin B sulfate and bacitracin zinc in a cholesterolized ointment* (moisturizer) base to help prevent infection. Formulated with a special blend of waxes and oils to help retain vital moisture needed to aid in healing.

**Uses:** First aid to help prevent infection in minor cuts, scrapes and burns.

**Directions:** Clean affected area. Apply small amount of this product (an amount equal to the surface area of the tip of the finger) on the area 1 to 3 times daily. May be covered with a sterile bandage.

**Warnings:** For External Use Only. Do not use in the eyes or apply over large areas of the body. In case of deep or puncture wounds, animal bites, or serious burns, consult a physician. Stop use and consult a physician if the condition persists or gets worse, or if a rash or other allergic reaction develops. Do not use this product if you are allergic to any of the ingredients. Do not use longer than 1

*Continued on next page*

## Betadine Ointment—Cont.

week unless directed by a physician. Keep this and all medications out of the reach of children. In case of accidental ingestion, seek professional assistance or contact a Poison Control Center immediately.

**Active Ingredients:** Per gram: Polymyxin B Sulfate (10,000 IU) and Bacitracin Zinc (500 IU).

**How Supplied:** 1/2 oz. plastic tube with applicator tip. Store at room temperature.
* Formulated with Aquaphor®—a registered trademark of Beiersdorf AG.

Copyright 1998, 2002g, The Purdue Frederick Company
*Shown in Product Identification Guide, page 523*

---

### BETADINE® BRAND PLUS
**First Aid Antibiotics + Pain Reliever Ointment**
[bā 'tăh-dīn" ]

**Actions:** Topical broad-spectrum antibiotics polymyxin B sulfate and bacitracin zinc plus topical anesthetic in a cholesterolized ointment* (moisturizer) base to help prevent infection and relieve pain.

**Uses:** First aid to help prevent infection and provide temporary pain relief in minor cuts, scrapes and burns.

**Directions:** Clean affected area. Apply small amount of this product (an amount equal to the surface area of the tip of the finger) on the area 1 to 3 times daily. May be covered with a sterile bandage. Children under 2 years of age: Consult a physician.

**Warnings:** For External Use Only. Do not use in the eyes or apply over large areas of the body. In case of deep or puncture wounds, animal bites, or serious burns, consult a physician. Stop use and consult a physician if the condition persists or gets worse, or if a rash or other allergic reaction develops. Do not use this product if you are allergic to any of the ingredients. Do not use longer than 1 week unless directed by a physician. Keep this and all medications out of the reach of children. In case of accidental ingestion, seek professional assistance or contact a Poison Control Center immediately.

**Active Ingredients:** Per gram: Polymyxin B Sulfate (10,000 IU), Bacitracin Zinc (500 IU), and Pramoxine HCl 10 mg.

**How Supplied:** 1/2 oz. plastic tube with an applicator tip. Store at room temperature.
*Formulated with Aquaphor® — a registered trademark of Beiersdorf AG.
Copyright 1998, 2002, The Purdue Frederick Company.
*Shown in Product Identification Guide, page 523*

---

### BETADINE® OINTMENT
**(povidone-iodine, 10%)**
### BETADINE® SOLUTION
**(povidone-iodine, 10%)**
### BETADINE ® SKIN CLEANSER
**(povidone-iodine, 7.5%)**
**Topical Antiseptic**
**Bactericide/Virucide**

**Action:** Topical microbicides active against organisms commonly encountered in minor skin wounds and burns.

**Uses:** **Ointment**—For the prevention of infection in minor burns, cuts and abrasions. Kills microorganisms promptly. **Solution**—Kills microorganisms in minor burns, cuts and scrapes. **Skin Cleanser**—Helps prevent infection in minor cuts, scrapes and burns. Use routinely for general hygiene.

**Directions:** **Ointment**—For the prevention of infection in minor burns, cuts and abrasions, apply directly to affected areas as needed. Nonocclusive: allows air to reach the wound. May be bandaged. **Solution**—For minor cuts, scrapes and burns, apply directly to affected area as needed. May be covered with gauze or adhesive bandage. **Skin Cleanser**—Wet skin and apply a sufficient amount to work up a rich, golden lather. Allow lather to remain about 3 minutes and rinse off. Repeat 2–3 times a day or as directed by physician.

**Warnings:** For External Use Only. Do not use in the eyes. Do not use if you are sensitive to iodine or other product ingredients. Do not use longer than one week unless directed by a doctor. In case of deep or puncture wounds or serious burns, consult physician. If redness, irritation, swelling or pain persists or increases, or if infection occurs, discontinue use and consult physician. If swallowed, get medical help or contact a Poison Control Center right away. Keep out of reach of children.

**How Supplied:**
**Ointment:** 1/32 oz. and 1/8 oz. packettes and 1 oz. tubes
**Solution:** 1/2 oz., 4 oz., 8 oz., 16 oz. (1 pt.), 32 oz. (1 qt.), and 1 gal. plastic bottles.
**Skin Cleanser:** 4 fl. oz. plastic bottles
Avoid storing at excessive heat.
Copyright 1991, 2002, The Purdue Frederick Company
*Shown in Product Identification Guide, page 523*

---

### BETADINE® PREPSTICK®
**APPLICATOR**
[bā' tăh-dīn'']
**[povidone-iodine, 10%]**
**Topical Antiseptic Bactericide/Virucide**
**Hospital Use Only**

Individually wrapped applicators are packaged dry with approximately 2.6 grams of microbicidal Betadine® Solution stored in the handle of the applica-

tor. Antiseptic solution is released into the $1^{3/8}$-inch-long, soft foam swab head by gently squeezing the 4-inch-long plastic handle.

**Actions:** Reduces bacterial load and the risk of infection.

**Uses:** For degerming skin and mucous membranes. Provides sufficient antiseptic solution for most kinds of site prepping—including prior to IM injections, venous punctures, and minor surgical procedures.

**Directions:** Tear wrapper on dotted line and discard top part of wrapper. With the tip still in the wrapper, gently squeeze plastic handle to break the seal. Release antiseptic solution into foam swab head by lightly squeezing handle. Apply to prep site with the moistened foam tip, working in a circular motion from inside to the outside. Apply as often as needed.

**Warnings:** For External Use Only. Do not use in the eyes. Do not use if you are sensitive to iodine or other product ingredients. Discontinue use if irritation and redness develop. **Do not heat prior to application.**

**How Supplied:** 150 individually packaged applicators per dispensing unit. Each applicator contains approximately 2.6 grams of solution.
Avoid storing at excessive heat.
Copyright 1999, 2002, The Purdue Frederick Company
*Shown in Product Identification Guide, page 523*

---

### BETADINE® PREPSTICK PLUS™
**applicator**
[ba'tah-dīn"]
**[povidone-iodine, 10%]**
**with alcohol for faster drying**
**Topical Antiseptic Bactericide/Virucide**
**Hospital Use Only**

Povidone-iodine with alcohol is stored in the 4-inch-long plastic handle of these individually wrapped applicators which are packaged dry. Antiseptic solution is released into the soft foam swab head by gently squeezing the handle.

**Actions:** Reduces bacterial load and the risk of infection.

**Uses:** For preparation of the skin prior to surgery. Helps reduce bacteria that potentially can cause skin infection. For preparation of the skin prior to an injection.

**Directions:** Gently squeeze plastic handle. This allows the release of the antiseptic solution into the foam swab head. Apply to prep site with the moistened foam tip, working in a circular motion from inside to outside. Apply as often as needed.

**Warnings:** For External Use Only. Do not use in the eyes. Do not use if you are sensitive to iodine or other product ingredients. Discontinue use if irritation and redness develop. **FLAMMABLE. KEEP AWAY FROM FIRE, FLAME OR ELECTRICAL SPARK.** Avoid storing at excessive heat.

**How Supplied:** 150 individually packaged applicators per dispensing unit. Each applicator contains approximately 2.6 grams of solution.
Copyright 2002, The Purdue Frederick Company
*Shown in Product Identification Guide, page 523*

---

**SENOKOT® Tablets/Granules**
**SenokotXTRA® Tablets**
**(standardized senna concentrate)**

**SENOKOT® Syrup**
**SENOKOT® Children's Syrup**
**(extract of senna concentrate)·**

**SENOKOT-S® Tablets**
**(standardized senna concentrate and docusate sodium)**

Natural Vegetable Laxative

**Actions:** Senna provides a colon-specific action which is gentle, effective, and predictable, generally producing bowel movement in 6 to 12 hours. Senokot-S tablets also contain a stool softener for smoother, easier evacuation.

**Uses:** For the relief of occasional constipation. Senokot products generally produce bowel movement in 6 to 12 hours.

**Directions:** Take according to product-package instructions or as directed by a doctor. Take preferably at bedtime. For use of Senokot Laxatives in children under 2 years of age, consult a doctor.

**Warnings:** Do not use a laxative product when abdominal pain, nausea or vomiting are present unless directed by a doctor. If you have noticed a sudden change in bowel movements that persists over a period of 2 weeks, consult a doctor before using a laxative. Do not use laxative products for longer than 1 week unless directed by a doctor. Rectal bleeding or failure to have a bowel movement after the use of a laxative may indicate a serious condition. Discontinue use and consult your doctor. As with any drug, if you are pregnant or nursing a baby, seek the advice of a health professional before using this product. In case of accidental overdose, seek professional assistance or contact a Poison Control Center immediately. Keep out of children's reach.
Senokot-S: Do not use if you are now taking mineral oil unless directed by a doctor.

**How Supplied:** Senokot Tablets: Boxes of 20; bottles of 50, 100, and 1000; Unit Strip Packs in boxes of 100 individually sealed tablets. Each Senokot Tablet contains 8.6 mg sennosides.
SenokotXTRA Tablets: Boxes of 12 and 36. Each SenokotXTRA Tablet contains 17.2 mg sennosides.

Senokot-S Tablets: Packages of 10; bottles of 30, 60 and 1000; Unit Strip boxes of 100. Each Senokot-S Tablet contains 8.6 mg sennosides and 50 mg docusate sodium.
Senokot Granules: 2, 6, and 12 oz. plastic containers. Each teaspoon of Senokot Granules contains 15 mg sennosides.
Senokot Syrup: 2 and 8 fl. oz. bottles.
Senokot Children's Syrup: Chocolate-flavored, alcohol-free syrup in 2.5 fl. oz. plastic bottle packaged with measuring cup. Each teaspoon of Senokot Syrup or Senokot Children's Syrup contains 8.8 mg sennosides.
Copyright 1991, 2002, The Purdue Frederick Company.
*Shown in Product Identification Guide, page 523*

---

**EDUCATIONAL MATERIAL**

Samples Available:
1) Senokot-S® Tablets Samples– 1 display of 12 (4 tablets per packette)
2) Betadine® Brand First Aid Antibiotics + Moisturizer Ointment Samples– 1 display of 48 packettes
3) Betadine® Brand Plus First Aid Antibiotics + Pain Reliever– 1 display of 48 packettes
4) **Up-to-date Information:**
**www.senokot.com** provides dosing information for the Senokot® products family of laxatives, as well as patient education about constipation and its causes. A special section on toilet training, written by a pediatrician, describes the popular child-centered approach.

---

**Richardson-Vicks Inc.**
**(See Procter & Gamble.)**

---

**Schering-Plough HealthCare Products**
**3 OAK WAY**
**BERKELEY HEIGHTS, NJ 07922**

**Direct Product Requests to:**
Schering-Plough HealthCare Products
Attn: Managed Care Department
3 Oak Way
Berkeley Heights, NJ 07922
**For Medical Emergencies Contact:**
Consumer Relations Department
(901) 320-2998 (Business Hours)
(901) 320-2364 (After Hours)

---

**A + D® Zinc Oxide Cream**

**Active Ingredients:** Dimethicone 1%, Zinc Oxide 10%.

**Inactive Ingredients:** Aloe Barbadensis Extract, Benzyl Alcohol, Coconut Oil, Cod Liver Oil (contains Vitamin A and Vitamin D), Fragrance, Glyceryl Oleate, Light Mineral Oil, Ozokerite, Paraffin, Propylene Glycol, Sorbitol, Synthetic Beeswax, Water.

**Indications:** Helps treat and prevent diaper rash. Protects chafed skin or minor skin irritation due to diaper rash and helps seal out wetness.

**Directions:** Change wet and soiled diapers promptly, cleanse the diaper area and allow to dry. Apply cream liberally as often as necessary with each diaper change especially at bedtime or anytime when exposure to wet diapers may be prolonged.

**Warnings:**
**For external use only**
**When using this product** avoid contact with the eyes
**Stop use and ask a doctor if** condition worsens or does not improve within 7 days
**Keep out of reach of children.** If swallowed, get medical help or contact a Poison Control Center right away.

**How Supplied:** A and D® Ointment with Zinc Oxide is available in a 3.6 oz (102g) pump and 1 $1/2$ ounce (42.5g) and 4-ounce (113g) tubes.
**Store between 15° and 30°C (59° and 86°F).**
*Shown in Product Identification Guide, page 523*

---

**A + D ® Original Ointment**

**Active Ingredients:** Petrolatum 53.4%, Lanolin 15.5%.

**Inactive Ingredients:** Cod Liver Oil (Contains Vitamin A and Vitamin D), Fragrance, Light Mineral Oil, Microcrystalline Wax, Paraffin.

**A+D Original Ointment for Diaper Rash:**

**Indications:** Helps treat and prevent diaper rash. Protects chafed skin or minor skin irritation due to diaper rash and helps seal out wetness.

**Directions:** Change wet and soiled diapers promptly, cleanse the diaper area, and allow to dry. Apply **A+D Original Ointment** liberally as often as necessary with each diaper change especially at bedtime or anytime when exposure to wet diapers may be prolonged.

**A+D Original Ointment for Skin Irritations:**

**Indications:** Helps prevent and temporarily protects chafed, chapped,

*Continued on next page*

---

*Information on Schering-Plough HealthCare Products appearing on these pages is effective as of November 2001.*

## A + D Ointment—Cont.

cracked or windburn skin and lips. Provides temporary protection of minor cuts, scrapes, burns and sunburn.

**Directions:** Apply **A+D Original Ointment** liberally as often as necessary.

**Warnings:**

**For external use only**

**Do not use** over deep or puncture wounds, infections or lacerations. Consult a doctor.

**When using this product** avoid contact with the eyes

**Stop use and ask a doctor if** condition worsens or does not improve within 7 days

**Keep out of reach of children.** If swallowed, get medical help or contact a Poison Control Center right away.

**How Supplied: A and D Ointment** is available in $1^1/_2$-ounce (42.5g) 3 ounce (81g) and 4-ounce (113g) tubes and 1-pound (454g) jars.

**Store between 15° and 30°C (59° and 86°F)**

*Shown in Product Identification Guide, page 523*

## AFRIN® 12 Hour
[á frin ]
**Original Nasal Spray**
**Original Pump Mist**
**Sinus Nasal Spray**
**Extra Moisturizing Nasal Spray**
**Severe Congestion Nasal Spray**

**Drug Facts:**

**Active Ingredient:**
Oxymetazoline hydrochloride 0.05%
**Purpose:**
Nasal decongestant

**Uses:**
• temporarily relieves nasal congestion due to:
  • common cold
  • hay fever
  • upper respiratory allergies
  • sinusitis
• shrinks swollen nasal membranes so you can breathe more freely

**Warnings:**

**Ask a doctor before use if you have**
• heart disease
• high blood pressure
• thyroid disease
• diabetes
• trouble urinating due to an enlarged prostate gland

**When using this product:**
• **do not use more than directed**
• do not use for more than 3 days. Use only as directed. Frequent or prolonged use may cause nasal congestion to recur or worsen.
• temporary discomfort such as burning, stinging, sneezing or an increase in nasal discharge may occur
• use of the container by more than one person may spread infection

**Stop use and ask a doctor if** symptoms persist.

**If pregnant or breast-feeding,** ask a health professional before use.

**Keep out of reach of children.** If swallowed, get medical help or contact a Poison Control Center right away.

**Directions:**
**Afrin Original Nasal Spray, Sinus Nasal Spray, Severe Congestion Nasal Spray and Extra Moisturizing Nasal Spray:**
• adults and children 6 to under 12 years of age (with adult supervision): 2 or 3 sprays in each nostril not more often than every 10 to 12 hours. Do not exceed 2 doses in any 24-hour period.
• children under 6 years of age: ask a doctor
To spray, squeeze bottle quickly and firmly. Do not tilt head backward while spraying. Wipe nozzle clean after use.

**Afrin Original Pump Mist:**
• adults and children 6 to under 12 years of age (with adult supervision): 2 or 3 sprays in each nostril not more often than every 10 to 12 hours. Do not exceed 2 doses in any 24-hour period.
• children under 6 years of age: ask a doctor
Before using the first time, remove the protective cap from the tip and prime metered pump by depressing pump firmly several times.
To spray, hold bottle with thumb at base and nozzle between first and second fingers. Without tilting head, insert nozzle into nostril. Fully depress rim with a firm, even stroke and sniff deeply. Wipe nozzle clean after use.

**Other Information:**
• store between 2° and 30°C (36° and 86°F)
• retain carton for future reference on full labeling

**Inactive Ingredients:**
**AFRIN® Original Nasal Spray and Pump Mist:** Benzalkonium chloride, edetate disodium, polyethylene glycol, povidone, propylene glycol, sodium phosphate dibasic, sodium phosphate monobasic, water
**AFRIN® Sinus Nasal Spray:** Benzalkonium chloride, benzyl alcohol, camphor, edetate disodium, eucalyptol, menthol, polysorbate 80, propylene glycol, sodium phosphate dibasic, sodium phosphate monobasic, water.
**AFRIN® Extra Moisturizing Nasal Spray:** Benzalkonium chloride, edetate disodium, glycerin, polyethylene glycol, povidone, propylene glycol, sodium phosphate dibasic, sodium phosphate monobasic, water.
**AFRIN® Severe Congestion Nasal Spray:** Benzalkonium chloride, benzyl alcohol, camphor, edetate disodium, eucalyptol, menthol, polysorbate 80, propylene glycol, sodium phosphate dibasic, sodium phosphate monobasic, water.

**How Supplied: AFRIN® Nasal Spray 0.05%**-15 ml and 30 ml plastic squeeze bottles.
**AFRIN® Pump Mist 0.05%**-15 ml pump bottle.
**AFRIN® Sinus Nasal Spray 0.05%**-15 ml plastic squeeze bottle.
**AFRIN® Extra Moisturizing Nasal Spray 0.05%**-15 ml plastic squeeze bottle.
**AFRIN® Severe Congestion Nasal Spray 0.05%**-15 ml plastic squeeze bottle.

*Shown in Product Identification Guide, page 523*

## AFRIN® No Drip Nasal Decongestant 12 Hour Pump Mist
**No Drip Original**
**No Drip Extra Moisturizing**
**No Drip Sinus**
**No Drip Severe Congestion**
Nonprescription Drugs
Oxymetazoline Hydrochloride

**Drug Facts:**

**Active Ingredient:**
Oxymetazoline hydrochloride 0.05%
**Purpose:**
Nasal decongestant

**Uses:**
• temporarily relieves nasal congestion due to:
  • common cold
  • hay fever
  • upper respiratory allergies
  • sinusitis
• shrinks swollen nasal membranes so you can breathe more freely

**Warnings:**
**Ask a doctor before use if you have**
• heart disease
• high blood pressure
• thyroid disease
• diabetes
• trouble urinating due to an enlarged prostate gland
**When using this product:**
• **do not use more than directed**
• do not use for more than 3 days. Use only as directed. Frequent or prolonged use may cause nasal congestion to recur or worsen.
• temporary discomfort such as burning, stinging, sneezing or an increase in nasal discharge may occur
• use of the container by more than one person may spread infection
**Stop use and ask a doctor if** symptoms persist
**If pregnant or breast-feeding,** ask a health professional before use.
**Keep out of reach of children.** If swallowed, get medical help or contact a Poison Control Center right away.

**Directions:**
• adults and children 6 to under 12 years of age (with adult supervision): 2 or 3 sprays in each nostril not more often than every 10 to 12 hours. Do not exceed 2 doses in any 24-hour period.
• children under 6 years of age: ask a doctor
Shake well before use. Before using the first time, remove the protective cap from the tip and prime metered pump by depressing pump firmly several times.
To spray, hold bottle with thumb at base and nozzle between first and second fingers. Without tilting head, insert nozzle into nostril. Fully depress rim with a firm, even stroke and sniff deeply. Wipe nozzle clean after use.

**Other Information:**
• store between 15° and 25°C (59° and 77°F)
• retain carton for future reference on full labeling

**Inactive Ingredients:**
**AFRIN® No Drip Original:** Benzalkonium chloride, benzyl alcohol, carboxymethylcellulose sodium, edetate disodium, flavor, microcrystalline cellulose,

polyethylene glycol, povidone, sodium phosphate dibasic, sodium phosphate monobasic, water.

**AFRIN® No Drip Extra Moisturizing:** Benzalkonium chloride, benzyl alcohol, carboxymethylcellulose sodium, edetate disodium, flavor, glycerin, microcrystalline cellulose, polyethylene glycol, povidone, sodium phosphate dibasic, sodium phosphate monobasic, water.

**AFRIN® No Drip Sinus:** Benzalkonium chloride, benzyl alcohol, camphor, carboxymethylcellulose sodium, edetate disodium, eucalyptol, menthol, microcrystalline cellulose, polyethylene glycol, povidone, sodium phosphate dibasic, sodium phosphate monobasic, water.

**AFRIN® No Drip Severe Congestion:** Benzalkonium chloride, benzyl alcohol, camphor, carboxymethylcellulose sodium, edetate disodium, eucalyptol, menthol, microcrystalline cellulose, polyethylene glycol, povidone, propylene glycol, sodium phosphate dibasic, sodium phosphate monobasic, water.

**How Supplied: Afrin® No Drip Pump Mist**—15 mL (0.5 fl. Oz.) pump bottle.

*Shown in Product Identification Guide, page 523*

---

## CHLOR–TRIMETON®

[klor-tri 'mĕ-ton ]
**4 Hour Allergy Tablets**
**8 Hour Allergy Tablets**
**12 Hour Allergy Tablets**

**Chlor–Trimeton® 4 Hour Allergy Tablets:**
**Drug Facts:**

**Active Ingredient:**
**(in each tablet)**                    **Purpose:**
Chlorpheniramine maleate
4 mg ..................................... Antihistamine
**Chlor–Trimeton® 8 Hour Allergy Tablets:**
**Drug Facts:**

**Active Ingredient:**
**(in each tablet)**                    **Purpose:**
Chlorpheniramine maleate
8 mg ..................................... Antihistamine
**Chlor–Trimeton® 12 Hour Allergy Tablets:**
**Drug Facts:**

**Active Ingredient:**
**(in each tablet)**                    **Purpose:**
Chlorpheniramine maleate
12 mg .................................. Antihistamine

**Inactive Ingredients:**
**Chlor-Trimeton® 4 Hour Allergy Tablets:** Corn Starch, D&C yellow No. 10 aluminum lake, lactose, magnesium stearate
**Chlor-Trimeton® 8 Hour Allergy Tablets:** Acacia, butylparaben, calcium phosphate tribasic, calcium sulfate, carnauba wax, corn starch, D&C yellow No. 10 aluminum lake, FD&C yellow No. 6, FD&C Yellow No. 6 aluminum lake, lactose, magnesium stearate, neutral soap, oleic acid, pharmaceutical ink, po-

tato starch, povidone, rosin, sugar, talc, titanium dioxide, white wax, zein
**Chlor-Trimeton® 12 Hour Allergy Tablets:** Acacia, butylparaben, calcium phosphate tribasic, calcium sulfate, carnauba wax, corn starch, D&C yellow No. 10 aluminum lake, FD&C blue No. 2 aluminum lake, FD&C yellow No. 6, FD&C yellow No. 6 aluminum lake, lactose, magnesium stearate, neutral soap, oleic acid, pharmaceutical ink, potato starch, povidone, rosin, sugar, talc, titanium dioxide, white wax, zein

**Uses:**
• temporarily relieves the following symptoms due to hay fever or other upper respiratory allergies:
  • sneezing
  • runny nose
  • itchy, watery eyes
  • itching of the nose or throat

**Warnings:**
**Ask a doctor before use if you have**
• a breathing problem such as emphysema or chronic bronchitis
• glaucoma
• trouble urinating due to an enlarged prostate gland
**Ask a doctor or pharmacist before use if you are** taking sedatives or tranquilizers
**When using this product:**
• excitability may occur, especially in children
• drowsiness may occur
• avoid alcoholic beverages
• alcohol, sedatives and tranquilizers may increase drowsiness
• use caution when driving a motor vehicle or operating machinery

**If pregnant or breast-feeding,** ask a health professional before use.
**Keep out of reach of children.** In case of overdose, get medical help or contact a Poison Control Center right away.

Applicable to CHLOR-TRIMETON 8 Hour Allergy Tablets and CHLOR-TRIMETON 12 Hour Allergy Tablets
Do not give to children under 12 years of age unless directed by a doctor.

**Directions:**
**Chlor-Trimeton® 4 Hour Allergy Tablets:**

| adults and children 12 years and over | 1 tablet every 4 to 6 hours, not to exceed 6 tablets in 24 hours |
|---|---|
| children 6 to under 12 years of age | ½ tablet (break tablet in half) every 4 to 6 hours, not to exceed 3 whole tablets in 24 hours |
| children under 6 years of age | ask a doctor |

**Chlor-Trimeton® 8 Hour Allergy Tablets:**
• adults and children 12 years and over: 1 tablet every 8 to 12 hours. Do not take more than 1 tablet every 8 hours or 3 tablets in 24 hours.
• children under 12 years of age: ask a doctor

**Chlor-Trimeton® 12 Hour Allergy Tablets:**
• adults and children 12 years and over: 1 tablet every 12 hours. Do not exceed 2 tablets in 24 hours.
• children under 12 years of age: ask a doctor
**Chlor-Trimeton® 4 Hour Allergy Tablets:**
store between 2° and 30°C (36° and 86°F).
**Other Information:**
**Chlor-Trimeton® 8 Hour Allergy Tablets:**
• **each tablet contains:** calcium 39 mg
• store between 2° and 30°C (36° and 86°F)
• Protect from excessive moisture
**Chlor-Trimeton® 12 Hour Allergy Tablets:**
• **each tablet contains:** calcium 36 mg
• store between 2° and 30°C (36° and 86°F)
• Protect from excessive moisture

**How Supplied:** CHLOR-TRIMETON 4 Hour Allergy Tablets, box of 24, bottles of 100.
CHLOR-TRIMETON 8 Hour Allergy Tablets, boxes of 15, bottles of 100.
CHLOR-TRIMETON 12 Hour Allergy Tablets, boxes of 10 and 24, bottles of 100.

*Shown in Product Identification Guide, page 523*

---

## CHLOR–TRIMETON®

[klortri 'mĕ-ton ]
**4 Hour Allergy/Decongestant Tablets**
**12 Hour Allergy/Decongestant Tablets**

**Chlor-Trimeton® 4 Hour Allergy/Decongestant Tablets:**

**Active Ingredients:**
**(in each tablet)**                    **Purpose:**
Chlorpheniramine
maleate 4 mg .................... Antihistamine
Pseudoephedrine
sulfate 60 mg .......... Nasal decongestant

**Chlor–Trimeton® 12 Hour Allergy/Decongestant Tablets:**

**Active Ingredients:**
**(in each tablet)**                    **Purpose:**
Chlorpheniramine
maleate 8 mg .................... Antihistamine
Pseudoephedrine
sulfate 120 mg ........ Nasal decongestant

**Inactive Ingredients:** (in each tablet)
**Chlor–Trimeton® 4 Hour Allergy/Decongestant Tablets:** Corn starch, FD&C blue No. 1, lactose, magnesium stearate, povidone.

*Continued on next page*

---

*Information on Schering-Plough HealthCare Products appearing on these pages is effective as of November 2001.*

## Chlor-Trimeton—Cont.

**Chlor–Trimeton® 12 Hour Allergy/ Decongestant Tablets:** Acacia, butylparaben, calcium sulfate, carnauba wax, corn starch, D&C yellow No. 10 aluminum lake, FD&C blue No. 1 aluminum lake, FD&C yellow No. 6 aluminum lake, gelatin, lactose, magnesium stearate, neutral soap, oleic acid, pharmaceutical ink, povidone, rosin, sugar, talc, titanium dioxide, white wax, zein.

**Uses:**
- Temporarily relieves the following symptoms due to hay fever or other upper respiratory allergies:
  - sneezing
  - runny nose
  - itchy, watery eyes
  - itching of the nose or throat
  - nasal congestion
- helps decongest sinus openings and passages
- reduces swelling of nasal passages, shrinks swollen membranes, and temporarily restores freer breathing through the nose

**Warnings:**

**Do not use** if you are now taking a prescription monoamine oxidase inhibitor (MAOI) (certain drugs for depression, psychiatric, or emotional conditions, or Parkinson's disease), or for 2 weeks after stopping the MAOI drug. If you do not know if your prescription drug contains an MAOI, ask a doctor or pharmacist before taking this product.

**Ask a doctor before use if you have**
- a breathing problem such as emphysema or chronic bronchitis
- glaucoma
- heart disease
- high blood pressure
- thyroid disease
- diabetes
- trouble urinating due to an enlarged prostate gland

**Ask a doctor or pharmacist before use if you are** taking sedatives or tranquilizers.

**When using this product**
- **do not use more than directed**
- excitability may occur, especially in children
- drowsiness may occur
- avoid alcoholic beverages
- alcohol, sedatives and tranquilizers may increase drowsiness
- use caution when driving a motor vehicle or operating machinery

**Stop use and ask a doctor if**
- nervousness, dizziness or sleeplessness occur
- symptoms do not improve within 7 days or occur with a fever

**If pregnant or breast-feeding,** ask a health professional before use.

**Keep out of reach of children.** In case of overdose, get medical help or contact a Poison Control Center right away.

Applicable to CHLOR-TRIMETON® 12 Hour Allergy/Decongestant Tablets: Do not give to children under 12 years of age unless directed by a doctor.

**Directions:**
**Chlor-Trimeton® 4 Hour Allergy/ Decongestant Tablets:**

| | |
|---|---|
| adults and children 12 years and over | 1 tablet every 4 to 6 hours, not to exceed 4 tablets in 24 hours |
| children 6 to under 12 years of age | ½ tablet (break tablet in half) every 4 to 6 hours, not to exceed 2 whole tablets in 24 hours |
| children under 6 years of age | ask a doctor |

**Chlor-Trimeton® 12 Hour Allergy/ Decongestant Tablets:**
- Adults and children 12 years and over: 1 tablet every 12 hours. Do not exceed 2 tablets in 24 hours.
- Children under 12 years of age: ask a doctor

**Other Information:**
- Store between 2° and 30°C (36° and 86°F)
- Protect from excessive moisture

Chlor-Trimeton® 12 Hour Allergy/ Decongestant Tablets:
- **each tablet contains:** calcium 92 mg

**How Supplied: Chlor-Trimeton** 4 Hour Allergy/Decongestant Tablets— boxes of 24. **Chlor-Trimeton** 12 Hour Allergy/Decongestant Tablets boxes of 10 and 24.

*Shown in Product Identification Guide, page 523*

---

## Clear Away®
## LIQUID WART REMOVER SYSTEM
## Clear Away®
## GEL with Aloe Wart Remover

| **Active Ingredient:** | **Purpose:** |
|---|---|
| Salicylic acid 17% (w/w) .. | Wart remover |

**Uses:**
- for removal of common and plantar warts
- common warts can be easily recognized by the rough cauliflower-like appearance of the surface
- plantar warts can be recognized by its location only on the bottom of the foot, its tenderness, and the interruption of the footprint pattern

**Warnings: For external use only**
**Flammable:** Keep away from fire or flame.
**Do not use:**
- if you are a diabetic
- if you have poor blood circulation
- on irritated skin or any area that is infected or reddened
- on moles, birthmarks, warts with hair growing from them, genital warts, or warts on the face or mucous membranes

**When using this product:**
- if product gets in eye, flush with water for 15 minutes
- do not inhale vapors
- cap bottle/tube tightly and store at room temperature away from heat

**Stop use and ask a doctor if** discomfort lasts
**Keep out of reach of children.** If swallowed, get medical help or contact a Poison Control Center right away.

**Directions:**
- wash affected area
- may soak wart in warm water for 5 minutes
- dry area thoroughly
- apply one drop of liquid or a thin layer of gel at a time to sufficiently cover each wart
- let dry
- self-adhesive cover-up discs may be used to conceal wart
- repeat procedure once or twice daily as needed (until wart is removed) for up to 12 weeks

**Inactive Ingredients:**
**(Clear Away Liquid Wart Remover):** acetone, alcohol SD-32 (17% w/w), balsam oregon, ether (52% w/w), flexible collodion.
**(Clear Away Gel with Aloe Wart Remover):** alcohol SD-40 (58% w/w), aloe barbadensis extract, ether (16% w/w), ethyl lactate, flexible collodion, hydroxypropyl cellulose, polybutene

**How Supplied:**
*Clear Away® Liquid Wart Remover System:* Available in a 1/3 fluid ounce liquid with dropper. Cover up discs help to hide wart while it is removed.
*Clear Away® Gel with Aloe Wart Remover:* Available in a ½ ounce tube. Cover up discs help to hide wart while it is removed.

---

## CLEAR AWAY®
## ONE STEP WART REMOVER
## CLEAR AWAY®
## ONE STEP WART REMOVER FOR KIDS
## CLEAR AWAY®
## ONE STEP PLANTAR WART REMOVER
## CLEAR AWAY® WART REMOVER SYSTEM
## CLEAR AWAY® WART REMOVER SYSTEM WITH INVISIBLE STRIP
## CLEAR AWAY® WART REMOVER SYSTEM PLANTAR

| **Active Ingredient:** | **Purpose:** |
|---|---|
| Salicylic Acid 40% ............ | Wart remover |

**Uses:**
- for removal of common plantar warts
- common warts can be easily recognized by the rough cauliflower-like appearance of the surface
- plantar warts can be recognized by its location only on the bottom of the foot, its tenderness, and the interruption of the footprint pattern

**Warnings: For external use only**
**Do not use:**
- on children under 2 years of age unless directed by a doctor
- if you are a diabetic
- if you have poor blood circulation
- on irritated skin or any area that is infected or reddened

- on moles, birthmarks, warts with hair growing from them, genital warts, or warts on the face or mucous membranes

**Stop use and ask a doctor if** discomfort lasts

**Keep out of reach of children.** If swallowed, get medical help or contact a Poison Control Center right away.

**Directions:**
- parents should supervise use by children
- wash affected area
- may soak wart in warm water for 5 minutes
- dry area thoroughly
- apply medicated disc/strip/cushioning pad directly over wart
- for Clear Away Wart Remover Systems, cover-up discs/adhesive strips/cushioning pads may be used to conceal medicated disc and wart
- repeat procedure every 48 hours as needed (until wart is removed) for up to 12 weeks

**Other Information:** Store between 15° and 30°C (59° and 86°F)

**Inactive Ingredients:** Antioxidant (CAS 991-84-4), iron oxides, mineral oil, petroleum hydrocarbon resin, silicon dioxide, synthetic polyisoprene rubber, talc

**How Supplied:** Clear Away One Step Wart Remover and Clear Away One Step Wart Remover for Kids contain 14 all-in-one medicated strips, Clear Away One Step Plantar Wart Remover contains 16 all-in-one medicated cushioning pads, Clear Away Wart Remover System contains 18 medicated discs and 20 cover-up pads, Clear Away Plantar Wart Remover System contains 24 medicated discs and 24 cushioning pads, Clear Away Wart Remover System with Invisible Strip contains 18 medicated discs and 18 cover-up pads that protect and conceal while treatment is ongoing. Conceals as it Heals™.

*Shown in Product Identification Guide, page 523*

---

## Coricidin D®
## Cold, Flu & Sinus Tablets
[kor-a-see'din]

**Active ingredients
(in each tablet):**      **Purpose:**
Acetaminophen
325 mg ......... Pain reliever/fever reducer
Chlorpheniramine maleate
2 mg ..................... Antihistamine
Pseudoephedrine sulfate
30 mg ........................ Nasal decongestant

**Inactive Ingredients:** Carnauba Wax, Hydroxypropyl Methylcellulose, Iron Oxide, Lactose, Magnesium Stearate, Microcrystalline Cellulose, Polyethylene Glycol, Polysorbate 80, Povidone, Pregelatinized Starch, Propylene Glycol, Shellac, Stearic Acid, Titanium Dioxide

**Uses:** Temporarily relieves these cold and flu symptoms: • runny nose • sneezing • nasal congestion • minor aches and pains • stuffy nose • headache • helps

decongest sinus openings and passages to temporarily relieve sinus congestion and pressure • temporarily reduces fever

**Warnings: Alcohol warning:** If you consume 3 or more alcoholic drinks every day, ask your doctor whether you should take acetaminophen or other pain relievers/fever reducers. Acetaminophen may cause liver damage.

**Do not use** if you are now taking a prescription monoamine oxidase inhibitor (MAOI) (certain drugs for depression, psychiatric or emotional conditions, or Parkinson's disease), or for 2 weeks after stopping the MAOI drug. If you do not know if your prescription drug contains an MAOI, ask a doctor or pharmacist before taking this product.

**Ask a doctor before use if you have:**
• a breathing problem such as emphysema or chronic bronchitis • glaucoma • heart disease • high blood pressure • thyroid disease • diabetes • trouble urinating due to an enlarged prostate gland

**Ask a doctor or pharmacist before use if you are** taking sedatives or tranquilizers
**When using this product**
• **do not use more than directed**
• drowsiness may occur
• excitability may occur, especially in children
• avoid alcoholic beverages
• alcohol, sedatives and tranquilizers may increase drowsiness
• use caution when driving a motor vehicle or operating machinery

**Stop use and ask a doctor if**
• symptoms last more than 7 days (for adults) or 5 days (for children 6 to under 12 years)
• nervousness, dizziness or sleeplessness occur
• symptoms do not improve
• new symptoms occur
• redness or swelling is present
• you also have a fever that lasts for more than 3 days

**If pregnant or breast-feeding,** ask a health professional before use.

**Keep out of reach of children.** In case of overdose, get medical help or contact a Poison Control Center right away. Prompt medical attention is critical for adults as well as children even if you do not notice any signs or symptoms.

**Directions:**

| Adults and children 12 years and over | 2 tablets every 4 to 6 hours, not more than 8 tablets in 24 hours |
|---|---|
| Children 6 to under 12 years | 1 tablet every 4 hours, not more than 4 tablets in 24 hours |
| Children under 6 years | ask a doctor |

CORICIDIN D® Decongestant Tablets—blisters of 24.
**Store between 15° and 25°C (59° and 77°F).**

PROTECT FROM EXCESSIVE MOISTURE.

*Shown in Product Identification Guide, page 523*

---

**CORICIDIN HBP® Brand**
[kor-a-see'din]
**Cold & Flu Tablets
Cough & Cold Tablets
Maximum Strength Flu Tablets**

**Cold and flu relief for people with high blood pressure.**

**CORICIDIN HBP® Cold & Flu Tablets:**

**Active Ingredients:**     **Purpose:**
**(in each tablet)**
Acetaminophen     Pain reliever/
325 mg ........................... fever reducer
Chlorpheniramine
maleate 2 mg ................. Antihistamine

**CORICIDIN HBP® Cough & Cold Tablets:**

**Active Ingredients:**     **Purpose:**
**(in each tablet)**
Chlorpheniramine
maleate 4mg ................. Antihistamine
Dextromethorphan
hydrobromide
30 mg .................... Cough suppressant

**CORICIDIN HBP® Maximum Strength Flu Tablets:**

**Active Ingredients:**     **Purpose:**
**(in each tablet)**
Acetaminophen     Pain reliever/
500 mg ........................... fever reducer
Chlorpheniramine
maleate 2 mg ................. Antihistamine
Dextromethorphan
hydrobromide
15 mg .................... Cough suppressant

**Inactive Ingredients:**
**CORICIDIN HBP® Cold & Flu Tablets:** Acacia, butylparaben, calcium sulfate, carnauba wax, corn starch, FD&C red No. 40 aluminum lake, FD&C yellow No. 6 aluminum lake, lactose, magnesium stearate, microcrystalline cellulose, pharmaceutical ink, povidone, sugar, talc, titanium dioxide, white wax
**CORICIDIN HBP® Cough & Cold Tablets:** Acacia, calcium sulfate, carnauba wax, croscarmellose sodium, D&C red No. 27 aluminum lake, FD&C yellow No. 6 aluminum lake, lactose, magnesium stearate, microcrystalline cellulose, pharmaceutical ink, povidone, sodium benzoate, sugar, talc, titanium dioxide, white wax
**CORICIDIN HBP® Maximum Strength Flu Tablets:** Carnauba Wax, FD&C red No. 40 aluminum lake, hydroxypropyl methylcellulose, lactose,

*Continued on next page*

---

*Information on Schering-Plough HealthCare Products appearing on these pages is effective as of November 2001.*

## Coricidin HBP—Cont.

magnesium stearate, microcrystalline cellulose, pharmaceutical ink, polyethylene glycol, povidone, pregelatinized starch, stearic acid, titanium dioxide

### Uses:
**CORICIDIN HBP® Cough and Cold**
- temporarily relieves cough due to minor throat irritations as may occur with a cold
- temporarily relieves runny nose and sneezing due to the common cold

**CORICIDIN HBP® Cold and Flu**
- temporarily relieves runny nose and sneezing due to the common cold
- temporarily relieves minor aches, pains and headache associated with a cold or flu
- temporarily reduces fever

**CORICIDIN HBP® Maximum Strength Flu**
- temporarily relieves cough, runny nose and sneezing associated with the common cold
- temporarily relieves minor aches and pains, headache, and muscular aches associated with a cold or flu
- temporarily reduces fever

### Warnings:
**CORICIDIN HBP® Cold & Flu**

**Alcohol warning:** If you consume 3 or more alcoholic drinks every day, ask your doctor whether you should take acetaminophen or other pain relievers/fever reducers. Acetaminophen may cause liver damage.

**Ask a doctor before use if you have**
- a breathing problem such as emphysema or chronic bronchitis
- glaucoma
- trouble urinating due to an enlarged prostate gland

**Ask a doctor or pharmacist before use if you are** taking sedatives or tranquilizers

**When using this product:**
- excitability may occur, especially in children
- drowsiness may occur
- avoid alcoholic beverages
- alcohol, sedatives and tranquilizers may increase drowsiness
- use caution when driving a motor vehicle or operating machinery

**Stop use and ask a doctor if:**
- pain lasts more than 10 days (adults) or 5 days (children 6 to under 12 years)
- fever lasts more than 3 days
- pain or fever persists or gets worse, if new symptoms occur or if redness or swelling is present. These could be signs of a serious condition.

**If pregnant or breast-feeding,** ask a health professional before use.

**Keep out of reach of children.** In case of overdose, get medical help or contact a Poison Control Center right away. Prompt medical attention is critical for adults as well as children even if you do not notice any signs or symptoms

**CORICIDIN HBP® Cough & Cold**

**Do not use** if you are now taking a prescription monoamine oxidase inhibitor (MAOI) (certain drugs for depression, psychiatric or emotional conditions, or Parkinson's disease), or for 2 weeks after stopping the MAOI drug. If you do not

know if your prescription drug contains an MAOI, ask a doctor or pharmacist before taking this product.

**Ask a doctor before use if you have**
- glaucoma
- trouble urinating due to an enlarged prostate gland
- cough that occurs with excessive phlegm (mucus)
- a breathing problem or persistent or chronic cough as occurs with smoking, asthma, chronic bronchitis, or emphysema

**Ask a doctor or pharmacist before use if you are** taking sedatives or tranquilizers

**When using this product:**
- excitability may occur, especially in children
- marked drowsiness may occur
- avoid alcoholic beverages
- alcohol, sedatives and tranquilizers may increase drowsiness
- use caution when driving a motor vehicle or operating machinery

**Stop use and ask a doctor if** cough lasts more than 7 days, reoccurs, or occurs with fever, rash or persistent headache. These could be signs of a serious condition.

**If pregnant or breast-feeding,** ask a health professional before use.

**Keep out of reach of children.** In case of overdose, get medical help or contact a Poison Control Center right away.

**CORICIDIN HBP® Maximum Strength Flu**

**Alcohol warning:** If you consume 3 or more alcoholic drinks every day, ask your doctor whether you should take acetaminophen or other pain relievers/fever reducers. Acetaminophen may cause liver damage.

**Do not use** if you are now taking a prescription monoamine oxidase inhibitor (MAOI) (certain drugs for depression, psychiatric or emotional conditions, or Parkinson's disease), or for 2 weeks after stopping the MAOI drug. If you do not know if your prescription drug contains an MAOI, ask a doctor or pharmacist before taking this product.

**Ask a doctor before use if you have:**
- glaucoma
- trouble urinating due to an enlarged prostate gland
- cough that occurs with excessive phlegm (mucus)
- a breathing problem or persistent or chronic cough as occurs with smoking, asthma, chronic bronchitis, or emphysema

**Ask a doctor or pharmacist before use if you are** taking sedatives or tranquilizers

**When using this product:**
- excitability may occur, especially in children
- marked drowsiness may occur
- avoid alcoholic beverages
- alcohol, sedatives and tranquilizers may increase drowsiness
- use caution when driving a motor vehicle or operating machinery

**Stop use and ask a doctor if:**
- pain lasts more than 10 days
- fever lasts more than 3 days
- pain or fever persists or gets worse, if new symptoms occur or if redness or swelling is present. These could be signs of a serious condition.

- cough lasts more than 7 days, reoccurs, or occurs with fever, rash or persistent headache. These could be signs of a serious condition.

**If pregnant or breast-feeding,** ask a health professional before use.

**Keep out of reach of children.** In case of overdose, get medical help or contact a Poison Control Center right away. Prompt medical attention is critical for adults as well as children even if you do not notice any signs or symptoms.

### Directions:
**CORICIDIN HBP® Cold & Flu Tablets:**

| Adults and children 12 years and over | 2 tablets every 4 to 6 hours, not more than 12 tablets in 24 hours |
| --- | --- |
| Children 6 to under 12 years of age | 1 tablet every 4 to 6 hours, not more than 5 tablets in 24 hours |
| Children under 6 years of age | ask a doctor |

**CORICIDIN HBP® Cough & Cold Tablets:**
- Adults and children 12 years and over: 1 tablet every 6 hours, not more than 4 tablets in 24 hours
- Children under 12 years of age: ask a doctor

**CORICIDIN HBP® Maximum Strength Flu Tablets:**
- Adults and children 12 years and over: 2 tablets every 6 hours, while symptoms persist, not more than 8 tablets in 24 hours
- Children under 12 years of age: ask a doctor

**CORICIDIN HBP® Maximum Strength Flu**

### Other Information:
- Store between 15° and 25°C (59° and 77°F)
- Protect from excessive moisture

**CORICIDIN HBP® Cough and Cold**
Store between 2° and 30°C (36° and 86°F)

**CORICIDIN HBP® Cold & Flu**
Store between 2° and 30°C (36° and 86°F)
Protect from excessive moisture.

**How Supplied: CORICIDIN HBP® Cold & Flu Tablets**—Bottles of 48, blisters of 12 and 24.
**CORICIDIN HBP® Cough & Cold Tablets**—blisters of 16.
**CORICIDIN HBP® Maximum Strength Flu Tablets**—blisters of 20.
*Shown in Product Identification Guide, page 524*

## CORRECTOL®
### Laxative Tablets and Caplets

**Active Ingredient:** Bisacodyl, 5 mg.

Correctol Tablets
**Inactive Ingredients:** Acacia, Calcium Carbonate, Calcium Sulfate, Carnauba Wax, Colloidal Silicon Dioxide, Confec-

tioner's Sugar, D&C Red No. 27 Aluminum Lake, FD&C Red No. 40 Aluminum Lake, Gelatin, Hypromellose, Kaolin, Lactose Monohydrate, Magnesium Stearate, Methacrylic Acid Copolymer, Microcrystalline Cellulose, Pharmaceutical Ink, Polyethylene Glycol, Polysorbate 80, Povidone, Pregelatinized Starch, Sodium Lauryl Sulfate, Sodium Starch Glycolate, Sucrose, Talc, Titanium Dioxide, Triacetin.

Correctol Caplets

**Inactive Ingredients:** Acetylated monoglycerides, calcium sulfate, carnauba wax, corn starch, D&C Red No. 7 calcium lake, gelatin, hydroxypropyl methylcellulose phthalate, lactose, magnesium stearate, povidone, sugar, talc, titanium dioxide, white wax.

**Indications:** For gentle, overnight relief of occasional constipation and irregularity. Correctol Laxative generally produces a bowel movement in 6 to 12 hours.

**Warnings:** Do not chew tablets or caplets. Do not give to children under 6 years of age, or to persons who cannot swallow without chewing, unless directed by a doctor. Do not take this product within 1 hour after taking an antacid or milk. Do not use laxative products when abdominal pain, nausea, or vomiting are present unless directed by a doctor. If you have noticed a sudden change in bowel habits that persists over a period of 2 weeks, consult a doctor before using a laxative. Laxative products should not be used for a period longer than 1 week unless directed by a doctor. Rectal bleeding or failure to have a bowel movement after use of a laxative may indicate a serious condition. Discontinue use and consult your doctor. All stimulant laxatives may cause abdominal discomfort, faintness, and cramps. As with any drug, if you are pregnant or nursing a baby, seek the advice of a health professional before using this product. Keep this and all drugs out of the reach of children. In case of accidental overdose, seek professional assistance or contact a Poison Control Center immediately. Store at temperatures not above 86°F (30°C). Protect from excessive moisture.

**Directions: Adults and children 12 years of age and older:** Take 1 to 3 tablets or caplets in a single dose once daily. **Children 6 to under 12 years of age:** Take 1 tablet or caplet once daily. **Children under 6 years of age:** consult a doctor. **Do not chew or crush tablets or caplets.**

Each laxative works differently. Adults and children over 12 may need fewer tablets or caplets of Correctol to get the same effect as more tablets or caplets of another brand. **We recommend you start with one Correctol tablet or caplet and take with water.** If one tablet or caplet does not produce desired results, then try two or three Correctol tablets or caplets daily. Do not take more than 3 tablets or caplets of Correctol daily.

**How Supplied:** Tablets: Individual foil-backed safety sealed blister packaging in boxes of 10, 30, 60, & 90 tablets. Caplets: Individual foil-backed safety sealed blister packaging in boxes of 30 caplets.

*Shown in Product Identification Guide, page 524*

---

## DRIXORAL® COLD & ALLERGY
[*dricks-or 'al* ]
**12 Hour Sustained-Action Tablets**

**Active Ingredients:**
**(in each tablet)**                    **Purpose:**
Dexbrompheniramine
  maleate 6 mg ................. Antihistamine
Pseudoephedrine
  sulfate 120 mg .... Nasal decongestant

**Inactive Ingredients:** Acacia, butylparaben, calcium sulfate, carnauba wax, corn starch, D&C yellow No. 10 aluminum lake, FD&C blue No. 1 aluminum lake, FD&C yellow No. 6 aluminum lake, gelatin, lactose, magnesium stearate, neutral soap, oleic acid, pharmaceutical ink, povidone, rosin, sugar, talc, titanium dioxide, white wax, zein.

**Uses:**
• temporarily relieves nasal congestion due to the common cold, hay fever or other upper respiratory allergies, and associated with sinusitis
• helps decongest sinus openings and sinus passages
• reduces swelling of nasal passages, shrinks swollen membranes, and temporarily restores freer breathing through the nose
• temporarily alleviates the following symptoms due to hay fever (allergic rhinitis):
  • runny nose
  • sneezing
  • itching of the nose or throat
  • itchy and watery eyes

**Warnings:**
**Do not use** if you are now taking a prescription monoamine oxidase inhibitor (MAOI) (certain drugs for depression, psychiatric or emotional conditions, or Parkinson's disease), or for 2 weeks after stopping the MAOI drug. If you do not know if your prescription drug contains an MAOI, ask a doctor or pharmacist before taking this product.
**Ask a doctor before use if you have**
• a breathing problem such as emphysema or chronic bronchitis
• glaucoma
• heart disease
• high blood pressure
• thyroid disease
• diabetes
• trouble urinating due to an enlarged prostate gland
**Ask a doctor or pharmacist before use if you are** taking sedatives or tranquilizers
**When using this product:**
• **do not use more than directed**
• excitability may occur, especially in children
• drowsiness may occur
• avoid alcoholic beverages
• alcohol, sedatives and tranquilizers may increase drowsiness

• use caution when driving a motor vehicle or operating machinery
**Stop use and ask a doctor if:**
• nervousness, dizziness or sleeplessness occur
• symptoms do not improve within 7 days or occur with a fever
Do not give to children under 12 years of age unless directed by a doctor.
**If pregnant or breast-feeding,** ask a health professional before use.
**Keep out of reach of children.** In case of overdose, get medical help or contact a Poison Control Center right away.

**Directions:**
• Adults and children 12 years and over: 1 tablet every 12 hours. Do not exceed 2 tablets in 24 hours.
• Children under 12 years of age: ask a doctor

**Other Information:**
• **Each tablet contains:** calcium 80 mg
• Store between 2° and 25°C (36° and 77°F)
• Protect from excessive moisture

**How Supplied:** Boxes of 10, 20, and 30.

*Shown in Product Identification Guide, page 524*

---

## DRIXORAL® NASAL DECONGESTANT
[*dricks-or'al*]
**12 Hour Sustained-Action Tablets**

**Active Ingredient:**                    **Purpose:**
**(in each tablet)**
Pseudoephedrine
  sulfate 120 mg ... Nasal decongestant

**Inactive Ingredients:** Acacia, butylparaben, calcium sulfate, carnauba wax, corn starch, FD&C blue No. 1 aluminum lake, gelatin, lactose, magnesium stearate, neutral soap, oleic acid, pharmaceutical ink, povidone, rosin, sugar, talc, titanium dioxide, white wax, zein.

**Uses:**
• temporarily relieves nasal congestion due to the common cold, hay fever or other upper respiratory allergies, and associated with sinusitis
• helps decongest sinus openings and sinus passages

**Warnings:**
**Do not use** if you are now taking a prescription monoamine oxidase inhibitor (MAOI) (certain drugs for depression, psychiatric or emotional conditions, or Parkinson's disease), or for 2 weeks after stopping the MAOI drug. If you do not know if your prescription drug contains an MAOI, ask a doctor or pharmacist before taking this product.
**Ask a doctor before use if you have**
• heart disease

*Continued on next page*

---

*Information on Schering-Plough HealthCare Products appearing on these pages is effective as of November 2001.*

## Drixoral Nasal Decong.—Cont.

- high blood pressure
- thyroid disease
- diabetes
- trouble urinating due to an enlarged prostate gland

**When using this product do not use more than directed.**

**Stop use and ask a doctor if:**
- nervousness, dizziness or sleeplessness occur
- symptoms do not improve within 7 days or occur with a fever

Do not give to children under 12 years of age, unless directed by a doctor.

**If pregnant or breast-feeding,** ask a health professional before use.

**Keep out of reach of children.** In case of overdose, get medical help or contact a Poison Control Center right away.

**Directions:**
- Adults and children 12 years and over: 1 tablet every 12 hours. Do not exceed 2 tablets in 24 hours.
- Children under 12 years of age: ask a doctor.

**Other Information:**
- **Each tablet contains:** calcium 93 mg
- Store between 2° and 25°C (36° and 77°F)
- Protect from excessive moisture

**How Supplied:** Boxes of 10's and 20's.

*Shown in Product Identification Guide, page 524*

---

## DRIXORAL® COLD & FLU

*[dricks-or 'al ]*
**12 Hour Sustained-Action Tablets**

**Active Ingredients:**      **Purpose:**
(in each tablet)
Acetaminophen      Pain reliever/
500 mg ............................ fever reducer
Dexbrompheniramine
maleate 3 mg ................ Antihistamine
Pseudoephedrine
sulfate 60 mg ...... Nasal decongestant

**Inactive Ingredients:**
Calcium phosphate dibasic, carnauba wax, D&C yellow No. 10 aluminum lake, FD&C blue No. 1 aluminum lake, FD&C yellow No. 6 aluminum lake, hydroxypropyl cellulose, hydroxypropyl methylcellulose, magnesium stearate, methylparaben, pharmaceutical ink, polyethylene glycol, pregelatinized starch, propylparaben, stearic acid, titanium dioxide.

**Uses:**
- temporarily relieves runny nose and sneezing due to the common cold
- temporarily relieves nasal congestion due to the common cold, hay fever or other upper respiratory allergies, and associated with sinusitis
- reduces swelling of nasal passages, shrinks swollen membranes, and temporarily restores freer breathing through the nose
- helps decongest sinus openings and sinus passages
- temporarily relieves minor aches, pains and headache and reduces fever due to the common cold

**Warnings:**

**Alcohol warning:** If you consume 3 or more alcoholic drinks every day, ask your doctor whether you should take acetaminophen or other pain relievers/fever reducers. Acetaminophen may cause liver damage.

**Do not use** if you are now taking a prescription monoamine oxidase inhibitor (MAOI) (certain drugs for depression, psychiatric or emotional conditions, or Parkinson's disease), or for 2 weeks after stopping the MAOI drug. If you do not know if your prescription drug contains an MAOI, ask a doctor or pharmacist before taking this product.

**Ask a doctor before use if you have:**
- a breathing problem such as emphysema or chronic bronchitis
- glaucoma
- heart disease
- high blood pressure
- thyroid disease
- diabetes
- trouble urinating due to an enlarged prostate gland

**Ask a doctor or pharmacist before use if you are** taking sedatives or tranquilizers

**When using this product:**
- **do not use more than directed**
- excitability may occur, especially in children
- drowsiness may occur
- avoid alcoholic beverages
- alcohol, sedatives and tranquilizers may increase drowsiness
- use caution when driving a motor vehicle or operating machinery

**Stop use and ask a doctor if**
- nervousness, dizziness or sleeplessness occur
- symptoms do not improve within 7 days
- fever lasts for more than 3 days, or recurs
- pain or fever persists or gets worse, if new symptoms occur or if redness or swelling is present. These could be signs of a serious condition.

Do not give to children under 12 years of age unless directed by a doctor.

**If pregnant or breast-feeding,** ask a health professional before use.

**Keep out of reach of children.** In case of overdose, get medical help or contact a Poison Control Center right away. Prompt medical attention is critical for adults as well as children even if you do not notice any signs or symptoms.

**Directions:**
- Adults and children 12 years and over: 2 tablets every 12 hours. Do not exceed 4 tablets in 24 hours.
- Children under 12 years of age: ask a doctor.

**Other Information:**
- **Each tablet contains:** calcium 23 mg
- Store between 2° and 25°C (36° and 77°F)
- Protect from excessive moisture

**How Supplied:** Boxes of 12's.

*Shown in Product Identification Guide, page 524*

---

## DRIXORAL® ALLERGY SINUS

*[dricks-or 'al ]*
**12 Hour Sustained-Action Tablets**

**Active Ingredients:**      **Purpose:**
(in each tablet)
Acetaminophen 500 mg ... Pain reliever
Dexbrompheniramine
maleate 3 mg ................ Antihistamine
Pseudoephedrine
sulfate 60 mg ...... Nasal decongestant

**Inactive Ingredients:** Calcium phosphate dibasic, carnauba wax, D&C yellow No. 10 aluminum lake, FD&C yellow No. 6 aluminum lake, hydroxypropyl cellulose, hydroxypropyl methylcellulose, magnesium stearate, methylparaben, pharmaceutical ink, polyethylene glycol, pregelatinized starch, propylparaben, stearic acid, titanium dioxide.

**Uses:**
- temporarily alleviates the following symptoms due to hay fever (allergic rhinitis)
  - runny nose
  - sneezing
  - itching of the nose or throat
  - itchy and watery eyes
- temporarily relieves headaches and minor aches and pains
- temporarily relieves nasal decongestion due to sinusitis, the common cold, and hay fever or other upper respiratory allergies
- helps decongest sinus openings and sinus passages and relieves sinus pressure
- reduces swelling of nasal passages, shrinks swollen membranes, and temporarily restores freer breathing through the nose

**Warnings:**

**Alcohol warning:** If you consume 3 or more alcoholic drinks every day, ask your doctor whether you should take acetaminophen or other pain relievers/fever reducers. Acetaminophen may cause liver damage.

**Do not use** if you are now taking a prescription monoamine oxidase inhibitor (MAOI) (certain drugs for depression, psychiatric or emotional conditions, or Parkinson's disease), or for 2 weeks after stopping the MAOI drug. If you do not know if your prescription drug contains an MAOI, ask a doctor or pharmacist before taking this product.

**Ask a doctor before use if you have:**
- a breathing problem such as emphysema or chronic bronchitis
- glaucoma
- heart disease
- high blood pressure
- thyroid disease
- diabetes
- trouble urinating due to an enlarged prostate gland

**Ask a doctor or pharmacist before use if you are** taking sedatives or tranquilizers

**When using this product:**
- **do not use more than directed**
- excitability may occur, especially in children
- drowsiness may occur
- avoid alcoholic beverages
- alcohol, sedatives and tranquilizers may increase drowsiness
- use caution when driving a motor vehicle or operating machinery

**Stop use and ask a doctor if:**
- nervousness, dizziness or sleeplessness occur
- symptoms do not improve within 7 days
- fever lasts for more than 3 days, or recurs
- pain or fever persists or gets worse, if new symptoms occur or if redness or swelling is present. These could be signs of a serious condition.

Do not give to children under 12 years of age unless directed by a doctor.

**If pregnant or breast-feeding,** ask a health professional before use.

**Keep out of reach of children.** In case of overdose, get medical help or contact a Poison Control Center right away. Prompt medical attention is critical for adults as well as children even if you do not notice any signs or symptoms.

**Directions:**
- Adults and children 12 years and over: 2 tablets every 12 hours. Do not exceed 4 tablets in 24 hours.
- Children under 12 years of age: ask a doctor

**Other Information:**
- **Each tablet contains:** calcium 23 mg
- Store between 2° and 25°C (36° and 77°F)
- Protect from excessive moisture

**How Supplied:** Boxes of 12's.

*Shown in Product Identification Guide, page 524*

---

**GYNE-LOTRIMIN 3®**
**3-Day Treatment**
**Clotrimazole Vaginal Cream (2%)**
**Vaginal Antifungal**
**3 Disposable Applicators**
**Vaginal Cream**

GYNE-LOTRIMIN 3® Vaginal Cream is a 3-day treatment that cures most vaginal yeast infections. **If this is the first time you have had vaginal itching and discomfort, talk to your doctor.** If you have had a doctor diagnose a vaginal yeast infection before and have the same symptoms now, use this cream as directed for 3 days in a row.

**Active Ingredient:** Clotrimazole 2% (100 mg per applicator).

**Use:**
- For the treatment of vaginal yeast infections *(candidiasis)*.

**Warnings:**
- **For vaginal use only. Do not use in eyes or take by mouth.**
- Do not use GYNE-LOTRIMIN 3 Vaginal Cream if you have any of the following symptoms:
  - fever (higher than 100°F).
  - pain in the lower abdomen, back, or either shoulder.
  - a foul-smelling vaginal discharge.
- While using GYNE-LOTRIMIN 3 Vaginal Cream, if you get a fever, abdominal pain, or a foul-smelling discharge, **stop the product** and contact your doctor right away. You may have a more serious illness.
- If your symptoms do not improve in 3 days, or you still have symptoms after 7 days, you should call your doctor.

- If your symptoms return within 2 months, you should talk to your doctor. You could be pregnant or there could be a serious underlying medical cause for your symptoms, including diabetes or a weakend immune system (which may be due to HIV-the virus that causes AIDS).
- Contact your doctor if you get hives or a skin rash while using this product.
- Do not use tampons, douches, or spermicides while using this product.
- Do not rely on condoms or diaphragms to prevent sexually transmitted diseases or pregnancy. This product may damage condoms and diaphragms and cause them to fail.
- If pregnant or breast-feeding, ask a health professional before use.
- Do not use in girls less than 12 years of age.
- **Keep this and all drugs out of the reach of children.** If swallowed, get medical help or contact a Poison Control Center right away.

**Directions:** Applicator and instructions are enclosed.
- Before using, read the enclosed brochure for complete instructions.
- To open: use cap to break seal.
- Insert one applicatorful of cream into the vagina at bedtime for 3 days in a row.

**Inactive Ingredients:** Benzyl alcohol, cetearyl alcohol, cetyl esters wax, octyldodecanol, polysorbate 60, purified water, sorbitan monostearate.
Store at room temperature 15°–30°C (59°–86°F). Avoid heat over 30°C or 86°F.
**Medical questions** should be answered by your doctor. If you have any other questions, or need more information on this product, call our **TOLL-FREE Number, at 1-877-496-3568**, between 8:00 a.m. and 5:00 p.m. Eastern Standard Time, Monday through Friday.

*Shown in Product Identification Guide, page 524*

---

**LOTRIMIN® AF ANTIFUNGAL**
[*lo-tre-min* ]
**Clotrimazole**
**Cream 1%**
**Solution 1%**
**Lotion 1%**
**Jock Itch Cream 1%**

**Description: Lotrimin® AF Cream 1%** is a white fully vanishing homogeneous cream containing 1% clotrimazole. The cream contains no sensitizing parabens and is totally grease free and nonstaining.
**Lotrimin® AF Solution** is a nonaqueous liquid, containing 1% clotrimazole. Also contains polyethylene glycol.
**Lotrimin® AF Lotion** is a light penetrating buffered emulsion containing 1% clotrimazole. Does not contain common sensitizing agents. Also is greaseless and nonstaining.
**Indications:** Lotrimin AF Cream, Solution and Lotion cure athlete's foot (tinea pedis), jock itch (tinea cruris) and ringworm (tinea corporis). For effective

relief of the itching, cracking, burning, scaling and discomfort which can accompany these conditions.

**Directions:** Cleanse skin with soap and water and dry thoroughly. Apply a thin layer over affected area morning and evening or as directed by a doctor. For athlete's foot, pay special attention to the spaces between the toes. It is also helpful to wear well-fitting, ventilated shoes and to change shoes and socks at least once daily. Best results in athlete's foot and ringworm are usually obtained with 4 weeks use of this product, and in jock itch with 2 weeks use. If satisfactory results have not occurred within these times, consult a doctor or pharmacist. Children under 12 years of age should be supervised in the use of this product. This product is not effective on the scalp or nails.

**Warnings:** For external use only. Avoid contact with the eyes. Do not use on children under 2 years of age except under the advice and supervision of a doctor. If irritation occurs or if there is no improvement within 4 weeks (for athlete's foot or ringworm) or within 2 weeks (for jock itch), discontinue use and consult a doctor or pharmacist. Keep this and all drugs out of the reach of children. In case of accidental ingestion, seek professional assistance or contact a Poison Control Center immediately.

**How Supplied: Lotrimin® AF Antifungal Cream** is available in a 0.42 oz. tube (12 grams) and a 0.84 oz. tube (24 grams). Lotrimin® AF Jock Itch Cream is available in a 0.42 oz tube (12 grams).
Inactive ingredients include: cetearyl alcohol, cetyl esters wax, octyldodecanol, polysorbate, sorbitan monostearate and water and as a preservative, benzyl alcohol (1%).

**Lotrimin® AF Antifungal Solution** is available in a 0.33 fl. oz. (10 milliliters) bottle. Inactive ingredient is PEG.

**Lotrimin® AF Antifungal Lotion** is available in a 0.66 fl. oz. (20 milliliters) bottle. Inactive ingredients include cetearyl alcohol, cetyl esters wax, octyldodecanol, polysorbate, sodium biphosphate, sodium phosphate dibasic, sorbitan monostearate and water and as a preservative, benzyl alcohol (1%).

**Storage:** Keep Lotrimin® AF Cream and Solution products between 2° and 30°C (36° and 86°F), and Lotrimin® AF Lotion product between 2° and 25°C (36° and 77°F).

*Shown in Product Identification Guide, page 524*

*Continued on next page*

---

*Information on Schering-Plough HealthCare Products appearing on these pages is effective as of November 2001.*

## LOTRIMIN® AF ANTIFUNGAL
**Miconazole Nitrate 2%**
**Athlete's Foot Spray Liquid**
**Athlete's Foot Spray Powder**
**Athlete's Foot Spray Deodorant**
**Powder**
**Athlete's Foot Powder**
**Jock Itch Spray Powder**

**Active Ingredients: SPRAY LIQUID** contains Miconazole Nitrate 2%. Also contains: Alcohol SD-40 (17% w/w), Cocamide DEA, Isobutane, Propylene Glycol, Tocopherol (vitamin E).
**SPRAY POWDER** (Athlete's Foot) contains Miconazole Nitrate 2%. Also contains: Alcohol SD-40 (10% w/w), Isobutane, Starch/Acrylates/Acrylamide Copolymer, Stearalkonium Hectorite, Talc.
**SPRAY POWDER** (Jock Itch) contains Miconazole Nitrate 2%. Also contains Alcohol SD-40 (10% w/w), Isobutane, Stearalkonium Hectorite, Talc.
**SPRAY DEODORANT POWDER** contains Miconazole Nitrate 2%. Also contains: Isobutane, Alcohol SD-40 (10% w/w), Talc, Starch/Acrylates/Acrylamide Copolymer, Stearalkonium Hectorite, Fragrance.
**POWDER** contains Miconazole Nitrate 2%. Also contains: Benzethonium Chloride, Corn Starch, Kaolin, Sodium Bicarbonate, Starch/Acrylates/Acrylamide Copolymer, Zinc Oxide.

**Indications: LOTRIMIN® AF Athlete's Foot Spray Liquid, Spray Powder, Spray Deodorant Powder and Powder** are proven clinically effective in the treatment of athlete's foot (tinea pedis), jock itch (tinea cruris) and ringworm (tinea corporis). For effective relief of the itching, cracking, burning, scaling and discomfort that can accompany these conditions.
LOTRIMIN AF Powder also aids in the drying of naturally moist areas.

**LOTRIMIN® AF Jock Itch Spray Powder** cures jock itch (tinea cruris). For effective relief of the itching, burning, scaling and discomfort associated with jock itch.

**Warnings: For Athlete's Foot Spray Powder, Spray Liquid, Spray Deodorant Powder and Jock Itch Spray Powder:** Do not use on children under 2 years of age unless directed by a doctor. For external use only. Avoid contact with the eyes. If irritation occurs or if there is no improvement within 4 weeks (for athlete's foot and ringworm) or 2 weeks (for jock itch), discontinue use and consult a doctor. Flammable. Do not use while smoking or near heat or flame. Avoid spraying in eyes. Contents under pressure. Do not puncture or incinerate. Do not store at temperature above 120°F. Use only as directed. Intentional misuse by deliberately concentrating and inhaling contents can be harmful or fatal. Keep this and all drugs out of the reach of children. In case of accidental ingestion, seek professional assistance or contact a Poison Control Center immediately.

**Lotrimin® AF Powder:** Do not use on children under 2 years of age unless directed by a doctor. For external use only. Avoid contact with the eyes. If irritation occurs, or if there is no improvement within 4 weeks (for athlete's foot or ringworm) or within 2 weeks (for jock itch), discontinue use and consult a doctor. Keep this and all drugs out of the reach of children. In case of accidental ingestion, seek professional assistance or contact a Poison Control Center immediately.

**Directions: For Athlete's Foot Spray Liquid, Spray Powder, Spray Deodorant Powder and Jock Itch Spray Powder:** Wash affected area and dry thoroughly. Shake can well. Spray a thin layer of product over affected area twice daily (morning and night) or as directed by a doctor. Supervise children in the use of this product. For athlete's foot, pay special attention to the spaces between the toes; wear well-fitting, ventilated shoes and change shoes and socks at least once daily. For athlete's foot and ringworm use daily for 4 weeks; for jock itch use daily for 2 weeks. If condition persists longer, consult a doctor. This product is not effective on the scalp or nails.
**Powder:** Wash affected area and dry thoroughly. Sprinkle a thin layer of product over affected area twice daily (morning and night) or as directed by a doctor. Supervise children in the use of this product. For athlete's foot, pay special attention to the spaces between the toes; wear well-fitting, ventilated shoes and change shoes and socks at least once daily. For athlete's foot and ringworm use daily for 4 weeks; for jock itch use daily for 2 weeks. If condition persists longer, consult a doctor. This product is not effective on the scalp or nails.
Store between 2° and 30° C (36° and 86°F).

**How Supplied:** LOTRIMIN® AF Athlete's Foot Spray Powder, Spray Deodorant Powder and Jock Itch Spray Powder—3.5 oz. cans. LOTRIMIN® AF Spray Liquid—4 oz. can. LOTRIMIN® AF Powder—3 oz. plastic bottle.
*Shown in Product Identification Guide, page 524*

---

## LOTRIMIN® ULTRA™
[lo-tre-min]
**Butenafine Hydrochloride Cream 1%**
**Antifungal**
**Athlete's Foot Cream**
**Jock Itch Cream**

**Drug Facts:**

| Active Ingredient: | Purpose: |
| --- | --- |
| Butenafine hydrochloride 1% .......... | Antifungal |

**Uses:**
**Athlete's Foot Cream:**
• cures most athlete's foot between the toes. Effectiveness on the bottom or sides of foot is unknown.

• cures most jock itch and ringworm
• relieves itching, burning, cracking, and scaling which accompany these conditions

**Jock Itch Cream:**
• cures most jock itch
• relieves itching, burning, cracking, and scaling which accompany this condition

**Warnings:**
**For external use only**
**Do not use**
• on nails or scalp
• in or near the mouth or the eyes
• for vaginal yeast infections
**When using this product** do not get into the eyes. If eye contact occurs, rinse thoroughly with water.
**Stop use and ask a doctor if** too much irritation occurs or gets worse
**Keep out of reach of children.** If swallowed, get medical help or contact a Poison Control Center right away.

**Directions:**
**Athlete's Foot Cream:**
• adults and children 12 years and older
  • use the tip of the cap to break the seal and open the tube
  • wash the affected skin with soap and water and dry completely before applying

Apply between and around the toes

1 week twice a day or 4 weeks once a day

  • **for athlete's foot between the toes:** apply to affected skin between and around the toes twice a day for 1 week (morning and night), or once a day for 4 weeks, or as directed by a doctor. Wear well-fitting, ventilated shoes. Change shoes and socks at least once daily.
  • **for jock itch and ringworm** apply once a day to affected skin for 2 weeks or as directed by a doctor
  • wash hands after each use
• children under 12 years: ask a doctor
**Jock Itch Cream:**
• adults and children 12 years and over
  • use the tip of the cap to break the seal and open the tube
  • wash the affected skin with soap and water and dry completely before applying
  • apply once a day to affected skin for 2 weeks or as directed by a doctor
  • wash hands after each use
• children under 12 years: ask a doctor

**Other Information:**
• do not use if seal on tube is broken or is not visible
• store at 5°–30°C (41°–86°F)

**Inactive Ingredients:** Benzyl alcohol, cetyl alcohol, diethanolamine, glycerin, glyceryl monostearate SE, polyoxyethylene (23) cetyl ether, propylene glycol dicaprylate, purified water, sodium benzoate, stearic acid, white petrolatum

**How Supplied:** Available in 0.42 oz (12 gram) tubes for both athlete's foot and jock itch. Also available in a 0.85 oz (24 gram) tube for athlete's foot.
*Shown in Product Identification Guide, page 524*

## SmithKline Beecham Consumer Healthcare, L.P.

For product information, please see GlaxoSmithKline.

---

## Standard Homeopathic Company

**210 WEST 131st STREET
BOX 61067
LOS ANGELES, CA 90061**

**Direct Inquiries to:**
Jay Borneman
(800) 624-9659 x20

### HYLAND'S ARNISPORT™

**Formula:** Arnica Montana 30X HPUS, Hypericum Perefoliatium 6X HPUS, Ruta Graveolens 6X HPUS, Ledum Palustre 6X HPUS, Bellis Perennis 6X HPUS, plus Hyland's Bioplasma™ in a base of Lactose, N.F.
Hyland's Bioplasma™ contains: Calcarea Fluorica 6X HPUS, Calcarea Phosphorica 3X HPUS, Calcarea Sulphurica 3X HPUS, Ferrum Phosphoricum 3X HPUS, Kali Muriaticum 3X HPUS, Kali Phosphoricum 3X HPUS, Kali Sulphuricum 3X HPUS, Magnesia Phosphorica 3X HPUS, Natrum Muriaticum 6X HPUS, Natrum Phosphoricum 3X HPUS, Natrum Sulphuricum 3X HPUS, Silicea 6X HPUS.

**Indications:** Natural relief for muscle pain and soreness from overexertion.

**Directions:** Adults: Dissolve 3–4 tablets in mouth every 2 hours until relieved. Children 2 years or older: Dissolve 1–2 tablets in mouth every 2 hours until relieved.

**Warnings:** Do not use if imprinted cap band is broken or missing. If symptoms persist for more than 7 days or worsen, contact a licensed health care professional. As with any drug, if you are pregnant or nursing a baby, consult a licensed health care professional before using this or any other medication. Keep this and all medications out of the reach of children. In case of accidental overdose, contact a poison control center immediately. In case of emergency, the manufacturer may be contacted 24 hours a day, 7 days a week by calling 800/624-9659.

**How Supplied:** Bottles of 50 three-grain sublingual tablets (NDC 54973-0232-01). Store at room temperature.

### HYLAND'S BACKACHE WITH ARNICA

**Active Ingredients:** BENZOICUM ACIDUM 3X HPUS, COLCHICUM AU-TUMNALE 3X HPUS, SULPHUR 3X HPUS, ARNICA MONTANA 6X HPUS, RHUS TOXICODENDRON 6X HPUS.

**Inactive Ingredients:** Lactose, N.F.

**Indications:** A homeopathic medicine for the temporary relief of symptoms of low back pain due to strain or overexertion.

**Directions:** Adults and children over 12 years of age: Take 1–2 caplets with water every 4 hours or as needed.

**Warnings:** Do not use if imprinted cap band is broken or missing. If symptoms persist for more than seven days or worsen, contact a licensed health care professional. As with any drug, if you are pregnant or nursing a baby, seek the advice of a licensed health care professional before using this product. Keep this and all medications out of the reach of children. In case of accidental overdose, contact a poison control center immediately. In case of emergency, the manufacturer may be reached 24 hours a day, 7 days a week at 800/624-9659.

**How Supplied:** Bottles of 40 5.5 grain caplets (NDC 54973-2965-2). Store at room temperature.

### HYLAND'S BUMPS 'N BRUISES™ TABLETS

**Active Ingredients:** Arnica Montana 6X HPUS, Hypericum Perforatum 6X HPUS, Bellis Perennis 6X HPUS, Ruta Graveolens 6X HPUS.

**Inactive Ingredients:** Lactose, N.F.

**Indications:** A homeopathic medicine for the temporary relief of symptoms of bruising and swelling from falls, trauma or overexertion. Easy to take soft tablets dissolve instantly in the mouth.

**Directions:** For over 1 year of age: Dissolve 3–4 tablets in a teaspoon of water or on the tongue at the time of injury. May be repeated as needed every 15 minutes until relieved.

**Warnings:** Do not use if imprinted cap band is broken or missing. If symptoms persist for more than 7 days or worsen, consult a licensed health care professional. As with any drug, if you are pregnant or nursing a baby, consult a health care professional before using this product. Keep this and all medications out of the reach of children. In case of accidental overdose, contact a poison control center immediately. In case of emergency, the manufacturer may be reached 24 hours a day, 7 days a week at 800/624-9659.

**How Supplied:** Bottles of 125 1-grain sublingual tablets (NDC 54973-7508-1). Store at room temperature.

### HYLAND'S CALMS FORTÉ™

**Active Ingredients:** *Passiflora* (Passion Flower) 1X triple strength HPUS, *Avena Sativa* (Oat) 1X double strength HPUS, *Humulus Lupulus* (Hops) 1X double strength HPUS, *Chamomilla* (Chamomile) 2X HPUS, *Calcarea Phosphorica* (Calcium Phosphate) 3X HPUS, *Ferrum Phosphorica* (Iron Phosphate) 3X HPUS, *Kali Phosphoricum* (Potassium Phosphate) 3X HPUS, *Natrum Phosphoricum* (Sodium Phosphate) 3X HPUS, *Magnesia Phosphoricum* (Magnesium Phosphate) 3X HPUS.

**Inactive Ingredients:** Lactose, N.F., Calcium Sulfate, Starch (Corn and Tapiocal), Magnesium Stearate.

**Indications:** Temporary symptomatic relief of simple nervous tension and sleeplessness.

**Directions:** Adults: As a relaxant: Swallow 1–2 tablets with water as needed, three times daily, preferably before meals. For insomnia: 1 to 3 tablets ½ to 1 hour before retiring. Repeat as needed without danger of side effects. Children: As a relaxant: Swallow 1 tablet with water as needed, three times daily, preferably before meals. For insomnia: 1 to 2 tablets ½ to 1 hour before retiring. Repeat as needed without danger of side effects.

**Warning:** Do not use if imprinted cap band is broken or missing. If symptoms persist for more than seven days or worsen, consult a licensed health care professional. As with any drug, if you are pregnant or nursing a baby, seek the advice of a licensed health care professional before using this product. Keep this and all medications out of the reach of children. In case of accidental overdose, contact a Poison Control Center immediately. In case of emergency, the manufacturer may be reached 24 hours a day, 7 days a week by calling 800/624-9659.

**How Supplied:** Bottles of 100 4-grain tablets (NDC 54973-1121-02), 50 4-grain tablets (NDC 54973-1121-01) and 32 5.5-grain caplets (NDC 54973-1121-48). Store at room temperature.

### HYLAND'S COLD TABLETS WITH ZINC

**Active Ingredients:** Aconitum Napellus 6X, HPUS; Allium Cepa 6X, HPUS; Gelsemium Sempervirens 6X, HPUS; Zinc Gluconate 2X, HPUS.

**Inactive Ingredients:** Lactose, NF

**Indications:** Temporary symptomatic treatment for the relief of the common cold.

**Directions:** Take 2 – 3 quick dissolving tablets under the tongue every 4 hours or as needed. Children 6 to 12 years old: ½ adult dose.

**Warnings:** Do not use if imprinted cap band is broken or missing. If symptoms persist for more than seven days or

*Continued on next page*

## Hyland's Cold w/Zinc—Cont.

worsen, contact a licensed health care professional. Discontinue if symptoms are accompanied by a high fever (over 101 °F) and contact a licensed health care professional. As with any drug, if you are pregnant or nursing a baby, seek the advice of a licensed health care professional before using this product. Keep this and all medications out of the reach of children. In case of accidental overdose, contact a poison control center immediately. In cases of emergency, the manufacturer may be contacted 24 hours a day, 7 days a week at 800/624-9659.

**How Supplied:** Bottles of 50 three-grain sublingual tablets (NDC 54973-3010-01). 60 three grain sublingual tablets (NDC 54973-2952-01). Store at room temperature.

---

## HYLAND'S COLIC TABLETS

**Active Ingredients:** *Disocorea* (Wild Yam) 3X HPUS, *Chamomilla* (Chamomile) 3X HPUS, *Colocynthinum* (Bitter Apple) 3X HPUS.

**Inactive Ingredients:** Lactose N.F.

**Indications:** A homeopathic combination for the temporary relief of symptoms of colic and gas pains caused by irritating food, feeding too quickly, swallowing air and similar conditions during teething, colds and other minor upset periods in children.

**Directions:** For children up to 2 years of age: Dissolve 2 tablets under the tongue every 15 minutes for up to 8 doses until relieved; then every 2 hours as required. If you prefer, tablets may first be dissolved in a teaspoon of water and then given to the child. Children over 2 years: Dissolve 3 tablets under the tongue as above; or as recommended by a licensed health care professional. Colic Tablets are very soft and dissolve almost instantly under the tongue. If your baby has been crying or has been very upset, your baby may fall asleep after using this product. This is because pain has been relieved and your child can rest.

**Warnings:** Do not use if imprinted cap band is broken or missing. If symptoms persist for more than seven days or worsen, consult a licensed health care professional. As with any drug, if you are pregnant or nursing a baby, seek the advice of a licensed health care professional before using this product. Keep this and all medications out of the reach of children. In case of accidental overdose, contact a poison control center immediately. In cases of emergency, the manufacturer may be contacted 24 hours a day, 7 days a week at 800/624-9659

**How Supplied:** Bottles of 125—one grain sublingual tablets (NDC 54973-7502-1). Store at room temperature.

## HYLAND'S EARACHE TABLETS

**Active Ingredients:** Pulsatilla (Wind Flower) 30C, HPUS; Chamomilla (Chamomile) 30C, HPUS; Sulphur 30C, HPUS; Calcarea Carbonica (Carbonate of Lime) 30C, HPUS; Belladonna 30C, HPUS; ($3 \times 10^{-60}$ % Alkaloids) and Lycopodium (Club Moss) 30C, HPUS.

**Inactive Ingredients:** Lactose NF

**Indications:** For the relief of symptoms of fever, pain, irritability and sleeplessness associated with earaches in children after diagnosis by a physician. If symptoms persist for more than 48 hours or if there is a discharge from the ear, discontinue use and contact your health care professional.

**Directions:** Dissolve 4 tablets under the tongue 3 times per day for 48 hours or until symptoms subside. If you prefer, tablets may be dissolved in a teaspoon of water and then given to the child. Earache Tablets are very soft and dissolve almost instantly under the tongue.

**Warnings:** Do not use if imprinted blisters are broken or damaged. If symptoms persist for more than 48 hours, or if there is a discharge from the ear, discontinue use and consult a licensed health care professional. As with any drug, if you are pregnant or nursing a baby, seek the advice of a licensed health care professional before using this product. Keep this and all medications out of the reach of children. In case of accidental overdose, contact a poison control center immediately. In cases of emergency, the manufacturer may be contacted 24 hours a day, 7 days a week at 800/624-9659.

**How Supplied:** Blister pack of 40 tablets (NDC 54973-7507-1). Store at room temperature.

---

## HYLAND'S LEG CRAMPS WITH QUININE

**Active Ingredients:** Cinchona Officinalis 3X, HPUS (Quinine), Viscum Album 3X, HPUS; Gnaphalium Polycephalum 3X, HPUS; Rhus Toxicodendron 6X, HPUS; Aconitum Napellus 6X, HPUS; Ledum Palustre 6X, HPUS; Magnesia Phosphorica 6X, HPUS.

**Inactive Ingredients:** Lactose, N.F.

**Indications:** Hyland's Leg Cramps is a traditional homeopathic formula for the relief of symptoms of cramps and pains in lower back and legs often made worse by damp weather. Working without contraindications or side effects, Hyland's Leg Cramps stimulates your body's natural healing response to relieve symptoms. Hyland's Leg Cramps is safe for adults and can be used in conjuction with other medications.

**Directions:** Adults: Dissolve 2–3 tablets under tongue every 4 hours as needed.

**Warnings:** Do not use if imprinted cap band is missing or broken. If symptoms persist for more than seven days or worsen, contact a licensed health care professional. As with any drug, if you are pregnant or nursing a baby, seek the advice of a licensed health care professional before using this product. Do not use if pregnant, sensitive to quinine or under 12 years of age. Keep this and all medications out of the reach of children. In case of accidental overdose, contact a poison control center immediately. In case of emergency, the manufacturer may be reached 24 hours a day, 7 days a week at 800-624-9659.

**How Supplied:** Bottles of 100 three-grain sublingual tablets (NDC 54973-2956-02), Bottles of 50 three-grain sublingual tablets (NDC 54973-2956-01), Bottles of 40 5.5 grain caplets (NDC 54973-2956-68). Store at room temperature.

---

## HYLAND'S MENOCALM™

**Ingredients:** AMYL NITROSUM 6X HPUS, SANGUINARIA CAN. 3X HPUS, LACHESIS MUTA 12X HPUS, CIMICIFUGA RACEMOSA 10MG RHIZOME (AS 40 MG CIMIPURE STANDARDIZED TO PROVIDE 4 MG TRITERPENE GLYCOSIDES DAILY), CALCIUM CITRATE USP 953 MG (TO PROVIDE 800MG CALCIUM PER DAY) EXCIPIENTS 5% (CELLULOSE, CROSCARMELLOSE SODIUM, VEGETABLE STEARIC ACID, SILICA, VEGETABLE MAGNESIUM STEARATE WITH A CELLULOSE COATING.)

**Indications:** Symptomatic relief for hot flashes, moodiness and irritability associated with menopause.

**Directions:** Take 2 tablets two times per day. Due to the calcium in MenoCalm™, the tablets are large. You may break the tablets along the score line without affecting the product's effectiveness. If symptoms persist for more than 14 days, discontinue use and contact your health care provider.

**Warnings:** Do not use if imprinted cap band is broken or missing. If symptoms persist for more than 14 days or worsen, consult a licensed health care practitioner. Do not use this product if your are pregnant or nursing. Keep this and all medications out of the reach of children. In case of accidental overdose, contact a poison control center immediately. In cases of emergency, the manufacturer may be contacted 24 hours a day, 7 days a week at 800/624-9659.

**How Supplied:** Bottles of 84 seven-grain tablets (NDC 54973-6056-1). Store at room temperature.

---

## HYLAND'S NERVE TONIC

**Active Ingredients:** Calcarea Phosphorica (Calcium Phosphate) 3X HPUS;

Ferrum Phosphorica (Iron Phosphate) 3X HPUS; Kali Phosphoricum (Potassium Phosphate) 3X HPUS; Natrum Phosphoricum (Sodium Phosphate) 3X HPUS; Magnesia Phosphoricum (Magnesium Phosphate) 3X HPUS.

**Inactive Ingredients:** Lactose, N.F.

**Indications:** Temporary symtomatic relief of simple nervous tension and stress.

**Directions:** Adults take 2–6 tablets before each meal and at bedtime. Children: 2 tablets. In severe cases take 3 tablets every 2 hours.

**Warnings:** Do not use if imprinted cap band is broken or missing. If symptoms persist for more than seven days or worsen, contact a licensed health care professional. As with any drug, if you are pregnant or nursing a baby, seek the advice of a licensed health care professional before using this product. Keep this and all medications out of the reach of children. In case of accidental overdose, contact a poison control center immediately. In cases of emergency, the manufacturer may be contacted 24 hours a day, 7 days a week at 800/624-9659.

**How Supplied:** Bottles of 32 caplets (NDC 54973-1129-68), Bottles of 500 tablets (NDC 54973-1129-1), Bottles of 1000 tablets (NDC 54973-1129-2)

## SMILE'S PRID ®

**Contains:** Acidum Carbolicum 2X HPUS, Ichthammol 2X HPUS, Arnica Montana 3X HPUS, Calendula Off 3X HPUS, Echinacea Ang 3X HPUS, Sulphur 12X HPUS, Hepar Sulph 12X HPUS, Silicea 12X HPUS, Rosin, Beeswax, Petrolatum, Stearyl Alcohol, Methyl & Propyl Paraben.

**Indications:** Temporary topical relief of pain symptoms associated with boils, minor skin eruptions, redness and irritation. Also aids in relieving the discomfort of superficial cuts, scratches and wounds.

**Directions:** Wash affected parts with hot water, dry and apply PRID® twice daily on clean bandage or gauze. Do not squeeze or pressure irritated skin area. After irritation subsides, repeat application once a day for several days. Children under two years: consult a physician. CAUTION: If symptoms persist for more than seven days or worsen, or if fever occurs, contact a licensed health care professional. Do not use on broken skin. Keep out of reach of children. In case of accidental ingestion, seek professional assistance or contact a poison control center. For external use only. Avoid contact with eyes.

**How Supplied:** 20GM tin (NDC 0619-4202-54). Keep in a cool dry place.

## HYLAND'S TEETHING GEL

**Active Ingredients:** Calcarea Phosphorica (Calcium Phosphate) 12X,

HPUS; Chamomilla (Chamomile) 6X, HPUS; Coffea Cruda (Coffee) 6X, HPUS; and Belladonna 6X, HPUS (Alkaloids 0.0000003%)

**Inactive Ingredients:** Deionized water, Vegetable Glycerin, Hydroxyethyl Cellulose, Methyl Paraben and Propyl Paraben.

**Indications:** A homeopathic combination for the temporary relief of symptoms of simple restlessness and wakeful irritability due to cutting teeth.

**Directions:** Apply to gums as necessary. If symptoms persist for more than seven days or worsen, discontinue use and contact your health care professional. Please note, if your baby has been crying or has been very upset, your baby may fall asleep after using this product because the pain has been relieved and your child can rest.

**Warnings:** Do not use if tube tip is broken or missing. If symptoms persist for more than seven days or if irritation persists, inflammation develops or fever or infection develop, discontinue use and consult a licensed health care professional. As with any drug, if you are pregnant or nursing a baby, seek the advice of a licensed health care professional before using this product. Keep this and all medications out of the reach of children. In case of accidental overdose, contact a poison control center immediately. In case of emergency, the manufacturer may be contacted 24 hours a day, 7 days a week at 800/624-9659.

**How Supplied:** Tubes of 1/3 OZ. (NDC 54973-7504-3). Store at room temperature.

## HYLAND'S TEETHING TABLETS

**Active Ingredients:** *Calcarea Phosphorica* (Calcium Phosphate) 3X HPUS, *Chamomilla* (Chamomile) 3X HPUS, *Coffea Cruda* (Coffee) 3X HPUS, *Belladonna* 3X HPUS (Alkaloids 0.0003%).

**Inactive Ingredients:** Lactose N.F.

**Indications:** A homeopathic combination for the temporary relief of symptoms of simple restlessness and wakeful irritability due to cutting teeth.

**Directions:** Dissolve 2 to 3 tablets under the tongue 4 times per day. If you prefer, tablets may first be dissolved in a teaspoon of water and then given to the child. If the child is restless or wakeful, 2 tablets every hour for 6 doses or as recommended by a licensed health care professional. Teething Tablets are very soft and dissolve almost instantly under the tongue. Please note, if your baby has been crying or has been very upset, your baby may fall asleep after using this product because the pain has been relieved and your child can rest.

**Warning:** Do Not use if imprinted cap band is broken or missing. If symptoms

persist for more than seven days, or if irritation persist, inflammation develops or fever or infection develop, discontinue use and consult a licensed health care professional. As with any drug, if you are pregnant or nursing a baby, seek the advice of a health care professional before using this product. Keep this and all medications out of the reach of children. In case of accidental overdose, contact a poison control center immediately. In case of emergency, the manufacturer may be contacted 24 hours a day, 7 days a week at 800/624-9659.

**How Supplied:** Bottles of 125—one grain sublingual tablets (NDC 54973-7504-01). Store at room temperature.

---

## EDUCATIONAL MATERIAL

Booklets—Brochures
"Homeopathy—What it is, How it Works," A Consumer's Guide to Homeopathic Medicine, Free
"Homeopathy—A Guide for Pharmacists," An ACPE (0.2 CEU) program on the basic principles of homeopathy.

## UAS Laboratories
**5610 ROWLAND RD #110**
**MINNETONKA, MN 55343**

**Direct Inquiries To:**
Dr. S.K. Dash: (952) 935-1707
(952) 935-1650

**Medical Emergency Contact:**
Dr. S.K. Dash: (952) 935-1707
Fax: (952) 935-1650

## DDS®-ACIDOPHILUS
**Capsule, Tablet & Powder free of dairy products, corn, soy, and preservatives**

**Description:** DDS®-Acidophilus is the source of a special strain of Lactobacillus acidophilus free of dairy products, corn, soy and preservatives. Each capsule or tablet contains one billion viable DDS®-1 L.acidophilus at the time of manufacturing. One gram of powder contains two billion viable DDS®-1 L.acidophilus.

**Indications and Usages:** An aid in implanting the gut with beneficial Lactobacillus acidophilus under conditions of digestive disorders, acne, yeast infections, and following antibiotic therapy.

**Administration:** One to two capsules or tablets twice daily before meals. One-fourth teaspoon powder can be substituted for two capsules or tablets.

*Continued on next page*

## DDS-Acidophilus—Cont.

**How Supplied:** Bottles of 100 capsules or tablets. 12 bottles per case. Powder is available in 2 oz. bottle; 12 bottles per case.

**Storage:** Keep refrigerated under 40°F.

---

### DDS®-Acidophilus
Booklet describing superior-strain Acidophilus without dairy products, corn, soy, or preservatives. Two billion viable DDS®-1. L.acidopohilus per gram.

---

## Upsher-Smith
## Laboratories, Inc.
**14905 23rd AVENUE N.**
**PLYMOUTH, MN 55447**

**Direct inquiries to:**
Professional Services
(763) 475-3023
Fax (763) 475-3410

### AMLACTIN® 12% Moisturizing Lotion and Cream
[ăm-lăk-tĭn]
Cosmetic Lotion and Cream

**Description:** AMLACTIN® Moisturizing Lotion and Cream are special formulations of 12% lactic acid neutralized with ammonium hydroxide to provide a lotion or cream pH of 4.5–5.5. Lactic acid, an alpha-hydroxy acid, is a naturally occurring humectant for the skin. AMLACTIN® moisturizes and softens rough, dry skin.

**How Supplied:** 225g (8oz) plastic bottle: List No. 0245-0023-22
400g (14oz) plastic bottle: List No. 0245-0023-40
140g (4.9oz) tube: List No. 0245-0024-14

---

### AMLACTIN® AP Anti-Itch Moisturizing Cream
[ăm-lăk'-tĭn]
1% Pramoxine HCl

**Description:** AMLACTIN® AP Anti-Itch Moisturizing Cream is a special formulation containing 12% lactic acid neutralized with ammonium hydroxide to provide a cream pH of 4.5–5.5 with pramoxine HCl. Lactic acid, an alpha-hydroxy acid, is a naturally occurring humectant which moisturizes and softens rough, dry skin. Promoxine HCl, USP,

1% is an effective antipruritic ingredient used to relieve itching associated with dry skin.
**How Supplied:** 140g (4.9oz) tube: NDC No. 0245-0025-14

---

## Wallace Pharmaceuticals
## MedPointe Healthcare Inc.
**CRANBURY, NJ 08512**

**Direct Inquiries to:**
Wallace Pharmaceuticals
MedPointe Healthcare Inc.
Cranbury, NJ 08512
609-655-6000

**For Medical Information, Contact:**
**Generally:**
**Professional Services**
800-526-3840

**After Hours and Weekend Emergencies**
609-655-6474

### MALTSUPEX®
(malt soup extract)
**Powder, Liquid, Tablets**

**Composition:** MALTSUPEX is a non-diastatic extract from barley malt, which is available in powder, liquid, and tablet form. Each MALTSUPEX product has a gentle laxative action and promotes soft, easily passed stools.
**Tablet:** Each tablet contains 750 mg of Malt Soup Extract. Other ingredients: D&C Yellow No. 10, FD&C Red No. 40, flavor (artificial), hydroxypropyl methylcellulose, methylparaben, polyethylene glycol, povidone, propylparaben, simethicone emulsion, stearic acid, talc, titanium dioxide. Sodium content: Each tablet contains approximately 1 mg of sodium.
**Powder:** Each level scoop provides approximately 8 g of Malt Soup Extract. Sodium content: Each scoopful contains approximately 5 mg of sodium.
**Liquid:** Each tablespoonful ($^1/_2$ fl. oz.) contains approximately the equivalent of

16 g Malt Soup Extract Powder. Other ingredients: Potassium sorbate and sodium propionate. Sodium content: Each tablespoon contains approximately 36 mg of sodium.

**EFFECTIVE, NON-HABIT-FORMING**

**Indications:** For relief of occasional constipation. This product generally produces a bowel movement in 12 to 72 hours.

**Warnings:** Do not use laxative products when abdominal pain, nausea or vomiting are present unless directed by a physician. If constipation persists, consult a physician.
If you have noticed a sudden change in bowel habits that persists over a period of 2 weeks, consult a physician before using a laxative.
Keep this and all medications out of the reach of children. In case of accidental overdose, seek professional assistance or contact a poison control center immediately.
Laxative products should not be used for a period longer than one week unless directed by a physician. Rectal bleeding or failure to have a bowel movement after use of a laxative may indicate a serious condition. Discontinue use and consult a physician.
As with any drug, if you are pregnant or nursing a baby, seek the advice of a health professional before using this product.
**MALTSUPEX Liquid only**—Do not use this product if you are on a sodium-restricted diet unless directed by a physician. Maltsupex Liquid contains approximately 1.58 mEq (36 mg) of sodium per tablespoon.
Maltsupex Tablets contain approximately 0.02 mEq (0.46 mg) of sodium per tablet.
Each scoop of Maltsupex Powder contains approximately 0.22 mEq (5 mg) of sodium per scoop.
**Note**: Allow for carbohydrate content in diabetic diets and infant formulas.
**Liquid:** (67%, 14 g/tablespoon, or 56 calories/tablespoon)
**Powder:** (83%, 6 g or 24 calories per scoop)
**Tablets:** (Approximately 83%, 0.5 g or 2.5 calories per tablet)

| MALTSUPEX Powder<br>AGE | CORRECTIVE* | MAINTENANCE |
|---|---|---|
| 12 years to ADULTS | Up to 4 scoops twice a day<br>(Take a full glass [8 oz.] of liquid with each dose.) | 2 to 4 scoops at bedtime |
| CHILDREN 6–12 years of age | Up to 2 scoops twice a day<br>(Take a full glass [8 oz.] of liquid with each dose.) | |
| CHILDREN 2–6 years of age | 1 scoop twice a day<br>(Take a full glass [8 oz.] of liquid with each dose.) | |
| INFANTS under 2 years of age | Consult a doctor. | |

* Full corrective dosage should be used for 3 or 4 days or until relief is noted. Then continue on maintenance dosage as needed. Use a clean, dry scoop to remove powder. Replace cover tightly to keep out moisture.

## MALTSUPEX Liquid

| AGE | CORRECTIVE* | MAINTENANCE |
|---|---|---|
| 12 years to ADULTS | 2 tablespoonfuls twice a day (Take a full glass [8 oz.] of liquid with each dose.) | 1 to 2 tablespoonfuls at bedtime |
| CHILDREN 6–12 years of age | 1 tablespoonful twice a day (Take a full glass [8 oz.] of liquid with each dose.) | |
| CHILDREN 2–6 years of age | ½ tablespoonful twice a day (Take a full glass [8 oz.] of liquid with each dose.) | |
| INFANTS under 2 years of age | Consult a doctor. | |

* Full corrective dosage should be used for 3 or 4 days or until relief is noted. Then continue on maintenance dosage as needed. Use a clean, dry spoon to remove the liquid. Replace cover tightly after use.

**Directions: General**—Drink a full glass (8 ounces) of liquid with each dose. The recommended daily dosage of MALTSUPEX may vary. Use the smallest dose that is effective and lower dosage as improvement occurs.

**MALTSUPEX Powder**—Each bottle contains a scoop. Each scoopful (which is the equivalent of a standard measuring tablespoon) should be leveled with a knife.

**MALTSUPEX Tablets:** Adult Dosage: Start with four tablets (3 g) four times daily (with meals and at bedtime) and adjust dosage according to response, not to exceed 48 tablets (36 g) daily. Drink a full glass (8 oz.) of liquid with each dose.

**Usual Dosage—Powder:**
[See table at bottom of previous page]

**Usual Dosage—Liquid:**
[See table above]

**Preparation Tips: Powder**—Add dosage to milk, water, or fruit juice and stir until dissolved. Mixing is easier if added to warm milk or warm water. May be flavored with vanilla or cocoa to make "malteds." Excellent with warm milk at bedtime. Also available in tablet and liquid forms.

**Note:** Although shade, texture, taste, and height of contents may vary between bottles, action remains the same.

**Liquid:** Mixing is easier if MALTSUPEX Liquid is added to an ounce or two of warm water and stirred. Then add milk, water, or fruit juice and stir until dissolved. May be flavored with vanilla or cocoa to make "malteds." Excellent with warm milk at bedtime. Also available in tablet and powder forms.

**Professional Labeling:** The dosage for children under 2 years of age is:

**Powder:** 2 to 3 level measuring teaspoonfuls, 3 to 4 times per day, in water, fruit juice, or formula.

**Liquid:** 1 to 2 measuring teaspoonfuls, 2 to 3 times per day, in water, fruit juice, or formula.

**How Supplied:** MALTSUPEX is supplied in 8 ounce (NDC 0037-9101-12) and 16 ounce (NDC 0037-9101-08) jars of MALTSUPEX Powder; 8 fluid ounce (NDC 0037-9051-12) and 1 pint (NDC 0037-9051-08) bottles of MALTSUPEX Liquid; and in bottles of 100 MALTSUPEX Tablets (NDC 0037-9201-01).

**Storage:** Store at controlled room temperature 20°–25°C (68°–77°F). Protect MALTSUPEX powder and tablets from moisture.

MALTSUPEX **Powder** and **Liquid** are

Distributed by
Wallace Pharmaceuticals
MedPointe Healthcare Inc.
Cranbury, NJ 08512

MALTSUPEX **Tablets** are

Manufactured by
Wallace Pharmaceuticals
MedPointe Healthcare Inc.
Cranbury, NJ 08512

Rev. 10/01
*Shown in Product Identification Guide, page 524*

---

## Wellness International Network, Ltd.
**5800 DEMOCRACY DRIVE PLANO, TX 75024**

**Direct Inquiries to:**
Product Coordinator
(972) 312-1100
FAX: (972) 943-5250

---

## BIO-COMPLEX 5000™
### Gentle Foaming Cleanser

**Uses:** BIO-COMPLEX 5000™ Gentle Foaming Cleanser, with alpha-hydroxy acids, aloe vera and botanical infusions, is an advanced cleansing gel designed for all skin types. BIO-COMPLEX 5000 Gentle Foaming Cleanser protects the skin and works to restore elasticity while gently removing surface impurities, make-up and pollution.

**Ingredients:** Water (Aqua), Ammonium Lauryl Sulfate, Lauramidopropyl Betaine, Salvia Officinalis (Sage) Leaf Extract, Anthemis Nobilis Flower Extract, Glycerin, Lauramide DEA, Cetyl Betaine, Tocopherol (Vitamin E), Ascorbic Acid (Vitamin C), Citric Acid, Methylchloroisothiazolinone, Methylisothia-

zolinone, Aloe Barbadensis Leaf Juice, Lactic Acid, Malic Acid, Propylparaben, Methylparaben.

**Directions:** Splash warm water onto face. Place a small amount of gel on fingertips. Apply evenly to face and neck in circular motions, massaging skin gently but thoroughly. Rinse completely and pat dry with a soft towel.

**How Supplied:** 8 fluid ounce/236 ml. bottle.

---

## BIO-COMPLEX 5000™
### Revitalizing Conditioner

**Uses:** BIO-COMPLEX 5000™ Revitalizing Conditioner, with vitamins, antioxidants, and sunscreen, helps restore moisture to dried-out, heat-styled hair. This advanced conditioner contains silkening agents which enhance the hair as well as detangle it after shampooing. Hair is left clean, soft, manageable, and protected against styling aids and environmental elements. BIO-COMPLEX 5000 Revitalizing Conditioner is excellent for all hair types, especially damaged or over-processed hair.

**Ingredients:** Water, Stearyl Alcohol, Propylene Glycol, Stearamidopropyl Dimethylamine, Cyclomethicone, Polyquaternium - 11, Stearalkonium Chloride, Cetearyl Alcohol, PEG - 40 Hydrogenated Castor Oil, Citric Acid, Tocopherol (Vitamin E), Ascorbic Acid (Vitamin C), Retinyl Palmitate (Vitamin A), Ethylhexyl Methoxycinnamate Fragrance (Parfum), Ceteth - 20, Hydrolyzed Keratin, Sodium Chloride, Imidazolidinyl Urea, Methylparaben, Propylparaben.

**Directions:** After shampooing with BIO-COMPLEX 5000™ Revitalizing Shampoo, apply to wet hair. Massage through hair, paying special attention to the ends. Leave on 2–3 minutes. Rinse thoroughly. Towel dry and style as usual.

**How Supplied:** 12 fluid ounce bottle.

---

## BIO-COMPLEX 5000™
### Revitalizing Shampoo

**Uses:** BIO-COMPLEX 5000™ Revitalizing Shampoo, with vitamins, antioxidants, and sunscreen, cleanses and moisturizes hair for excellent manageability. Specially formulated with the essence of awapuhi, a Hawaiian ginger plant extract known for its healing qualities, this formula contains the mildest blend of surfactants and a wealth of natural conditioning ingredients to provide body, luster and healthier-looking hair.

**Ingredients:** Water, Ammonium Lauryl Sulfate, Tea Lauryl Sulfate, Cocamidopropyl Betaine, Lauramide DEA, Cetyl Betaine, Glycerin, Ascorbic Acid

*Continued on next page*

## Bio-Complex 5000—Cont.

(Vitamin C), Tocopherol (Vitamin E), Retinyl Palmitate (Vitamin A), Citric Acid, Hydrolyzed Wheat Protein, Fragrance (Parfum), Ethylhexyl Methoxycinnamate, PEG - 7 Glyceryl Cocoate, Methylchloroisothiazolinone, Methylisothiazolinone, Caramel.

**Directions:** Apply a small amount to wet hair and massage gently into scalp, creating a generous lather. Rinse and repeat if necessary. To further intensify this reconstructive process, follow with BIO-COMPLEX 5000™ Revitalizing Conditioner.

**How Supplied:** 12 fluid ounce bottle.

---

## STEPHAN™ BIO-NUTRITIONAL
### Daytime Hydrating Creme

**Uses:** Hypo-allergenic STEPHAN™ BIO-NUTRITIONAL Daytime Hydrating Creme hydrates the skin and preserves the moisture level of the upper layers of the epidermis. It is an excellent day cream for both men and women who wish to combat the visible signs of aging skin, the appearance of wrinkles or lines, and the inelastic look of facial features and contours. These light emulsions are absorbed rapidly, leaving an invisible protective film which hydrates the epidermis, regulates moisture levels and leaves skin feeling supple and soft.

**Ingredients:** Water (Aqua), Stearic Acid, Isodecyl Neopentanoate, Isostearyl Stearoyl Stearate, DEA-Cetyl Phosphate, C12-15 Alkyl Benzoate, Tocopherol (Vitamin E), Aloe Barbadensis Leaf Juice, Squalane, Cetyl Esters, Benzophenone-3, Dimethicone, Fragrance (Parfum), Carbomer, Triethanolamine, Imidazolidinyl Urea, Methylparaben, Propylparaben, Annatto.

**Directions:** Apply in the morning and during the day to clean skin. May be used around the eye area, avoiding direct contact with the eyes. Suitable for all skin types. For best results, use in conjunction with the complete STEPHAN BIO-NUTRITIONAL Skin Care line.

**Warnings:** For external use only. Avoid contact with eyes.

**How Supplied:** Net Wt. 1.75 oz.

---

## STEPHAN™ BIO-NUTRITIONAL
### Eye-Firming Concentrate

**Uses:** Hypo-allergenic STEPHAN™ BIO-NUTRITIONAL Eye-Firming Concentrate is specially formulated to revitalize the delicate area around the eyes. This non-oily fluid pampers sensitive eyes while reducing the look of puffiness and dark circles, and smoothing and softening the appearance of fine lines in the eye area.

**Ingredients:** Water (Aqua), Centaurea Cyanus Flower Extract, Methylsilanol Hydroxyproline Aspartate, Methyl Gluceth-20, Dimethicone Copolyol, PEG-30 Glyceryl Laurate, Equisetum Arvense Extract, Panthenol, Propylene Glycol, Carbomer, Disodium EDTA, Triethanolamine, Xanthan Gum, Diazolidinyl Urea, Methylparaben, Propylparaben.

**Directions:** Apply in the morning, or any time of the day, in small quantities to the skin around the eyes with light, tapping motions, avoiding direct contact with the eyes. In the evening, apply gently to the entire eye contour area. For best results, use in conjunction with the complete STEPHAN BIO-NUTRITIONAL Skin Care line.

**Warnings:** For external use only. Avoid direct contact with eyes.

**How Supplied:** 1 fl. oz.

---

## STEPHAN™ BIO-NUTRITIONAL
### Nightime Moisture Creme

**Uses:** Hypo-allergenic STEPHAN™ BIO-NUTRITIONAL Nightime Moisture Creme is a heavier, richer cream for mature, dry or sun-damaged skin. This advanced formula is excellent for dehydrated skin, promoting suppleness and moisture, while improving the appearance of fine lines and wrinkles.

**Ingredients:** Water (Aqua), Caprylic/Capric Triglyceride, Propylene, Glycol/Dicaprylate/Dicaprate, Stearic Acid, Polysorbate 60, Cetyl Alcohol, Ethylhexyl Palmitate, Cera Alba (Beeswax), Sorbitan Stearate, Canola Oil, Persea Gratissima (Avocado) Oil, Carthamus Tinctorius (safflower) Seed Oil, Squalane, Lecithin (Liposomes), Soluble Collagen, Dimethicone, Bisabolol, Aloe Barbadensis Leaf Juice, Fragrance (Parfum), C12–15 Alkyl Benzoate, Hydroxyethylcellulose, Alcohol, Ethylhexyl Methoxycinnamate, Disodium EDTA, Sodium Borate, Benzophenone-3, Allantoin, Potassium Sorbate, Phenoxyethanol, Methylparaben, Propylparaben, Butylparaben, Ethylparaben, Yellow 10, Caramel.

**Directions:** In the evening, apply by lightly massaging onto a thoroughly cleansed face and neck. Avoid direct contact with eyes. For drier skin, it may be used during the day as a moisturizer, under make-up or after sun bathing. For best results, use in conjunction with the complete STEPHAN BIO-NUTRITIONAL Skin Care line.

**Warning:** For external use only. Avoid contact with eyes.

**How Supplied:** Net Wt. 1.75 oz.

---

## STEPHAN™ BIO-NUTRITIONAL
### Refreshing Moisture Gel

**Uses:** Hypo-allergenic STEPHAN™ BIO-NUTRITIONAL Refreshing Moisture Gel is specially formulated to refine pores and promote a clear, clean and smooth-looking complexion. It is designed to deeply cleanse and super-stimulate the skin. This gel is suitable for all skin types, especially problem areas. A quick "pick-me-up," STEPHAN BIO-NUTRITIONAL Refreshing Moisture Gel immediately restores the radiant, firm and youthful appearance of the face while acting as a cumulative, revitalizing beauty treatment.

**Ingredients:** Water (Aqua), Propylene Glycol, Glycerin, Hydroxyethylcellulose, Saccharum Officinarum (Sugar Cane) Extract, Citrus Unshiu Extract, Pyrus Malus (Apple) Extract, Camellia Oleifera Leaf Extract, Hydrolyzed Wheat Protein, Yeast Extract, Saccharomyces Lysate Extract, Panthenol, Aloe Barbadensis Leaf Juice, Phenethyl Alcohol, Laureth-4, Magnesium Aluminum Silicate, Tetrasodium EDTA, Benzophenone-3, Imidazolidinyl Urea, Methylchloroisothiazolinone, Methylisothiazolinone, Methylparaben, Propylparaben, Yellow 10, Red 40, Yellow 5.

**Directions:** Apply to clean skin at anytime. Remove after 20 minutes with warm water. Can be used around the eye area, avoiding direct contact with the eyes. Suitable for all skin types. For best results, use in conjunction with the complete STEPHAN BIO-NUTRITIONAL Skin Care line.

**Warnings:** For external use only. Avoid contact with eyes.

**How Supplied:** Net Wt. 1.75 oz.

---

## STEPHAN™ BIO-NUTRITIONAL
### Ultra Hydrating Fluid

**Uses:** Hypo-allergenic STEPHAN™ BIO-NUTRITIONAL Ultra Hydrating Fluid is a complete treatment formulated to soften fine lines and preserve youthful-looking, radiant skin. By utilizing ingredients focused on revitalization, STEPHAN BIO-NUTRITIONAL Ultra Hydrating Fluid possesses a progressive firming effect, helping to combat the aged look of skin due to external negative conditions.

**Ingredients:** Water (Aqua), Methylsilanol Hydroxyproline Aspar, Methyl Gluceth-20, Dimethicone Copolyol, Peg-30 Glyceryl Laurate, Panthenol Saccharum Officinarum (Sugar Cane) Extract, Citrus Unshiu Extract, Pyrus Malus (Apple) Extract, Cammelia Oleifera Leaf Extract, Saccharomyces Lysate Extract, Laureth-4, Yeast Extract, Hydrolyzed Wheat Protein, Methylchloroisothiazolinone, Methylisothiazolinone, Phenethyl Alcohol, 2-Bromo-2-Nitropropane-1, 3-Diol, Xanthan Gum, Disodium EDTA, Methylparaben, Propylparaben.

**Directions:** Gently apply all over the face, neck and eye contour area, preferably in the morning. Make-up can be applied afterwards. Use as a part of a regular daily skin care routine or as an occasional preventive treatment. For best results, use in conjunction with the complete STEPHAN BIO-NUTRITIONAL Skin Care line.

**Warnings:** For external use only. Avoid direct contact with eyes.

**How Supplied:** 1 fl. oz.

---

# Whitehall-Robins Healthcare American Home Products Corporation
**FIVE GIRALDA FARMS MADISON, NJ 07940**

**Direct Inquiries to:**
Whitehall Consumer Product Information 800-322-3129
Robins Consumer Product Information 800-762-4672

## ADVIL®
[ad 'vil ]
**Ibuprofen Tablets, USP**
**Ibuprofen Caplets (Oval-Shaped Tablets)**
**Ibuprofen Gel Caplets (Oval-Shaped Gelatin Coated Tablets)**
**Ibpurofen Liqui-Gel Capsules**

**Active Ingredient:** Each tablet, caplet, or liquigel capsule contains Ibuprofen 200 mg

**Inactive Ingredients:**
**Tablets and Caplets:** Acetylated Monoglyceride, Beeswax and/or Carnauba Wax, Croscarmellose Sodium, Iron Oxides, Lecithin, Methylparaben, Microcrystalline Cellulose, Pharmaceutical Glaze, Povidone, Propylparaben, Silicon Dioxide, Simethicone, Sodium Benzoate, Sodium Lauryl Sulfate, Starch, Stearic Acid, Sucrose, Titanium Dioxide.
**Gel Caplets:** Croscarmellose Sodium, FD&C Red 40, FD&C Yellow 6, Gelatin, Glycerin Hydroxypropyl Methylcellulose, Iron Oxides, Lecithin, Pharmaceutical Glaze, Propyl Gallate, Silicon Dioxide, Simethicone, Sodium Lauryl Sulfate, Starch, Stearic Acid, Titanium Dioxide, Triacetin.
**Liqui-Gels:** FD&C Green No. 3, Gelatin, Pharmaceutical Ink, Polyethylene Glycol, Potassium Hydroxide, Purified Water, Sorbitan, Sorbitol.

**Indications:** temporarily relieves minor aches and pains due to the common cold, headache, toothache, muscular aches, backache, minor pain of arthritis, menstrual cramps; and temporarily reduces fever.

**Dosage and Administration:**
*Directions*—Do not take more than directed
**Adults:**
• take 1 tablet, caplet, gelcap or liquigel capsule every 4 to 6 hours while symptoms occur
• if pain or fever does not respond to 1 tablet, caplet, gelcap, or liquigel capsule, 2 tablets, caplets, gelcaps or liquigel capsules may be used, but do not exceed 6 tablets, caplets, gelcaps or liquigel capsules in 24 hours, unless directed by a doctor
• the smallest effective dose should be used
**Children:** do not give to children under 12 unless directed by a doctor

**Warnings**
**Allergy alert:** ibuprofen may cause a severe allergic reaction which may include:
• hives
• facial swelling
• asthma (wheezing)
• shock
**Alcohol warning:** if you consume 3 or more alcoholic drinks every day, ask your doctor whether you should take ibuprofen or other pain relievers/fever reducers. Ibuprofen may cause stomach bleeding.
**Do not use** if you have ever had an allergic reaction to any other pain reliever/fever reducer
**Ask a doctor before use if you have** had problems or side effects with any pain reliever/fever reducer
**Ask a doctor or pharmacist before use if you are**
• under a doctor's care for any continuing medical condition
• taking other drugs on a regular basis
• taking any other product containing ibuprofen, or any other pain reliever/fever reducer
**Stop use and ask a doctor if**
• an allergic reaction occurs. Seek medical help right away.
• fever gets worse or lasts more than 3 days
• pain gets worse or lasts more than 10 days
• stomach pain occurs with the use of this product
• the painful area is red or swollen
• any new or unexpected symptoms occur
**If pregnant or breast-feeding,** ask a health professional before use. It is especially important not to use ibuprofen during the last 3 months of pregnancy unless definitely directed to do so by a doctor because it may cause problems in the unborn child or complications during delivery.
**Keep out of reach of children.** In case of overdose, get medical help or contact a Poison Control Center right away.

**How Supplied:**
Coated tablets in bottles of 6, 8, 24, 50, 72 (non-child resistant E-Z open cap), 100, 165, and 250. Coated caplets in bottles of 24, 50, 72 (non-child resistant E-Z Cap) 100, 165, and 250.
Gel caplets in bottles of 24, 50, 100, 165 and 250.
Liqui-Gels in bottles of 20, 40, 80, 135 and 200.

**Storage:** Store at 20–25°C (68–77°F) Avoid excessive heat 40°C (above 104°F)

---

## ADVIL® COLD and SINUS
**Ibuprofen/Pseudoephedrine HCl Caplets* and Tablets**
**Pain Reliever/Fever Reducer/Nasal Decongestant**

---

*Oval-Shaped tablets

**Active Ingredients:**
**(in each tablet)**                    **Purposes:**
Ibuprofen
   200 mg ... Pain reliever/fever reducer
Pseudoephedrine HCl
   30 mg .................... Nasal decongestant

**Inactive Ingredients:** Carnauba or Equivalent Wax, Croscarmellose Sodium, Iron Oxides, Methylparaben, Microcrystalline Cellulose, Propylparaben, Silicon Dioxide, Sodium Benzoate, Sodium Lauryl Sulfate, Starch, Stearic Acid, Sucrose, Titanium Dioxide

**Uses:** Temporarily relieves these symptoms associated with the common cold, sinusitis or flu:
• headache • fever • nasal congestion
• minor body aches and pains

**Directions:**
• adults and children 12 years of age and over:
   • take 1 tablet every 4 to 6 hours while symptoms persist. If symptoms do not respond to 1 tablet, 2 tablets may be used.
   • do not use more than 6 tablets in any 24-hour period unless directed by a doctor
   • the smallest effective dose should be used
• children under 12 years of age: consult a doctor

**Warnings:**
**Allergy Alert:** Ibuprofen may cause a severe allergic reaction which may include: • hives • facial swelling • asthma (wheezing) • shock

**Alcohol warning:** If you consume 3 or more alcoholic drinks every day, ask your doctor whether you should take ibuprofen or other pain relievers/fever reducers. Ibuprofen may cause stomach bleeding.
**Do not use:**
• if you have ever had an allergic reaction to any other pain reliever/fever reducer
• if you are now taking a prescription monoamine oxidase inhibitor (MAOI) (certain drugs for depression, psychiatric, or emotional conditions, or Parkinson's disease), or for 2 weeks after stopping the MAOI drug. If you do not know if your prescription drug contains an MAOI, ask a doctor or pharmacist before taking this product
**Ask a doctor before use if you have:**
• heart disease • high blood pressure • thyroid disease • diabetes
• trouble urinating due to an enlarged prostate gland
• stomach pain
• had serious side effects from any pain reliever/fever reducer

*Continued on next page*

## Advil Cold/Sinus—Cont.

**Ask a doctor or pharmacist before use if you are:**
- taking any other product that contains ibuprofen or pseudoephedrine
- taking any other pain reliever/fever reducer or nasal decongestant
- under a doctor's care for any continuing medical condition
- taking other drugs on a regular basis

**When using this product:**
- do not use more than directed
- take with food or milk if stomach upset occurs

**Stop use and ask a doctor if:**
- an allergic reaction occurs. Seek medical help right away.
- you get nervous, dizzy, or sleepless
- nasal congestion lasts more than 7 days
- fever lasts for more than 3 days
- symptoms continue or get worse
- new or unexpected symptoms occur
- stomach pain occurs with use of this product or if even mild symptoms persist

**If pregnant or breast-feeding,** ask a health professional before use. It is especially important not to use this product during the last 3 months of pregnancy unless definitely directed to do so by a doctor because it may cause problems in the unborn child or complications during delivery.

**Keep out of reach of children.** In case of overdose, get medical help or contact a Poison Control Center right away.

**Other Information:**
- store at 20–25°C (68–77°F). Avoid excessive heat above 40°C (104°F).
- read all warnings and directions before use. Keep carton.

**How Supplied:** Advil® Cold and Sinus is an oval-shaped, tan-colored caplet, or tan-colored tablet. The caplet is supplied in blister packs of 20 and 40. The tablet is available in blister packs of 20.

**Storage:** Store at 20–25°C (68–77°F); avoid excessive heat 40°C, (above 104°F).

---

## ADVIL®
## FLU & BODY ACHE Caplets

**Uses:**
- temporarily relieves these symptoms associated with the common cold, sinusitis, or flu
  - headache
  - fever
  - nasal congestion
  - minor body aches and pains

**Active Ingredients**
| (In each caplet): | Purpose: |
|---|---|
| Ibuprofen 200 mg .... | Pain reliever/fever reducer |
| Pseudoephedrine HCl 30 mg ........ | Nasal decongestant |

**Inactive Ingredients:** Carnauba or equivalent wax, croscarmellose sodium, iron oxide, methylparaben, microcrystalline cellulose, propylparaben, silicon dioxide, sodium benzoate, sodium lauryl sulfate, starch, stearic acid, sucrose, titanium dioxide

**Directions:**
- Adults and children 12 years of age and over: Take 1 caplet every 4 to 6 hours while symptoms persist. If symptoms do not respond to 1 caplet, 2 caplets may be used.
- do not use more than 6 caplets in any 24-hour period unless directed by a doctor
- the smallest effective dose should be used
- Children under 12 years of age: consult a doctor

**Warnings:**
**Allergy alert:** ibuprofen may cause a severe allergic reaction which may include: • hives • facial swelling • asthma (wheezing) • shock
**Alcohol warning:** if you consume 3 or more alcoholic drinks every day, ask your doctor whether you should take ibuprofen or other pain relievers/fever reducers. Ibuprofen may cause stomach bleeding.
**Do not use:**
- if you have ever had an allergic reaction to any other pain reliever/fever reducer
- if you are now taking a prescription monoamine oxidase inhibitor (MAOI) (certain drugs for depression, psychiatric, or emotional conditions, or Parkinson's disease), or for 2 weeks after stopping the MAOI drug. If you do not know if your prescription drug contains an MAOI, ask a doctor or pharmacist before taking this product.

**Ask a doctor before use if you have**
- heart disease • high blood pressure
- thyroid disease • diabetes
- trouble urinating due to an enlarged prostate gland
- stomach pain
- had serious side effects from any pain reliever/fever reducer

**Ask a doctor or pharmacist before use if you are**
- taking any other product that contains ibuprofen or pseudoephedrine
- taking any other pain reliever/fever reducer or nasal decongestant
- under a doctor's care for any continuing medical condition
- taking other drugs on a regular basis

**When using this product**
- do not use more than directed
- take with food or milk if stomach upset occurs

**Stop use and ask a doctor if**
- an allergic reaction occurs. Seek medical help right away.
- you get nervous, dizzy, or sleepless
- nasal congestion lasts more than 7 days
- fever lasts for more than 3 days
- symptoms continue or get worse
- new or unexpected symptoms occur
- stomach pain occurs with use of this product or if even mild symptoms persist

**If pregnant or breast-feeding,** ask a health professional before use. It is especially important not to use this product during the last 3 months of pregnancy unless definitely directed to do so by a doctor because it may cause problems in the unborn child or complications during delivery.

**Keep out of reach of children.** In case of overdose, get medical help or contact a Poison Control Center right away.
- do not use if blister unit is broken or open
- store at 20–25°C (68–77°F); Avoid excessive heat above 40°C (104°F)
- read all warnings and directioons before use. Keep carton.

**How Supplied:**
Blister packs of 20 caplets.

---

## ADVIL®
## MIGRAINE Liquigels

**Use:** Treats migraine

**Active Ingredient:**
Each brown, oval capsule contains solubilized ibuprofen, a pain reliever, equal to 200 mg ibuprofen (present as the free acid and potassium salt)

**Inactive Ingredients:**
D&C yellow no. 10, FD&C green no. 3, FD&C red no. 40, gelatin, light mineral oil, pharmaceutical ink, polyethylene glycol, potassium hydroxide, purified water, sorbitan, sorbitol

**Directions:**

| Adults: | • take 2 capsules with a glass of water<br>• if symptoms persist or worsen, ask your doctor<br>• do not take more than 2 capsules in 24 hours, unless directed by a doctor |
|---|---|
| Under 18 years of age: | • ask a doctor |

**Warnings:**
**Allergy alert:** Ibuprofen may cause a severe allergic reaction which may include:
- hives
- facial swelling
- asthma (wheezing)
- shock

**Alcohol warning:** If you consume 3 or more alcoholic drinks every day, ask your doctor whether you should take ibuprofen or other pain relievers/fever reducers. Ibuprofen may cause stomach bleeding.
**Do not use** if you have ever had an allergic reaction to any other pain reliever/fever reducer

**Ask a doctor before use if you have:**
- never had migraines diagnosed by a health professional
- a headache that is different from your usual migraines
- the worse headache of your life
- fever and stiff neck
- headaches beginning after, or caused by head injury, exertion, coughing or bending
- experienced your first headache after the age of 50
- daily headaches
- a migraine so severe as to require bed rest
- problems or serious side effects from taking pain relievers or fever reducers
- stomach pain

## Ask a doctor or pharmacist before use if you are:

- under a doctor's care for any continuing medical condition
- taking other drugs on a regular basis
- taking another product containing ibuprofen, or any other pain reliever/fever reducer

## Stop use and ask a doctor if:

- an allergic reaction occurs. Seek medical help right away.
- migraine headache pain is not relieved or gets worse after first dose
- stomach pain occurs with the use of this product
- new or unexpected symptoms occur

**If pregnant or breast-feeding,** ask a health professional before use. It is especially important not to use ibuprofen during the last 3 months of pregnancy unless definitely directed to do so by a doctor because it may cause problems in the unborn child or complications during delivery.

**Keep out of reach of children.** In case of overdose, get medical help or contact a Poison Control Center right away.

## Other information:

- read all directions and warnings before use. Keep carton.
- store at 20–25°C (68–77°F)
- avoid excessive heat 40°C (above 104°F)

**How Supplied:** Bottles of 20, 40, & 80 liquigels.

---

## INFANTS' ADVIL CONCENTRATED DROPS
[ad' vil]

## Active Ingredient:
**(in each 1.25 mL)**          **Purposes:**
Ibuprofen
50 mg .......... Fever reducer/pain reliever

**Uses:**   Temporarily:
- reduces fever
- relieves minor aches and pains due to the common cold, flu, headaches and toothaches

## Warnings:
**Allergy Alert:**  Ibuprofen may cause a severe allergic reaction which may include:
- hives • asthma (wheezing)
- facial swelling • shock

**Do not use** if the child has ever had an allergic reaction to any other fever reducer/pain reliever

**Ask a doctor before use if the child has:**
- not been drinking fluids
- lost a lot of fluid due to continued vomiting or diarrhea
- stomach pain
- problems or serious side effects from taking fever reducers or pain relievers

**Ask a doctor or pharmacist before use if the child is:**
- under a doctor's care for any serious condition
- taking any other drug
- taking any other product that contains ibuprofen, or any other pain reliever/fever reducer

**When using this product** give with food or milk if upset stomach occurs

**Stop use and ask a doctor if:**
- an allergic reaction occurs. Seek medical help right away.

---

- fever or pain gets worse or lasts more than 3 days
- the child does not get any relief within first day (24 hours) of treatment
- stomach pain or upset gets worse or lasts
- redness or swelling is present in the painful area
- any new symptoms appear

**Keep out of reach of children.** In case of overdose, get medical help or contact a Poison Control Center right away.

## Directions:
- do not give more than directed
- shake well before using
- find right dose on chart below. If possible, use weight to dose; otherwise use age.
- repeat dose every 6–8 hours, if needed
- do not use more than 4 times a day
- measure with the dosing device provided. Do not use with any other device.

[See table above]

## Other Information:
- one dose lasts 6–8 hours

**Inactive Ingredients:**  (FRUIT FLAVOR) Artificial flavors, caroboxymethylcellulose sodium, citric acid, edetate disodium, FD&C red no. 40, glycerin, microcrystalline cellulose, polysorbate 80, purified water, sodium benzoate, sorbitol solution, sucrose, xanthan gum

**Inactive Ingredients:**  (GRAPE FLAVOR) Artificial flavor, caroboxymethylcellulose sodium, citric acid, edetate disodium, FD&C blue no. 1, FD&C red no. 40, glycerin, microcrystalline cellulose, polysorbate 80, purified water, sodium benzoate, sorbitol solution, sucrose, xanthan gum

**How Supplied:**  Bottles of ½ fl. oz. in grape and fruit flavors.

---

## CHILDREN'S ADVIL CHEWABLE TABLETS
[ad' vil]

## Active Ingredient:
**(in each tablet)**          **Purposes:**
Ibuprofen 50 mg ............. Fever reducer/pain reliever

---

**Uses:**   Temporarily:
- reduces fever
- relieves minor aches and pains due to the common cold, flu, sore throat, headaches and toothaches

## Warnings:
**Allergy alert:**  Ibuprofen may cause a severe allergic reaction which may include:
- hives • asthma (wheezing)
- facial swelling • shock

**Sore throat warning:**  Severe or persistent sore throat or sore throat accompanied by high fever, headache, nausea, and vomiting may be serious. Consult doctor promptly. Do not use more than 2 days or administer to children under 3 years of age unless directed by doctor.

**Do not use** if the child has ever had an allergic reaction to any other fever reducer/pain reliever

**Ask a doctor before use if the child has:**
- not been drinking fluids
- lost a lot of fluid due to continued vomiting or diarrhea
- stomach pain
- problems or serious side effects from taking fever reducers or pain relievers

**Ask a doctor or pharmacist before use if the child is:**
- under a doctor's care for any serious condition
- taking any other drug
- taking any other product that contains ibuprofen, or any other pain reliever/fever reducer

**When using this product** give with food or milk if stomach upset occurs

**Stop use and ask a doctor if:**
- an allergic reaction occurs. Seek medical help right away.
- fever or pain gets worse or lasts more than 3 days
- the child does not get any relief within first day (24 hours) of treatment
- stomach pain or upset gets worse or lasts

*Continued on next page*

### Dosing Chart (top)

| Weight (lb) | Age (mos) | Dose (mL) |
|---|---|---|
| under 6 mo | | ask a doctor |
| 12–17 lb | 6–11 mos | 1.25 mL |
| 18–23 lb | 12–23 mos | 1.875 mL |

### Dosing Chart (bottom)

| Weight (lb) | Age (yr) | Dose (tablets) |
|---|---|---|
| under 24 lb | under 2 yr | ask a doctor |
| 24–35 lb | 2–3 yr | 2 tablets |
| 36–47 lb | 4–5 yr | 3 tablets |
| 48–59 lb | 6–8 yr | 4 tablets |
| 60–71 lb | 9–10 yr | 5 tablets |
| 72–95 lb | 11 yr | 6 tablets |

## Children's Advil—Cont.

- redness or swelling is present in the painful area
- any new symptoms appear

**Keep out of reach of children.** In case of overdose, get medical help or contact a Poison Control Center right away.

### Directions:
- do not give more than directed
- find right dose on chart below. If possible, use weight to dose; otherwise use age.
- repeat dose every 6–8 hours, if needed
- do not use more than 4 times a day [See table at bottom of previous page]

### Other Information:
- **Phenylketonurics:** contains phenylalanine 2.1 mg per tablet
- one dose last 6–8 hours
- store at 20–25°C (68–77°F) (for bottles and pouches)
- store in a dry place at 20–25°C (68–77°F) (for blisters)

**Inactive Ingredients:** (GRAPE FLAVOR) Artificial flavor, aspartame, cellulose acetate phthalate, D&C red no. 30 lake, FD&C blue no. 2 lake, gelatin, magnasweet, magnesium stearate, mannitol, microcrystalline cellulose, silicon dioxide, sodium starch glycolate

**Inactive Ingredients:** (FRUIT FLAVOR) Aspartame, cellulose acetate phthalate, D&C red no. 27 lake, FD&C red no. 40 lake, gelatin, magnasweet, magnesium stearate, mannitol, microcrystalline cellulose, natural and artifical flavors, silicon dioxide, sodium starch glycolate

**How Supplied:** Blister of 24 (fruit and grape flavors). Store at 20–25°C (68–77°F)

---

## CHILDREN'S ADVIL SUSPENSION
*[ad' vil]*

### Active Ingredient:
**(in each 5 mL)**      **Purposes:**
Ibuprofen 100 mg ............ Fever reducer/pain reliever

**Uses:** Temporarily:
- reduces fever
- relieves minor aches and pains due to the common cold, flu, sore throat, headaches and toothaches

### Warnings:
**Allergy alert:** Ibuprofen may cause a severe allergic reaction which may include:
- hives • asthma (wheezing)
- facial swelling • shock

**Sore throat warning:** Severe or persistent sore throat or sore throat accompanied by high fever, headache, nausea, and vomiting may be serious. Consult doctor promptly. Do not use more than 2 days or administer to children under 3 years of age unless directed by doctor.

**Do not use** if the child has ever had an allergic reaction to any other fever reducer/pain reliever

**Ask a doctor before use if the child has:**
- not been drinking fluids
- lost a lot of fluid due to continued vomiting or diarrhea
- stomach pain
- problems or serious side effects from taking fever reducers or pain relievers

**Ask a doctor or pharmacist before use if the child is:**
- under a doctor's care for any serious condition
- taking any other drug
- taking any other product that contains ibuprofen, or any other pain reliever/fever reducer

**When using this product** give with food or milk if stomach upset occurs

**Stop use and ask a doctor if:**
- an allergic reaction occurs. Seek medical help right away.
- fever or pain gets worse or lasts more than 3 days
- the child does not get any relief within first day (24 hours) of treatment
- stomach pain or upset gets worse or lasts
- redness or swelling is present in the painful area
- any new symptoms appear

**Keep out of reach of children.** In case of overdose, get medical help or contact a Poison Control Center right away.

### Directions:
- do not give more than directed
- shake well before using
- find right dose on chart below. If possible, use weight to dose; otherwise use age.
- repeat dose every 6–8 hours, if needed
- do not use more than 4 times a day
- measure only with the blue dosing cup provided. Blue dosing cup to be used with Children's Advil Suspension only. Do not use with other products. Dose lines account for product remaining in cup due to thickness of suspension.

[See table below]

### Other Information:
- one dose lasts 6–8 hours
- store at 20–25°C (68–77°F)

**Inactive Ingredients:** (FRUIT FLAVOR) Artifical flavors, carboxymethylcellulose sodium, citric acid, edetate disodium, FD&C red no. 40, glycerin, microcrystalline cellulose, polysorbate 80, purified water, sodium benzoate, sorbitol solution, sucrose, xanthan gum

**Inactive Ingredients:** (GRAPE FLAVOR) Artifical flavor, carboxymethylcellulose sodium, citric acid, edetate disodium, FD&C blue no. 1, FD&C red no. 40, glycerin, microcrystalline cellulose, polysorbate 80, purified water, sodium benzoate, sorbitol solution, sucrose, xanthan gum

**Inactive Ingredients:** (BLUE RASPBERRY FLAVOR) Carboxymethylcellulose sodium, citric acid, edetate disodium, FD&C blue no. 1, flavors, glycerin, microcrystalline cellulose, polysorbate 80, purified water, sodium benzoate, sodium citrate, sorbitol solution, sucrose, xanthan gum

**How Supplied:** Bottles of 2 fl. oz. and 4 fl. oz. in grape, fruit, and blue raspberry flavors.

---

## JUNIOR STRENGTH ADVIL CHEWABLE TABLETS
*[ad' vil]*

### Active Ingredient:
**(in each tablet)**      **Purposes:**
Ibuprofen 100 mg ..... Fever reducer/pain reliever

**Uses:** Temporarily:
- reduces fever
- relieves minor aches and pains due to the common cold, flu, sore throat, headaches and toothaches

### Warnings:
**Allergy alert:** Ibuprofen may cause a severe allergic reaction which may include:
- hives • asthma (wheezing)
- facial swelling • shock

**Sore throat warning:** Severe or persistent sore throat or sore throat accompanied by high fever, headache, nausea, and vomiting may be serious. Consult doctor promptly. Do not use more than 2 days or administer to children under 3 years of age unless directed by doctor.

**Do not use** if the child has ever had an allergic reaction to any other fever reducer/pain reliever

**Ask a doctor before use if the child has:**
- not been drinking fluids
- lost a lot of fluid due to continued vomiting or diarrhea
- stomach pain
- problems or serious side effects from taking fever reducers or pain relievers

**Ask a doctor or pharmacist before use if the child is:**
- under a doctor's care for any serious condition
- taking any other drug
- taking any other product that contains ibuprofen, or any other pain reliever/fever reducer

**When using this product** give with food or milk if stomach upset occurs

### Dosing Chart

| Weight (lb) | Age (yr) | Dose (tsp) |
|---|---|---|
| under 24 lb | under 2 yr | ask a doctor |
| 24–35 lb | 2–3 yr | 1 tsp |
| 36–47 lb | 4–5 yr | 1½ tsp |
| 48–59 lb | 6–8 yr | 2 tsp |
| 60–71 lb | 9–10 yr | 2½ tsp |
| 72–95 lb | 11 yr | 3 tsp |

## Dosing Chart

| Weight (lb) | Age (yr) | Dose (tablets) |
|---|---|---|
| under 48 lb | under 6 yr | ask a doctor |
| 48–59 lb | 6–8 yr | 2 tablets |
| 60–71 lb | 9–10 yr | 2 ½ tablets |
| 72–95 lb | 11 yr | 3 tablets |

### Stop use and ask a doctor if:
- an allergic reaction occurs. Seek medical help right away.
- fever or pain gets worse or lasts more than 3 days
- the child does not get any relief within first day (24 hours) of treatment
- stomach pain or upset gets worse or lasts
- redness or swelling is present in the painful area
- any new symptoms appear

**Keep out of reach of children.** In case of overdose, get medical help or contact a Poison Control Center right away.

### Directions:
- do not give more than directed
- find right dose on chart below. If possible, use weight to dose; otherwise use age.
- repeat dose every 6–8 hours, if needed
- do not use more than 4 times a day
[See table above]

### Other Information:
- **Phenylketonurics:** contains phenylalanine 4.2 mg per tablet
- one dose lasts 6–8 hours
- store in a dry place at 20–25°C (68–77°F) (for blisters)
- store at 20–25°C (68–77°F) (for bottles and pouches)

**Inactive Ingredients:** (GRAPE FLAVOR) Artificial flavor, aspartame, cellulose acetate phthalate, D&C red no. 30 lake, FD&C blue no. 2 lake, gelatin, magnasweet, magnesium stearate, mannitol, microcrystalline cellulose, silicon dioxide, sodium starch glycolate

**Inactive Ingredients:** (FRUIT FLAVOR) Aspartame, cellulose acetate phthalate, D&C red no. 27 lake, FD&C red no. 40 lake, gelatin, magnasweet, magnesium stearate, mannitol, microcrystalline cellulose, natural and artificial flavors, silicon dioxide, sodium starch glycolate

### How Supplied:
Chewable Tablets: bottles of 24 (fruit and grape flavors).

---

## JUNIOR STRENGTH ADVIL SWALLOW TABLETS
[ad' vil]

**Active Ingredient:**
**(in each tablet)** **Purposes:**
Ibuprofen
100 mg ............................ Fever reducer/
pain reliever

**Uses:** Temporarily:
- reduces fever
- relieves minor aches and pains due to the common cold, flu, sore throat, headaches and toothaches

### Warnings:
**Allergy alert:** Ibuprofen may cause a severe allergic reaction which may include:
- hives • asthma (wheezing)
- facial swelling • shock

**Sore throat warning:** Severe or persistent sore throat or sore throat accompanied by high fever, headache, nausea, and vomiting may be serious. Consult doctor promptly. Do not use more than 2 days or administer to children under 3 years of age unless directed by doctor.

**Do not use** if the child has ever had an allergic reaction to any other fever reducer or pain reliever

**Ask a doctor before use if the child has:**
- not been drinking fluids
- lost a lot of fluid due to continued vomiting or diarrhea
- stomach pain
- problems or serious side effects from taking fever reducers or pain relievers

**Ask a doctor or pharmacist before use if the child is:**
- under a doctor's care for any serious condition
- taking any other drug
- taking any other product that contains ibuprofen, or any other pain reliever/fever reducer

**When using this product** give with food or milk if stomach upset occurs

**Stop use and ask a doctor if**
- an allergic reaction occurs. Seek medical help right away.
- fever or pain gets worse or lasts more than 3 days
- the child does not get any relief within first day (24 hours) of treatment
- stomach pain or upset gets worse or lasts
- redness or swelling is present in the painful area
- any new symptoms appear

**Keep out of reach of children.** In case of overdose, get medical help or contact a Poison Control Center right away.

### Directions:
- do not give more than directed
- find right dose on chart below. If possible, use weight to dose; otherwise use age.
- repeat dose every 6–8 hours, if needed
- do not use more than 4 times a day

### Dosing Chart

| Weight (lb) | Age (yr) | Dose (tablets) |
|---|---|---|
| under 48 lb | under 6 yr | ask a doctor |
| 48–71 lb | 6–10 yr | 2 tablets |
| 72–95 lb | 11 yr | 3 tablets |

### Other Information:
- one dose lasts 6–8 hours
- store at 20–25°C (68–77°F)
- avoid excessive heat 40°C (104°F) – (for blisters and pouches only)

**Inactive Ingredients:** acetylated monoglycerides, carnauba wax, colloidal silicon dioxide, croscarmellose sodium, iron oxides, methylparaben, microcrystalline cellulose, povidone, pregelatinized starch, propylene glycol, propylparaben, shellac, sodium benzoate, starch, stearic acid, sucrose, titanium dioxide

**How Supplied:** Coated Tablets in bottles of 24.

---

## MAXIMUM STRENGTH
### ANBESOL® Gel and Liquid
[an 'ba-sol"]
**Oral Anesthetic**

### ANBESOL JUNIOR® Gel
**Oral Anesthetic Gel**

### BABY ANBESOL®
**Grape Flavor**
**Oral Anesthetic Gel**

**Description:** Anbesol is an oral anesthetic which is available in a Maximum Strength gel and liquid. Anbesol Junior, available in a gel, is an oral anesthetic. Baby Anbesol, available in a grape-flavored gel, is an oral anesthetic and is alcohol-free. Maximum Strength formulations contain Benzocaine 20%.
Anbesol Junior Gel contains Benzocaine 10%.
Baby Anbesol Gel contains Benzocaine 7.5%.

**Indications:** Maximum Strength Anbesol is indicated for the temporary relief of pain associated with toothache, canker sores, minor dental procedures, sore gums, braces, and dentures. Anbesol Junior is indicated for the temporary relief of braces, sore gums, canker sores, toothaches, and minor dental procedures. Baby Anbesol Gel is indicated for the temporary relief of sore gums due to teething in infants and children 4 months of age and older.

**Warnings: Allergy alert:** Do not use this product if you have a history of allergy to local anesthetics such as procaine, butacaine, benzocaine, or other "caine" anesthetics.
Baby Anbesol: **Do not use** to treat fever and nasal congestion. These are not symptoms of teething and may indicate the presence of infection. If these symptoms persist, consult your doctor.
**When using this product**
- avoid contact with the eyes
- do not exceed recommended dosage
- do not use for more than 7 days unless directed by a doctor/dentist
**Stop use and ask a doctor if**
- sore mouth symptoms do not improve in 7 days

*Continued on next page*

## Anbesol—Cont.

- irritation, pain, or redness persists or worsens
- swelling, rash, or fever develops

**Keep out of reach of children.** If more than used for pain is accidentally swallowed, get medical help or contact a Poison Control Center right away.

**Dosage and Administration:** Maximum Strength Anbesol: Gel—
- to open tube, cut tip of the tube on score mark with scissors
- adults and children 2 years of age and older: apply to the affected area up to 4 times daily or as directed by a doctor/dentist
- children under 12 years of age: adult supervision should be given in the use of this product
- children under 2 years of age: consult a doctor/dentist
- for denture irritation:
  - apply thin layer to the affected area
  - do not reinsert dental work until irritation/pain is relieved
  - rinse mouth well before reinserting

Liquid—
- adults and children 2 years of age and older:
  - wipe liquid on with cotton, or cotton swab, or fingertip
  - apply to the affected area up to 4 times daily or as directed by a doctor/dentist
- children under 12 years of age: adult supervision should be given in the use of this product
- children under 2 years of age; consult a doctor/dentist

Anbesol Junior:
- to open tube, cut tip of the tube on score mark with scissors
- adults and children 2 years of age and older: apply to the affected area up to 4 times daily or as directed by a doctor/dentist
- children under 12 years of age: adult supervision should be given in the use of this product
- children under 2 years of age: consult a doctor/dentist

Grape Baby Anbesol Gel:
- to open tube, cut tip of the tube on score mark with scissors
- children 4 months of age and older: apply to the affected area not more than 4 times daily or as directed by a doctor/dentist
- infants under 4 months of age: no recommended treatment except under the advice and supervision of a doctor/dentist

**Inactive Ingredients:**

**Maximum Strength Gel:** Carbomer 934P, D&C Yellow No. 10, FD&C Blue No. 1, FD&C Red No. 40, Flavor, Glycerin, Methylparaben, Phenylcarbinol, Polyethylene Glycol, Propylene Glycol, Saccharin.

**Maximum Strength Liquid:** D&C Yellow No. 10, FD&C Blue No. 1, FD&C Red No. 40, Flavor, Methylparaben, Polyethylene Glycol, Propylene Glycol, Saccharin.

**Junior Gel:** Artificial flavor, benzyl alcohol, carbomer 934P, D&C red no. 33, glycerin, methylparaben, polyethylene glycol, potassium acesulfame

**Grape Baby Gel:** Benzoic acid, carbomer 934P, D&C red no. 33, edetate disodium, FD&C blue no. 1, flavor, glycerin, methylparaben, polyethylene glycol, propylparaben, saccharin, water

**How Supplied:** All Gels in .25 oz (7.1 g) tubes, Maximum Strength Liquid in .31 fl oz (9 mL) bottle. Store at 20–25°C (68–77°F)

---

## ANBESOL COLD SORE THERAPY

**Uses:**
- temporarily relieves pain associated with fever blisters and cold sores
- relieves dryness and softens fever blisters and cold sores

| **Active ingredients:** | **Purpose:** |
|---|---|
| Allantoin 1% | Skin protectant |
| Benzocaine 20% | Fever blister/cold sore treatment |
| Camphor 3% | Fever blister/cold sore treatment |
| White petrolatum 64.9% | Skin protectant |

**Inactive Ingredients:** Aloe extract, benzyl alcohol, butylparaben, glyceryl stearate, isocetyl stearate, menthol, methylparaben, propylparaben, sodium lauryl sulfate, vitamin E, white wax

**Directions:**
- to open tube, cut tip of the tube on score mark with scissors
- adults and children 2 years of age and older: apply to the affected area not more than 3 to 4 times daily
- children under 2 years of age: consult a doctor

**Warnings: For external use only**
**Allergy Alert:** Do not use this product if you have a history of allergy to local anesthetics such as procaine, butacaine, benzocaine, or other "caine" anesthetics.
**Do not use** over deep or puncture wounds, infections, or lacerations. Consult a doctor.
**When using this product** avoid contact with the eyes
**Stop use and ask a doctor if:**
- condition worsens
- symptoms persist for more than 7 days
- symptoms clear up and occur again within a few days

**Keep out of reach of children.** If swallowed, get medical help or contact a poison control center right away.
**Other Information**
- store at 20–25°C (68–77°F)

**How Supplied:** 0.25 oz Tube

---

## DIMETAPP® Infant Drops Decongestant
[dī 'mĕ-tap ]
**Nasal Decongestant**

Alcohol-Free

**Active Ingredients:** Each 0.8 mL (1 dropperful) contains: 7.5 mg Pseudoephedrine Hydrochloride, USP.

**Inactive Ingredients:** caramel, citric acid, D&C red no. 33, FD&C blue no. 1, flavors, glycerin, high fructose corn syrup, maltol, menthol, polyethylene glycol, propylene glycol, sodium benzoate, sorbitol, sucrose, water

**Uses:** For temporary relief of nasal congestion due to the common cold, hay fever, other upper respiratory allergies, or associated with sinusitis.

**Warnings:**
**Do not use** in a child who is taking a prescription monoamine oxidase inhibitor (MAOI) (certain drugs for depression, psychiatric, or emotional conditions, or Parkinson's disease), or for 2 weeks after stopping the MAOI drug. If you do not know if your child's prescription drug contains an MAOI, ask a doctor or pharmacist before giving this product.
**Ask a doctor before use if your child has:**
- heart disease
- high blood pressure
- thyroid disease
- diabetes

**When using this product:**
- do not use more than directed
- give by mouth only; not for nasal use

**Stop use and ask a doctor if:**
- your child gets nervous, dizzy, or sleepless
- symptoms do not get better within 7 days or are accompanied by fever

**Keep out of reach of children.** In case of overdose, get medical help or contact a Poison Control Center right away.

**Directions:**
- do not give more than 4 doses in any 24-hour period
- children 2 to 3 years: 2 dropperfuls (1.6 mL) every 4 to 6 hours or as directed by a physician
- children under 2 years: ask a doctor

**Storage:** Store at Controlled Room Temperature, between 20°C and 25°C (68°F and 77°F).

**How Supplied:** $^1/_4$ oz (8 mL) bottle with dropper.

---

## DIMETAPP® DM COLD & COUGH Elixir
[dī 'mĕ-tap ]
**Nasal Decongestant, Antihistamine, Cough Suppressant**

**Active Ingredients:** Each 5 mL (1 teaspoonful) of DIMETAPP DM Elixir contains:

| | |
|---|---|
| Brompheniramine Maleate, USP | 1 mg |
| Pseudoephedrine Hydrochloride | 15 mg |
| Dextromethorphan Hydrobromide, USP | 5 mg |

**Inactive Ingredients:** artificial flavor, citric acid, FD&C blue no. 1, FD&C red no. 40, glycerin, high fructose corn syrup, propylene glycol, saccharin sodium, sodium benzoate, sorbitol, water

**Uses:**
- temporarily relieves cough due to minor throat and bronchial irritation occurring with a cold, and nasal conges-

tion due to the common cold, hay fever or other upper respiratory allergies, or associated with sinusitis
- temporarily relieves these symptoms due to hay fever (allergic rhinitis):
  - runny nose
  - sneezing
  - itchy, watery eyes
  - itching of the nose or throat
  - temporarily restores freer breathing through the nose

**Warnings:**
**Do not use** if you are now taking a prescription monoamine oxidase inhibitor (MAOI) (certain drugs for depression, psychiatric, or emotional conditions, or Parkinson's disease), or for 2 weeks after stopping the MAOI drug. If you do not know if your prescription drug contains an MAOI, ask a doctor or pharmacist before taking this product.

**Ask a doctor before use if you have**
- heart disease
- high blood pressure
- thyroid disease
- diabetes
- trouble urinating due to an enlarged prostate gland
- glaucoma
- cough that occurs with too much phlegm (mucus)
- a breathing problem or persistent or chronic cough that lasts or as occurs with smoking, asthma, chronic bronchitis, or emphysema

**Ask a doctor or pharmacist before use if you are** taking sedatives or tranquilizers.

**When using this product**
- **do not use more than directed**
- marked drowsiness may occur
- avoid alcoholic beverages
- alcohol, sedatives, and tranquilizers may increase drowsiness
- be careful when driving a motor vehicle or operating machinery
- excitability may occur, especially in children

**Stop use and ask a doctor if**
- you get nervous, dizzy, or sleepless
- symptoms do not get better within 7 days or are accompanied by fever
- cough lasts more than 7 days, comes back, or is accompanied by fever, rash, or persistent headache. These could be signs of a serious condition

**If pregnant or breast-feeding,** ask a health professional before use.

**Keep out of reach of children.** In case of overdose, get medical help or contact a Poison Control Center right away.

**Directions:**
- do not take more than 4 doses in any 24-hour period

| Age | Dose |
|---|---|
| adults and children 12 years and over | 4 tsp every 4 hours |
| children 6 to under 12 years | 2 tsp every 4 hours |
| children under 6 years | ask a doctor |

Store at Controlled Room Temperature, Between 20°C and 25°C (68°F and 77°F)

---

**How Supplied (DIMETAPP DM ELIXIR):** Red, grape-flavored liquid in bottles of 4 fl oz, 8 fl oz and 12 fl oz. Not a USP Elixir. Dosage cup provided.

---

### DIMETAPP®
### Infant Drops Decongestant Plus Cough
**Nasal decongestant/cough suppressant**
**Alcohol-Free/non-staining**

**Active Ingredient:** Each 0.8 mL (1 dropperful) contains: 7.5 mg Pseudoephedrine Hydrochloride, USP; 2.5 mg Dextromethorphan Hydrobromide, USP.
**Inactive Ingredients:** Citric Acid, Flavors, Glycerin, High Fructose Corn Syrup, Maltol, Menthol, Polyethylene Glycol, Propylene Glycol, Sodium Benzoate, Sorbitol, Sucrose, Water.

**Indications:** Temporarily relieves cough occurring with the common cold and temporarily relieves nasal congestion due to a cold, hay fever, or other upper respiratory allergies.

**Warnings:**
**Do not use** in a child who is taking a prescription monoamine oxidase inhibitor (MAOI) (certain drugs for depression, psychiatric, or emotional conditions, or Parkinson's disease), or for 2 weeks after stopping the MAOI drug. If you do not know if your child's prescription drug contains an MAOI, ask a doctor or pharmacist before giving this product.

**Ask a doctor before use if your child has**
- heart disease
- high blood pressure
- thyroid disease
- diabetes
- cough that occurs with too much phlegm (mucus)
- cough that lasts or is chronic such as occurs with asthma

**When using this product**
- **do not use more than directed**
- give by mouth only; not for nasal use

**Stop use and ask a doctor if**
- your child gets nervous, dizzy, or sleepless
- symptoms do not get better within 7 days or are accompanied by fever
- cough lasts more than 7 days, comes back, or is accompanied by fever, rash, or persistent headache. These could be signs of a serious condition

**Keep out of reach of children.** In case of overdose, get medical help or contact a Poison Control Center right away.

**Directions:** do not give more than 4 doses in any 24-hour period

| Age | Dose |
|---|---|
| children 2-3 years | 2 dropperfuls (1.6 mL) every 4-6 hours or as directed by a physician |
| children under 2 years | ask a doctor |

**Storage:** Store at Controlled Room Temperature, between 20°C and 25°C (68°F and 77°F).

---

**How Supplied:** Infant Drops ¼ fl oz (8mL). Oral Dropper Provided

---

### DIMETAPP®
### NIGHTTIME FLU SYRUP

**Active Ingredients:**
(in each 5 mL tsp):          **Purpose:**
Acetaminophen, USP
160 mg ......... Pain reliever/fever reducer
Brompheniramine maleate,
USP 1 mg ......................... Antihistamine
Dextromethorphan HBr,
USP 5 mg ................. Cough suppressant
Pseudoephedrine HCl,
USP 15 mg ............... Nasal decongestant

**Inactive Ingredients:** citric acid, FD&C red no. 40, flavor, glycerin, high fructose corn syrup, polyethylene glycol, povidone, saccharin sodium, sodium benzoate, sodium citrate, sorbitol, water.

**Uses:** Temporarily relieves these symptoms associated with a cold or flu: headache, sore throat, fever, muscular aches, minor aches and pains. Temporarily relieves nasal congestion, and cough due to minor throat and bronchial irritation occurring with a cold. Temporarily relieves these symptoms due to hay fever or other respiratory allergies: sneezing; itching of the nose or throat; itchy, watery eyes, runny nose. Temporarily restores freer breathing through the nose.

**Warnings:**
**Alcohol warning:** if you consume 3 or more alcoholic drinks every day, ask your doctor whether you should take acetaminophen or other pain relievers/fever reducers. Acetaminophen may cause liver damage.
**Sore throat warning:** if sore throat is severe, persists for more than two days, is accompanied or followed by fever, headache, rash, nausea, or vomiting, consult a doctor promptly.
**Do not use** if you are now taking a prescription monoamine oxidase inhibitor (MAOI) (certain drugs for depression, psychiatric, or emotional conditions, or Parkinson's disease), or for 2 weeks after stopping the MAOI drug. If you do not know if your prescription drug contains an MAOI, ask a doctor or pharmacist before taking this product. Do not use with any other product containing acetaminophen as this may lead to an overdose. Overdose requires prompt medical attention even if you do not notice any signs or symptoms.
**Ask a doctor before use if you have:**
- heart disease
- high blood pressure
- thyroid disease
- diabetes
- trouble urinating due to an enlarged prostate gland
- glaucoma
- cough that occurs with too much phlegm (mucus)
- a breathing problem or persistent or chronic cough that lasts or as occurs with smoking, asthma, chronic bronchitis, or emphysema

*Continued on next page*

## Dimetapp Nighttime Flu—Cont.

**Ask a doctor or pharmacist before use if you are taking sedatives or tranquilizers.**

**When using this product:**
- do not use more than directed
- marked drowsiness may occur
- avoid alcoholic beverages
- alcohol, sedatives, and tranquilizers may increase drowsiness
- be careful when driving a motor vehicle or operating machinery
- excitability may occur, especially in children

**Stop use and ask a doctor if:**
- you get nervous, dizzy, or sleepless
- new symptoms occur
- you need to use for more than 7 days (adults) or 5 days (children)
- symptoms do not get better, get worse, or are accompanied by fever more than 3 days
- redness or swelling is present
- cough lasts more than 7 days, comes back, or is accompanied by fever, rash, or persistent headache. These could be signs of a serious condition.

**If pregnant or breast-feeding,** ask a health professional before use. **Keep out of reach of children.** In case of overdose, get medical help or contact a Poison Control Center right away. Quick medical attention is critical for adults as well as for children, even if you do not notice any signs or symptoms.

**Directions:**
- do not use more than 4 doses in any 24-hour period
- do not exceed recommended dosage. Taking more than the recommended dose (overdose) may cause serious liver damage.

| Age | Dose |
|---|---|
| adults and children 12 years and over | 4 teaspoonfuls every 4 hours |
| children 6 to under 12 years | 2 teaspoonfuls every 4 hours |
| children under 6 years | ask a doctor |

**Other information:**
- store at 20–25°C (68–77°F) • not USP. Meets specifications when tested with a validated non-USP assay method.

**How Supplied:** 4 oz bottle with dosage cup.

---

## DIMETAPP® NON-DROWSY FLU Syrup

**Active Ingredients:**
| (in each 5 mL tsp): | Purpose: |
|---|---|

Acetaminophen, USP
160 mg ..................... Pain reliever/fever reducer
Dextromethorphan HBr, USP
5 mg ........................... Cough suppressant
Pseudoephedrine HCl, USP
15 mg ....................... Nasal decongestant

**Inactive Ingredients:** Citric acid, FD&C red no. 40, FD&C yellow no. 6, flavor, glycerin, high fructose corn syrup, polyethylene glycol, povidone, saccharin sodium, sodium benzoate, sodium citrate, sorbitol, water.

**Uses:** Temporarily relieves these symptoms associated with a cold, or flu: headache, sore throat, fever, muscular aches, minor aches and pain Temporarily relieves nasal congestion, and cough due to minor throat and bronchial irritation occurring with a cold. Temporarily restores freer breathing through the nose

**Warnings:**
**Alcohol warning:** if you consume 3 or more alcoholic drinks every day, ask your doctor whether you should take acetaminophen or other pain relievers/fever reducers. Acetaminophen may cause liver damage

**Sore throat warning:** if sore throat is severe, persists for more than two days, is accompanied or followed by fever, headache, rash, nausea, or vomiting, consult a doctor promptly

**Do not use** if you are now taking a prescription monoamine oxidase inhibitor (MAOI) (certain drugs for depression, psychiatric, or emotional conditions, or Parkinson's disease), or for 2 weeks after stopping the MAOI drug. If you do not know if your prescription drug contains an MAOI, ask a doctor or pharmacist before taking this product. Do not use with any other product containing acetaminophen as this may lead to an overdose. Overdose requires prompt medical attention even if you do not notice any signs or symptoms.

**Ask a doctor before use if you have:** heart disease, high blood pressure, thyroid disease, diabetes, trouble urinating due to an enlarged prostate gland, cough that occurs with too much phlegm (mucus), or cough that lasts or is chronic such as occurs with smoking, asthma, or emphysema

**When using this product do not use more than directed.**

**Stop use and ask a doctor if:** you get nervous, dizzy, or sleepless; new symptoms occur; you need to use for more than 7 days (adults) or 5 days (children); symptoms do not get better, get worse, or are accompanied by fever more than 3 days; redness or swelling is present; or if cough lasts more than 7 days, comes back, or is accompanied by fever, rash, or persistent headache These could be signs of a serious condition.

**If pregnant or breast-feeding,** ask a health professional before use. **Keep out of reach of children.** In case of overdose, get medical help or contact a Poison Control Center right away. Quick medical attention is critical for adults as well as for children, even if you do not notice any signs or symptoms

**Directions:**
- do not use more than 4 doses in any 24-hour period
- do not exceed recommended dosage. Taking more than the recommended dose (overdose) may cause serious liver damage.

| Age | Dose |
|---|---|
| adults and children 12 years and over | 4 tsp every 4 hours |
| children 6 to under 12 years | 2 tsp every 4 hours |
| children 2 to under 6 years | 1 tsp every 4 hours |
| children under 2 years | consult a doctor |

**Other information:**
- store at 20–25°C (68–77°F)
- not USP. Meets specifications when tested with a validated non-USP assay method

**How Supplied:** 4 oz bottle with dosage cup.

---

## DIMETAPP® Elixir
## Nasal Decongestant, Antihistamine

**Active Ingredients:**
Each 5 mL (1 teaspoonful) contains:
Brompheniramine
Maleate, USP .................................. 1 mg
Pseudoephedrine
Hydrochloride, USP ................... 15 mg

**Inactive ingredients:** Artificial Flavor, Citric Acid, FD&C Blue No. 1, FD&C Red No. 40, Glycerin, High Fructose Corn Syrup, Propylene Glycol, Saccharin Sodium, Sodium Benzoate, Sorbitol, Water

**Uses:**
- temporarily relieves nasal congestion due to the common cold, hay fever or other upper respiratory allergies, or associated with sinusitis
- temporarily relieves these symptoms due to hay fever (allergic rhinitis):
  - runny nose
  - sneezing
  - itchy, watery eyes
  - itching of the nose or throat
- temporarily restores freer breathing through the nose

**Warnings:**
**Do not use** if you are now taking a prescription monoamine oxidase inhibitor (MAOI) (certain drugs for depression, psychiatric, or emotional conditions, or Parkinson's disease), or for 2 weeks after stopping the MAOI drug. If you do not know if your prescription drug contains an MAOI, ask a doctor or pharmacist before taking this product.

**Ask a doctor before use if you have:**
- heart disease
- high blood pressure
- thyroid disease
- diabetes
- trouble urinating due to an enlarged prostate gland
- glaucoma
- a breathing problem such as emphysema or chronic bronchitis

**Ask a doctor or pharmacist before use if you are** taking sedatives or tranquilizers.

**When using this product:**
- **do not use more than directed**
- drowsiness may occur
- avoid alcoholic beverages
- alcohol, sedatives, and tranquilizers may increase drowsiness
- be careful when driving a motor vehicle or operating machinery
- excitability may occur, especially in children

**Stop use and ask a doctor if:**
- you get nervous, dizzy, or sleepless
- symptoms do not get better within 7 days or are accompanied by fever

**If pregnant or breast-feeding,** ask a health professional before use.

**Keep out of reach of children.** In case of overdose, get medical help or contact a Poison Control Center right away.

**Directions:**
- do not take more than 4 doses in any 24-hour period

| age | dose |
|---|---|
| adults and children 12 years and over | 4 tsp every 4 hours |
| children 6 to under 12 years | 2 tsp every 4 hours |
| children under 6 years | ask a doctor |

Store at Controlled Room Temperature, between 20°C and 25°C (68°F and 77°F).

**How Supplied:** Purple, grape-flavored liquid in bottles of 4 fl oz, 8 fl oz, and 12 fl oz. Not a USP elixir.

---

**PREPARATION H®**
[prep-e 'rā-shen-āch ]
**Hemorrhoidal Ointment and Cream**
**PREPARATION H®**
**Hemorrhoidal Suppositories**
**PREPARATION H®**
**Hemorrhoidal Cooling Gel**

**Description:** Preparation H is available in ointment, cream, gel, and suppository product forms. The **Ointment** contains Petrolatum 71.9%, Mineral Oil 14%, Shark Liver Oil 3% and Phenylephrine HCl 0.25%.
The **Cream** contains Petrolatum 18%, Glycerin 12%, Shark Liver Oil 3% and Phenylephrine HCl 0.25%.
The **Suppositories** contain Hard Fat 91.3% and Phenylephrine HCL 0.25%.
The **Cooling Gel** contains Phenylephrine HCl 0.25% and Witch Hazel 50%.

**Indications:** Preparation H Ointment, Cream, and Suppositories help
- relieve the local itching and discomfort associated with hemorrhoids
- temporarily shrink hemorrhoidal tissue and relieve burning
- temporarily provide a coating for relief of anorectal discomforts
- temporarily protect the inflamed, irritated anorectal surface to help make bowel movements less painful

Cooling Gel helps
- relieve the local itching and discomfort associated with hemorrhoids
- temporarily relieves irritation and burning
- temporarily shrinks hemorrhoidal tissue
- aids in protecting irritated anorectal areas

**Warnings:**
**Ask a doctor before use if you have:**
- heart disease
- high blood pressure
- thyroid disease
- diabetes
- difficulty in urination due to enlargement of the prostate gland

**Ask a doctor or pharmacist before use if you** are presently taking a prescription drug for high blood pressure or depression.

**When using this product** do not exceed the recommended daily dosage unless directed by a doctor.

**If pregnant or breast-feeding,** ask a health professional before use.

**Keep out of reach of children.** If swallowed, get medical help or contact a Poison Control Center right away.

**Cream/Cooling Gel:** For external use only. Do not put into the rectum by using fingers or any mechanical device or applicator.

**Stop use and ask a doctor if:**
- bleeding occurs
- condition worsens or does not improve within 7 days

**Ointment:** Stop use and ask a doctor if introduction of applicator into the rectum causes additional pain. For external and/or intrarectal use only.

**Suppositories:** For rectal use only.

**Dosage and Administration:**
**Ointment—**
- adults: when practical, cleanse the affected area by patting or blotting with an appropriate cleansing wipe. Gently dry by patting or blotting with a tissue or a soft cloth before applying ointment.
- when first opening the tube, puncture foil seal with top end of cap
- apply to the affected area up to 4 times daily, especially at night, in the morning or after each bowel movement
- intrarectal use:
  - remove cover from applicator, attach applicator to tube, lubricate applicator well and gently insert applicator into the rectum
  - thoroughly cleanse applicator after each use and replace cover
- also apply ointment to external area
- regular use provides continual therapy for relief of symptoms
- children under 12 years of age: ask a doctor

Tamper-Evident: Do Not Use if tube seal under cap embossed with "H" is broken or missing.

**Cream—**
- adults: when practical, cleanse the affected area by patting or blotting with an appropriate cleansing wipe. Gently dry by patting or blotting with a tissue or a soft cloth before applying cream.
- when first opening the tube, puncture foil seal with top end of cap
- apply externally or in the lower portion of the anal canal only

- apply externally to the affected area up to 4 times daily, especially at night, in the morning or after each bowel movement
- for application in the lower anal canal: remove cover from dispensing cap. Attach dispensing cap tube. Lubricate dispensing cap well, then gently insert dispensing cap partway into the anus.
- thoroughly cleanse dispensing cap after each use and replace cover
- children under 12 years of age: ask a doctor

Tamper-Evident: Do Not Use if tube seal under cap embossed with "H" is broken or missing.

**Suppositories—**
- adults: when practical, cleanse the affected area by patting or blotting with an appropriate cleansing wipe. Gently dry by patting or blotting with a tissue or a soft cloth before insertion of this product.
- detach one suppository from the strip; remove wrapper before inserting into the rectum as follows:
  - as shown, hold suppository upright (with tabs labeled "pull apart" at top)
  - slowly and evenly pull tabs apart (do not tear) separating wrapper down both sides to expose the suppository
  - remove exposed suppository from wrapper
  - insert one suppository into the rectum up to 4 times daily, especially at night, in the morning or after each bowel movement
- children under 12 years of age: ask a doctor

Tamper-Evident: Individually quality sealed for your protection. Do Not Use if foil imprinted "PREPARATION H" is torn or damaged (appears on end flap).

**Cooling Gel—**
- adults: when practical, cleanse the affected area by patting or blotting with an appropriate cleansing wipe. Gently dry by patting or blotting with a tissue or a soft cloth before applying gel.
- when first opening the tube, puncture foil seal with top end of cap
- apply externally to the affected area up to 4 times daily, especially at night, in the morning or after each bowel movement
- children under 12 years of age: ask a doctor

Tamper-Evident: Do Not Use if tube seal under cap embossed with "H" is broken or missing.

**Inactive Ingredients: Ointment—** Benzoic Acid, BHA, BHT, Corn Oil, Glycerin, Lanolin, Lanolin Alcohol, Methylparaben, Paraffin, Propylparaben, Thyme Oil, Tocopherol, Water, Wax
**Cream—** BHA, Carboxymethylcellulose Sodium, Cetyl Alcohol, Citric Acid, Edetate Disodium, Glyceryl Oleate, Glyceryl Stearate, Lanolin, Methylparaben, Propyl Gallate, Propylene Glycol, Propylparaben, Simethicone, Sodium Benzoate, Sodium Lauryl Sulfate, Stearyl Alcohol, Tocopherol, Water, Xanthan Gum.
**Suppositories—** aloe extract, beta carotene, methylparaben, petrolatum, propylparaben, tocopheryl acetate (Vitamin E)
**Cooling Gel—** aloe barbadensis gel, benzophenone-4, edetate disodium, hydroxy-

*Continued on next page*

## Preparation H—Cont.

ethylcellulose, methylparaben, polysorbate 80, propylene glycol, propylparaben, sodium citrate, vitamin E, water

**How Supplied:** <u>Ointment:</u> Net Wt. 1 oz and 2 oz **Cream:** Net Wt. 0.9 oz and 1.8 oz **Suppositories:** 12's, 24's and 48's. **Cooling Gel:** Net Wt. 0.9 oz and 1.8 oz

**Storage:** Store at 20–25°C (68–77°F).

---

## PREPARATION H HYDROCORTISONE CREAM
### Anti-itch cream

**Active ingredient:** **Purpose:**
Hydrocortisone 1% ..................... Anti-itch

**Inactive Ingredients:** BHA, carboxymethylcellulose sodium, cetyl alcohol, citric acid, edetate disodium, glycerin, glyceryl oleate, glyceryl stearate, lanolin, methylparaben, petrolatum, propyl gallate, propylene glycol, propylparaben, simethicone, sodium benzoate, sodium lauryl sulfate, stearyl alcohol, water, xanthan gum.

**Uses:**
- temporary relief of external anal itching
- temporary relief of itching associated with minor skin irritations and rashes
- other uses of this product should be only under the advice and supervision of a doctor

**Warnings:**
**For external use only**
**Do not use** for the treatment of diaper rash. Consult a doctor.
**When using this product:**
- avoid contact with the eyes
- do not exceed the recommended daily dosage unless directed by a doctor
- do not put into the rectum by using fingers or any mechanical device or applicator

**Stop use and ask a doctor if**
- bleeding occurs
- condition worsens
- symptoms persist for more than 7 days or clear up and occur again within a few days. Do not begin use of this or any other hydrocortisone product unless you have consulted a doctor.
**Keep out of reach of children.** If swallowed, get medical help or contact a Poison Control Center right away.

**Directions:**
- adults: when practical, cleanse the affected area by patting or blotting with an appropriate cleansing wipe. Gently dry by patting or blotting with a tissue or soft cloth before application of this product.
- when first opening the tube, puncture foil seal with top end of cap
- adults and children 12 years of age and older: apply to the affected area not more than 3 to 4 times daily
- children under 12 years of age: do not use, consult a doctor

**How Supplied:** 0.9 oz. tubes
*Storage:* Store at 20–25 °C (68–77 °F)

---

## PREPARATION H®
## MEDICATED WIPES

**Uses:**
- helps relieve the local itching and discomfort associated with hemorrhoids
- temporary relief of irritation and burning
- aids in protecting irritated anorectal areas
- **for vaginal care**—cleanse the area by gently wiping, patting or blotting. Repeat as needed.
- **for use as a moist compress**—if necessary, first cleanse the area as previously described. Fold wipe to desired size and place in contact with tissue for a soothing and cooling effect. Leave in place for up to 15 minutes and repeat as needed.

**Active Ingredients:** Soft pads are pre-moistened with a solution containing Witch Hazel 50%.

**Inactive ingredients:** Aloe barbadensis gel, capryl/capramidopropyl betaine, citric acid, diazolidinyl urea, glycerin, methylparaben, propylene glycol, propylparaben, sodium citrate, water.

**Directions:**
- remove tab on right side of wipes pouch label and peel back to open
- grab the top wipe at the edge of the center fold and pull out of pouch
- carefully reseal label on pouch after each use to retain moistness
- adults: unfold wipe and cleanse the area by gently wiping, patting or blotting. If necessary, repeat until all matter is removed from the area.
- use up to 6 times daily or after each bowel movement and before applying topical hemorrhoidal treatments
- children under 12 years of age: consult a doctor

**Warnings:**
**For external use only**
**When using this product**
- do not exceed the recommended daily dosage unless directed by a doctor
- do not put this product into the rectum by using fingers or any mechanical device or applicator

**Stop use and ask a doctor if**
- bleeding occurs
- condition worsens or does not improve within 7 days
**If pregnant or breast-feeding,** ask a health professional before use. **Keep out of reach of children.** If swallowed, get medical help or contact a Poison Control Center right away.
- store at 20–25°C (68–77°F)
- for best results, flush only one or two wipes at a time

**How Supplied:** Containers of 48 wipes. Refills of 48 wipes.

---

## PRIMATENE®
[*prīm 'a-tēn* ]
### Mist
**(Epinephrine Inhalation Aerosol Bronchodilator)**

**Active Ingredient:**
*(in each inhalation)*
Epinephrine ................................. 0.22 mg

**Indications:** For temporary relief of shortness of breath, tightness of chest, and wheezing due to bronchial asthma. Eases breathing for asthma patients by reducing spasms of bronchial muscles.

**Directions:**
- **do not use more often or at higher doses unless directed by a doctor**
- supervise children using this product
- adults and children 4 years and over: start with one inhalation, then wait at least 1 minute. If not relieved, use once more. Do not use again for at least 3 hours.
- children under 4 years of age: ask a doctor

**Warnings:**
**For inhalation only**
**Do not use**
- unless a doctor has said you have asthma
- if you are now taking a prescription monoamine oxidase inhibitor (MAOI) (certain drugs for depression, psychiatric, or emotional conditions, or Parkinson's disease), or for 2 weeks after stopping the MAOI drug If you do not know if your prescription drug contains an MAOI, ask a doctor or pharmacist before taking this product
**Ask a doctor before use if you have**
- heart disease
- thyroid disease
- diabetes
- high blood pressure
- ever been hospitalized for asthma
- trouble urinating due to an enlarged prostate gland
**Ask a doctor or pharmacist before use if you are** taking any prescription drug for asthma
**When using this product:**
- overuse may cause nervousness, rapid heart beat, and heart problems
- **do not continue to use, but seek medical assistance immediately if symptoms are not relieved within 20 minutes or become worse**
- do not puncture or throw into incinerator. Contents under pressure.
- do not use or store near open flame or heat above 120°F (49°C). May cause bursting.
**Contains CFC 12, 114,** substances which harm public health and environment by destroying ozone in the upper atmosphere.
**If pregnant or breast-feeding,** ask a health professional before use.
Keep out of reach of children. In case of overdose, get medical help or contact a Poison Control Center right away.

**Directions For Use of Mouthpiece:**
The Primatene Mist mouthpiece, which is enclosed in the Primatene Mist 15 mL size (not the refill size), should be used for inhalation only with Primatene Mist.
1. Take plastic cap off mouthpiece. (For refills, use mouthpiece from previous purchase.)
2. Take plastic mouthpiece off bottle.
3. Place other end of mouthpiece on bottle.
4. Turn bottle upside down. Place thumb on bottom of mouthpiece over circular button and forefinger on top of vial. Empty the lungs as completely as possible by exhaling.
5. Place mouthpiece in mouth with lips closed around opening. Inhale deeply

while squeezing mouthpiece and bottle together. Release immediately and remove unit from mouth. Complete taking the deep breath, drawing the medication into your lungs and holding breath as long as comfortable.
6. Exhale slowly keeping lips nearly closed. This helps distribute the medication in the lungs.
7. Replace plastic cap on mouthpiece.

### Care of the Mouthpiece:
The Primatene Mist mouthpiece should be washed once daily with soap and hot water, and rinsed thoroughly. Then it should be dried with a clean, lint-free cloth.
If the unit becomes clogged and fails to spray, please send the clogged unit to:
Whitehall Laboratories
5 Giralda Farms
Madison, N.J. 07940

**Inactive Ingredients:** Alcohol 34%, Ascorbic Acid, Fluorocarbons (Propellant), Water. Contains No Sulfites.
**Storage:** Store at room temperature, between 20–25°C (68–77°F).

### How Supplied:
$^1/_2$ Fl oz (15 mL) With Mouthpiece.
$^1/_2$ Fl oz (15 mL) Refill
$^3/_4$ Fl oz (22.5 mL) Refill
*Questions or comments?* Call weekdays from 9 AM to 5 PM EST at 1-8PRIMATENE (1-877-462-8363)
www.Primatene.com

---

### PRIMATENE®
[prīm 'a-tēn ]
**Tablets**

### Active Ingredients:
*(in each tablet)*
Ephedrine HCl, USP .................. 12.5 mg
Guaifenesin ..................................... 200 mg

**Indications:** For temporary relief of shortness of breath, tightness of chest, and wheezing due to bronchial asthma. Eases breathing for asthma patients by reducing spasms of bronchial muscles. Helps loosen phlegm (mucus) and thin bronchial secretions to rid bronchial passageways of bothersome mucus, and to make coughs more productive.

### Directions:
• do not use more than dosage below unless directed by a doctor
• adults and children 12 years and over: take 2 tablets initially, then 2 tablets every 4 hours, as needed, not to exceed 12 tablets in 24 hours
• children under 12 years: ask a doctor

### Warnings:
**Do not use**
• unless a diagnosis of asthma has been made by a doctor
• if you are now taking a prescription monoamine oxidase inhibitor (MAOI) (certain drugs for depression, psychiatric, or emotional conditions, or Parkinson's disease), or for 2 weeks after stopping the MAOI drug  If you do not know if your prescription drug contains an MAOI, ask a doctor or pharmacist before taking this product

**Ask a doctor before use if you have**
• heart disease
• high blood pressure
• thyroid disease
• diabetes
• trouble urinating due to an enlarged prostate gland
• ever been hospitalized for asthma
• cough that occurs with too much phlegm (mucus)
• cough that lasts or is chronic such as occurs with smoking, asthma, chronic bronchitis, or emphysema

**Ask a doctor or pharmacist before use if you are** taking any prescription drug for asthma

**When using this product** some users may experience nervousness, tremor, sleeplessness, nausea, and loss of appetite

**Stop use and ask a doctor if**
• symptoms are not relieved within 1 hour or become worse
• nervousness, tremor, sleeplessness, nausea, and loss of appetite persist or become worse
• cough lasts more than 7 days, comes back, or occurs with fever, rash, or persistent headache  These could be signs of a serious condition

**If pregnant or breast-feeding,** ask a health professional before use

**Keep out of reach of children.** In case of overdose, get medical help or contact a Poison Control Center right away.

**Inactive ingredients:** crospovidone, D&C yellow No. 10 aluminum lake, FD&C yellow No. 6 aluminum lake, magnesium stearate, microcrystalline cellulose, povidone, silicon dioxide (colloidal)
**Storage:**  store at 20–25°C (68–77°F)

**How Supplied:**  Available in 24 and 60 tablet thermoform blister cartons.
*Questions or comments?* Call weekdays from 9 AM to 5 PM EST at 1-8PRIMATENE (1-877-462-8363)
www.Primatene.com

---

### ROBITUSSIN® COLD
### COLD & CONGESTION
### SOFTGELS, CAPLETS
[ro "bĭ-tuss 'in ]
**Nasal Decongestant, Expectorant, Cough Suppressant**

### Active Ingredients
**(in each softgel, caplet):**
Dextromethorphan HBr,
USP ...................................... 10 mg
Guaifenesin, USP ........................ 200 mg
Pseudoephedrine HCl,
USP ...................................... 30 mg

**Inactive    Ingredients:    Softgels:** FD&C Blue No. 1, FD&C Red No. 40, Gelatin, Glycerin, Mannitol, Pharmaceutical Glaze, Polyethylene Glycol, Povidone, Propylene Glycol, Sorbitan, Sorbitol, Titanium Dioxide, Water.

**Inactive Ingredients, Caplets:**  Calcium Stearate, Croscarmellose Sodium, FD&C Red No. 40 Aluminum Lake, Hydroxypropyl Methylcellulose, Maltodextrin, Microcrystalline Cellulose, Polydextrose, Polyethylene Glycol, Povidone, Pregelatinized Starch, Silicon Dioxide, Stearic Acid, Titanium Dioxide, Triacetin.

### Indications:
• temporarily relieves nasal congestion, and cough due to minor throat and bronchial irritation occurring with the common cold
• helps loosen phlegm (mucus) and thin bronchial secretions to make coughs more productive
• temporarily relieves nasal congestion associated with hay fever or other upper respiratory allergies, or associated with sinusitis

### Warnings:
**Do not use** if you are now taking a prescription monoamine oxidase inhibitor (MAOI) (certain drugs for depression, psychiatric, or emotional conditions, or Parkinson's disease), or for 2 weeks after stopping the MAOI drug. If you do not know if your prescription drug contains an MAOI, ask a doctor or pharmacist before taking this product.

**Ask a doctor before use if you have:**
• heart disease
• high blood pressure
• thyroid disease
• diabetes
• trouble urinating due to an enlarged prostate gland
• cough that occurs with too much phlegm (mucus)
• cough that lasts or is chronic such as occurs with smoking, asthma, chronic bronchitis, or emphysema

**When using this product do not use more than directed.**

**Stop use and ask a doctor if:**
• you get nervous, dizzy, or sleepless
• symptoms do not get better within 7 days or are accompanied by fever
• cough lasts more than 7 days, comes back, or is accompanied by fever, rash, or persistent headache. These could be signs of a serious condition.

**If pregnant or breast-feeding,** ask a health professional before use.

**Keep out of reach of children.** In case of overdose, get medical help or contact a Poison Control Center right away.

**Directions:**  Follow dosage below: Do Not Exceed 4 Doses in any 24-Hour Period. Adults and children 12 years of age and over: 2 softgels or caplets every 4 hours. Children 6 to under 12 years: 1 softgel or caplet every 4 hours. Children under 6: Ask a doctor.

**How Supplied:**  Softgels in consumer packages of 12 and 20 (individually packaged). Red caplets imprinted CC in consumer packages of 20 (individually packaged).

**Storage:**  Store at Controlled Room Temperature, between 20°C and 25°C (68°F and 77°F)

*Continued on next page*

## ROBITUSSIN® COLD MULTI-SYMPTOM COLD & FLU SOFTGELS, CAPLETS

[ro "bĭ-tuss 'ĭn ]

**Pain Reliever, Fever Reducer, Cough Suppressant, Nasal Decongestant, Expectorant**

**Active Ingredients Softgels:**
Acetaminophen, USP ................... 250 mg
Guaifenesin, USP ......................... 100 mg
Pseudoephedrine HCL, USP ........ 30 mg
Dextromethorphan HBr, USP ..... 10 mg

**Active Ingredients Caplets:**
Acetaminophen, USP ................... 325 mg
Guaifenesin, USP ......................... 200 mg
Pseudoephedrine HCL, USP ........ 30 mg
Dextromethorphan HBr, USP ..... 10 mg

**Inactive Ingredients Softgels:** D&C Yellow No. 10, FD&C Red No. 40, Gelatin, Glycerin, Iron Oxides, Lecithin, Mannitol, Pharmaceutical Glaze, Polyethylene Glycol, Povidone, Propylene Glycol, Simethicone, Sorbitan, Sorbitol, Water.

**Inactive Ingredients Caplets:** Calcium Stearate, Croscarmellose Sodium, D&C Yellow No. 10 Aluminum Lake, FD&C Yellow No. 6 Aluminum Lake, Hydroxypropyl Methylcellulose, Maltodextrin, Microcrystalline Cellulose, Polydextrose, Polyethylene Glycol, Povidone, Pregelatinized Starch, Silicon Dioxide, Stearic Acid, Titanium Dioxide, Triacetin.

**Indications:** For the temporary relief of minor aches and pains, headache, muscular aches and sore throat associated with cold or flu, and to reduce fever. Temporarily relieves cough due to minor throat and bronchial irritation and nasal congestion as may occur with a cold. Helps loosen phlegm (mucus) and thin bronchial secretions to make coughs more productive.

**Warnings:**
**Alcohol warning:** if you consume 3 or more alcoholic drinks every day, ask your doctor whether you should take acetaminophen or other pain relievers/fever reducers. Acetaminophen may cause liver damage.
**Sore throat warning:** if sore threat is severe, persists for more than two days, is accompanied or followed by fever, headache, rash, nausea, or vomiting, consult a doctor promptly.
**Do not use**
• if you are now taking a prescription monoamine oxidase inhibitor (MAOI) (certain drugs for depression, psychiatric, or emotional conditions, or Parkinson's disease), or for 2 weeks after stopping the MAOI drug. If you do not know if your prescription drug contains an MAOI, ask a doctor or pharmacist before taking this product.
• with any other product containing acetaminophen as this may lead to an overdose. Overdose requires prompt medical attention even if you do not notice any signs or symptoms.
**Ask a doctor before use if you have:**
• heart disease
• high blood pressure

• thyroid disease
• diabetes
• trouble urinating due to an enlarged prostate gland
• cough that occurs with too much phlegm (mucus)
• cough that lasts or is chronic such as occurs with smoking, asthma, chronic bronchitis, or emphysema
**When using this product do not use more than directed.**
**Stop use and ask a doctor if:**
• you get nervous, dizzy, or sleepless
• new symptoms occur
• you need to use for more than 7 days (adults) or 5 days (children)
• symptoms do not get better, get worse, or are accompanied by fever more than 3 days
• redness or swelling is present
• cough lasts more than 7 days, comes back, or is accompanied by fever, rash, or persistent headache. These could be signs of a serious condition.
**If pregnant or breast-feeding,** ask a health professional before use.
**Keep out of reach of children.** In case of overdose, get medical help or contact a Poison Control Center right away. Prompt medical attention is critical for adults as well as for children, even if you do not notice any signs or symptoms.

**Directions:** Multi-Symptom Cold & Flu **Softgels:** Follow dosage below:
• do not use more than 4 doses in any 24-hour period
• do not exceed recommended dosage. Taking more than the recommended dose (overdose) may cause serious liver damage.

| age | dose |
| --- | --- |
| adults and children 12 years and over | 2 softgels every 4 hours |
| children under 12 years | ask a doctor |

**Directions:** Multi-Symptom Cold & Flu **Caplets:** Follow dosage below:
• do not use more than 4 doses in any 24-hour period
• do not exceed recommended dosage. Taking more than the recommended dose (overdose) may cause serious liver damage.

| age | dose |
| --- | --- |
| adults and children 12 years and over | 2 caplets every 4 hours |
| children 6 to under 12 years | 1 caplet every 4 hours |
| children under 6 years | ask a doctor |

**How Supplied:** Blister Packs of 12's and 20's.

**Storage:** Store at Controlled Room Temperature, between 20°C and 25°C (68°F and 77°F).

## ROBITUSSIN® COUGH DROPS

[ro "bĭ-tuss 'ĭn]

**Menthol Eucalyptus, Cherry, and Honey-Lemon Flavors**

**Active Ingredient:**

| (in each drop) | Purposes: |
| --- | --- |

*Menthol Eucalyptus:*
Menthol, USP ................................ 10 mg
*Cherry and Honey-Lemon:*
Menthol, USP ................................ 5 mg

**Inactive Ingredients:**
*Menthol Eucalyptus:* Corn Syrup, Eucalyptus Oil, Flavor, Sucrose.
*Cherry:* Corn Syrup, FD&C Red #40, Flavor, Methylparaben, Propylparaben, Sodium Benzoate, Sucrose.
*Honey-Lemon:* Citric Acid, Corn Syrup, D&C Yellow #10, FD&C Yellow #6, Honey, Lemon Oil, Methylparaben, Povidone, Propylparaben, Sodium Benzoate, Sucrose.

**Uses:**
• temporarily relieves
  • occasional minor irritation, pain, sore mouth, and sore throat
  • cough associated with a cold or inhaled irritants

**Warnings:**
**Sore throat warning:** severe or persistent sore throat or sore throat accompanied by high fever, headache, nausea, and vomiting may be serious. Consult a doctor right away. Do not use more than 2 days or give to children under 3 years of age unless directed by a doctor
**Ask a doctor before use if you have**
• cough that occurs with too much phlegm (mucus)
• cough that lasts or is chronic such as occurs with smoking, asthma, or emphysema
**Stop use and ask a doctor if**
• cough lasts more than 7 days, comes back, or is accompanied by fever, rash, or persistent headache. These could be signs of a serious condition.
**If pregnant or breast-feeding,** ask a health professional before use.
**Keep out of reach of children.**

**Directions:**
• adults and children 4 years and over: allow 1 drop to dissolve slowly in the mouth
  • for sore throat: may be repeated every 2 hours, as needed, or as directed by a doctor
  • for cough: may be repeated every hour, as needed, or as directed by a doctor
• children under 4 years of age: ask a doctor
**Storage:** Store at 20–25°C (68–77°F).

**How Supplied:** All 3 flavors of Robitussin Cough Drops are available in bags of 25 drops.

---

## ROBITUSSIN® COLD SEVERE CONGESTION SOFTGELS

[ro "bĭ-tuss 'ĭn ]

**Nasal Decongestant, Expectorant**

**Active Ingredients:**
Each Robitussin Severe Congestion Softgel contains:

Guaifenesin, USP ...................... 200 mg
Pseudoephedrine Hydrochloride,
USP ............................................. 30 mg

**Inactive Ingredients:** FD&C Green No. 3, Gelatin, Glycerin, Mannitol, Pharmaceutical Glaze, Polyethylene Glycol, Povidone, Propylene Glycol, Sorbitan, Sorbitol, Titanium Dioxide, Water.

**Indications:** For the temporary relief of nasal congestion due to the common cold, hay fever or other upper respiratory allergies, or associated with sinusitis. Helps loosen phlegm (mucus) and thin bronchial secretions to make coughs more productive.

**Warnings:**

**Do not use** if you are now taking a prescription monoamine oxidase inhibitor (MAOI) (certain drugs for depression, psychiatric, or emotional conditions, or Parkinson's disease), or for 2 weeks after stopping the MAOI drug. If you do not know if your prescription drug contains an MAOI, ask a doctor or pharmacist before taking this product.

**Ask a doctor before use if you have:**
- heart disease
- high blood pressure
- thyroid disease
- diabetes
- trouble urinating due to an enlarged prostate gland
- cough that occurs with too much phlegm (mucus)
- cough that lasts or is chronic such as occurs with smoking, asthma, chronic bronchitis, or emphysema

**When using this product**
- do not use more than directed.

**Stop use and ask a doctor if:**
- you get nervous, dizzy, or sleepless
- symptoms do not get better within 7 days or are accompanied by fever
- cough lasts more than 7 days, comes back, or is accompanied by fever, rash, or persistent headache. These could be signs of a serious condition.

**If pregnant or breast-feeding,** ask a health professional before use.

**Keep out of reach of children.** In case of overdose, get medical help or contact a Poison Control Center right away.

**Directions:** Do Not Exceed 4 Doses in any 24-Hour Period. Adults and children 12 years of age and over: 2 softgels every 4 hours. Children 6 to under 12 years: 1 softgel every 4 hours. Children under 6, ask a doctor.

**How Supplied:** Blister Packs of 12's and 20's.

**Storage:** Store at 20–25°C (68°F and 77°F).

---

## ROBITUSSIN COUGH & COLD INFANT DROPS
[ro "bĭ-tuss 'ĭn ]
**Nasal Decongestant, Cough Suppressant, Expectorant**
**Alcohol-Free Cough & Cold Formula**

**Active Ingredients:**
Each half teaspoonful (2.5 mL) contains:

Guaifenesin, USP ........................ 100 mg
Pseudoephedrine HCl, USP ......... 15 mg
Dextromethorphan HBr, USP ........ 5 mg

**Inactive Ingredients:** Citric Acid, FD&C Red No. 40, Flavors, Glycerin, High Fructose Corn Syrup, Maltitol, Maltol, Polyethylene Glycol, Povidone, Propylene Glycol, Saccharin Sodium, Sodium Benzoate, Sodium Citrate, Water.

**Indications:** Temporarily relieves cough due to minor throat and bronchial irritation, and nasal congestion due to a cold. Helps loosen phlegm (mucus) and thin bronchial secretions to make coughs more productive.

**Warnings:**

**Do not use** in a child who is taking a prescription monoamine oxidase inhibitor (MAOI) (certain drugs for depression, psychiatric, or emotional conditions, or Parkinson's disease), or for 2 weeks after stopping the MAOI drug. If you do not know if your child's prescription drug contains an MAOI, ask a doctor or pharmacist before giving this product.

**Ask a doctor before use if your child has:**
- heart disease
- high blood pressure
- thyroid disease
- diabetes
- cough that occurs with too much phlegm (mucus)
- cough that lasts or is chronic such as occurs with asthma

**When using this product do not use more than directed.**

**Stop use and ask a doctor if:**
- your child gets nervous, dizzy, or sleepless
- symptoms do not get better within 7 days or are accompanied by fever
- cough lasts more than 7 days, comes back, or is accompanied by fever, rash, or persistent headache. These could be signs of a serious condition.

**Keep out of reach of children.** In case of overdose, get medical help or contact a Poison Control Center right away.

**Directions:** Follow dosage below. Oral dosing syringe provided. Do not use more than 4 doses in any 24-Hour Period. Repeat every 4 hours.

**Dosage:** Choose dosage by weight. (If weight is not known, choose by age). Measure with the dosing device provided. Do not use with any other device.

| Age | Weight | Dose |
|---|---|---|
| Under 2 yrs. | Under 24 lbs. | Consult doctor |
| 2 to under 6 yrs. | 24–47 lbs. | 2.5 mL |

**How Supplied:** 1 fluid oz bottle with dosing syringe.

**Storage:** Store at 20°C–25°C (68°F and 77°F).

---

## ROBITUSSIN® SINUS & CONGESTION CAPLETS
**Pain Reliever/Fever Reducer, Nasal Decongestant, Expectorant**

**Active Ingredients (in each caplet):**
Acetaminophen, USP ................... 325 mg
Guaifenesin, USP ........................ 200 mg
Pseudoephedrine
hydrochloride, USP ................... 30 mg

**Inactive ingredients:** calcium stearate, croscarmellose sodium, FD&C blue no. 2 aluminum lake, hydroxypropyl methylcellulose, lactose, microcrystalline cellulose, povidone, pregelatinized starch, silicon dioxide, stearic acid, titanium dioxide, triacetin.

**Indications:**
- temporarily relieves these symptoms associated with a cold, or flu:
  - headache
  - sore throat
  - fever
  - muscular aches
  - minor aches and pains
- temporarily relieves nasal congestion occurring with a cold
- helps loosen phlegm (mucus) and thin bronchial secretions to make coughs more productive

**Warnings:**

**Alcohol warning:** If you consume 3 or more alcoholic drinks every day, ask your doctor whether you should take acetaminophen or other pain relievers/fever reducers. Acetaminophen may cause liver damage.

**Sore throat warning:** If sore throat is severe, persists for more than 2 days, is accompanied or followed by fever, headache, rash, nausea, or vomiting, consult a doctor promptly.

**Do not use:**
- if you are now taking a prescription monoamine oxidase inhibitor (MAOI) (certain drugs for depression, psychiatric, or emotional conditions, or Parkinson's disease), or for 2 weeks after stopping the MAOI drug. If you do not know if your prescription drug contains an MAOI, ask a doctor or pharmacist before taking this product.
- with any other product containing acetaminophen as this may lead to an overdose. Overdose requires prompt medical attention even if you do not notice any signs or symptoms.

**Ask a doctor before use if you have:**
- heart disease
- high blood pressure
- thyroid disease
- diabetes
- trouble urinating due to an enlarged prostate gland
- cough that occurs with too much phlegm (mucus)
- cough that lasts or is chronic such as occurs with smoking, asthma, chronic bronchitis, or emphysema

**When using this product do not use more than directed.**

**Stop use and ask a doctor if**
- you get nervous, dizzy, or sleepless
- new symptoms occur

*Continued on next page*

## Robitussin Sinus/Cong.—Cont.

- you need to use for more than 7 days (adults) or 5 days (children)
- symptoms do not get better, get worse, or are accompanied by fever more than 3 days
- redness or swelling is present
- cough lasts more than 7 days, comes back, or is accompanied by fever, rash, or persistent headache. These could be signs of a serious condition.

**If pregnant or breast-feeding,** ask a health professional before use.

**Keep out of reach of children.** In case of overdose, get medical help or contact a Poison Control Center right away. Prompt medical attention is critical for adults as well as for children, even if you do not notice any signs or symptoms.

**Directions:**
- do not use more than 4 doses in any 24-hour period
- do not exceed recommended dosage. Taking more than the recommended dose (overdose) may cause serious liver damage.

| age | dose |
| --- | --- |
| adults and children 12 years and over | 2 caplets every 4 hours |
| children 6 to under 12 years | 1 caplet every 4 hours |
| children under 6 years | ask a doctor |

**How Supplied: Packages of 12 and 24**
**Storage:** Store at 20–25°C (68–77°F)

## ROBITUSSIN®
[ro "bĭ-tuss 'ĭn ]
**Alcohol-Free Cough Formula**
**Expectorant**

**Active Ingredients:** Each teaspoonful (5 mL) contains:
Guaifenesin, USP ...................... 100 mg

**Inactive Ingredients:** Caramel, Citric Acid, FD&C Red No. 40, Flavors, Glucose, Glycerin, High Fructose Corn Syrup, Menthol, Saccharin Sodium, Sodium Benzoate, Water.

**Indications:** Helps loosen phlegm (mucus) and thin bronchial secretions to make coughs more productive.

**Warnings:**
**Ask a doctor before use if you have**
- cough that occurs with too much phlegm (mucus)
- cough that lasts or is chronic such as occurs with smoking, asthma, chronic bronchitis, or emphysema

Stop use and ask a doctor if cough lasts more than 7 days, comes back, or is accompanied by fever, rash, or persistent headache. These could be signs of a serious condition.

If pregnant or breast-feeding, ask a health professional before use.

Keep out of reach of children. In case of overdose, get medical help or contact a Poison Control Center right away.

**Directions:** Follow dosage below. Dosage cup provided (except for the 16 oz size).
Do not take more than 6 doses in any 24-hour period.
**ADULT DOSE** (and children 12 years and over): 2–4 teaspoonfuls every 4 hrs.
**CHILD DOSE**
**6 yrs. to under 12 yrs.** 1–2 teaspoonfuls every 4 hrs.
**2 yrs. to under 6 yrs.** 1/2–1 teaspoonful every 4 hrs.
**Under 2:** ask a doctor.

**How Supplied:** Robitussin (wine-colored) in bottles of 4 fl oz, 8 fl oz, 16 fl oz. Store at 20°C–25°C (68°F and 77°F).

## ROBITUSSIN® ALLERGY & COUGH

**Active Ingredients**
**(in each 5 mL tsp)**      **Purpose:**
Brompheniramine maleate,
USP 2 mg ...................... Antihistamine
Dextromethorphan HBr,
USP 10 mg ........... Cough suppressant
Pseudoephedrine HCl,
USP 30 mg ........... Nasal decongestant

**Uses:**
- temporarily relieves these symptoms due to hay fever (allergic rhinitis):
- runny nose
- sneezing
- itchy, watery eyes
- itching of the nose or throat
- nasal congestion
- temporarily controls cough due to minor throat and bronchial irritation associated with inhaled irritants
- temporarily restores freer breathing through the nose

**Warnings:**
**Do not use** if you are now taking a prescription monoamine oxidase inhibitor (MAOI) (certain drugs for depression, psychiatric, or emotional conditions, or Parkinson's disease), or for 2 weeks after stopping the MAOI drug. If you do not know if your prescription drug contains an MAOI, ask a doctor or pharmacist before taking this product.

**Ask a doctor before use if you have:**
- heart disease
- high blood pressure
- thyroid disease
- diabetes
- trouble urinating due to an enlarged prostate gland
- glaucoma
- cough that occurs with too much phlegm (mucus)
- cough that lasts or is chronic such as occurs with smoking, asthma, chronic bronchitis or emphysema

**Ask a doctor or pharmacist before use if you are** taking sedatives or tranquilizers.

**When using this product:**
- **do not use more than directed**
- marked drowsiness may occur
- avoid alcoholic beverages
- alcohol, sedatives, and tranquilizers may increase drowsiness

- be careful when driving a motor vehicle or operating machinery
- excitability may occur, especially in children

**Stop use and ask a doctor if**
- you get nervous, dizzy, or sleepless
- symptoms do not get better within 7 days or are accompanied by fever
- cough lasts more than 7 days, comes back, or is accompanied by fever, rash, or persistent headache. These could be signs of a serious condition.

**If pregnant or breast-feeding,** ask a health professional before use.

**Keep out of reach of children.** In case of overdose, get medical help or contact a Poison Control Center right away.

**Directions:**
- do not take more than 4 doses in any 24-hour period

| age | dose |
| --- | --- |
| adults and children 12 years and over | 2 teaspoonfuls every 4 hours |
| children 6 years to under 12 years | 1 teaspoonful every 4 hours |
| under 6 years | ask a doctor |

**Inactive Ingredients:** Artificial flavor, citric acid, glycerin, propylene glycol, saccharin sodium, sodium benzoate, sorbitol, water

**Other Information:**
- store at 20–25°C (68–77°F)
- alcohol free
- dosage cup provided

**How Supplied:** Bottles of 4 fl. oz.

## ROBITUSSIN®–CF
[ro "bĭ-tuss 'ĭn ]
**Alcohol-Free Cough Formula**
**Nasal Decongestant, Cough**
**Suppressant, Expectorant**

**Active Ingredients:** Each teaspoonful (5 mL) contains:
Guaifenesin, USP ...................... 100 mg
Pseudoephedrine
Hydrochloride, USP ............... 30 mg
Dextromethorphan
Hydrobromide, USP ............... 10 mg

**Inactive Ingredients:** Citric Acid, FD&C Red No. 40, Flavors, Glycerin, Propylene Glycol, Saccharin Sodium, Sodium Benzoate, Sorbitol, Water.

**Indications:** Temporarily relieves cough due to minor throat and bronchial irritation and nasal congestion as may occur with a cold. Helps loosen phlegm (mucus) and thin bronchial secretions to make coughs more productive.

**Warnings:**

**Do not use** if you are now taking a prescription monoamine oxidase inhibitor (MAOI) (certain drugs for depression, psychiatric, or emotional conditions, or Parkinson's disease), or for 2 weeks after stopping the MAOI drug. If you do not know if your prescription drug contains an MAOI, ask a doctor or pharmacist before taking this product.

**Ask a doctor before use if you have**
- heart disease
- high blood pressure
- thyroid disease
- diabetes
- trouble urinating due to an enlarged prostate gland
- cough that occurs with too much phlegm (mucus)
- cough that lasts or is chronic such as occurs with smoking, asthma, chronic bronchitis or emphysema

**When using this product do not use more than directed.**

**Stop use and ask a doctor if**
- you get nervous, dizzy, or sleepless
- symptoms do not get better within 7 days or are accompanied by fever
- cough lasts more than 7 days, comes back, or is accompanied by fever, rash, or persistent headache. These could be signs of a serious condition.

**If pregnant or breast-feeding,** ask a health professional before use.

**Keep out of reach of children.** In case of overdose, get medical help or contact a Poison Control Center right away.

**Directions:** Follow dosage below. Dosage cup provided. Do not take more than 4 doses in any 24-hour period.
**ADULT DOSE** (and children 12 years and over): 2 teaspoonfuls every 4 hrs.
**CHILD DOSE**
**6 yrs. to under 12 yrs.**
1 teaspoonful every 4 hrs.
**2 yrs. to under 6 yrs.**
$1/_2$ teaspoonful every 4 hrs.
**Under 2: Ask a doctor.**

**How Supplied:** Robitussin-CF (red-colored) in bottles of 4 fl oz, 8 fl oz, and 12 fl oz.
Store at 20°C–25°C (68°F and 77°F).

---

## ROBITUSSIN®-DM
## ROBITUSSIN DM INFANT DROPS
[ro "bĭ-tuss 'ĭn ]
**Cough suppressant, Expectorant Alcohol-Free Cough Formula**

**Active Ingredients:** Each teaspoonful of **Robitussin DM** (5 mL) contains:
Dextromethorphan Hydrobromide, USP ........................................... 10 mg
Guaifenesin, USP ....................... 100 mg

**Inactive Ingredients (Robitussin DM):** Citric Acid, FD&C Red No. 40, Flavors, Glucose, Glycerin, High Fructose Corn Syrup, Menthol, Saccharin Sodium, Sodium Benzoate, Water.

**Active Ingredients:**
Each 2.5 mL ($1/_2$ teaspoonful) of **Robitussin DM Infant Drops** contains:
Dextromethorphan Hydrobromide, USP ......................................... 5 mg
Guaifenesin, USP ....................... 100 mg
Alcohol-Free Cough Formula

**Inactive Ingredients (Robitussin DM Infant Drops):**

**Inactive Ingredients:** Citric Acid, FD&C Red No. 40, Flavors, Glycerin, High Fructose Corn Syrup, Maltitol, Maltol, Polyethylene Glycol, Povidone, Propylene Glycol, Saccharin Sodium, Sodium Benzoate, Sodium Chloride, Sodium Citrate, Water.

**Indications:** Temporarily relieves cough due to minor throat and bronchial irritation as may occur with a cold and helps loosen phlegm (mucus) and thin bronchial secretions to make coughs more productive.

**Warnings:**
**Do not use** if you or your child are now taking a prescription monoamine oxidase inhibitor (MAOI) (certain drugs for depression, psychiatric, or emotional conditions, or Parkinson's disease), or for 2 weeks after stopping the MAOI drug. If you do not know if you or your child's prescription drug contains an MAOI, ask a doctor or pharmacist before taking this product.

**Ask a doctor before use if you have:**
- cough that occurs with too much phlegm (mucus)
- cough that lasts or is chronic such as occurs with smoking, asthma, chronic bronchitis, or emphysema

**Stop use and ask a doctor if:**
- cough lasts more than 7 days, comes back, or is accompanied by fever, rash, or persistent headache. These could be signs of a serious condition.

**If pregnant or breast-feeding,** ask a health professional before use.

**Keep out of reach of children.** In case of overdose, get medical help or contact a Poison Control Center right away.

**Directions Robitussin DM:** Follow dosage below. Dosage cup provided (except for the 16 oz size). Do not exceed 6 doses in a 24-hour period. Adults and children 12 years and over: 2 teaspoonfuls every 4 hours; children 6 years to under 12 years, 1 teaspoonful every 4 hours; children 2 years to under 6 years, $1/_2$ teaspoonful every 4 hours; children under 2 years: ask a doctor.

**Directions Robitussin DM Infant Drops:** Oral dosing syringe provided. Do not use more than 6 doses in any 24-hour period. Repeat every 4 hours. Choose dosage by weight (if weight not known, choose by age). Measure with the dosing device provided. Do not use with any other device. 2 years to under 6 years (24–47 lbs.) 2.5 mL; under 2 yrs (under 24 lbs.): ask a doctor.

**How Supplied: Robitussin-DM** (cherry-colored) in bottles of 4 fl oz, 8 fl oz, 12 fl oz, 16 fl oz and single doses: premeasured doses—$1/_3$ fl oz each.

**How Supplied (Robitussin DM Infant Drops):** (berry flavor) in 1 fl oz bottles with oral syringe.

**Storage:** Store at 20°C–25°C (68°F and 77°F).

---

## ROBITUSSIN®-PE SYRUP
[ro "bĭ-tuss 'ĭn ]
**Nasal Decongestant, Expectorant Alcohol-Free Cough Formula**

**Active Ingredients:**
Each teaspoonful of Robitussin-PE (5 mL) contains:
Guaifenesin, USP ...................... 100 mg
Pseudoephedrine Hydrochloride, USP ............................................. 30 mg

**Inactive Ingredients:**
**Robitussin-PE:** Citric Acid, FD&C Red No. 40, Flavors, Glucose, Glycerin, High Fructose Corn Syrup, Maltol, Menthol, Propylene Glycol, Saccharin Sodium, Sodium Benzoate, Water.

**Indications:** Temporarily relieves nasal congestion due to a cold. Helps loosen phlegm (mucus) and thin bronchial secretions to make coughs more productive.

**Warnings:**
**Do not use** if you are now taking a prescription monoamine oxidase inhibitor (MAOI) (certain drugs for depression, psychiatric, or emotional conditions, or Parkinson's disease), or for 2 weeks after stopping the MAOI drug. If you do not know if your prescription drug contains an MAOI, ask a doctor or pharmacist before taking this product.

**Ask a doctor before use if you have:**
- heart disease
- high blood pressure
- thyroid disease
- diabetes
- trouble urinating due to an enlarged prostate gland
- cough that occurs with too much phlegm (mucus)
- cough that lasts or is chronic such as occurs with smoking, asthma, chronic bronchitis, or emphysema

**When using this product**
- do not use more than directed.

**Stop use and ask a doctor if:**
- you get nervous, dizzy, or sleepless
- symptoms do not get better within 7 days or are accompanied by fever
- cough lasts more than 7 days, comes back, or is accompanied by fever, rash, or persistent headache. These could be signs of a serious condition.

**If pregnant or breast-feeding,** ask a health professional before use.

**Keep out of reach of children.** In case of overdose, get medical help or contact a Poison Control Center right away.

**Directions: Robitussin-PE:** Dosage cup provided. Follow dosage below:
Do Not Exceed 4 Doses in any 24-Hour Period.
**ADULT DOSE** (and children 12 years and over): 2 teaspoonfuls every 4 hrs.
**CHILD DOSE**
**6 yrs. to under 12 yrs.** 1 teaspoonful every 4 hrs.
**2 yrs. to under 6 yrs.** 1/2 teaspoonful every 4 hrs.
**Under 2—Ask a Doctor.**

**How Supplied:** Robitussin-PE (orange-red) in bottles of 4 fl oz, and 8 fl oz.

**Storage:** Store at 20°C and 25°C (68°F and 77°F).

*Continued on next page*

## ROBITUSSIN®
## HONEY CALMERS THROAT
## DROPS (BERRY)

**Use:** Temporarily relieves occasional minor irritation, pain, sore mouth, and sore throat.

**Active ingredient
(in each drop):**     **Purpose:**
Menthol,
USP 1 mg .................... Oral pain reliever

**Warnings**
**Sore throat warning:** Severe or persistent sore throat or sore throat accompanied by high fever, headache, nausea, and vomiting may be serious. Consult a doctor right away. Do not use more than 2 days or give to children under 3 years of age unless directed by a doctor.
**If pregnant or breast-feeding,** ask a health professional before use.
**Keep out of reach of children.**

**Inactive Ingredients** Carmine, citric acid, cochineal extract, corn syrup, glycerin, natural flavor blend, natural grade A wildflower honey, sucrose

**Directions**
- adults and children 4 years and over: allow 2 drops to dissolve slowly in the mouth. May be repeated every 2 hours, as needed, or as directed by a doctor.
- children under 4 years of age: ask a doctor

**Storage:** Store at 20–25°C (68–77°F)

**How Supplied:** Packages of 25 drops.

---

## ROBITUSSIN® FLU

**Active Ingredients:
(in each 5 mL tsp)**     **Purposes:**
Acetaminophen,
USP 160 mg ............ Pain reliever/fever
reducer
Chlorpheniramine maleate,
USP 1 mg ........................ Antihistamine
Dextromethorphan HBr,
USP 5 mg ............... Cough suppressant
Pseudoephedrine HCl,
USP 15 mg ............ Nasal decongestant

**Uses:**
- temporarily relieves these symptoms occurring with a cold or flu, hay fever, or other upper respiratory allergies:
  - headache
  - cough
  - runny nose
  - itching of the nose or throat
  - nasal congestion
  - muscular aches
  - sneezing
  - sore throat
  - minor aches and pains
  - itchy, watery eyes
  - fever

**Warnings:**
**Alcohol warning:** If you consume 3 or more alcoholic drinks every day, ask your doctor whether you should take acetaminophen or other pain relievers/fever re-

ducers. Acetaminophen may cause liver damage.

**Sore throat warning:** If sore throat is severe, persists for more than 2 days, is accompanied or followed by fever, headache, rash, nausea, or vomiting, consult a doctor promptly.

**Do not use:**
- if you are now taking a prescription monoamine oxidase inhibitor (MAOI) (certain drugs for depression, psychiatric, or emotional conditions, or Parkinson's disease), or for 2 weeks after stopping the MAOI drug. If you do not know if your prescription drug contains an MAOI, ask a doctor or pharmacist before taking this product.
- with any other product containing acetaminophen as this may lead to an overdose. Overdose requires prompt medical attention even if you do not notice any signs or symptoms.

**Ask a doctor before use if you have:**
- heart disease
- trouble urinating due to an enlarged prostate gland
- cough that occurs with too much phlegm (mucus)
- a breathing problem or chronic cough that lasts or as occurs with smoking, asthma, chronic bronchitis, or emphysema
- high blood pressure
- thyroid disease
- diabetes
- glaucoma

**Ask a doctor or pharmacist before use if you are** taking sedatives or tranquilizers.

**When using this product:**
- **do not use more than directed**
- marked drowsiness may occur
- alcohol, sedatives, and tranquilizers may increase drowsiness
- be careful when driving a motor vehicle or operating machinery
- excitability may occur, especially in children
- avoid alcoholic drinks

**Stop use and ask a doctor if:**
- you get nervous, dizzy, or sleepless
- new symptoms occur
- symptoms do not get better within 7 days or are accompanied by fever
- symptoms do not get better, get worse, or are accompanied by fever more than 3 days
- redness or swelling is present
- cough lasts more than 7 days, comes back, or is accompanied by fever, rash, or persistent headache. These could be signs of a serious condition.

**If pregnant or breast-feeding,** ask a health professional before use.

**Keep out of reach of children.** In case of overdose, get medical help or contact a Poison Control Center right away. Quick medical attention is critical for adults as well as for children, even if you do not notice any signs or symptoms.

**Directions:**
- do not take more than 4 doses in any 24-hour period
- do not exceed recommended dosage. Taking more than the recommended dose (overdose) may cause serious liver damage.

| age | dose |
|---|---|
| adults and children 12 years and over | 4 teaspoonfuls every 4 hours |
| children 6 years to under 12 years | 2 teaspoonfuls every 4 hours |
| under 6 years | ask a doctor |

**Inactive Ingredients:** Citric acid, D&C red no. 33, FD&C yellow no. 6, flavor, glycerin, high fructose corn syrup, polyethylene glycol, purified water, sodium benzoate, sodium citrate, sorbitol solution, sucralose

**Other Information:**
- store at 20–25°C (68–77°F)
- alcohol free

**How Supplied:** Bottles of 4 fl. oz.

---

## ROBITUSSIN®
## HONEY COUGH™
**Alcohol-Free Cough Formula
Cough Suppressant**

**Active Ingredient:**
Each teaspoonful (5 mL) contains:
Dextromethorphan HBr, USP ..... 10 mg

**Inactive Ingredients:** Flavors, Glucose, Glycerin, Honey, Maltol, Methylparaben, Propylene Glycol, Sodium Benzoate, Water.

**Indications:** Temporarily relieves cough due to minor throat and bronchial irritation as may occur with a cold.

**Directions:** Follow dosage below. Dosage cup provided. Do not take more than 4 doses in any 24-hour period.

| age | dose |
|---|---|
| adults and children 12 years and older | 3 teaspoonfuls every 6 to 8 hours |
| children 6 to under 12 years | 1.5 teaspoonfuls every 6 to 8 hours |
| children under 6 years | not recommended |

**Warnings:**
**Do not use** if you are now taking a prescription monoamine oxidase inhibitor (MAOI) (certain drugs for depression, psychiatric, or emotional conditions, or Parkinson's disease), or for 2 weeks after stopping the MAOI drug. If you do not know if your prescription drug contains an MAOI, ask a doctor or pharmacist before taking this product.
**Ask a doctor before use if you have:**
- cough that occurs with too much phlegm (mucus)
- cough that lasts or is chronic such as occurs with smoking, asthma, or emphysema

**Stop use and ask a doctor if:** cough lasts more than 7 days, comes back, or is accompanied by fever, rash, or persistent headache. These could be signs of a serious condition

**If pregnant or breast-feeding,** ask a health professional before use.

**Keep out of reach of children.** In case of overdose, get medical help or contact a Poison Control Center right away.

**How Supplied:** Bottles of 4 fl. oz. and 8 fl. oz.

**Storage:** Store at 20–25°C (68°–77°F).

---

## ROBITUSSIN®
## HONEY COUGH Drops
**Honey-Lemon Tea, Herbal Honey Citrus, Herbal with Natural Honey Center, and Herbal Almond with Natural Honey Center**

### Uses
• Temporarily relieves
  • occasional minor irritation, pain, sore mouth, and sore throat
  • cough associated with a cold or inhaled irritants

**Active Ingredients:**
**(in each drop)**
*Herbal with Natural Honey Center* and *Honey-Lemon Tea:*

|  | Purposes |
|---|---|
| Menthol, USP 5 mg | Oral pain reliever/cough suppressant |

*Herbal Honey Citrus* and *Herbal Almond with Natural Honey Center:*

|  | Purposes |
|---|---|
| Menthol, USP 2.5 mg | Oral pain reliever/cough suppressant |

**Inactive Ingredients:**
*Herbal with Natural Honey Center:* Caramel, corn syrup, glycerin, high fructose corn syrup, honey, natural herbal flavor, sorbitol, sucrose
*Honey Lemon Tea:* Caramel, citric acid, corn syrup, honey, natural flavor, sucrose, tea extract
*Herbal Honey Citrus:* Citric acid, corn syrup, flavors, honey, sucrose
*Herbal Almond with Natural Honey Center:* Caramel, corn syrup, glycerin, honey, natural almond flavor, natural anise flavor, natural coriander flavor, natural fennel flavor, natural honey flavor and other natural flavors, sorbitol, sucrose.

### Directions:
• adults and children 4 years and over:
  • for sore throat: allow 1 drop to dissolve slowly in the mouth. May be repeated every 2 hours, as needed, or as directed by a doctor.
  • for cough: *Honey-Lemon Tea and Herbal with Natural Honey Center*— allow 1 drop to dissolve slowly in mouth.
  *Herbal Honey Citrus and Herbal Almond with Natural Honey Center*—allow 2 drops to dissolve slowly in mouth.

May be repeated every hour, as needed, or as directed by a doctor.
• children under 4 years: ask a doctor

### Warnings
**Sore throat warning:** severe or persistent sore throat or sore throat accompanied by high fever, headache, nausea, and vomiting may be serious. Consult a doctor right away. Do not use more than 2 days or give to children under 3 years of age unless directed by a doctor.

**Ask a doctor before use if you have**
• cough that occurs with too much phlegm (mucus)
• cough that lasts or is chronic such as occurs with smoking, asthma, or emphysema

**Stop use and ask a doctor if** cough lasts more than 7 days, comes back, or is accompanied by fever, rash, or persistent headache. These could be signs of a serious condition.

**If pregnant or breast-feeding,** ask a health professional before use.

**Keep out of reach of children.**

**Storage:** Store at 20–25°C (68–77°F).

**How Supplied:** Packages of 20 drops.

---

## ROBITUSSIN® MAXIMUM STRENGTH COUGH SUPPRESSANT
## ROBITUSSIN® PEDIATRIC COUGH SUPPRESSANT
[ro "bĭ-tuss 'ĭn ]

**Active Ingredients:**
*Robitussin Maximum Strength Cough Suppressant:* Each teaspoonful [5 mL] contains Dextromethorphan Hydrobromide, USP .......................................... 15 mg
*Robitussin Pediatric Strength Cough Suppressant:* Each teaspoonful [5 mL] contains Dextromethorphan Hydrobromide, USP ........................................ 7.5 mg

**Inactive Ingredients (Robitussin Maximum Strength Cough Suppressant):** Alcohol, Citric Acid, FD&C Red No. 40, Flavors, Glucose, Glycerin, High Fructose Corn Syrup, Menthol, Saccharin Sodium, Sodium Benzoate, Water.

**Inactive Ingredients (Robitussin Pediatric Cough Suppressant):** Citric Acid, FD&C Red No. 40, Flavor, Glycerin, High Fructose Corn Syrup, Saccharin Sodium, Sodium Benzoate, Sodium Chloride, Sodium Citrate, Water.

**Indications:** Temporarily relieves cough due to minor throat and bronchial irritation as may occur with a cold.

**Warnings:**
**Do not use** if you are now taking a prescription monoamine oxidase inhibitor (MAOI) (certain drugs for depression, psychiatric, or emotional conditions, or Parkinson's disease), or for 2 weeks after stopping the MAOI drug. If you do not know if your prescription drug contains an MAOI, ask a doctor or pharmacist before taking this product.

**Ask a doctor before use if you have:**
• cough that occurs with too much phlegm (mucus)
• cough that lasts or is chronic such as occurs with smoking, asthma, or emphysema

**Stop use and ask a doctor if:** cough lasts more than 7 days, comes back, or is accompanied by fever, rash, or persistent headache  These could be signs of a serious condition.

**If pregnant or breast-feeding,** ask a health professional before use.

**Keep out of reach of children.** In case of overdose, get medical help or contact a Poison Control Center right away.

**Directions:** Follow dosage below. Dosage cup provided. Do not exceed 4 doses in any 24-hour period. **Robitussin Maximum Strength Cough Suppressant ADULT DOSE** (and children 12 yrs. and over): 2 teaspoonfuls every 6–8 hours, in dosage cup. **CHILD DOSE** (under 12 yrs.): Ask a doctor.
**Robitussin Pediatric Cough Suppressant** Repeat every 6 to 8 hours. Dosage: choose by weight, if known; if weight is not known, choose by age.
[See table above]

| Age | Weight | Dose |
|---|---|---|
| Under 2 yrs. | Under 24 lbs. | Ask a doctor |
| 2 to under 6 yrs. | 24–47 lbs. | 1 Teaspoonful |
| 6 to under 12 yrs. | 48–95 lbs. | 2 Teaspoonfuls |
| 12 yrs. and older | 96 lbs. and over | 4 Teaspoonfuls |

**How Supplied:** Robitussin Maximum Strength (dark red-colored) in bottles of 4 and 8 fl oz. Store at 20–25°C (68–77°F).

**How Supplied:** Robitussin Pediatric (cherry-colored) in bottles of 4 fl oz.

**Storage:** Store at 20–25°C (68–77°F).

---

## ROBITUSSIN® MAXIMUM STRENGTH COUGH& COLD
## ROBITUSSIN® PEDIATRIC COUGH & COLD FORMULA
[ro "bĭ-tuss 'ĭn ]
**Cough Suppressant, Nasal Decongestant**

**Active Ingredients:** Each teaspoonful (5 mL) of **Robitussin Maximum Strength Cough & Cold** contains:
Dextromethorphan Hydrobromide, USP ............................................. 15 mg
Pseudoephedrine Hydrochloride, USP ............................................. 30 mg

*Continued on next page*

## Robitussin Cough/Cold—Cont.

**Active Ingredients:** Each teaspoonful (5 mL) of **Robitussin Pediatric Cough & Cold Formula** contains:
Dextromethorphan Hydrobromide,
USP ................................. 7.5 mg
Pseudoephedrine Hydrochloride,
USP ................................. 15 mg

**Inactive Ingredients (Robitussin Maximum Strength Cough & Cold):** Alcohol, Citric Acid, FD&C Red No. 40, Flavors, Glucose, Glycerin, High Fructose Corn Syrup, Menthol, Saccharin Sodium, Sodium Benzoate, Water.

**Inactive Ingredients (Robitussin Pediatric Cough & Cold Formula):** Citric Acid, FD&C Red No. 40, Flavor, Glycerin, High Fructose Corn Syrup, Saccharin Sodium, Sodium Benzoate, Sodium Chloride, Sodium Citrate, Water.

**Indications:** Temporarily relieves cough due to minor throat and bronchial irritation and nasal congestion as may occur with a cold.

**Warnings:**
**Do not use** if you are now taking a prescription monoamine oxidase inhibitor (MAOI) (certain drugs for depression, psychiatric, or emotional conditions, or Parkinson's disease), or for 2 weeks after stopping the MAOI drug. If you do not know if your prescription drug contains an MAOI, ask a doctor or pharmacist before taking this product.
**Ask a doctor before use if you have:**
• heart disease
• high blood pressure
• thyroid disease
• diabetes
• trouble urinating due to an enlarged prostate gland
• cough that occurs with too much phlegm (mucus)
• cough that lasts or is chronic such as occurs with smoking, asthma, or emphysema
**When using this product do not use more than directed.**
**Stop use and ask a doctor if:**
• you get nervous, dizzy, or sleepless
• symptoms do not get better within 7 days or are accompanied by fever
• cough lasts more than 7 days, comes back, or is accompanied by fever, rash, or persistent headache. These could be signs of a serious condition.
**If pregnant or breast-feeding,** ask a health professional before use.
**Keep out of reach of children.** In case of overdose, get medical help or contact a Poison Control Center right away.

**Directions:** Follow dosage (dosage cup provided). Do Not Exceed 4 Doses in any

24-Hour Period. **Robitussin Maximum Strength Cough & Cold.** Adults and children 12 years and over: 2 teaspoonfuls every 6 hours, as needed. Children under 12 years: Ask a doctor.
**Robitussin Pediatric Cough & Cold Formula** Repeat every 6 hours. Dosage: choose by weight, if known; if weight is not known, choose by age. [See table below]

**How Supplied Robitussin Maximum Strength Cough & Cold:** Red syrup in bottles of 4 fl oz and 8 fl oz.
**How Supplied:** Robitussin Pediatric Cough & Cold formula (bright red) in bottles of 4 fl oz.
**Storage:** Store at 20°C–25°C (68°F and 77°F).

---

## ROBITUSSIN® MULTI SYMPTOM HONEY FLU™
**Non-Drowsy Cough Formula**
**Cough Suppressant, Nasal Decongestant, Pain Reliever/Fever Reducer**

**Active Ingredients:**
Each teaspoonful (5 mL) contains:
Acetaminophen, USP ............... 166.6 mg
Dextromethorphan HBr, USP .... 6.6 mg
Pseudoephedrine HCl, USP ......... 20 mg

**Inactive Ingredients:** Citric Acid, Flavors, Glucose, Glycerin, High Fructose Corn Syrup, Menthol, Natural Grade A Honey, Polyethylene Glycol, Propylene Glycol, Saccharin Sodium, Sodium Benzoate, Water

**Indications** For the temporary relief of these symptoms associated with a cold or flu: nasal congestion, minor aches and pains, sore throat, cough, fever, headache, muscular aches.

**Directions:** Do not take more than 4 doses in any 24-hour period. Follow dosage below. Dosage cup provided.
**Adults and children over 12 years of age:** Take 3 teaspoons every 4 hours, as needed.
**Children:** Children under 12 years: not recommended. Do not use in children under 2 years of age.
Do not exceed recommended dosage. Taking more than the recommended dose (overdose) may cause serious liver damage.

**Warnings:**
**Alcohol warning:** if you consume 3 or more alcoholic drinks every day, ask your doctor whether you should take acetaminophen or other pain relievers/fever reducers. Acetaminophen may cause liver damage.

**Sore throat warning:** if sore throat is severe, persists for more than two days, is accompanied or followed by fever, headache, rash, nausea, or vomiting, consult a doctor promptly.
**Do not use**
• if you are now taking a prescription monoamine oxidase inhibitor (MAOI) (certain drugs for depression, psychiatric, or emotional conditions, or Parkinson's disease), or for 2 weeks after stopping the MAOI drug. If you do not know if your prescription drug contains an MAOI, ask a doctor or pharmacist before taking this product.
• with any other product containing acetaminophen as this may lead to an overdose. Overdose requires prompt medical attention even if you do not notice any signs or symptoms.
**Ask a doctor before use if you have:**
• heart disease
• high blood pressure
• thyroid disease
• diabetes
• trouble urinating due to an enlarged prostate gland
• cough that occurs with too much phlegm (mucus)
• a breathing problem or chronic cough that lasts or as occurs with smoking, asthma, or emphysema
**When using this product**
• do not use more than directed
**Stop use and ask a doctor if:**
• you get nervous, dizzy, or sleepless
• new symptoms occur
• you need to use for more than 7 days
• symptoms do not get better, get worse, or are accompanied by fever more than 3 days
• redness or swelling is present
• cough lasts more than 7 days, comes back, or is accompanied by fever, rash, or persistent headache. These could be signs of a serious condition.
**If pregnant or breast-feeding,** ask a health professional before use.
**Keep out of reach of children.** In case of overdose, get medical help or contact a Poison Control Center right away. Quick medical attention is critical for adults as well as for children, even if you do not notice any signs or symptoms.

**How Supplied:** Bottles of 4 fl. oz. (118 mL).
Not labeled USP due to microbial content of natural honey.

**Storage:** Store at 20–25°C (68–77°F).

---

## ROBITUSSIN® HONEY FLU NIGHTTIME FORMULA

**Active Ingredients:**
**(in each pouch = 15 mL):**     **Purposes:**
Acetaminophen,
USP 500 mg .................... Pain reliever/
fever reducer
Chlorpheniramine maleate,
USP 4 mg ........................ Antihistamine
Dextromethorphan HBr,
USP 20 mg ............ Cough suppressant
Pseudoephedrine HCl,
USP 60 mg ............ Nasal decongestant

| Age | Weight | Dose |
|---|---|---|
| Under 2 yrs. | Under 24 lbs. | Ask a doctor |
| 2 to under 6 yrs. | 24–47 lbs. | 1 Teaspoonful |
| 6 to under 12 yrs. | 48–95 lbs. | 2 Teaspoonfuls |
| 12 yrs. and older | 96 lbs. and over | 4 Teaspoonfuls |

## Uses:

- temporarily relieves these symptoms associated with a cold, or flu, hay fever, or other upper respiratory allergies:
  - headache
  - nasal congestion
  - sore throat
  - fever
  - cough
  - muscular aches
  - minor aches and pains
  - runny nose
  - sneezing
  - itchy, watery eyes
  - itching of the nose or throat

## Warnings:

**Alcohol warning:** If you consume 3 or more alcoholic drinks every day, ask your doctor whether you should take acetaminophen or other pain relievers/fever reducers. Acetaminophen may cause liver damage.

**Sore throat warning:** If sore throat is severe, persists for more than two days, is accompanied or followed by fever, headache, rash, nausea, or vomiting, consult a doctor promptly.

**Do not use:**

- if you are now taking a prescription monoamine oxidase inhibitor (MAOI) (certain drugs for depression, psychiatric, or emotional conditions, or Parkinson's disease), or for 2 weeks after stopping the MAOI drug. If you do not know if your prescription drug contains an MAOI, ask a doctor or pharmacist before taking this product.
- with any other product containing acetaminophen as this may lead to an overdose. Overdose requires prompt medical attention even if you do not notice any signs or symptoms.

**Ask a doctor before use if you have:**

- heart disease
- high blood pressure
- thyroid disease
- diabetes
- trouble urinating due to an enlarged prostate gland
- glaucoma
- cough that occurs with too much phlegm (mucus)
- a breathing problem or chronic cough that lasts or as occurs with smoking, asthma, chronic bronchitis, or emphysema

**Ask a doctor or pharmacist before use if you are** taking sedatives or tranquilizers.

**When using this product:**

- **do not use more than directed**
- marked drowsiness may occur
- avoid alcoholic drinks
- alcohol, sedatives, and tranquilizers may increase drowsiness
- be careful when driving a motor vehicle or operating machinery
- excitability may occur, especially in children

**Stop use and ask a doctor if:**

- you get nervous, dizzy, or sleepless
- new symptoms occur
- you need to use for more than 7 days
- symptoms do not get better, get worse, or are accompanied by fever more than 3 days
- redness or swelling is present
- cough lasts more than 7 days, comes back, or is accompanied by fever, rash, or persistent headache. These could be signs of a serious condition.

**If pregnant or breast-feeding,** ask a health professional before use.

**Keep out of reach of children.** In case of overdose, get medical help or contact a Poison Control Center right away. Prompt medical attention is critical for adults as well as for children, even if you do not notice any signs or symptoms.

## Directions:

- do not take more than 4 doses in any 24-hour period
- adults and children 12 years and over: empty entire pouch into a 4–6 oz cup of hot beverage (tea). Repeat every 4 hours, as needed.
- children under 12 years: not recommended
- do not use in children under 2 years
- do not exceed recommended dosage. Taking more than the recommended dose (overdose) may cause serious liver damage.

**Inactive Ingredients:** Citric acid, flavors, glucose, glycerin, high fructose corn syrup, natural grade A honey, polyethylene glycol, propylene glycol, saccharin sodium, sodium benzoate, water

## How Supplied:

Each box contains 6 honey syrup pouches (15 mL each)

**Other Information:** Store at 20–25°C (68–77°F). Not labeled USP due to microbial content of natural honey.

---

## ROBITUSSIN® SUGAR FREE COUGH

### Active Ingredients:

| (in each 5 mL tsp) | Purpose: |
|---|---|
| Dextromethorphan HBr, USP 10 mg ............. | Cough suppressant |
| Guaifenesin, USP 100 mg ....................... | Expectorant |

### Uses:

- temporarily relieves cough due to minor throat and bronchial irritation as may occur with a cold
- helps loosen phlegm (mucus) and thin bronchial secretions to make coughs more productive

### Warnings:

**Do not use** if you are now taking a prescription monoamine oxidase inhibitor (MAOI) (certain drugs for depression, psychiatric, or emotional conditions, or Parkinson's disease), or for 2 weeks after stopping the MAOI drug. If you do not know if your prescription drug contains an MAOI, ask a doctor or pharmacist before taking this product.

**Ask a doctor before use if you have:**

- cough that occurs with too much phlegm (mucus)
- cough that lasts or is chronic such as occurs with smoking, asthma, chronic bronchitis, or emphysema

**Stop use and ask a doctor if** cough lasts more than 7 days, comes back, or is accompanied by fever, rash, or persistent headache. These could be signs of a serious condition.

**If pregnant or breast-feeding,** ask a health professional before use.

**Keep out of reach of children.** In case of overdose, get medical help or contact a Poison Control Center right away.

### Directions:

- do not take more than 6 doses in any 24-hour period

| age | dose |
|---|---|
| adults and children 12 years and over | 2 teaspoonfuls every 4 hours |
| children 6 years to under 12 years | 1 teaspoonful every 4 hours |
| children 2 years to under 6 years | 1/2 teaspoonful every 4 hours |
| under 2 years | ask a doctor |

**Inactive Ingredients:** Acesulfame potassium, citric acid, flavors, glycerin, methylparaben, polyethylene glycol, povidone, propylene glycol, saccharin sodium, sodium benzoate, water

**Other Information:**

- store at 20–25°C (68–77°F)
- alcohol-free
- dosage cup provided

**How Supplied:** Bottles of 4 fl. oz.

---

## ROBITUSSIN® SUGAR FREE Throat Drops (Natural Citrus and Tropical Fruit Flavors)

### Active Ingredient:

| (in each drop) | Purposes: |
|---|---|
| Menthol, USP 2.5 mg ................................ | Oral pain reliever/cough suppressant |

### Uses:

- temporarily relieves
  - occasional minor irritation, pain, sore mouth, and sore throat
  - cough associated with a cold or inhaled irritants

**Inactive Ingredients:** Aspartame, canola oil, citric acid, D&C Yellow No. 10 aluminum lake (Natural Citrus only), FD&C blue No. 1 (Natural Citrus only), FD&C Yellow No. 6 (Tropical Fruit only), isomalt, maltilol, natural flavor.

### Directions:

- adults and children 4 years and over: allow 2 drops to dissolve slowly in the mouth
  - for sore throat: may be repeated every 2 hours, as needed, up to 9 drops per day, or as directed by a doctor
  - for cough: may be repeated every hour, as needed, up to 9 drops per day, as or as directed by a doctor
- children under 4 years: ask a doctor

### Warnings:

**Sore throat warning:** severe or persistent sore throat or sore throat accom-

*Continued on next page*

## Robitussin S.F. Throat—Cont.

panied by high fever, headache, nausea, and vomiting may be serious. Consult a doctor right away. Do not use more than 2 days or give to children under 3 years of age unless directed by a doctor.

**Ask a doctor before use if you have:**
- cough that occurs with too much phlegm (mucus)
- cough that lasts or is chronic such as occurs with smoking, asthma, or emphysema

**When using this product** excessive use may have a laxative effect.

**Stop use and ask a doctor if** cough lasts more than 7 days, comes back, or is accompanied by fever, rash, or persistent headache. These could be signs of a serious condition.

**If pregnant or breast-feeding,** ask a health professional before use.

**Keep out of reach of children.**

**Other Information:**
- each drop contains: **phenylalanine 3.37 mg**
- store at 20–25°C (68–77°F)
- does not promote tooth decay
- product may be useful in a diabetic's diet on the advice of a doctor. Exchange information*:

   3 Drops = FREE Exchange
   9 Drops = 1 Fruit

*The dietary exchanges are based on Exchange Lists for Meal Planning. Copyright 1995 by the American Diabetes Association Inc. and the American Dietetic Association.

**How Supplied:** Packages of 18 drops.

---

## ROBITUSSIN SUNNY ORANGE VITAMIN C SUPPLEMENT DROPS

**Each soothing, refreshing drop provides a great tasting and convenient way to get 100% of the Daily Value of Vitamin C.**
**Made with 5% real orange juice.**

**Supplement Facts:**
**Serving Size: 1 drop**

| Amount Per Drop | | % Daily Value |
|---|---|---|
| Calories | 15 | |
| Total Carbohydrate | 3 g | 1%* |
| Sugars | 3 g | + |
| Vitamin C (as sodium ascorbate and ascorbic acid) | 60 mg | 100% |
| Sodium | 10 mg | <1% |

*Daily Value (%DV) not established.
+Percent Daily Values are based on a 2,000 calorie diet.

**Other Ingredients:** Corn syrup, sucrose.
**Contains less than 2 % of the following:** ascorbyl palmitate, beta carotene, citric acid, citrus aurantium dulcis (orange) juice (concentrate), corn oil, gelatin, menthol, methylparaben, natural flavor, phosphoric acid, potassium sorbate, propylparaben, sodium benzoate, sorbitol, tocopherols.

**Directions:** Take a minimum of 3 to 4 drops a day, not to exceed 15 drops per day. Allow drop to dissolve fully in mouth and swallow. Not formulated for use in children.

**Warnings: Keep out of reach of children.**
If you are pregnant or nursing a baby, contact your physician before taking this product.
**Storage:** Store at 20–25°C (68–77°F)

**How Supplied:** 25 Drops

---

## Zila Pharmaceuticals, Inc.

**5227 NORTH 7th STREET
PHOENIX, AZ 85014-2800**

**Direct Inquiries to:**
Diane Hammond
Associate Marketing Manager
(602) 266-6700
World Wide Web Address
www.zila.com

**ZILACTIN® Cold Sore Gel**
**ZILACTIN®-L Cold Sore Liquid**
**ZILACTIN®-B Canker Sore Gel**

**Indication:**
**Zilactin** Medicated Gel stops pain and speeds healing of fever blisters and cold sores. Zilactin forms a tenacious, occlusive film which holds the medication in place while controlling pain. Intra-orally, the film can last up to 6 hours, usually allowing pain-free eating and drinking. Extra-orally, the film will last much longer. May also be used for canker sores.

**Zilactin-L** is a non film-forming liquid that treats and relieves the pain, itching and burning of developing and existing cold sores and fever blisters. Zilactin-L is specially formulated to treat the initial signs of tingling, itching or burning that signal an oncoming cold sore or fever blister.

**Zilactin-B** is a medicated gel containing benzocaine that forms a smooth, flexible and occlusive film on the oral mucosa. It's specially formulated to control pain and shield the mouth sores, canker sores, cheek bites and gum sores that occur from dental appliances from the environment of the mouth. The film can last up to 6 hours. *Clinical studies on the effectiveness of Zila's products are available on request.*

**Active Ingredients: Zilactin**—Benzyl Alcohol (10%); **Zilactin-L**—Lidocaine (2.5%); **Zilactin-B**—Benzocaine (10%);

**Directions:**
**Zilactin:** FOR USE IN THE MOUTH AND ON LIPS. Apply every four hours for the first three days and then as needed. Dry the affected area. Apply a thin coat of Zilactin and allow 60 seconds for the gel to dry into a film. Outside the mouth, Zilactin forms a transparent film. Inside the mouth, the film is white.

**Zilactin-L:** FOR USE ON THE LIPS AND AROUND THE MOUTH. Moisten a cotton swab with several drops of Zilactin-L. Apply on lip area where symptoms are noted or directly on existing cold sore or fever blister and allow to dry for 15 seconds. Do not apply more than 3 to 4 times daily. For optimal effectiveness use at first signs of tingling or itching.

**Zilactin-B:** FOR USE IN THE MOUTH. Apply every four hours for the first three days and then as needed. Dry the affected area. Apply a thin coat of Zilactin-B and allow 60 seconds for the gel to dry into a film.

**Warning:** A mild, temporary stinging sensation may be experienced when applying Zilactin, Zilactin-L or Zilactin-B to an open cut, sore or blister. This may be minimized by first applying ice for a minute before application of the medication. **Do not peel off protective film.** Attempting to peel off film may result in skin irritation or tenderness. To remove film, first apply another coat of Zilactin-B to film, and immediately wipe the area with a moist gauze pad or tissue. DO NOT USE IN OR NEAR EYES. In the event of accidental contact with the eye, flush with water immediately and continuously for ten minutes. Seek immediate medical attention if pain or irritation persists. For temporary relief only. As with all medications, keep out of the reach of children. Do not use Zilactin-L or Zilactin-B if you have a history of allergy to local anesthetics such as benzocaine, lidocaine or other "caine" anesthetics. If condition worsens, or if symptoms persist for more than 7 days or clear up and occur again within a few days, discontinue use of this product and consult a physician.

**How Supplied:** Zila products are non-prescription and carried by most drug wholesalers, retail chains and independent pharmacies. Each product is available to physicians and dentists directly from Zila in single use packages.

For further information call or write:

**Zila Consumer Pharmaceuticals, Inc.**

5227 N. 7th Street, Phoenix, AZ 85014-2800, (602) 266-6700

U.S. patent numbers 4,285,934; 4,381,296; and 5,081,158

## ZILACTIN® BABY Teething Gel
**Oral Pain Reliever Gel**
**Alcohol-Free**

### Indication:
**Zilactin-Baby** medicated gel is uniquely formulated to temporarily relieve sore gums caused by teething in infants and children 4 months of age and older. The extra strength level of medication in Zilactin-Baby begins relieving the discomfort of teething pain in seconds. This specially developed gel combines a pleasant grape flavor with an advanced ingredient that imparts a cooling sensation.

**Active Ingredient:** Benzocaine (10%)

**Inactive Ingredients:** PEG-8, PEG-75, Glycerin, Water, Potassium Acesulfame, Flavor, Menthyl Lactate, Glycine, Methylparaben, Propylparaben, Sorbic Acid.

**Directions: Wash hands. Apply small amount to the affected gum area with fingertip or cotton applicator. Apply to affected area not more than 4 times daily or as directed by a dentist or physician.** For infants under 4 months of age, there is no recommended dosage or treatment except under the advice and supervision of a physician.

**Warning:** DO NOT USE THIS PRODUCT FOR MORE THAN 7 DAYS UNLESS DIRECTED BY A DENTIST OR PHYSICIAN. If sore mouth symptoms do not improve in 7 days, or if irritation, pain, rash or fever develops, see a dentist or physician promptly. Do not exceed the recommended dosage. Do not use this product if there is a history of allergy to topical anesthetics such as procaine, butacaine, benzocaine or other "caine" anesthetics. Fever and nasal congestion are not symptoms of teething and may indicate the presence of infection. If these symptoms persist consult your physician. Keep this and all drugs out of the reach of children. In case of accidental overdose, seek professional assistance or contact a Poison Control Center immediately.

---

### EDUCATIONAL MATERIAL

Samples and literature are available to medical professionals on request.

# DIETARY SUPPLEMENT INFORMATION

This section presents information on natural reme- dies and nutritional supplements marketed under the Dietary Supplement Health and Education Act of 1994. It is made possible through the courtesy of the manufacturers whose products appear on the fol- lowing pages. The information concerning each product has been prepared, edited, and approved by professional staff of the manufacturer.

Products to be found in this section include vitamins, minerals, herbs and other botanicals, amino acids, other substances intended to supplement the diet, and concentrates, metabolites, constituents, extracts, and combinations of these ingredients. The descriptions of these products are designed to provide all information necessary for informed use, including, when applicable, active ingredients, inac- tive ingredients, actions, warnings, cautions, interac- tions, symptoms and treatment of oral overdosage, dosage and directions for use, and how supplied.

Descriptions in this section must be in full compli- ance with the Dietary Supplement Health and Education Act, which permits claims regarding a product's effect on the structure or functioning of the body, but forbids claims regarding a product's ability to treat, diagnose, cure, or prevent any spe- cific disease. Descriptions of products marketed under the act do not receive formal evaluation or approval from the Food and Drug Administration.

In compiling this section, the publisher has empha- sized the necessity of describing products compre- hensively. The descriptions seen here include all information made available by the manufacturer. The publisher does not warrant or guarantee any product described here, and does not perform any independent analysis of the information provided. Inclusion of a product in this book does not repre- sent an endorsement, and the publisher does not necessarily advocate the use of any product listed.

# A & Z Pharmaceutical Inc.

**180 OSER AVENUE, SUITE 300
HAUPPAUGE, NY 11788**

**Direct Inquiries to:**
Customer Service
(631) 952-3800
Fax: (631) 952-3900

## D-CAL™
### Calcium Supplement with Vitamin D
### Chewable Caplets

**Ingredients:** Calcium Carbonate, Vitamin D, Sorbitol, Flavor, D&C Red #27 Lake, Magnesium Stearate. No sugar, No salt, No lactose, No preservative.

**Supplement Facts**

| Serving Size One Caplet | | |
| --- | --- | --- |
| Each Caplet Contains | % Daily Value | |
| Calcium (as calcium carbonate) | 300 mg | 30% |
| Vitamin D | 100 IU | 25% |

**Recommended Intake:** Take two caplets daily for adult and one caplet for child, or as directed by your physician.

**Warnings:** KEEP OUT OF REACH OF CHILDREN. Do not accept if safely seal under cap is broken or missing.

**Actions:** D-Cal™ provides a concentrated form of calcium to help build healthy bones. It contains Vitamin D to help the body absorb calcium. D-Cal™ can also help prevent osteoporosis. It is helpful to pregnant and nursing women, children's growth, and calcium deficiency at all ages.

**How Supplied:** Bottles of 30 and 60 caplets
*Shown in Product Identification Guide, page 503*

---

# AkPharma Inc.

**P.O. BOX 111
PLEASANTVILLE, NJ
08232-0111**

**Direct Inquiries To:**
Elizabeth Klein: (609) 645-5100
FAX: (609) 645-0767

**Medical Emergency Contact:**
Alan E. Kligerman: (609) 645-5100

## PRELIEF®

PRODUCT OVERVIEW
**Key Facts:** Prelief is AkPharma's brand name for calcium glycerophos-

phate. It is used to remove acid from acidic foods and beverages when acidic foods are to be avoided for more tolerable ingestion. Prelief tablets are swallowed with the food or beverage. Prelief granulate is added to each serving of acidic food or beverage.

**Major Uses:** Takes acid out of acidic foods such as tomato sauce, citrus, fruit drinks, coffee, wine, beer and colas. Acid foods are now established as problematic for persons with Interstitial Cystitis, urinary urgency and are suspect in some intestinal irritation. Those with Interstitial Cystitis or incontinence, whose symptoms may be exacerbated by acidic foods, may particularly benefit.

**Safety Information:** Prelief is made from an FDA Generally Recognized as Safe (GRAS)[1] dietary supplement ingredient and is also listed as a food ingredient in the US Government Food Chemicals Codex (FCC)[2]

PRODUCT INFORMATION
**Prelief®**

**Description:** Prelief Tablets: Each tablet contains 333 mg of calcium glycerophosphate. The tablets also contain 0.5% magnesium stearate as a processing aid. Two or three tablets should be swallowed with the food or beverage. (See chart)

Prelief Granulate: Each packet contains 333 mg of calcium glycerophosphate. Add 2 packets of granulate to each serving of acidic food or beverage. Except for alcoholic beverages, the granulate dissolves rapidly in the acidic food or beverage. An additional 1–2 tablets or packets may be needed on foods that may be particularly high in acid. (See chart)

Each tablet or packet of granulate supplies 6% (65 mg) of the US Recommended Daily Allowance (USRDA) for

calcium and 5% (50 mg) of the USRDA for phosphorus. No sodium; no aluminum; no sugar.

---

[1]reference 21 CFR §184.1201
[2]reference Food Chemicals Codex, 3rd Edition, pp 51–52

**Reasons for Use:** Prelief is a dietary supplement for use with acidic foods and beverages. It is a dietary intervention used to take acid out of these ingestibles for persons who identify acid discomfort with the ingestion of acidic foods and beverages.

**Action:** Prelief neutralizes the acid found in a large number of foods which many people find cause them discomfort. See Table.

**Usage:** 2 tablets or 2 granulate packets per serving of acidic food or beverage.

**How Supplied:** Prelief is supplied in both tablet form (30, 60 and 120 tablet bottle sizes and 24 tablets in 12–2 tablet packets), and granulate form (36 packets and 50 serving granulate shaker).

**Kosher:** Prelief is Kosher and Pareve.
**Use Limitations:** None, except as may apply below.

**Adverse Reactions:** None known
**Toxicity:** None known
**Lead Content:** There is no practical upper limit for tablet or packet consumption regarding California Proposition 65 on lead content.

**Interactions with Drugs:** Calcium may interfere with efficacy of some medications. If a medication is being taken, check with physician, pharmacist or other health professional about the possible interactions of calcium with that medication. No other drug interactions known.

**Precautions:** People who have been advised by their physician not to take

| Typical Food Acid Removal by Prelief | | | |
| --- | --- | --- | --- |
| Product | 1 Packet or 1 Tablet | 2 Packets or 2 Tablets | 3 Packets or 3 Tablets |
| Pepsi Cola® – 8 oz. | 98% | 99.8% | – |
| Mott's® 100% Apple Juice – 4 oz. | 49.8% | 74.9% | 90% |
| Tropicana® Orange Juice – 4 oz. | 20.6% | 36.9% | 60% |
| Coors Light® Beer – 12 oz. | 80.1% | 95% | 96.8% |
| Monty's Hill® Chardonnay – 4 oz. | 37% | 60.1% | 80% |
| Ireland® Coffee – 6 oz. | 93.7% | 96.8% | 98% |
| Tetley® Iced Tea – 8 oz. | 99% | 99.5% | – |
| Seven Seas® Red Wine & Vinegar Salad Dressing – 31 gm | 90% | 95% | 98% |
| Old El Paso® Thick'n Chunky Salsa Medium – 2 Tbsp. | 80.1% | 95% | 97.5% |
| Heinz® Tomato Ketchup – 1 Tbsp. | 68.4% | 87.4% | 92.1% |
| Kraft® Original Barbeque Sauce 2 Tbsp. | 60.2% | 80% | 90% |
| Ragu® Old World Style Traditional Sauce – 125 gm | 20.6% | 36.9% | 60.2% |
| Dannon® Strawberry Lowfat Yogurt (fully mixed) – 116 gm | 49.9% | 68.4% | 80.1% |
| Grapefruit Sections – 150 gm | 36.9% | 50% | 68.3% |
| Sauerkraut – 2 Tbsp. | 60.3% | 80% | 92.1% |
| Red Cabbage – 130 gm | 49.7% | 68.3% | 74.8% |

calcium, phosphorus or glycerin/glycerol should consult with their physician before using Prelief.

Prelief is classified as a dietary supplement, not a drug.

For more information and samples, please write or call toll-free 1-800-994-4711.

[See table at bottom of previous page]

*Shown in Product Identification Guide, page 503*

---

## American Longevity
**2400 BOSWELL ROAD
CHULA VISTA, CA 91914**

**Direct Inquiries to:**
Customer Service
800-982-3189
Fax:
619-934-3205
www.americanlongevity.net

### Plant Derived Minerals

**Description:** Minerals which are so important to our health are not so readily available. Minerals never occured in a uniform blanket on the crust of the Earth. Therefore, unless you supplement with minerals, you can't guarantee that you will get all you need through the 4 food groups. Our Plant Derived Mineral products are liquid concentrates containing a natural assortment of up to 77 minerals from prehistoric plants in their unaltered colloidal form. A mineral deficiency can lead to disease or even death. Plant Derived Minerals can help you in your fight against deficiencies. Now, it even comes in a great tasting cherry flavor.

**Supplement Facts:**
Calories <5
Majestic Earth Plant          600mg *
   Derived Minerals
*daily value not established

**Directions:**
1) Store in cool environment after opening
2) Suggested as a dietary supplement. For adults, mix 1 or 2 ounces in a small glass of fruit or vegetable juice of your choice. Drink during or after meals, 1 to 3 times a day or as desired. For children reduce amount by two-thirds

**Other Ingredients:** Calcium, Chlorine, Magnesium, Phosphorus, Potassium, Sodium, Sulfur, Antimony, Arsenic, Aluminum Hydroxide, Barium, Beryllium, Bismuth, Boron, Bromine, Cadmium, Carbon, Cerium Cesium, Chromium, Cobalt, Copper, Dysprosium, Erbium, Europium, Fluorine, Gadolinium, Gallium, Germanium, Gold, Hafnium, Holmium Hydrogen, Indium, Iodine, Iridium, Iron, Lanthanum, Lead, Lithium, Lutetium, Manganese, Mercury, Molybdenum, Neodymium, Nickel,

| | | |
|---|---|---|
| Calories 40 | | |
| Total Fat 0 | | |
| Total Carbohydrates | 9g | |
|    Dietary Fibers | 0 | |
|    Sugars | 9g | |
| Sodium | 0g | |
| Protein | 0g | |
| Vitamin A (as palmitate beta carotene) | 10,000 IU | 200% |
| Vitamin C (as ascorbic acid) | 1,000 mg | 1667% |
| Vitamin D3 (as cholecalciferol) | 200 IU | 50% |
| Vitamin E (as d-alphatocopheryl) | 200 IU | 667% |
| Vitamin K (as menadione) | 30mg | 38% |
| Thiamin (as mononitrate) | 30mg | 2000% |
| Riboflavin (as 5-phosphate) | 30mg | 1765% |
| Niacin (as niacinamide) | 30mg | 150% |
| Vitamin B-6 (as pyridoxine hydrochloride) | 30mg | 1500% |
| Floic Acid | 400 mcg | 100% |
| Vitamin B-12 (as cyanocobalamin) | 500mcg | 8333% |
| Biotin | 300mcg | 100% |
| Pantothenic Acid (as pantothenol) | 150 mg | 1000% |
| Calcium | 600 mg | 60% |
|    (as citrate, di calcium phosphate dihydrate) | | |
| Iron (as gluconate) | 4mg | 22% |
| Magnesium (as citrate) | 300mg | 75% |
| Zinc (as gluconate) | 15mg | 100% |
| Selenium (as methionine) | 100mcg | 143% |
| Copper (as gluconate) | 1mg | 50% |
| Manganese (as gluconate) | 5mg | 250% |
| Chromium (as polynicotinate) | 200mcg | 167% |
| Potassium (as citrate) | 100mg | 3% |
| Choline (as pitartrate) | 30mg | * |
| Inositol | 30mg | * |
| Boron (as amino acid complex) | 1mg | * |
| Amino Acid Mix | 125 mg | * |
|    (proprietary Formula-alanine, arginine, aspartic acid, cystine, glutamic acid, glycine, histidine, isoleucine, leucine, lysine, methionine, phenylalanine, proline, serine, threonine, tryptophan, tyrosine, valine) | | |
| Grape Seed (vitis vinifera)    p.e.**4:1 | 25 mg | * |
| CoEnzyme Q-10 | 5mg | * |
| Dimethylglycine | 25mg | * |
| Para-Amino Benzoic Acid | 30mg | * |
| Bioflavonids | 13mg | * |
| Plant Derived Minerals | 14.175mL | * |
| GDL (glucono delta lactone) | 150mg | * |

. percent daily value based on 2000 calorie diet
* daily value not established.
** standardized plant extract.

---

Niobium, Nitrogen, Osmium, Oxygen, Palladium, Platinum, Praseodymium, Rhenium, Rhodium, Rubidium, Ruthenium, Samarium, Scandium, Selenium, Silicon, Silver, Strontium, Tantalum, Tellurium, Terbium, Thallium, Thorium, Thulium, Tin, Titanium, Tungsten, Vanadium, Ytterbium, Yttrium, Zinc, Zirconium.

---

### Ultimate Classic

**Description:** With today's active lifestyle, almost all of us are lacking essential nutrients such as amino acids, vitamins and minerals. American Longevity's Majestic Earth Ultimate line of liquids is formulated to feed your body those vital nutrients. The unique properties of Majestic Earth Ultimate make it the ultimate in absorption and completeness. It's so completely loaded with up to 77 minerals and other nutrients such as bioflavinoids and grape seed extract that virtually no other supplementation is needed. This great product is available in the Classic or great tasting Tangy Tangerine flavor. Give your body the ultimate fuel with that Majestic Earth Ultimate line of liquids.

**Supplement Facts:**
[See table above]

**Other Ingredients:** Purified water, vegetable glycerin, sodium, erythorbate, citrate acid, malic acid, span 60, tween 80, natural orange flavor, natural berry flavor, potassium sorbate, sodium benzoate.

**Directions:**
1) Store in cool environment after opening.
2) As with any nutritional supplement program, seek advice of your health care professional.

**Warnings:**

Keep out of reach of children

For dietary supplement use only

Refrigerate after opening

*Continued on next page*

## Ultimate Classic—Cont.

**Suggested Use:**
Adults mix 1 fluid ounce per of 100 lbs body weight, 1 to 2 times daily. Children 1 teaspoon daily per 20lbs body weight. Not to exceed 1 fluid ounce.

---

## Awareness Corporation

**1201 SOUTH ALMA SCHOOL ROAD**
**SUITE 4750**
**MESA, AZ 85210-1112**

**Direct Inquiries to:**
1-800-69AWARE
www.awarenesshealth.com

### AWARENESS CLEAR™

**\*Description:** Helps with Candida, mold, and general microbial conditions.

**Ingredients:** Proprietary blend of Green Hull Black Walnut, Cloves, Pumpkin Seed, Gentian Root, Hyssop, Black Seed, Cramp Bark, Peppermint Leaf, Thyme Leaf, Fennel, Grapefruit Seed

**Directions:** Take 2 capsules each morning on an empty stomach, 1–2 hours before eating with 1 glass of water, for a minimum of 90 days.

**Warnings:** Do not use if Pregnant or Breastfeeding. Stop product if you experience allergic reaction. Keep out of reach of children.

**How Supplied:** 30 Capsules (Vegetarian) per Bottle

*These statements have not been evaluated by the Food and Drug Administration. These products are not intended to diagnose, treat, cure, or prevent any disease.
*Shown in Product Identification Guide, page 503*

---

### AWARENESS FEMALE BALANCE™

**\*Description:** To help with symptoms from Menopause and PMS. 75 year old Mediterranean product.

**Ingredients:** Black Cohosh Root, Cramp Bark, Squaw Vine, King Solomon Seed, Valerian Root, Dandelion Root, Chaste Tree Berry, Rosemary Leaves Caraway Seeds (Black Seed), Queen of the Meadow, Epimedium Leaf, Chuanxiong Rhizome, Schizandra Berry, Peppermint leaves, Red Raspberry leaves.

**Directions:** Menopause: take 1 or 2 capsules morning and evening with 1 glass of water PMS: take approx 7 days before and during menstruation.

**Warning:** Do not use this product if you are pregnant or breastfeeding. Consult your doctor prior to using this product if you are taking any medication. Keep out of reach of children.

**How Supplied:** 90 Capsules (Vegetarian) per Bottle

*These statements have not been evaluated by the Food and Drug Administration. These products are not intended to diagnose, treat, cure, or prevent any disease.
*Shown in Product Identification Guide, page 503*

---

### DIABETIC BALANCE™

**\*Description:** a 100% natural dietary supplement formulated to nourish the body

**Ingredients:** Proprietary blend of Sage Leaves, Horsetail, Mullein, Coriander Seed, Black Seed, Corn Silk, Neem Leaves, Gymnema Sylvestre, Bitter Melon, Fenugreek, Guava Leaves, Bilberry, Mulberry Leaves, Olive Leaves

**Directions:** Only take this product with water. Take 1 or 2 capsules in the morning, and 1 or 2 capsules before bed time. Monitor your blood sugar level on a daily basis to adjust your dosage accordingly. Contact your healthcare practitioner for further advice.

**Warning:** Do not use if pregnant or breast-feeding. Keep out of reach of children. Consult your doctor prior to using this product if you are taking any medication.

**How Supplied:** 60 Capsules (Vegetarian) per Bottle.

*These statements have not been evaluated by the Food and Drug Administration. This product is not intended to diagnose, treat, cure, or prevent any disease.
European Nutraceuticals Research
1-800-726-1569
550 W. Baseline Road
Suite 102-347
Mesa, Arizona 85210
www.diabeticbalance.com

---

### EXPERIENCE™

**\*Description:** Known to help with weight loss, energy, known to improve overall digestions and regularity. 100 year old Mediterranean Natural Product.

**Ingredients:** Proprietary blend of psyllium seed husk, king solomon seed, rhubarb, fennel seed, corn silk, and kelp

**Directions:** Take 1 to 3 Capsules before bedtime with a full glass of water. Or for faster results take 20 minutes after each meal.

**Warning:** Do not use if pregnant or breast-feeding or if you have colitis. Keep out of reach of children.

**How Supplied:** 90 Capsules (Vegetarian) per Bottle

*These statements have not been evaluated by the Food and Drug Administration. These products are not intended to diagnose, treat, cure, or prevent any disease.
*Shown in Product Identification Guide, page 503*

---

## Bayer Corporation Consumer Care Division

**36 COLUMBIA ROAD**
**P.O. BOX 1910**
**MORRISTOWN, NJ 07962-1910**

**Direct Inquiries to:**
Consumer Relations
(800) 331-4536
www.bayercare.com

**For Medical Emergency Contact:**
Bayer Corporation
Consumer Care Division
(800) 331-4536

### FERGON®
**Ferrous Gluconate**
**Iron Supplement**
**High Potency**

Fergon Tablets are for use as a dietary iron supplement.

**Directions:** Adults: One tablet daily, with food.

Serving Size: One tablet

|  | Amount Per Serving | % Daily Value |
|---|---|---|
| Iron | 27 mg | 150% |

**Ingredients:** Ferrous Gluconate Sucrose, Corn Starch, Hydroxypropyl Methylcellulose, Talc, Maltodextrin, Magnesium Stearate, Silicon Dioxide, Titanium Dioxide, Polyethylene Glycol, FD&C Yellow #5 Aluminum Lake (tartrazine), FD&C Blue #1 Aluminum Lake, Polysorbate 80, Carnauba Wax.
**AVOID EXCESSIVE HEAT**
**USP:** Fergon meets the USP standards for strength, quality, and purity.

**Warning:** Accidental overdose of iron-containing products is a leading cause of fatal poisoning in children under 6. Keep this product out of reach of children. In case of accidental overdose, call a doctor or Poison Control Center immediately.

**If pregnant or breast feeding, ask a health professional before use.**

**How Supplied:** Bottle of 100 Easy to Swallow Tablets
*USE ONLY IF SEAL UNDER BOTTLE CAP WITH BLUE "Bayer Corporation" PRINT IS INTACT*
**Questions? Comments?**
Please call 1-800-331-4536.
**Visit our website at**
**www.bayercare.com**
Bayer Corporation
Consumer Care Division
Morristown, NJ 07960 USA
*Shown in Product Identification Guide, page 504*

---

## FLINTSTONES® COMPLETE
**Children's Chewable Multivitamin/ Multimineral Supplement**

**Directions:** 2 & 3 years of age —**Chew** one-half tablet daily. Adults and children 4 years of age and older—**Chew** one tablet daily.

Serving Size: $1/2$ tablet (2 & 3 years of age); 1 tablet (4 years of age and older)

| Amount Per Tablet | % Daily Value for Children 2 & 3 Years of Age ($^1/_2$ Tablet) | % Daily Value for Adults and Children 4 Years of Age and older (1 Tablet) |
|---|---|---|
| Vitamin A | | |
| 5000 IU | 100% | 100% |
| Vitamin C 60 mg | 75% | 100% |
| Vitamin D 400 IU | 50% | 100% |
| Vitamin E 30 IU | 150% | 100% |
| Thiamin (B₁) | | |
| 1.5 mg | 107% | 100% |
| Riboflavin (B₂) | | |
| 1.7 mg | 106% | 100% |
| Niacin 20 mg | 111% | 100% |
| Vitamin B₆ 2 mg | 143% | 100% |
| Folic Acid | | |
| 400 mcg | 100% | 100% |
| Vitamin B₁₂ | | |
| 6 mcg | 100% | 100% |
| Biotin 40 mcg | 13% | 13% |
| Pantothenic Acid | | |
| 10 mg | 100% | 100% |
| Calcium | 6% | 10% |
| (elemental) | | |
| 100 mg | | |
| Iron | | |
| 18 mg | 90% | 100% |
| Phosphorus | | |
| 100 mg | 6% | 10% |
| Iodine 150 mcg | 107% | 100% |
| Magnesium | | |
| 20 mg | 5% | 5% |
| Zinc 15 mg | 94% | 100% |
| Copper 2 mg | 100% | 100% |

**Ingredients:**
Dicalcium Phosphate, Sorbitol, Magnesium Phosphate, Sodium Ascorbate, Gelatin, Ferrous Fumarate, Natural and Artificial Flavors (including fruit acids), Starch, Stearic Acid, Vitamin E Acetate, Carrageenan, Magnesium Stearate, Niacinamide, Zinc Oxide, Hydrogenated Vegetable Oil, Calcium Pantothenate, FD&C Red #40 Lake, FD&C Yellow #6 Lake, Xylitol, Aspartame* (a sweetener), FD&C Blue #2 Lake, Cupric Oxide, Pyridoxine Hydrochloride, Vitamin A Acetate, Riboflavin, Thiamine Mononitrate, Monoammonium Glycyrrhizinate, Beta Carotene, Folic Acid, Potassium Iodide, Vitamin D, Biotin, Magnesium Oxide, Vitamin B₁₂. **PHENYLKETONURICS: CONTAINS PHENYLALANINE.**

> **Warning:** Accidental overdose of iron-containing products is a leading cause of fatal poisoning in children under 6. Keep this product out of reach of children. In case of accidental overdose, call a doctor or Poison Control Center immediately.

**KEEP OUT OF REACH OF CHILDREN.**

**How Supplied:** Bottles of 60s.
THE FLINTSTONES and all related characters and elements are trademarks of Hanna-Barbera © 2000.
*Shown in Product Identification Guide, page 504*

---

## MY FIRST FLINTSTONES®
**Children's Multivitamin Supplement**

#1 Pediatricians' Choice
For children's chewable vitamins
• Specially formulated for children 2 and 3 years of age.
• Provides 10 essential vitamins, including A, D, and C, important for your child's healthy growth and development.
• Small, easy to chew tablets
• **GREAT TASTING** flavors
• **FUN CHARACTER SHAPES**
**THE NUTRIENTS NEEDED TO GROW-UP STRONG AND HEALTHY.**
**B VITAMINS**
Aid in the release of energy from food*.
**VITAMIN C**
Helps support the immune system.*
**VITAMIN D**
Helps absorption of Calcium for strong bones and teeth.*

---

*These statements have not been evaluated by the FDA. This product is not intended to diagnose, treat, cure, or prevent any disease.

**Directions:** Children 2–3 years of age – **Chew** one tablet daily. Tablet should be fully chewed or crushed for children who cannot chew.

Serving Size: One tablet

| | Amount Per Tablet | % Daily Value for Children 2 & 3 Years of Age |
|---|---|---|
| Vitamin A | 2500 IU | 100% |
| Vitamin C | 60 mg | 150% |
| Vitamin D | 400 IU | 100% |
| Vitamin E | 15 IU | 150% |
| Thiamin (B₁) | 1.05 mg | 150% |
| Riboflavin (B₂) | 1.2 mg | 150% |
| Niacin | 13.5 mg | 150% |
| Vitamin B₆ | 1.05 mg | 150% |
| Folic Acid | 300 mcg | 150% |
| Vitamin B₁₂ | 4.5 mcg | 150% |

**Ingredients:** Sucrose (a natural sweetener), Sodium Ascorbate, Stearic Acid, Invert Sugar, Artificial Flavors (including fruit acids), Gelatin, Vitamin E Acetate, Niacinamide, FD&C Red #40 Lake, FD&C Yellow #6 Lake, FD&C Blue #2 Lake, Pyridoxine Hydrochloride, Riboflavin, Thiamine Mononitrate, Vitamin A Acetate, Folic Acid, Beta Carotene, Vitamin D, Vitamin B₁₂.
**USP:** My First Flintstones formula meets the USP standards for strength, quality, and purity for Oil- and Water-soluble Vitamins Tablets. Complies with USP Method 2: Vitamins A, D, E, B12, Thiamin, Riboflavin, Niacin, and B6.
**Keep out of reach of children.**

**How Supplied:** Flintstones in bottles of 60 Chewable Tablets.
THE FLINTSTONES and all related characters and elements are trademarks of and © Hanna-Barbera.
(s01)
*Questions or comments?*
Please call 1-800-800-4793.
**Visit our website at**
**www.bayercare.com**
Bayer Corporation Consumer Care Division
36 Columbia Road
P.O. Box 1910
Morristown, NJ 07962-1910
*Shown in Product Identification Guide, page 504*

---

## ONE-A-DAY® ACTIVE DIETARY SUPPLEMENT
**Energy enhancing multivitamin tailored for active lifestyles—Feel your best**

*Complete with 32 ingredients formulated to help you keep up with your active lifestyle.*
• More Ginseng than any leading multivitamin.
• More cell protective antioxidants Vitamin C and E plus Beta Carotene and Selenium.*
• More essential B vitamins for energy metabolism plus Chromium to help your body regulate fuel stores for energy.*

---

*These statements have not been evaluated by the Food and Drug Administration. This product is not intended to diagnose, treat, cure, or prevent any disease.

**Directions:** Adults: One tablet daily, with food.

*Continued on next page*

## One-A-Day Active—Cont.

Serving Size: One tablet

| | Amount Per Serving | % Daily Value |
|---|---|---|
| Vitamin A | 5000 IU | 100% |
| Vitamin C | 120 mg | 200% |
| Vitamin D | 400 IU | 100% |
| Vitamin E | 60 IU | 200% |
| Vitamin K | 25 mcg | 31% |
| Thiamin ($B_1$) | 4.5 mg | 300% |
| Riboflavin ($B_2$) | 5.1 mg | 300% |
| Niacin | 40 mg | 200% |
| Vitamin $B_6$ | 6 mg | 300% |
| Folic Acid | 400 mcg | 100% |
| Vitamin $B_{12}$ | 18 mcg | 300% |
| Biotin | 40 mcg | 13% |
| Pantothenic Acid | 10 mg | 100% |
| Calcium (elemental) | 110 mg | 11% |
| Iron | 9 mg | 50% |
| Phosphorus | 48 mg | 4% |
| Iodine | 150 mcg | 100% |
| Magnesium | 40 mg | 10% |
| Zinc | 15 mg | 100% |
| Selenium | 45 mcg | 64% |
| Copper | 2 mg | 100% |
| Manganese | 2 mg | 100% |
| Chromium | 100 mcg | 83% |
| Molybdenum | 25 mcg | 33% |
| Chloride | 180 mg | 5% |
| Potassium | 200 mg | 5% |
| Nickel | 5 mcg | * |
| Tin | 10 mcg | * |
| Silicon | 6 mg | * |
| Vanadium | 10 mcg | * |
| Boron | 150 mcg | * |
| American Ginseng Standardized Extract (Panax quinquefolius) (root) | 55 mg | * |

*Daily Value not established

**Ingredients:** Potassium Chloride, Dicalcium Phosphate, Ascorbic Acid, Calcium Carbonate, Cellulose, Gelatin, Magnesium Oxide, dl-alpha Tocopheryl Acetate, American Ginseng Extract, Niacinamide, Ferrous Fumarate, Croscarmellose Sodium, Silicon Dioxide, Zinc Oxide, Stearic Acid, Hydroxypropyl Methylcellulose, Dextrin, d-Calcium Pantothenate, Pyridoxine Hydrochloride, Magnesium Stearate, Acacia, Manganese Sulfate, Riboflavin, Titanium Dioxide, Thiamine Mononitrate, Polyethylene Glycol, FD&C Yellow #6 Lake, Starch, FD&C Red #40 Lake, Mannitol, Cupric Oxide, Resin, Dextrose, Lecithin, Beta Carotene, Vitamin A Acetate, Sodium Borate, Potassium Borate, Chromium Chloride, FD&C Blue #2 Lake, Folic Acid, Potassium Iodide, Sodium Selenate, Sodium Molybdate, Sodium Metavanadate, d-Biotin, Sodium Metasilicate, Phytonadione, Nickelous Sulfate, Cyanocobalamin, Stannous Chloride, Ergocalciferol.

**USP:** One-A-Day Active formula meets the USP standards of strength, quality, and purity for Oil- and Water-Soluble Vitamins with Minerals Tablets.†

---

**WARNING:** Accidental overdose of iron-containing products is a leading cause of fatal poisoning in children under 6. Keep this product out of reach of children. In case of accidental overdose, call a doctor or Poison Control Center immediately.

**If pregnant or breast-feeding, ask a health professional before use.**
†Complies with USP-Method 2: Vitamins A, D, E, Biotin, Ascorbic Acid, $B_{12}$, Thiamin, Riboflavin, Niacin, and $B_6$; Method 3: Pantothenic Acid.

**How Supplied:** Bottle of 50 Tablets.
Questions? Comments?
Please call 1-800-800-4793.
Visit out website at www.oneaday.com
Distributed by:
Bayer Corporation
P.O. Box 1910
Morristown, NJ 07962-1910
*Shown in Product Identification Guide, page 504*

---

## ONE-A-DAY® ENERGY FORMULA
**Dietary Supplement**

**Directions:** Adults (18 years and older): Take one tablet daily, with food.

Serving Size: One Tablet

| | AMOUNT PER SERVING | % DAILY VALUE |
|---|---|---|
| Thiamin ($B_1$) | 2.25 mg | 150% |
| Niacin | 20 mg | 100% |
| Vitamin $B_6$ | 3 mg | 150% |
| Folic Acid | 200 mcg | 50% |
| Pantothenic Acid | 10 mg | 100% |
| Chromium (as Picolinate) | 100 mcg | 83% |
| American Ginseng Standardized Extract (Panax quinquefolius) (root) | 200 mg | * |

*Daily Value not established.

**Ingredients:** Calcium Carbonate, American Ginseng Extract, Cellulose, Maltodextrin, Hydroxypropyl Methylcellulose, Nicotinic Acid, Croscarmellose Sodium, d-Calcium Pantothenate, Crospovidone, Stearic Acid, Silicon Dioxide, Titanium Dioxide, Pyridoxine Hydrochloride, Magnesium Stearate, Starch, Thiamine Mononitrate, Hydroxypropyl Cellulose, Acacia, Polyethylene Glycol, FD&C Yellow #6 Lake, Chromium Picolinate, FD&C Blue #1 Lake, Folic Acid, Polysorbate 80.

**Warnings:** Seek the advice of a health professional before use if you are taking medication for high blood pressure or anticoagulation (blood-thinning) or if you have diabetes. **Do Not Use If Pregnant or Breast-feeding.** If using for more than 6 months, consult your doctor. Before any surgery, ask your doctor about continued use of this product. Keep out of reach of children.

**How Supplied:** Bottles of 30.

---

## ONE-A-DAY® KIDS COMPLETE
**BUGS BUNNY AND FRIENDS SUGAR FREE**
**CHILDREN'S MULTIVITAMIN/MULTIMINERAL SUPPLEMENT**

**Complete with 19 essential vitamins and minerals, including Vitamin C, Iron, and Calcium for your child's healthy growth and development.**

**Directions:** 2 & 3 years of age—**Chew** one-half tablet daily. Adults and children 4 years of age and older—**Chew** one tablet daily.

Serving Size: ½ tablet – (2 & 3 years of age); 1 tablet – (4 years of age and older)
[See table at top of next page]

**Ingredients:** Dicalcium Phosphate, Sorbitol, Magnesium Phosphate, Sodium Ascorbate, Gelatin, Ferrous Fumarate, Natural and Artificial Flavors (including fruit acids), Starch, Stearic Acid, FD&C Red #40 Lake, Vitamin E Acetate, Carrageenan, Niacinamide, Magnesium Stearate, Hydrogenated Vegetable Oil, Zinc Oxide, FD&C Yellow #6 Lake, FD&C Blue #2 Lake, Calcium Pantothenate, Aspartame** (a sweetener), Cupric Oxide, Pyridoxine Hydrochloride, Vitamin A Acetate, Riboflavin, Thiamine Mononitrate, Beta Carotene, Folic Acid, Potassium Iodide, Vitamin D, Biotin, Magnesium Oxide, Vitamin $B_{12}$.

** PHENYLKETONURICS: CONTAINS PHENYLALANINE**

WARNING: Accidental overdose of iron-containing products is a leading cause of fatal poisoning in children under 6. Keep this product out of reach of children. In case of accidental overdose, call a doctor or Poison Control Center immediately.

**USP:** Bugs Bunny Complete formula meets the USP standards for strength, quality, and purity for Oil- and Water-soluble Vitamins and Minerals Tablets.†

†Complies with USP Method 2: Vitamins A, D, E, Biotin, B12, Thiamin, Riboflavin, Niacin, and B6; Method 3: Pantothenic Acid.

**How Supplied:** Contains 60 chewable tablets

Cartoon Network and logo are trademarks of Cartoon Network ©2001

LOONEY TUNES, characters, names and all related indicia are trademarks of Warner Bros. ©2001.

| Amount Per Tablet | % Daily Value for Children 2 & 3 Years of Age (½ Tablet) | % Daily Value for Adults and Children 4 Years of Age and Older (1 Tablet) |
|---|---|---|
| Calories 3 | | |
| Total Carbohydrates <1g | † | 4%* |
| Sugars <1g | † | † |
| Vitamin A 5000 IU | 100% | 100% |
| Vitamin C 60 mg | 75% | 100% |
| Vitamin D 400 IU | 50% | 100% |
| Vitamin E 30 IU | 150% | 100% |
| Thiamin (B₁) 1.5 mg | 107% | 100% |
| Riboflavin (B₂) 1.7 mg | 106% | 100% |
| Niacin 20 mg | 111% | 100% |
| Vitamin B₆ 2 mg | 143% | 100% |
| Folic Acid 400 mcg | 100% | 100% |
| Vitamin B₁₂ 6 mcg | 100% | 100% |
| Biotin 40 mcg | 13% | 13% |
| Pantothenic Acid 10 mg | 100% | 100% |
| Calcium (elemental) 100 mg | 6% | 10% |
| Iron 18 mg | 90% | 100% |
| Phosphorus 100 mg | 6% | 10% |
| Iodine 150 mcg | 107% | 100% |
| Magnesium 20 mg | 5% | 5% |
| Zinc 15 mg | 94% | 100% |
| Copper 2 mg | 100% | 100% |

\* Percent Daily Values are based on a 2,000 calorie diet.
† Daily Value not established.

WARNING: Accidental overdose of iron-containing products is a leading cause of fatal poisoning in children under 6. Keep this product out of reach of children. In case of accidental overdose, call a doctor or Poison Control Center immediately.

Scooby-Doo Complete formula meets the USP standards for strength, quality, and purity for Oil- and Water-soluble Vitamins and Minerals Tablets.†
**KEEP OUT OF THE REACH OF CHILDREN**

**How Supplied:** ONE-A-DAY® KIDS COMPLETE SCOOBY-DOO contains 50 chewable tablets.
SCOOBY-DOO, characters, names and all related indicia are trademarks of Hanna-Barbera © 2001.
CARTOON NETWORK and logo are trademarks of Cartoon Network © 2001

† Complies with USP Method 2: Vitamins A, D, E, Biotin, B12, Thiamin, Riboflavin, Niacin, and B6; Method 3: Pantothenic Acid.

*Shown in Product Identification Guide, page 504*

## ONE-A-DAY® KIDS COMPLETE SCOOBY-DOO!™
### CHILDREN'S MULTIVITAMIN/ MULTIMINERAL SUPPLEMENT

**Provides 19 essential vitamins and minerals, including Vitamin C, Iron, and Calcium for your child's healthy growth and development.**

**Directions:** 2 & 3 years of age—**Chew** one-half tablet daily. Adults and children 4 years of age and older—**Chew** one tablet daily.
Serving Size: ½ tablet (2 & 3 years of age); 1 tablet (4 years of age and older) [See table below]

**Ingredients:** Dicalcium Phosphate, Sorbitol, Magnesium Phosphate, Sodium Ascorbate, Gelatin, Ferrous Fumarate, Natural and Artificial Flavors (including fruit acids), Starch, Stearic Acid, Vitamin E Acetate, Carrageenan, Magnesium Stearate, Niacinamide, Zinc Oxide, Hydrogenated Vegetable Oil, Calcium Pantothenate, FD&C Red #40 Lake, FD&C Yellow #6 Lake, Xylitol, Aspartame* (a sweetener), FD&C Blue #2 Lake, Cupric Oxide, Pyridoxine Hydrochloride, Vitamin A Acetate, Riboflavin, Thiamine Mononitrate, Monoammonium Glycyrrhizinate, Beta Carotene, Folic Acid, Potassium Iodide, Vitamin D, Biotin, Magnesium Oxide, Vitamin B₁₂.

**\*PHENYLKETONURICS: CONTAINS PHENYLALANINE**

| Amount Per Tablet | % Daily Value for Children 2 & 3 Years of Age (½ Tablet) | % Daily Value for Adults and Children 4 Years of Age and older (1 Tablet) |
|---|---|---|
| Vitamin A 5000 IU | 100% | 100% |
| Vitamin C 60 mg | 75% | 100% |
| Vitamin D 400 IU | 50% | 100% |
| Vitamin E 30 IU | 150% | 100% |
| Thiamin (B₁) 1.5 mg | 107% | 100% |
| Riboflavin (B₂) 1.7 mg | 106% | 100% |
| Niacin 20 mg | 111% | 100% |
| Vitamin B₆ 2 mg | 143% | 100% |
| Folic Acid 400 mcg | 100% | 100% |
| Vitamin B₁₂ 6 mcg | 100% | 100% |
| Biotin 40 mcg | 13% | 13% |
| Pantothenic Acid 10 mg | 100% | 100% |
| Calcium (elemental) 100 mg | 6% | 10% |
| Iron 18 mg | 90% | 100% |
| Phosphorus 100 mg | 6% | 10% |
| Iodine 150 mcg | 107% | 100% |
| Magnesium 20 mg | 5% | 5% |
| Zinc 15 mg | 94% | 100% |
| Copper 2 mg | 100% | 100% |

## ONE-A-DAY® KIDS PLUS CALCIUM SCOOBY-DOO
### CHILDREN'S MULTIVITAMIN SUPPLEMENT

**Provides 10 essential vitamins plus calcium for your child's healthy growth and development. Contains as much calcium as one 5 oz glass of milk.**

**Directions:** Adults and children 2 years of age and older—**Chew** one tablet daily.

Serving Size: One tablet

| Amount Per Tablet | % Daily Value for Children 2 & 3 Years of Age | % Daily Value for Adults and Children 4 Years of Age and older |
|---|---|---|
| Vitamin A 2500 IU | 100% | 50% |
| Vitamin C 60 mg | 150% | 100% |
| Vitamin D 400 IU | 100% | 100% |
| Vitamin E 15 IU | 150% | 50% |
| Thiamin (B₁) 1.05 mg | 150% | 70% |
| Riboflavin (B₂) 1.2 mg | 150% | 70% |
| Niacin 13.5 mg | 150% | 67% |
| Vitamin B₆ 1.05 mg | 150% | 52% |

*Continued on next page*

## One-A-Day Kids Plus—Cont.

| | | |
|---|---|---|
| Folic Acid | | |
| 300 mcg | 150% | 75% |
| Vitamin B$_{12}$ | | |
| 4.5 mcg | 150% | 75% |
| Calcium (elemental) | | |
| 200 mg | 25% | 20% |

**Ingredients:** Calcium Carbonate, Sorbitol, Starch, Sodium Ascorbate, Natural and Artificial Flavors (including fruit acids), Stearic Acid, Gelatin, Magnesium Stearate, Vitamin E Acetate, Niacinamide, FD&C Red #40 Lake, FD&C Yellow #6 Lake, Aspartame* (a sweetener), FD&C Blue #2 Lake, Pyridoxine Hydrochloride, Riboflavin, Thiamine Mononitrate, Vitamin A Acetate, Monoammonium Glycyrrhizinate, Folic Acid, Beta Carotene, Vitamin D, Vitamin B$_{12}$.

* **PHENYLKETONURICS: CONTAINS PHENYLALANINE**
**Keep out of reach of children**
USP: Scooby-Doo Plus Calcium formula meets the USP standards for strength, quality, and purity for Oil- and Water-soluble Vitamins and Minerals Tablets.†

† Complies with USP Method 2: Vitamins A, D, E, B12, Thiamin, Riboflavin, Niacin, and B6.

**How Supplied:** Contains 50 Chewable Tablets.
SCOOBY-DOO, characters, names and all related indicia are trademarks of Hanna-Barbera ©2001.
CARTOON NETWORK and logo are trademarks of Cartoon Network ©2001
*Questions or comments?*
Please call 1-800-800-4793.
Visit our website at www.oneaday.com
Made in U.S.A.
Bayer Corporation
Consumer Care Division
P.O. Box 1910
Morristown, NJ 07962-1910 USA
*Shown in Product Identification Guide, page 504*

## ONE-A-DAY® MEMORY & CONCENTRATION
**Dietary Supplement**

**Directions:** Adults (18 years and older): Take one to two tablets daily, with food.

Serving Size: 1 Tablet

| | Amount Per Serving | % Daily Value |
|---|---|---|
| Vitamin B$_6$ | 1 mg | 50% |
| Vitamin B$_{12}$ | 3 mcg | 50% |
| Choline | 30 mg | * |
| Ginkgo Biloba Extract (*Ginkgo biloba*) (leaf) | 60 mg | * |

(Standardized to 24% Ginkgo Flavone Glycosides and 6% Terpene Lactones)

*Daily Value (DV) not established.

**Ingredients:** Calcium Carbonate, Cellulose, Choline Bitartrate, Ginkgo Biloba Leaf Extract, Maltodextrin, Hydroxypropyl Methylcellulose, Polyethylene Glycol, Silicon Dioxide, Croscarmellose Sodium, Magnesium Stearate, Acacia, Titanium Dioxide, Crospovidone, FD&C Yellow #5 (Tartrazine) Lake, Starch, Hydroxypropyl Cellulose, Pyridoxine Hydrochloride, Resin, FD&C Yellow #6 Lake, Polysorbate 80, Cyanocobalamin.

**Warnings:** Do not take this product, without first consulting a health professional, if you are taking medication for anticoagulation (thinning the blood). **If you are pregnant or breast-feeding, ask a health professional before use.** Before any surgery ask your doctor about continued use of this product. Keep out of reach of children.

**How Supplied:** Bottles of 30.

## ONE-A-DAY® MEN'S MULTIVITAMIN/MULTIMINERAL SUPPLEMENT

**Directions:** Adults: One tablet daily with food.

**Serving Size: One Tablet**

| | AMOUNT PER SERVING | | % DAILY VALUE |
|---|---|---|---|
| Vitamin A | 5000 | IU | 100% |
| Vitamin C | 90 | mg | 150% |
| Vitamin D | 400 | IU | 100% |
| Vitamin E | 45 | IU | 150% |
| Thiamin (B$_1$) | 2.25 | mg | 150% |
| Riboflavin (B$_2$) | 2.55 | mg | 150% |
| Niacin | 20 | mg | 100% |
| Vitamin B$_6$ | 3 | mg | 150% |
| Folic Acid | 400 | mcg | 100% |
| Vitamin B$_{12}$ | 9 | mcg | 150% |
| Pantothenic Acid | 10 | mg | 100% |
| Iodine | 150 | mcg | 100% |
| Magnesium | 100 | mg | 25% |
| Zinc | 15 | mg | 100% |
| Selenium | 87.5 | mcg | 125% |
| Copper | 2 | mg | 100% |
| Manganese | 3.5 | mg | 175% |
| Chromium | 150 | mcg | 125% |
| Molybdenum | 42 | mcg | 56% |
| Chloride | 34 | mg | 1% |
| Potassium | 37.5 | mg | 1% |

**Ingredients:** Magnesium Oxide, Dicalcium Phosphate, Niacinamide Ascorbate, Potassium Chloride, Gelatin, dl-Alpha Tocopheryl Acetate, Zinc Sulfate, Cellulose, Ascorbic Acid, Croscarmellose Sodium, Crospovidone, d-Calcium Pantothenate, Manganese Sulfate, Starch, Dextrin, Magnesium Stearate, Silicon Dioxide, Hydroxypropyl Methylcellulose, Titanium Dioxide, Cupric Sulfate, Pyridoxine Hydrochloride, Stearic Acid, Riboflavin, Polyethylene Glycol, Thiamine Mononitrate, Vitamin A Acetate, Dextrose, FD&C Yellow #6 Lake, Resin, Lecithin, Chromium Chloride, Beta Carotene, FD&C Yellow #5 (tartrazine) Lake, Folic Acid, Sodium Selenate, Potassium Iodide, Sodium Molybdate, FD&C Blue #2 Lake, Cholecalciferol, Cyanocobalamin.

**KEEP OUT OF REACH OF CHILDREN**

**How Supplied:** Bottles of 60's & 100's.

**USP:** One-A-Day Men's formula meets the USP standards of strength, quality, and purity for Oil- and Water-Soluble Vitamins with Minerals Tablets.†

*Questions or comments?*
Please call 1-800-800-4793.
Visit our website at www.oneaday.com
Distributed by:
Bayer Corporation
Consumer Care Division
P.O. Box 1910
Morristown, NJ 07962-1910 USA

## ONE-A-DAY® PROSTATE HEALTH
**Dietary Supplement**

**Directions:** Adults (18 years and older): Take two softgels daily, with food.

Serving Size: Two softgels

| | AMOUNT PER SERVING | % DAILY VALUE |
|---|---|---|
| Vitamin E | 9 IU | 30% |
| Zinc | 15 mg | 100% |
| Selenium | 35 mcg | 50% |
| Saw Palmetto Standardized Extract (*Serenoa repens*) (fruit) | 320 mg | * |
| Lycopene (*Lycoperiscon esculentum*) (fruit) | 3 mg | * |

*Daily Value not established.

**Ingredients:** Saw Palmetto Berry Extract, Gelatin, Glycerin, Zinc Gluconate Chelate, Soybean Oil, Yellow Beeswax, Tomato Oleoresin, Dicalcium Phosphate, Lecithin, dl-Alpha Tocopheryl, Titanium Dioxide, FD&C Yellow #5 (tartrazine), FD&C Red #40, Sodium Selenate, FD&C Blue #1, FD&C Yellow #6

**Warnings:** If you are experiencing urinary problems, or are being treated for prostate problems, consult your doctor. Keep out of reach of children.

**How Supplied:** Bottles of 30.

## ONE-A-DAY® TENSION & MOOD
**Dietary Supplement**

**Directions:** Adults (18 years and older): Take one to two tablets daily with food. Do not exceed recommended dosage.

Serving Size: One Tablet

| | AMOUNT PER SERVING | % DAILY VALUE |
|---|---|---|
| Vitamin C | 60 mg | 100% |
| Thiamin (B1) | 1.125 mg | 75% |
| Niacin | 10 mg | 50% |
| Folic Acid | 100 mcg | 25% |
| Pantothenic Acid | 5 mg | 50% |
| Lecithin | 15 mg | * |
| Kava Kava Standardized Extract (*Piper methysticum*) (rhizome and root) | 100 mg | * |
| St. John's Wort Standardized Extract (*Hypericum perforatum*) (leaves and flowers) | 225 mg | * |

*Daily Value not established.

**Ingredients:** Dicalcium Phosphate, St. John's Wort Extract, Cellulose, Kava Kava Extract, Ascorbic Acid, Croscarmellose Sodium, Hydroxypropyl Methylcellulose, Crospovidone, Stearic Acid, Lecithin, Niacin, Silicon Dioxide, Magnesium Stearate, d-Calcium Pantothenate, Titanium Dioxide, Pharmaceutical Glaze, Polyethylene Glycol, Thiamine Mononitrate, Starch, Hydroxypropyl Cellulose, FD&C Yellow #5 (Tartrazine) Lake, FD&C Yellow #6 Lake, Polysorbate 80, Folic Acid, FD&C Blue #1 Lake, FD&C Red #40 Lake.

**Warnings:** Ask a doctor before use if you are presently or have been taking a monoamine oxidase inhibitor (MAOI) (certain drugs for depression, psychiatric or emotional conditions, or Parkinson's disease) in the past 2 weeks, or if you are taking any other prescription drug. May cause drowsiness. Do not take with alcohol, sedatives or tranquilizers. Use caution when driving a motor vehicle or operating machinery.

Before any surgery ask your doctor about continued use of this product. **Do not use if pregnant or breast-feeding.** Keep out of reach of children.

**How Supplied:** Bottles of 30.

---

**ONE-A-DAY® TODAY**
**Specially designed for ACTIVE WOMEN 50 and over**
**Dietary Supplement**

**Directions:** Adults: One tablet daily, with food.

Serving Size: One Tablet

| | Amount Per Serving | % Daily Value* |
|---|---|---|
| Vitamin A | 3000 IU | 129% |
| Vitamin C | 75 mg | 100% |
| Vitamin D† | 400 IU | 100% |
| Vitamin E | 33 IU | 100% |
| Vitamin K | 20 mcg | 22% |
| Thiamin (B₁) | 1.1 mg | 100% |
| Riboflavin (B₂) | 1.7 mg | 154% |
| Niacin | 14 mg | 100% |
| Vitamin B₆ | 3 mg | 200% |
| Folic Acid | 400 mcg | 100% |
| Vitamin B₁₂ | 18 mcg | 750% |
| Biotin | 30 mcg | 100% |
| Pantothenic Acid | 5 mg | 100% |
| Calcium (elemental) | 240 mg | 20% |
| Magnesium | 120 mg | 38% |
| Zinc | 15 mg | 187% |
| Selenium | 70 mcg | 127% |
| Copper | 2 mg | 222% |
| Manganese | 2 mg | 111% |
| Chromium | 120 mcg | 600% |
| Potassium | 100 mg | 3% |
| Soy Extract (*Glycine max.*) (Standardized to 40% Isoflavones) | 10 mg | ** |

*Percentages based upon Dietary Reference Intakes (DRIs) for women over 50, Food and Nutrition Board of the Institute of Medicine, 2001
†DRI for women over 70 is 600 IU.
**Daily Value not established

**Ingredients:** Calcium Carbonate, Magnesium Oxide, Potassium Chloride, Cellulose, Ascorbic Acid, dl-alpha Tocopheryl Acetate, Acacia, Croscarmellose Sodium, Zinc Oxide, Dicalcium Phosphate, Stearic Acid, Dextrin, Titanium Dioxide, Niacinamide, Silicon Dioxide, Hydroxypropyl Methylcellulose, Gelatin, Soy Extract, Magnesium Stearate, Calcium Silicate, d-Calcium Pantothenate, Manganese Sulfate, Polyethylene Glycol, Starch, Pyridoxine Hydrochloride, Mannitol, Cupric Oxide, Resin, Lecithin, Riboflavin, Thiamine Mononitrate, Vitamin A Acetate, Chromium Chloride, Folic Acid, Dextrose, Beta Carotene, FD&C Red #40 Lake, FD&C Blue #2 Lake, Sodium Selenate, Biotin, Phytonadione, Cyanocobalamin, Ergocalciferol.

**If pregnant or breast-feeding, ask a health professional before use.**

**USP:** One-A-Day Today Formula meets the USP standards of strength, quality, and purity for Oil- and Water-Soluble Vitamins with Minerals Tablets.†

**KEEP OUT OF REACH OF CHILDREN**
CHILD RESISTANT CAP
Do not use this product if safety seal bearing *SEALED for YOUR PROTECTION* under cap is torn or missing.

**How Supplied:** Bottles of 55 Tablets.

---

†Complies with USP-Method 2: Vitamins A, D, E, Ascorbic Acid, Biotin, B₁₂, Thiamin, Riboflavin, Niacin, and B₆; Method 3: Pantothenic Acid.

---

Questions or comments?
Please call 1-800-800-4793.
Visit our website at www.oneaday.com
Made in the U.S.A.
Distributed by:
Bayer Corporation
Consumer Care Division
P.O. Box 1910
Morristown, NJ 07962-1910 USA
*Shown in Product Identification Guide, page 504*

**ONE-A-DAY® WOMEN'S**
**Multivitamin/Multimineral Supplement**

**Directions:** Adults: One tablet daily with food.
Serving Size: One tablet

| | AMOUNT PER SERVING | | % DAILY VALUE |
|---|---|---|---|
| Vitamin A | 2500 | IU | 50% |
| Vitamin C | 60 | mg | 100% |
| Vitamin D | 400 | IU | 100% |
| Vitamin E | 30 | IU | 100% |
| Thiamine (B₁) | 1.5 | mg | 100% |
| Riboflavin (B₂) | 1.7 | mg | 100% |
| Niacin | 10 | mg | 50% |
| Vitamin B₆ | 2 | mg | 100% |
| Folic Acid | 400 | mcg | 100% |
| Vitamin B₁₂ | 6 | mcg | 100% |
| Pantothenic Acid | 5 | mg | 50% |
| Calcium (elemental) | 450 | mg | 45% |
| Iron | 18 | mg | 100% |
| Magnesium | 50 | mg | 12% |
| Zinc | 15 | mg | 100% |

**Ingredients:** Calcium Carbonate, Magnesium Oxide, Ascorbic Acid, Acacia, Ferrous Fumarate, Cellulose, dl-alpha Tocopheryl Acetate, Croscarmellose Sodium, Zinc Oxide, Magnesium Stearate, Titanium Dioxide, Dextrin, Hydroxypropyl Methylcellulose, Niacinamide, Gelatin, Starch, d-Calcium Pantothenate, Calcium Silicate, Polyethylene Glycol, Silicon Dioxide, Dextrose, Pyridoxine Hydrochloride, Lecithin, Riboflavin, Thiamine Mononitrate, Vitamin A Acetate, Resin, Folic Acid, Beta Carotene, FD&C Yellow #5 (tartrazine) Lake, FD&C Yellow #6 Lake, FD&C Blue #2 Lake, Cholecalciferol, Cyanocobalamin.

**USP:** One-A-Day Women's formula meets the USP standards of strength, quality, and purity for Oil- and Water-Soluble Vitamins with Minerals Tablets.

**Warning:** Accidental overdose of iron-containing products is a leading cause of fatal poisoning in children under 6. Keep this product out of reach of children. In case of accidental overdose, call a doctor or Poison Control Center immediately.

**KEEP OUT OF REACH OF CHILDREN**
**How Supplied:** Bottles of 60 and 100.

*Continued on next page*

## One-A-Day Women's—Cont.

Questions or comments?
Please call 1-800-800-4793.
Visit our website at www.oneaday.com
Distributed by:
Bayer Corporation
Consumer Care Division
P.O. Box 1910
Morristown, NJ 07962-1910 USA

---

## Beach Pharmaceuticals

**Division of Beach Products, Inc.**
**5220 SOUTH MANHATTAN AVE.**
**TAMPA, FL 33611**

**Direct Inquiries to:**
Richard Stephen Jenkins, Exec. V.P.:
(813) 839-6565

**BEELITH Tablets**
**MAGNESIUM SUPPLEMENT with PYRIDOXINE HCL**

**Description:** Each tablet contains magnesium oxide 600 mg and pyridoxine hydrochloride (Vitamin $B_6$) 25 mg equivalent to Vitamin $B_6$ 20 mg.

**Supplement Facts**
Serving Size: 1 Tablet

|  | Amount Per Tablet | % Daily Value |
|---|---|---|
| Magnesium | 362 mg | 90% |
| Vitamin $B_6$ | 20 mg | 1000% |

**Inactive Ingredients:** D&C Yellow No. 10, FD&C Yellow No. 6 (Sunset Yellow), hydroxypropylmethylcellulose, magnesium stearate, microcrystalline cellulose, polyethylene glycol, sodium starch glycolate, titanium dioxide, and water.

**Indications:** As a dietary supplement for patients with magnesium and/or Vitamin $B_6$ deficiencies resulting from malnutrition, alcoholism, magnesium depleting drugs, chemotherapy, and inadequate nutritional intake or absorption. Also, increases urinary magnesium levels.

**Dosage:** One tablet daily or as directed by a physician.

**Warnings:** Do not take this product if you are presently taking a prescription drug without consulting your physician or other health professional. If you have kidney disease, take only under the supervision of a physician. Excessive dosage may cause laxation. If pregnant or breast-feeding, ask a health professional before use. **KEEP OUT OF THE REACH OF CHILDREN.**

**How Supplied:** Golden yellow, film-coated tablet with the letters **BP** and the number **132** imprinted on each tablet. Packaged in bottles of 100 (NDC 0486-1132-01) tablets.

---

## Body Wise International Inc

**2802 DOW AVENUE**
**TUSTIN, CA 92780**

**For direct inquiries contact:**
Wellness Research Center:
Phone# (714) 505-6121
Fax# (714) 832-7247
Email: wellness@bodywise.com

**PRODUCT LISTING:**
**BETA-C™**

---
**CoENZYME Q10+™**

---
**FEMALE ADVANTAGE™**

---
**GLUCOMINE™**

---
**LEAN INDEX™ BARS AND SHAKES**

---
**MALE ADVANTAGE™**

---
**MEM X²™**

---
**OMEGA COMPLETE™**

---
**OXY-G²®**

---
**SUPER RESHAPE FORMULA®**

---
**St. JOHN'S COMPLEX™**

---
**SUPER CELL™**

---
**TIGER VITES™**

---
**WORKOUT FORMULA™**

---
**XTREME™**

---

**AG-IMMUNE™ CAPSULES**

We at Body Wise® believe this is the most powerful product ever created for the immune system. AG-Immune contains Ai/E10™, a patented and proprietary antigen infused bovine colostrum/whey extract. In addition, AG-Immune contains three important herbs: arabinogalactan, astragalus, and maitake mushroom D-fraction. This amazing product was designed to give your immune system the support it needs to deal with the poor nutrition, infections, trauma, toxins, and stress we encounter every day. When you support your immune system, you support your overall health.

**Highlighted Ingredients:**
**Ai/E¹⁰™**
**Chemistry**
Antigen Infused Bovine Colostrum/Whey Extract (Ai/E¹⁰™) is a complex extract that requires highly controlled conditions in order to attain the desired product. The process of extraction uses breakthrough technology to recover key immune factors to get the communication molecules. This is designed to maintain communication pathways the way no other product on the market can. Specific immune supporting molecules are extracted from the antigen infused material, creating a very powerful and concentrated product unlike anything else available. It is highly absorbable. Regular bovine colostrum is of limited nutritional value and varies widely in quality and consistency. Ai/E comes from "clean" herds of cows, which are raised drug-and-hormone free.

**Mechanism of Action**
Antigen infused bovine colostrum/whey extract plays an important role in modulating the immune system via multiple mechanisms.

**Research**
- *May increase natural killer cell activity in healthy people.* In one unpublished clinical study and one unpublished, double-blind, placebo-controlled study, antigen infused bovine colostrum/whey extract was able to increase natural killer (NK) cell activity in healthy people. The double-blind placebo-controlled study also showed that this special extract was able to increase the levels of other important immune-system components.

**Safety**
No side effects were reported in the studies discussed above. Since none of the milk proteins remain, this product is even tolerated by people with a dairy allergy.

**Conclusion**
Antigen infused bovine colostrum/whey extract is definitely the breakthrough product of the 21st century. Unpublished research suggests that this special extract increases NK-cell activity as well as other immune-system components in healthy people.

**Arabinigalactan**
Larch arabinogalactan is a polysaccharide with health-supporting properties. Preliminary studies suggest that larch arabinogalactan increases NK-cell activity and other immune-system functions. It also helps to support healthy levels of gut microflora.

**Astragalus**
Astragalus has been traditionally used by the Chinese for hundreds of years. It has been shown to have strong antioxidant properties. Preliminary research suggests that it may help support the immune system and maintain liver, mental, and cardiovascular health.

**Maitake D-Fraction**

The main active ingredient in maitake is D-fraction, a polysaccharide. Preliminary research has shown that maitake helps to support a healthy immune system, maintains cardiovascular health, and helps to support healthy blood sugar levels.

### Ingredients: (Each 2 capsules contain):

| | |
|---|---|
| Arabinogalactan | 300mg |
| Ai/E$^{10}$ | 100mg |
| Astragalus Root | 50mg |
| Maitake Mushroom Extract 4:1 | 50mg |

**Directions:** 1 to 2 capsules can be taken from 2 to four times daily.

## ALLER WISE™

**Description:**
Homeopathic remedy designed to provide relief from the symptoms of airborne allergens such as pollens, molds, dusts, and danders. Supplies six homeopathic remedies that, according to homeopathic provings, collectively cover the most common symptoms of respiratory allergy. Symptoms such as sneezing, itchy eyes/ears/throat, watery eyes, and nasal discharge can all be alleviated with Aller Wise. This great product also contains, a special allergen-infused form of Ai/E10™ (see complete description under AG-Immune). Contains no stimulants such as ephedrine, pseudoephedrine, or phenlypropanolamine (PPA). Aller Wise can be used with AG-Immune to support a healthy immune system.

### Active Homeopathic Ingredients:

| | |
|---|---|
| Apis Melifica | 30X |
| Alium Cepa | 6X |
| Euphrasia | 6X |
| Histaminium | 6X |
| Natrum Muriaticum | 6X |
| Sabidilla | 6X |

**Inactive Ingredients:** Lactose, **allergen-infused bovine colostrum/whey extract (Ai/E$^{10}$)**, Silicon Dioxide, Lactase, and Magnesium Stearate.

**Directions:** Take one tablet twice daily (dissolved under the tongue). For acute conditions can be used hourly until improved. Can also be chewed or swallowed.

## BETA-C Tablets

**Description:**
**Beta-C is your sunshine connection!**

Its remarkable nutrient matrix is composed of beta carotene, an antioxidant, plus an exclusive, esterified form of vitamin C. We've also added the nutritional benefits of cruciferous vegetables, bilberry and garlic-a powerful combination of life-affirming nutrients!

### Highlighted Ingredients:
**Vitamin C**
Essential for collagen formation, and helps to support a healthy immune system.
**Natural Mixed Carotenoids**
Plant-based compounds which fight free radicals and promote a strong immune system
**Cruciferous Vegetables**
Rich in antioxidants and a great source of fiber.
**Garlic**
Helps to support healthy cholesterol levels and maintain cardiovascular health.

### Beta-C
**Supplement facts**

Serving Size 4 Tablets

| Amount per 4 Tablets | | % Daily Value |
|---|---|---|
| Beta Carotene (Dunaliella salina algae) | 3 mg | |
| Equivalent to Vitamin A | 5000 IU | 100% |

Contains other naturally occurring carotenoids in D. salina; Alpha Carotene, Cryptoxanthin, Zeaxanthin and Lutein.

| | | |
|---|---|---|
| Vitamin C (Esterified) | 2000 mg | 3333% |
| Calcium (from Dicalcium Phosphate) | 96 mg | 10% |
| Cruciferous Vegetable Concentrate | 500 mg | * |
| Deodorized Garlic Bulb | 400 mg | * |
| Mixed Bioflavonoid Complex | 200 mg | * |
| Bilberry Fruit Extract 4:1 | 100 mg | * |
| Acerola Cherry Fruit Extract 4:1 | 40 mg | * |
| Rose Hips | 40 mg | * |
| Grapefruit Bioflavonoid Complex | 40 mg | * |
| Hesperidin Fruit Citrus Complex | 40 mg | * |
| Red Clover Blossoms | 40 mg | * |
| Rutin Flower Buds | 40 mg | * |

*Daily Value not established.

**Directions:** As a dietary supplement, adults take four tablets daily with food.

**How Supplied:** Bottles of 120 Tablets.

## RELIEF™

**Description:**
Homeopathic nasal and throat spray designed to work in the upper respiratory tract where the body first comes in contact with foreign particles in the air. Relief is designed to alleviate the symptoms associated with the common cold, flu, sinusitis, and minor earache. The four homeopathic remedies contained in Relief are described in homeopathic findings to cover such symptoms as sore throat/pain with swallowing, runny nose, yellow and green mucous, cough, ear pain, low-grade fever, and painful/throbbing sinuses. Relief also contains Ai/E10™ (see full description under AG-Immune), the patented and proprietary antigen infused bovine colostrum/whey extract found in the entire Body Wise immune family of products.

### Active Homeopathic Ingredients:

| | |
|---|---|
| Lachesis Mutus | 12X |
| Mercurius Vivus | 12X |
| Hepar Sulphuris Calcareum | 8X |
| Belladonna | 4X |

**Inactive Ingredients:**
Benzalkonium chloride, 2-deoxy-d-glucose, **antigen-infused bovine colostrum/whey extract (Ai/E10™)**, disodium EDTA, eucalyptus oil, filtered water, sodium hydroxide, thimerosal.

**Directions:** (Adults and children over 3): Shake well before using. Keep head upright; spray 1 to four times in each nostril and/or in throat 1–6 times daily as needed. Consult physician if symptoms persist for more than 5 days. If you are pregnant or nursing a baby, consult your physician before using.

## RIGHT CHOICE® A.M. MULTI FORMULA

**Description:** Body Wise Right Choice® A.M. formula is focused on B-vitamins, antioxidants, and nutrients that promote efficient energy utilization such as chromium and alpha-ketoglutarate. These nutrients support you through the active phase of your day.

**Each three caplets contain:**

| | Amount | %RDA |
|---|---|---|
| **Vitamins** | | |
| Beta Carotene | 6 mg | |

*Continued on next page*

## Right Choice A.M.—Cont.

(Dunaliella salina algae)
equivalent to   10,000 IU    200
Vitamin A
(contains other naturally occurring
carotenoids in D. salina: Alpha
Carotene, Cryptoxanthin, Zeaxanthin,
Lutein and Lycopene)

| | | |
|---|---|---|
| Vitamin A | | |
| (palmitate) | 5,000 IU | 100 |
| Vitamin C | 1,000 mg | 1667 |
| Ascorbyl | | |
| Palmitate | 50 mg | ** |
| Vitamin B1 | 25 mg | 1667 |
| (thiamine mononitrate) | | |
| Vitamin B2 | | |
| (riboflavin) | 15 mg | 882 |
| Niacinamide | 50 mg | 250 |
| Vitamin B6 | | |
| (pyridoxine | | |
| HCL) | 25 mg | 1250 |
| Folic Acid | 800 mcg | 200 |
| Vitamin B12 | 200 mcg | 3333 |
| (cobalamin concentrate) | | |
| Pantothenic | | |
| Acid | 50 mg | 500 |
| (d-cal pantothenate) | | |
| Biotin | 300 mcg | 100 |

**Vitamin E Complex**

| | | |
|---|---|---|
| Vitamin E | 200 IU | 667 |

(d-alpha tocopherol acid succinate
and mixed tocopherols beta, gamma
and delta)

**PhytoNutrients/Food Factors**

| | | |
|---|---|---|
| Green Barley | 50 mg | ** |
| Chlorella | 50 mg | ** |
| Spirulina | 50 mg | ** |
| Lemon | | |
| Bioflavonoid | | |
| Complex | 50 mg | ** |

**Additional Constituents**

| | | |
|---|---|---|
| Chromium*** | 100 mcg | ** |
| L-Glutamine | 50 mg | ** |
| Alpha | | |
| Ketoglutarate | 200 mg | ** |
| Ginkgo Biloba | 50 mg | ** |
| Orchard Blend | 100 mg | ** |

**No nutritional requirement
established.
***Krebs Cycle Chelate.

**Inactive Ingredients:** Cellulose, vegetable stearine, magnesium stearate, silicon dioxide, and aqueous base white filmcoat.

**Recommended Adult Use:** As a dietary supplement, take three caplets with your morning meal.

**How Supplied/Availability:** Supplied in bottles of 90 or 270. Available through Body Wise International.

*These Statements have not been evaluated by the U.S. FDA. This product is not intended to diagnose treat, cure or prevent any disease.

---

## RIGHT CHOICE® P.M. MULTI FORMULA

**Description:** Body Wise Right Choice* P.M. Provides meaningful levels of essen-

tial minerals and more to help your body replenish and rebuild. Fortified with hydrochloric acid to help with nutrient uptake, and green foods such as barley grass and chlorella that may further enhance absorption.

**Each three caplets contain:**

| | Amount | %RDA |
|---|---|---|
| **Minerals** | | |
| Calcium** | 500 mg | 50 |
| Magnesium** | 250 mg | 63 |
| Zinc** | 15 mg | 100 |
| Copper** | 2 mg | 100 |
| Manganese** | 5 mg | 250 |
| Chromium** | 100 mcg | 83 |
| Selenium | | |
| (1-selenomethionine) | 50 mcg | 71 |
| Molybdenum** | 100 mcg | 133 |
| Vanadium** | 50 mcg | *** |
| Potassium** | 99 mg | *** |
| Phytonutrient | | |
| Multimins™*** | 25 mg | |
| **Lipotropic Complex** | | |
| Inositol | 50 mg | |
| Betaine HCl | 100 mg | **** |
| Choline (bitartrate) | 50 mg | **** |
| **Amino Acid/Antioxidant** | | |
| L-Glutathione | 15 mg | **** |
| **PhytoNutrients/Food Factors** | | |
| Green Barley | 50 mg | **** |
| Chlorella | 50 mg | **** |
| Spirulina | 50 mg | **** |
| **Additional Constituents** | | |
| Vitamin D3 | | |
| (ergocalciferol) | 400 IU | 100 |
| Iodine (kelp) | 150 mcg | 100 |

**Krebs Cycle Chelated* Mineral Replenishment Factors are uniquely formulated with Citrates, Aspartates, Fumarates, Succinates and Malates.
***Determined to be essential nutrient but actual requirements have not been established.
****No nutritional requirement established.

**Inactive Ingredients:** Cellulose, vegetable stearine, magnesium stearate, silicon dioxide, and an aqueous base green film coating.

**Recommended Adult Use:** As a dietary supplement, take three caplets with your evening meal.

**How Supplied/Availability:** Supplied in bottles of 90 or 270. Available through Body Wise International.

*These Statements have not been evaluated by the U.S. FDA. This product is not intended to diagnose treat, cure or prevent any disease.

---

## Covex

SECTOR OFICIOS 33, 1-3
28760 TRES CANTOS
MADRID SPAIN

**For direct inquiries contact:**
+34-91-804-4545
Fax +34-91-804-3030
vinpocetin@covex.es

### INTELECTOL™ MEMORY ENHANCER VINPOCETINE TABLETS COVEX

**Description:** Intelectol® is a powerful memory enhancer. Scientific studies have shown that its ingredient vinpocetine helps the body to maintain healthy circulation in the brain by decreasing cerebral vascular resistance, improving cerebral blood flow and cerebral oxygen and glucose utilization, and that vinpocetine increases the concentration of some neurotransmitters involved in the process of memory formation. Intelectol™ can be taken for enhancing the following cognitive functions: memory, attention, orientation, perception, information fixation, judgment. Clinical studies have also shown that vinpocetine helps to maintain healthy microcirculation in the inner ear and eyes.

**Active ingredients:** Vinpocetine 5mg (No U.S. RDA established)
**Inactive ingredients:** Lactose, Hydropropylcellulose, Magnesium Stearate, Talc.

**Recommended Use:** 1 to 2 tablets × 3 times daily with meals.

**Warning:** Keep out of reach of children. Do not take if you are pregnant or lactating. If you have hemophilia or are on blood thinning medication, please consult your physician before taking this product.
**Interactions:** Not known.

**How Supplied:** packs of 50 tablets.
**Availability:** Available at Web Site http://www.intelectol.com, http://www.the-memory-pill.com, toll free number 1 888 613 9920.

**References/Function Claim:**
Visit Web Site http://www.intelectol.com
*Shown in Product Identification Guide, page 506*

---

**IF YOU SUSPECT
AN INTERACTION. . .**
The 1,800-page
*PDR Companion Guide*™ can help.
Use the order form
in the front of this book.

**IF YOU SUSPECT
AN INTERACTION. . .**
The 1,800-page
*PDR Companion Guide*™ can help.
Use the order form
in the front of this book.

## Fleming & Company
**1600 FENPARK DR.**
**FENTON, MO 63026**

**Direct Inquiries to:**
Tom Fleming
636 343-8200
FAX (636) 343-9865
e-mail: info@flemingcompany.com

**MAGONATE® Tablets**
**MAGONATE® Liquid**
**MAGONATE NATAL Liquid**
**Magnesium Gluconate (Dihydrate), USP**
**(Dietary Supplement)**

**Description:** Each 2 tablets contain magnesium 54 mgs (from 1000 mg magnesium gluconate dihydrate) calcium 175 mg and phosphorous 182 mg (from 752 mgs dibasic calcium phosphate dihydrate). Each 5 mL of MAGONATE® liquid contains magnesium (elemental) 54 mgs. (Each 5 ml contains the same amount of magnesium as contained in 1000 mgs of magnesium gluconate dihydrate). Each ml of MAGONATE NATAL Liquid (magnesium gluconate) contains 3.52 mg (0.29 mEq) of magnesium as the gluconate in a sugarless and flavor free isotonic base.

**Suggested Uses:** Magonate® Tablets and Liquid are indicated to maintain magnesium levels when the dietary intake of magnesium is inadequate or when excretion and loss are excessive. Magonate® is recommended during and for three weeks after a course in chemotherapy, then monitored regularly. MAGONATE NATAL Liquid is indicated for newborns with magnesium deficiency and for the restoration of magnesium in infants.

**Precautions:** Excessive dosage may cause loose stools.

**Contraindications:** Patients with kidney disease should not take magnesium supplements without the supervision of a physician.

**Dosages And Administration:** Two Magonate® tablets or 1 teaspoon Magonate® Liquid three times a day (midmorning, mid-afternoon and bedtime) on an empty stomach with a glass of water. MAGONATE Natal Liquid usual dose is 1 ml per kg of body weight daily, divided into two doses or 10 drops per kg twice a day.

**How Supplied:** Magonate® Tablets are orange scored, and supplied in bottles of 100 (NDC 256-0172-01), and 1000 (NDC 256-0172-02) tablets. Magonate® Liquid is supplied in pints, (NDC 256-0184-01). MAGONATE NATAL Liquid is supplied 90 mL bottles.

Rev. 7/00

---

**NICOTINEX Elixir**
**Niacin Dietary Supplement**

**Composition:** Contains niacin 50 mg./ tsp. in a sherry wine base (amber color).

**Action and Uses:** Produces peripheral flushing. To increase micro-circulation of inner-ear in Meniere's, tinnitus and labyrinthine syndromes. For 'cold hands & feet', and as a vehicle for additives.

**Administration and Dosage:** One or two teaspoonsful on fasting stomach, or as directed by physician.

**Side Effects:** Patients should be warned of dermal flush. Ulcer and gout patients may be affected by 10% alcoholic content.

**Contraindications:** Severe hypotension and hemorrhage.

**How Supplied:** Plastic pints.

---

## GlaxoSmithKline Consumer Healthcare, L.P.

**P.O. BOX 1467**
**PITTSBURGH, PA 15230**

**Direct Inquiries to:**
Consumer Affairs
1-800-245-1040

**For Medical Emergencies Contact:**
Consumer Affairs
1-800-245-1040

**ALLUNA™ SLEEP**
**Herbal Supplement Tablet**

**Use:** **Alluna Sleep** is an herbal supplement that can relieve occasional sleeplessness.* It works by helping you relax, so you can drift off to sleep naturally.*
Alluna Sleep has been clinically tested and shown to be effective in actually promoting your body's own natural sleep pattern – safely and gently.* This is a natural process. Depending upon your particular circumstances, benefits are typically seen within a few nights with more consistent results within two weeks.
**Alluna Sleep** is not habit forming and is safe to take over time. You can expect to wake up refreshed, with no groggy side effects, because you experience a natural, healthy sleep through the night.*

**Supplement Facts:**
Serving Size: 2 Tablets

|  | Amount Per 2 Tablets | % Daily Value |
| --- | --- | --- |
| **Calories** | 5 | |
| Valerian Root Extract | 500 mg | † |
| Hops Extract | 120 mg | † |

†Daily Value Not Established

**Other Ingredients:** microcrystalline cellulose, soy polysaccharide, hydrogenated castor oil, hydroxypropyl methylcellulose. Contains less than 2% of titanium dioxide, propylene glycol, magnesium stearate, silica, polyethylene glycol (400, 6,000 and 20,000), blue 2 lake, artificial flavoring.

**Directions:** Take **two** (2) tablets one hour before bedtime with a glass of water.

**Warning:** As with all dietary supplements, contact your doctor before use if you are pregnant or lactating. Keep this and all dietary supplements out of the reach of children. Driving or operating machinery while using this product is not recommended. Chronic insomniacs should consult their doctor before using this product.
**Please Note:** The herbs in this product have a distinct natural aroma.
**Store in a cool, dry place. Avoid temperatures above 86°F.**

**How Supplied:** Packets of 28 and 56 Tablets

---

**BEANO®**
[bēan ō]
**Food Enzyme Dietary Supplement**

**PRODUCT INFORMATION**
**Description:**
*Beano drops*: each 5 drop dosage follows Food Chemical Codex (FCC) standards for activity and contains 150 GalU (galactosidase units) of alpha-D-galactosidase derived from *Aspergillus niger* mold. The enzyme is in a liquid carrier of water and xylitol. Add about 5 drops on the first bite of food serving, but remember a normal meal has 2-3 servings of the problem foods.
*Beano tablets*: each tablet follows Food Chemical Codex (FCC) standards for activity and contains 150 GalU (galactosidase units) of alpha-D-galactosidase derived from *Aspergillus niger* mold. The enzyme is in a carrier of cellulose gel, mannitol, invertase, potato starch, magnesium stearate, gelatin (fish), colloidal silica. 3 tablets swallowed, chewed, or crumbled onto food should be enough for a normal meal of 3 servings of problem foods (1 tablet per serving). Beano® will hydrolyze complex sugars, raffinose, stachyose and verbascose, into the simple sugars - glucose, galactose and fructose, and the easily digestible disaccharide, sucrose. (Sucrose hydrolysis happens simultaneously with normal digestion.) In some cases, more enzyme than 5 drops or 3 tablets will be re-

*Continued on next page*

## Beano—Cont.

quired, and this is a function of the quantity of food eaten, the levels of alpha-linked sugars in the food, and the gas-producing propensity of the person.

**Action:** Hydrolysis converts raffinose, stachyose and verbascose into their monosaccharide components: glucose, galactose, fructose and sucrose. Raffinose yields sucrose + galactose; stachyose yields sucrose + galactose; verbascose yields glucose + fructose + galactose.

**Indications:** Helps prevent flatulence and/or bloat from a variety of grains, cereals, nuts, seeds, and vegetables containing the sugars raffinose, stachyose and/or verbascose. This includes all or most legumes and all or most cruciferous vegetables. Examples of such foods are oats, wheat, beans of all kinds, chickpeas, peas, lentils, peanuts, soy-content foods, broccoli, brussel sprouts, cabbage, carrots, corn, leeks, onions, parsnips, squash. Note: Most vegetables and beans also contain fiber, which is gas productive in some people, but usually far less so than the alpha-linked sugars. Beano® has no effect on fiber.

**Usage:** About 5 drops per food serving or 3 tablets per meal (1 tablet per serving) of 3 servings of problem foods; higher levels depending on symptoms.

**Adverse Reactions:** Reports to date include gastroenterological symptoms, such as cramping and diarrhea as well as allergic-type reactions including rash and pruritus. Rare reports of more serious allergic reactions have been received.

**Precautions:** If you are pregnant or nursing, ask your doctor before product use. Galactosemics should not use without physician's advice, since one of the breakdown sugars is galactose.

**How Supplied:** Beano® is supplied in both a liquid form (30 and 75 serving sizes, at 5 drops per serving), and a tablet form (30, 60, and 100 tablet sizes as well as 24 tablets in packets of 3). These statements have not been evaluated by the Food and Drug Administration. This product is not intended to diagnose, treat, cure or prevent any disease.
For more information and free samples, please write or call toll-free 1-800-257-8650 or visit www.beano.net.

---

**FEOSOL® Caplets**
**Hematinic**
**Iron Supplement**

**Description:** FEOSOL Caplets contain pure iron micro particles called carbonyl iron. Replacing FEOSOL Capsules, this advanced formula is specially designed to be well absorbed, gentle on the stomach and offers enhanced safety in the event of an accidental overdose. Each FEOSOL carbonyl iron caplet delivers 45 mg of pure elemental iron, the same amount of elemental iron contained in the 225 mg ferrous sulfate capsule. At equivalent doses, carbonyl iron and ferrous sulfate were shown to be equally efficacious in correcting hemoglobin, hematocrit and serum iron levels in iron-deficient patients[1].

**Safety:** According to the American Association of Poison Control Centers, iron containing supplements are the leading cause of pediatric poisoning deaths for children under six in the United States[2]. Widely used as a food additive, carbonyl iron must be gastrically solubilized before it can be absorbed, giving it lower toxicity and enhancing its safety versus any of the ferrous salts[3]. As a result, carbonyl iron presents less chance of harm from accidental overdose. In addition, at equivalent doses, carbonyl iron side effects are no greater than those experienced with ferrous sulfate[4].

**Warnings:** Do not exceed recommended dosage. The treatment of any anemic condition should be under the advice and supervision of a physician. Since oral iron products interfere with absorption of oral tetracycline antibiotics, these products should not be taken within two hours of each other. Occasional gastrointestinal discomfort (such as nausea) may be minimized by taking with meals. Iron containing medication may occasionally cause constipation or diarrhea. If you are pregnant or nursing a baby, seek the advice of a health professional before using this product.
**WARNING:** **Accidental overdose of iron-containing products is a leading cause of fatal poisoning in children under 6. Keep this product out of reach of children. In case of accidental overdose, call a doctor or poison control center immediately.**

---

**SUPPLEMENT FACTS**
Serving Size: 1 Caplet

| Amount per Caplet | % Daily Value |
|---|---|
| Iron 45 mg | 250% |

---

**Ingredients:** Lactose, Sorbitol, Carbonyl Iron, Hydroxypropyl Methylcellulose. Contains 1% or less of the following ingredients: Carnauba Wax, Crospovidone, FD&C Blue #2 Al Lake, FD&C Red #40 Al Lake, FD&C Yellow #6 Al Lake, Magnesium Stearate, Polydextrose, Polyethylene Glycol, Polyethylene Glycol 8000 (Powder), Stearic Acid, Titanium Dioxide, Triacetin.

**Directions:** Adults—one caplet daily or as directed by a physician. Children under 12 years: Consult a physician.

**Tamper-Evident Feature:** Each caplet is encased in a plastic cell with a foil back; do not use if cell or foil is broken.

**References:** [1]Devasthali SD, Gordeuk VR, Brittenham GM, et al, "Bioavailability of Carbonyl Iron: A randomized, double-blind study." Eur J Haematology, 1991; 46:272–278.

[2]FDA Consumer; March 1996:7
[3]Heubers, JA, Brittenham GM, Csiba E and Finch CA. "Absorption of carbonyl iron." J Lab Clin Med 1986; 108:473–78.
[4]Devasthali SD, Gordeuk VR, Brittenham GM, et al, "Bioavailability of a Carbonyl Iron: A randomized, double-blind study." Eur J Haematology, 1991; 46:272–278.

**Store at room temperature, avoid excessive heat (greater than 100°F) or humidity.**

**How Supplied:** Boxes of 30 and 60 caplets in blisters. Also available in single unit packages of 100 caplets intended for institutional use
Also available: Feosol Tablets.
Comments or Questions? Call Toll-Free 1-800-245-1040 Weekdays.
SmithKline Beecham Consumer Healthcare, L.P.
Pittsburgh, PA 15230    Made in USA
*Shown in Product Identification Guide, page 507*

---

## FEOSOL® TABLETS
**Hematinic**
**Iron Supplement**

**Description:** Feosol tablets provide the body with ferrous sulfate—an iron supplement for iron deficiency and iron deficiency anemia when the need for such therapy has been determined by a physician.

---

**SUPPLEMENT FACTS**
Serving Size: 1 Tablet

| Amount per Tablet | % Daily Value |
|---|---|
| Iron 65 mg | 360% |

---

**Ingredients:** Dried ferrous sulfate 200 mg (65 mg of elemental iron) equivalent to 325 mg of ferrous sulfate per tablet. Lactose, Sorbitol, Crospovidone, Magnesium Stearate, Carnauba Wax. Contains 2% or less of the following ingredients: FD&C Blue #1, FD&C Yellow #6, Hydroxypropyl Methylcellulose, Polydextrose, Polyethylene Glycol, Titanium Dioxide, Triacetin.

**Directions:** Adults and children 12 years and over—One tablet daily or as directed by a physician. Children under 12 years—Consult a physician.

**Tamper-Evident Feature:** Each tablet is encased in a plastic cell with a foil back; do not use if cell or foil is broken.

**Warnings: Do not exceed recommended dosage.** The treatment of any anemic condition should be under the advice and supervision of a physician. Since oral iron products interfere with absorption of oral tetracycline antibiotics, these products should not be taken within two hours of each other. Occasional gastrointestinal discomfort (such as nausea) may be minimized by taking with meals. Iron containing medication may occassionally cause constipation or diarrhea.

**Supplement Facts**
Serving Size 1 Tablet

| Amount Per Serving | % Daily Value for Pregnant or Lactating Women | % Daily Value for Adults and Children 4 or more years of age |
|---|---|---|
| Calories 5 | | |
| Calcium 500 mg | 38% | 50% |

If you are pregnant or nursing a baby, seek the advice of a health professional before using this product.
**WARNING: Accidental overdose of iron-containing products is a leading cause of fatal poisoning in children under 6. Keep this product out of reach of children. In case of accidental overdose, call a doctor, or poison control center immediately.**
Store at room temperature (59–86°F). Not USP for dissolution.

**How Supplied:** Cartons of 100 tablets in child-resistant blisters.
Previously packaged in bottles.
Also available: Feosol caplets.
**Comments or Questions?**
**Call toll-free 800-245-1040 weekdays.**
SmithKline Beecham Consumer Healthcare, L.P.
Pittsburgh, PA 15230     Made in USA
*Shown in Product Identification Guide, page 507*

---

## OS-CAL® CHEWABLE
**Calcium Supplement**

**Description:** Calcium supplement to help reduce the risk of osteoporosis. Osteoporosis affects middle-aged and older persons, especially Caucasian and Asian women, and those whose families tend to have fragile bones in later years. A lifetime of regular exercise and eating a healthful diet that includes enough calcium, especially during teen and early adult years, builds and maintains good bone health and may reduce the risk of osteoporosis in later life. Adequate calcium intake is important, but daily intakes above 2000 mg are not likely to provide any additional benefit. [See table above]

**Ingredients:** Calcium carbonate, dextrose monohydrate, maltodextrin, microcrystalline cellulose, magnesium stearate, artificial flavors, sodium chloride. Each tablet provides 500 mg of elemental calcium

**Directions:** One tablet two to three times a day with meals, or as recommended by your physician.

**How Supplied:** Bottle of 60 tablets
Store at room temperature.
Keep out of reach of children.
*Shown in Product Identification Guide, page 508*

---

## OS-CAL® 250 + D
**Calcium with Vitamin D Supplement**

**Description:** Calcium supplement to help reduce the risk of osteoporosis (see below*). Also contains Vitamin D.

---

**Supplement Facts**
Serving Size 1 Tablet
[See first table below]

**Ingredients:** Oyster shell powder, corn syrup solids, talc, corn starch, hydroxypropyl methylcellulose. Contains less than 1% of calcium stearate, polysorbate 80, titanium dioxide, polyethylene glycol, Vitamin D, propylparaben and methylparaben (preservative), simethicone, yellow 5 lake, blue 1 lake, carnauba wax, edetate sodium.

**Directions:** One tablet three times a day with meals, or as recommended by your physician.

**How Supplied:** Bottle of 100 and 240 tablets
Store at room temperature.
Keep out of reach of children.
*Osteoporosis affects middle-aged and older persons, especially Caucasian and Asian women, and those whose families tend to have fragile bones in later years. A lifetime of regular exercise and eating a healthful diet that includes enough calcium, especially during teen and early adult years, builds and maintains good bone health and may reduce the risk of osteoporosis in later life. Adequate calcium intake is important, but daily intakes above 2000 mg are not likely to provide any additional benefit.
*Shown in Product Identification Guide, page 508*

---

## OS-CAL® 500
**Calcium Supplement**

**Description:** Calcium supplement to help reduce the risk of osteoporosis.

| Amount Per Tablet | % Daily Value for Pregnant or Lactating Women | % Daily Value for Adults and Children 4 or More Years of Age |
|---|---|---|
| Vitamin D 125 IU | 31% | 31% |
| Calcium 250 mg | 19% | 25% |

| Amount Per Tablet | % Daily Value for Pregnant or Lactating Women | % Daily Value for Adults and children 4 or more years of age |
|---|---|---|
| Calcium 500 mg | 38% | 50% |

**Supplement Facts**
Serving Size 1 Tablet

| Amount Per Tablet | % Daily Value for Pregnant or Lactating Women | % Daily Value for Adults and Children 4 or more years of age |
|---|---|---|
| Vitamin D 200 IU | 50% | 50% |
| Calcium 500 mg | 38% | 50% |

Osteoporosis effects middle-aged and older persons, especially Caucasian and Asian women, and those whose families tend to have fragile bones in later years. A lifetime of regular exercise and eating a healthful diet that includes enough calcium, especially during teen and early adult years, builds and maintains good bone health and may reduce the risk of osteoporosis in later life. Adequate calcium intake is important, but daily intakes above 2000 mg are not likely to provide any additional benefit.

**Supplement Facts**
Serving Size 1 Tablet
[See second table below]

**Ingredients:** Oyster shell powder, corn syrup solids, talc, corn starch. Contains less than 1% of sodium starch glycolate, calcium stearate, polysorbate 80, hydroxypropyl methylcellulose, polydextrose, titanium dioxide, propylparaben and methylparaben (preservative), triacetin, yellow 5 lake, blue 1 lake, polyethylene glycol, carnauba wax.

**Directions:** One tablet two to three times a day with meals, or as recommended by your physician.

**How Supplied:** Bottles of 75 and 160 tablets
Store at room temperature.
Keep out of reach of children.
*Shown in Product Identification Guide, page 508*

---

## OS-CAL® 500 + D
**Calcium with Vitamin D Supplement**

**Description:** Calcium supplement to help reduce the risk of osteoporosis (see below*). Also contains Vitamin D.
[See third table below]

**Ingredients:** Oyster shell powder, corn syrup solids, talc, corn starch. Contains less than 1% of sodium starch glycolate, calcium stearate, polysorbate 80, hydrox-

*Continued on next page*

## Os-Cal 500+D—Cont.

ypropyl methylcellulose, polydextrose, titanium dioxide, Vitamin D, propylparaben and methylparaben (preservative), triacetin, yellow 5 lake, blue 1 lake, polyethylene glycol, carnauba wax.

**Directions:** One tablet two to three times a day with meals, or as recommended by your physician.

**How Supplied:** Bottle of 75 and 160 tablets
Store at room temperature.
Keep out of reach of children.
*Osteoporosis affects middle-aged and older persons, especially Caucasian and Asian women, and those whose families tend to have fragile bones in later years. A lifetime of regular exercise and eating a healthful diet that includes enough calcium, especially during teen and early adult years, builds and maintains good bone health and may reduce the risk of osteoporosis in later life.
Adequate calcium intake is important, but daily intakes above 2000 mg are not likely to provide any additional benefit.
*Shown in Product Identification Guide, page 508*

---

**REMIFEMIN Menopause**
Drug Free
Herbal Supplement
A safe, natural, effective way to help ease the physical and emotional symptoms of menopause*

*Remifemin Menopause* is a unique, natural formula. For over 40 years in Europe, it has helped reduce the unpleasant physical and emotional symptoms associated with menopause, such as hot flashes, night sweats and mood swings. Clinically shown to be safe and effective. Not a drug.
*Remifemin Menopause* helps you approach menopause with confidence – naturally.*

**Supplement Facts**
Serving Size 1 tablet

| Ingredients: | Amount Per Tablet: | % Daily Value: |
|---|---|---|
| Black Cohosh Extract (Root and Rhizome) Equivalent to | 20 mg | † |

†Daily Value Not Established.

**Other Ingredients:** Lactose, Cellulose, Potato Starch, Magnesium Stearate, and Natural Peppermint Flavor. Standardized to be equivalent to 20 mg Black Cohosh (*Cimicifuga racemosa*) root and rhizome.
Contains no salt, yeast, wheat, gluten, corn, soy, coloring, or preservatives.

**Directions:** Take one tablet in the morning and one tablet in the evening, with water. You can expect to notice improvements within a few weeks with full benefits after using Remifemin twice a day for 4 to 12 weeks. This product is intended for use by women who are experiencing menopausal symptoms. Does not contain estrogen. Remifemin is not meant to replace any drug therapy.

**Warnings:** This product should not be used by women who are pregnant or considering becoming pregnant or are nursing. As with any dietary supplement, always keep out of reach of children. For a few consumers, gastric discomfort may occur but should not be persistent. If gastric discomfort persists, discontinue use and see your health care practitioner. As part of an overall good health care program, we encourage you to see your health care practitioner on a regular basis.

### Making Sense Out of Menopause with Remifemin Menopause
Today, women are leading very dynamic and diverse lifestyles. Despite this diversity, there is one constant. They are all experiencing physiological changes. They will all experience menopause. The time when you have menopausal symptoms is a multiphasic period. Technically, the change or transitional process of menopause is known as the *"Climacteric"*. There are different phases of the climacteric that a woman experiences:

*1. Perimenopause* is the transitional phase when hormone levels begin to drop. This phase lasts typically 3 to 5 years but can last up to 10 years. This gradual decline in estrogen levels causes the troublesome effects of menopause.

*2. Menopause* is the permanent cessation of menstruation. The average age at menopause is 51, but there is considerable variation in this timing among women. Menopause is medically defined as one year without menstruation.

*3. Postmenopause* is the phase following menopause. During this phase, your body gets used to the loss of estrogen and eventually the symptoms such as hot flashes go away.

### Some Commonly Asked Questions Regarding Remifemin Menopause
*1. What is Remifemin Menopause?* Remifemin Menopause is a uniquely formulated natural herbal supplement derived from the black cohosh plant. It is formulated to work with your body to promote physical and emotional balance during menopause. Over 40 years of clinical research has shown Remifemin Menopause helps reduce hot flashes, night sweats, related occasional sleeplessness, irritability and mood swings. In a recent clinical study, on average, women experienced the following overall improvements:
[See chart at top of next column]

*2. What makes Remifemin Menopause so special?* Remifemin Menopause contains an *exclusive* extract of black cohosh. It is developed with specific modern analytical techniques which produce a standardized extract of the black cohosh root and rhizome.

*3. With so many products out there claiming to be "natural," how can I be sure that this product is safe and effec-*

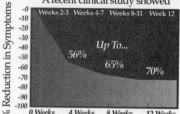

A recent clinical study showed

Up To...
56%  65%  70%

Weeks of use of Remifemin Menopause

*tive?* Remifemin's Menopause formulation is supported by over 40 years of clinical research, and millions of women in Europe have safely used it. Remifemin Menopause is drug free and estrogen free. And it is brought to you from a world-renowned health care company.

*4. How does Remifemin Menopause work?* Remifemin Menopause contains a proprietary standardized extract taken from the rootstock of the black cohosh plant. Studies have shown that the compounds found within this standardized herbal extract seem to interact with certain hormone receptors – without influencing hormone levels.*

*5. How long does it take for Remifemin Menopause to work?* Remifemin Menopause is a natural herbal supplement, not a drug. It will take time for your body's cycles to respond to its gentle onset. Personally, you may notice improvements within a few weeks. But for some women, it may take 4 to 12 weeks to benefit fully from Remifemin Menopause. Since the effects of Remifemin Menopause increase after extended twice daily use, we recommend that you take Remifemin Menopause for at least 12 weeks. If you do not find any difference in your well being after 12 weeks, please consult your physician to discuss other options.

*6. Can I take it over a long period of time, since the menopausal period lasts for years?* We recommend that you take Remifemin Menopause twice daily for up to 6 months continuously. If, after discontinuing use, your symptoms return, you may start taking Remifemin Menopause again. Keep in mind that Remifemin Menopause is a natural herbal supplement that supports a natural change that may take you years to go through.* As part of an overall good health care program, we encourage you to see your health care practitioner on a regular basis.

*7. Are there any known side effects?* When used properly following the package directions, Remifemin Menopause has few side effects, if any. In clinical research, there was a small percentage of gastric discomfort complaints. If you have been taking Remifemin Menopause and find that this or any other condition develops and persists, please discontinue use and see your physician.

*8. Is there a certain time of the day when I should take this product? Do I*

**need to take it with food?** You can take Remifemin Menopause with or without food. We recommend that you take one tablet in the morning with your breakfast and one tablet in the evening with water for relief from day and nighttime effects of menopause.

**9. Can I chew a tablet?** While they do have a mild peppermint flavor, Remifemin Menopause tablets are purposely made to be swallowed with water. They could be chewed, but some women may find the taste unpleasant.

**10. Can I take my herbal tea, vitamins, or other dietary supplements with Remifemin Menopause?** Typically, dietary supplements can be taken with other dietary supplements. Always follow package directions. If you should notice any undesirable effects, discontinue taking them together.

**Expiration and Storage Information**
The expiration date of this package is printed on the side panel flap of the outer carton as well as on the blister packs. Do not use this product after this date.
**Store this product in a cool, dry place. Keep out of the reach of children. Avoid storing at temperatures above 86°F.**

---

**\*These statements have not been evaluated by the Food and Drug Administration. This product is not intended to diagnose, treat, cure, or prevent any disease.**

---

Questions or Comments? Call toll-free 1-800-965-8804 weekdays, or visit www.remifemin.com anytime.

Remifemin ® is a trademark of Schaper & Brümmer GmbH & Co. KG, licensed to SmithKline Beecham.
© 2000 SmithKline Beecham 59175XA

---

# Kyowa Engineering-Sundory

**6-964 NAKAMOZU-CHO, SAKAI-CITY, OSAKA, JAPAN**

**Direct Inquiries to:**
Consumer Relations
Tel: 81-72-257-8568
Osaka
Fax: 81-722-57-8655
MRL: http://www.sundory.jp

**SEN-SEI-RO LIQUID GOLD™**
Kyowa's *Agaricus blazei Murill*
Mushroom Extract
100 ml liquid
Dietary Supplement

**Description:** Sen-Sei-Ro Liquid Gold™, a dietary supplement containing an exclusive all-natural, standardized extract of the Kyowa's cultured *Agaricus*

*blazei Murill* mushroom is primarily used to reduce symptoms of fatigue, to promote vitality, overall well-being, and to support immune functions.[†] Normal immune function can decline with age, and are necessary for maintenance of vitality, energy, good health, and quality of life. A few major biomarkers for decreased immune functions are decreased natural killer cell (NK) activity, and the number of lymphocytes and macrophage cells. These cells, primarily attack diseased cells and thereby, maintain body homeostasis, promote health and quality of life. For the past half a century in Brazil and other countries, *Agaricus blazei Murill* mushroom has been used to restore vitality, and energy, and to serve as a potent tonic conducive to general health and aging concerns.[†]

**Clinical Trials:** The effectiveness of ABMK22 in Sen-Sei-Ro Gold™ for health benefits were tested in several controlled pre- and clinical trials in animals and in humans.[†] Recent studies in Japan led researchers to report that in humans, ABMK22 in Sen-Sei-Ro Gold™ enhanced NK cell activity, promoted maturation and activation of dendritic cells indicated by increased cell kill, elevated expression of CD80 and CD83 expressions (Biotherapy 15(4): 503–507, 2001), increased the number of macrophage (Anticancer Research 17(1A): 274–284, 1997; Japanese Association of Cancer Research, no. 2268, 1999) and tumor necrosis factor α (TNF-α)(Japanese Association of Cancer Research, no. 1406, 1999; Japanese J. Veterinary Clin. Medicine 17(2):31–42, 1998).[†] Further clinical studies with Sen-Sei-Ro Gold™ among 100 cancer patients undergoing chemotherapy in Korea have shown that NK cell activity were significantly enhanced, while NK cell activity in the placebo group was markedly diminished.[†] Earlier and recent both pre- and clinical studies in Japan, and Korea, led researchers to report that Kyowa's *Agaricus blazei Murill* mushroom extract can be part of an effective treatment for supporting the immune systems of cancer patients by stimulating host defense system (Biotherapy 15(4): 503–507, 2001; Carbohydrate Res. 186(2): 267–273, 1989; Japanese J. Pharmacology 662: 265–271, 1994; Agricultural and Biological Chemistry 54: 2889–2905, 1990).[†]

**Ingredients:** Each 100ml heat-treated high pressure pack of all natural Kyowa's *Agaricus blazei Murill* water extract is scientifically standardized to contain 300mg% carbohydrate, 700mg% protein, 0mg% fat,; 1.4mg% sodium, 0% food quality cellulose, and 4 Kcal energy.

Molecular weights of polysaccharopeptides ranges between 600∼8,000. Water: 99.2g%,; includes a variety of amino acids and vitamins (arginine 12mg%, lysine 6mg%, histidine 2mg%, phenylalanine 4mg%, tyrosine 4mg%, leucine 5mg%, isoleucine 3mg%, methionine 1mg%, valine 5mg%, alanine 13mg%,

glycine 7mg%, proline 13mg%, glutamic acid 53mg%, serine 6mg%, threonine 5mg%, and asparagine 10mg%.

**Recommended Use:** As a dietary supplement, take 1∼3 packs per day. Pour the liquid content into a cup or drink directly from the pack. Do not heat the pack either in a microwave oven or heating range or leave the pack open since the product does not contain any preservatives. If warming is necessary, place the pack in warm to mildly hot water for desired length of time. Once the pack is open, drink immediately.

**Adverse Reactions:** No subjects have reported any side effects since the dietary supplement was placed for consumers in Japan, and Korea for the past 8, and 3 years, respectively. The use of this dietary supplement is generally safe based on two-year chronic toxicity studies of the product carried out by the Good Laboratory Practice (GLP) and American Association of Accreditation of Laboratory Animal Certification (AAALAC) certified Toxicology Research Center. No toxicity of general, CNS, reproductive and developmental, cardiovascular, immunology, and the two-year bioassay for carcinogenicity was negative. Recent clinical studies with 100 cancer patients undergoing chemotherapy in Korea have shown no known side effects or contraindications.[†]

**Warnings:** Sen-Sei-Ro Liquid Gold™ has not been evaluated in pregnant and breast feeding mothers or children and should consult a physician prior to use. Also consult a physician prior to use if taking a prescription medication. **Keep this product out of the reach of children. Do not use if you are pregnant, can become pregnant or breast feeding.**

**How Supplied:** Sen-Sei-Ro Liquid Gold™ 100ml water extract is high pressure heat sealed. A box contains 30, 100ml packs, and can be purchased directly from company representatives, health food stores, and independent pharmacies. Storage condition keep at room temperature and avoid any direct heat or sun light.

---

[†]**These statements have not been evaluated by the Food and Drug Administration. These products are not intended to diagnose, treat, cure or prevent any disease.**
*Shown in Product Identification Guide, page 509*

---

**SEN-SEI-RO POWDER GOLD™**
KYOWA'S *Agaricus blazei Murill*
Mushroom
1800mg standard granulated powder
Dietary Supplement

**Description:** Sen-Sei-Ro Powder Gold™ slim pack, a dietary supplement

*Continued on next page*

## Sen-Sei-Ro Powder—Cont.

containing an exclusively all natural and prepared from Kyowa's *Agaricus blazei Murill* mushroom is primarily used to reduce symptoms of fatigue, to promote vitality, overall well-being, and to support immune functions.[†] Normal immune function can decline with age, and are necessary for maintenance of vitality, energy, good health, and quality of life. A few major biomarkers for decreased immune functions are decreased natural killer cell (NK) activity, and the number of lymphocytes and macrophage cells. These cells, primarily attack diseased cells and thereby, maintain body homeostasis, promote health and quality of life. For the past half a century in Brazil and other countries, *Agaricus blazei Murill* mushroom has been used to restore vitality, and energy, and to serve as a potent tonic conducive to general health and aging concerns.[†]

**Clinical Trials:** The effectiveness of Sen-Sei-Ro Powder Gold™ for health benefits were tested in several controlled pre- and clinical trials in animals and in humans.[†] Recent studies in Japan, and Korea led researcher to report that in humans, Sen-Sei-Ro Powder Gold™ enhanced NK cell activity, increased the number of macrophage cells (Anticancer Research 17 (1A): 274–284, 1997; Japanese Association of Cancer Research, no. 2268, 1999) and tumor necrosis factor α (TNF-α)(Japanese Association of Cancer Research, no. 1406, 1999).[†] Antitumor effects of Sen-Sei-Ro against various murine and dog tumors were thought to be mediated by stimulation of NK cell activity, increased number of macrophage cells, and increased activity of tumor necrosis factor α (TNF-α)(Japanese J. Veterinary Clin. Medicine 17(2):31–42, 1998).[†] Recent clinical studies in Japan, and Korea, led researchers to report that *Agaricus blazei Murill* mushroom extract can be part of an effective treatment for supporting the immune systems of cancer patients by stimulating host defense system (Biotherapy 15(4): 503–507, 2001; Carbohydrate Res. 186(2): 267–273, 1989; Japanese J. Pharmacology 662: 265–271, 1994; Agricultural and Biological Chemistry 54: 2889–2905, 1990).[†]

**Ingredients:** Each 1800mg granulated powder in a slim pack contains 488 mg protein, 820 mg carbohydrate, 47 mg fat, 0.19 mg Sodium; 284 mg food grade cellulose; 5.7 kcal energy.

Water: 68mg, includes 0.1 mg Fe, 0.24 mg Ca, 37 mg K, 0.01mg thiamine, 0.04mg ergosterol, 0.59mg niacin.

**Recommended use:** As a dietary supplement, take 1~3 packs per day. Pour the content into a cup containing warm water or other desirable beverage and mix and drink. Do not heat the pack either in a microwave oven or heating range or leave the pack open since the product does not contain any preservatives. Once the pack is open, drink immediately.

**Adverse Reactions:** No subjects have reported any side effects since the dietary supplement was placed for consumers in Japan and Korea for the past 8, and 3 years, respectively. The use of this dietary supplement is generally safe based on two-year chronic toxicity studies of the product by the Good Laboratory Practice (GLP) and American Association of Accreditation of Laboratory Animal Certification (AAALAC) certified Toxicology Research Center. Toxicity evaluation of general, CNS, reproductive and developmental, cardiovascular, immunology, and the two-year bioassay for carcinogenicity was negative.[†]

**Warnings:** Sen-Sei-Ro Powder Gold™ has not been evaluated in pregnant and breast feeding mothers or children and should consult a physician prior to use. Also consult a physician prior to use if taking a prescription medications.. **Keep this product out of the reach of children. Do not use if you are pregnant, can become pregnant or breast feeding.** Quality of the dietary supplement is guaranteed for 2 years from the manufactured date, but for more information, please write or call 81-72-257-8568 or 81-3-3512-5032.

**How Supplied:** Sen-Sei-Ro Powder Gold™ is high pressure heat sealed. A box contains 30 slim packs of each with 1800mg per pack, and can be purchased directly from company representatives, health food stores, and independent pharmacies. Storage condition keep at room temperature and avoid any direct heat or sun light.

---

[†]**These statements have not been evaluated by the Food and Drug Administration. These products are not intended to diagnose, treat, cure or prevent any disease.**

*Shown in Product Identification Guide, page 509*

---

# Lederle Consumer Health

**A Division of Whitehall-Robins Healthcare**
**FIVE GIRALDA FARMS**
**MADISON, NJ 07940**

**Direct Inquiries to:**
Lederle Consumer Product Information (800) 282-8805

**CALTRATE® 600**
**CALTRATE® 600 + D**
**CALTRATE® 600 + SOY**
[căl-trāte ]

**Description:** CALCIUM SUPPLEMENT WITHOUT/WITH VITAMIN D,

NATURE'S MOST CONCENTRATED FORM OF CALCIUM® NO SALT, NO LACTOSE; TABLET SHAPE SPECIALLY DESIGNED FOR EASIER SWALLOWING
CALTRATE 600 + SOY CONTAINS SOY ISOFLAVONES

**SUPPLEMENT FACTS:**
Serving Size 1 Tablet

| AMOUNT PER SERVING | | % DAILY VALUE |
|---|---|---|
| **CALTRATE® 600** | Calcium 600 mg | 60% |
| **CALTRATE® 600 + D** | Vitamin D 200 IU | 50% |
| | Calcium 600 mg | 60% |
| **CALTRATE® 600 + SOY** | Vitamin D 200 IU | 50% |
| | Calcium 600 mg | 60% |
| | Soy Isoflavones 25 mg | * |

*Daily Value Not Established

**Ingredients:** *CALTRATE® 600:* Calcium Carbonate, Maltodextrin, Cellulose, Mineral Oil, Hydroxypropyl Methylcellulose, Titanium Dioxide, Light Mineral Oil, Polysorbate 80, Sodium Lauryl Sulfate, Carnauba Wax, Crospovidone, Magnesium Stearate, Stearic Acid.
*CALTRATE® 600 + D:* Calcium Carbonate, Maltodextrin, Cellulose, Hydroxypropyl Methylcellulose, Mineral Oil, Titanium Dioxide, Polysorbate 80, Polyethylene Glycol, Gelatin, Sucrose, Corn Starch, Canola Oil, Carnauba Wax, FD&C Yellow #6 Aluminum Lake, Crospovidone, Magnesium Stearate, Stearic Acid, Cholecalciferol (Vit. D), dl-Alpha Tocopherol (Vit. E).
*CALTRATE® 600 + SOY:* Calcium Carbonate, Maltodextrin, Soy Isoflavones Extract, Cellulose, Mineral Oil, Soy Polysaccharides, Hydroxypropyl Methylcellulose, Gelatin, Sucrose, Corn Starch, Polyethylene Glycol, Canola Oil, Carnauba Wax, Crospovidone, Magnesium Stearate, Stearic Acid, Cholecalciferol (Vit. D), dl-Alpha Tocopherol (Vit. E).

**Warnings:**
Caltrate® 600
Caltrate® 600 + D
As with any supplement, if you are pregnant or nursing a baby, contact your healthcare professional.
Caltrate® 600 + Soy
Use only as directed. Do not exceed recommended dosage. As with any supplement, if you are taking a prescription medication, or if you are pregnant or nursing a baby, contact your physician before using this product.
**Keep out of reach of children.**

**Suggested Use:** Take one tablet twice daily with food or as directed by your physician. Not formulated for use in children.
Bottle sealed with printed foil under cap. Do not use if foil is torn.

**How Supplied:** Caltrate 600, Bottles of 60, 150 tablets

Caltrate 600 + D, Bottles of 60, 120, 180 tablets

Caltrate 600 + SOY, Bottle of 60 tablets

Storage: Store at Room temperature. Keep bottle tightly closed.

---

## CALTRATE® 600 PLUS™ Tablets, CALTRATE® 600 PLUS™ Chewables
[căl-trāte]
Calcium Carbonate

**Calcium Supplement With Vitamin D & Minerals**
**No Salt, No Lactose**

### SUPPLEMENT FACTS
Serving Size: 1 Tablet
AMOUNT PER SERVING:

| | | % Daily Value |
|---|---|---|
| Vitamin D | 200 IU | 50% |
| Calcium | 600 mg | 60% |
| Magnesium | 40 mg | 10% |
| Zinc | 7.5 mg | 50% |
| Copper | 1 mg | 50% |
| Manganese | 1.8 mg | 90% |
| Boron | 250 mcg | * |

Chewables only:
Calories 10

| Total | | |
|---|---|---|
| Carbohydrate | 2 g | <1%† |
| Sugars | 2 g | * |

\* Daily Value not established.
† Percent daily value based on a 2000 calorie diet.

**Ingredients (Tablets):** Calcium Carbonate, Maltodextrin, Magnesium Oxide, Cellulose, Hydroxypropyl Methylcellulose, Mineral Oil, Zinc Oxide, Soy Polysaccharides, Titanium Dioxide, Manganese Sulfate, Polysorbate 80, Sodium Borate, Cupric Oxide, Polyethylene Glycol, Gelatin, Sucrose, FD&C Yellow No. 6 Aluminum Lake, Corn Starch, Canola Oil, Carnauba Wax, FD&C Red No. 40 Aluminum Lake, FD&C Blue No. 1 Aluminum Lake, Crospovidone, Magnesium Stearate, Stearic Acid, Cholecalciferol (Vit D), dl-Alpha Tocopherol (Vit. E).

**Ingredients (Chewables): Assorted Fruit Flavors (• Cherry • Orange • Fruit Punch):** Dextrose, Calcium Carbonate, Maltodextrin, Magnesium Stearate, Magnesium Oxide, Adipic Acid, Natural and Artificial Flavors, Cellulose, Mineral Oil, Zinc Oxide, Manganese Sulfate, FD&C Red #40 Aluminum Lake, FD&C Yellow #6 Aluminum Lake, Sodium Borate, FD&C Blue #2 Aluminum Lake, Cupric Oxide, Gelatin, Sucrose, Cornstarch, Canola Oil, Crospovidone, Hydroxypropyl Methylcellulose, Stearic Acid, Cholecalciferol (Vit. D), dl-Alpha Tocopherol (Vit. E).

**Suggested Use:** Take one tablet twice daily with food or as directed by your physician. Not formulated for use in children.

Bottle sealed with printed foil under cap. Do not use if foil is torn.

**Warnings:** As with any supplement, if you are pregnant or nursing a baby, contact your healthcare professional.

**Keep out of reach of children.**

**How Supplied:** Caltrate® 600 Plus™ Chewables, Bottles of 60 with Assorted Fruit Flavors. Caltrate® 600 Plus™ Tablets, Bottles of 60 & 120 tablets.

**Storage:** Store at room temperature. Keep bottle tightly closed.

© 1999

---

## CENTRUM®
[sĕn-trŭm ]
**High Potency Multivitamin-Multimineral Supplement, Advanced Formula From A to Zinc®**

## CENTRUM CHEWABLE
(Orange Flavor)
**Multivitamin-Multimineral Supplement**

### Centrum

**Supplement Facts:**
**Serving Size 1 Tablet**

| Each Tablet Contains | %DV |
|---|---|
| Vitamin A 5000 IU (20% as Beta Carotene) | 100% |
| Vitamin C 60 mg | 100% |
| Vitamin D 400 IU | 100% |
| Vitamin E 30 IU | 100% |
| Vitamin K 25 mcg | 31% |
| Thiamin 1.5 mg | 100% |
| Riboflavin 1.7 mg | 100% |
| Niacin 20 mg | 100% |
| Vitamin B$_6$ 2 mg | 100% |
| Folic Acid 400 mcg | 100% |
| Vitamin B$_{12}$ 6 mcg | 100% |
| Biotin 30 mcg | 10% |
| Pantothenic Acid 10 mg | 100% |
| Calcium 162 mg | 16% |
| Iron 18 mg | 100% |
| Phosphorus 20 mg | 2% |
| Iodine 150 mcg | 100% |
| Magnesium 100 mg | 25% |
| Zinc 15 mg | 100% |
| Selenium 20 mcg | 29% |
| Copper 2 mg | 100% |
| Manganese 2 mg | 100% |
| Chromium 120 mcg | 100% |
| Molybdenum 75 mcg | 100% |
| Chloride 72 mg | 2% |
| Potassium 80 mg | 2% |
| Boron 150 mcg | * |
| Nickel 5 mcg | * |
| Silicon 2 mg | * |
| Tin 10 mcg | * |
| Vanadium 10 mcg | * |
| Lutein 250 mcg | * |

*Daily Value (%DV) not established.

---

### Centrum Chewable

**Supplement Facts:**
**Serving Size 1 Tablet**

| Each Tablet Contains | %DV |
|---|---|
| Total Carbohydrate <1g | <1%+ |
| Vitamin A 5000 IU (20% as Beta Carotene) | 100% |
| Vitamin C 60 mg | 100% |
| Vitamin D 400 IU | 100% |
| Vitamin E 30 IU | 100% |
| Vitamin K 10 mcg | 13% |
| Thiamin 1.5 mg | 100% |
| Riboflavin 1.7 mg | 100% |
| Niacin 20 mg | 100% |
| Vitamin B$_6$ 2 mg | 100% |
| Folic Acid 400 mcg | 100% |
| Vitamin B$_{12}$ 6 mcg | 100% |
| Biotin 45 mcg | 15% |
| Pantothenic Acid 10 mg | 100% |
| Calcium 108 mg | 11% |
| Iron 18 mg | 100% |
| Phosphorus 50 mg | 5% |
| Iodine 150 mcg | 100% |
| Magnesium 40 mg | 10% |
| Zinc 15 mg | 100% |
| Copper 2 mg | 100% |
| Manganese 1 mg | 50% |
| Chromium 20 mcg | 17% |
| Molybdenum 20 mcg | 27% |

+Percent Daily Values based on a 2,000 calorie diet.

**CONTAINS ASPARTAME. PHENYLKETONURICS: CONTAINS PHENYLALANINE.**
**Centrum:**
**Ingredients:** Calcium Carbonate, Magnesium Oxide, Potassium Chloride, Microcrystalline Cellulose, Dibasic Calcium Phosphate, Ascorbic Acid (Vit. C), Ferrous Fumarate, Starch, dl-Alpha Tocopheryl Acetate (Vit. E), Gelatin, Crospovidone, Niacinamide, Zinc Oxide, Calcium Pantothenate, Manganese Sulfate, Silicon Dioxide, Pyridoxine Hydrochloride (Vit. B$_6$), Cupric Oxide, Vitamin A Acetate (Vit. A), Riboflavin (Vit. B$_2$), Thiamin Mononitrate (Vit. B$_1$), Beta Carotene, Chromium Chloride, Folic Acid, Lutein, Sodium Molybdate, Potassium Iodide, Borates, Sodium Selenate, Nickelous Sulfate, Phytonadione (Vit. K), Biotin, Sodium Metavanadate, Stannous Chloride, Ergocalciferol (Vit. D), Cyanocobalamin (Vit. B$_{12}$). **Contains less than 2% of the following:** Acacia Gum, Ascorbyl Palmitate, Butylated Hydroxytoluene (BHT), Calcium Stearate, Citric Acid, dl-Alpha Tocopherol, FD&C Yellow No. 6 Aluminum Lake, Hydroxypropyl Methylcellulose, Magnesium Stearate, Polysorbate 80, Potassium Sorbate, Sodium Aluminum Silicate, Sodium Ascorbate, Sodium Benzoate, Sodium Citrate, Sorbic Acid, Sucrose, Titanium Dioxide, Triethyl Citrate. **May also contain:** Lactose.
**Centrum Chewable**
**Ingredients:** Sucrose, Dibasic Calcium Phosphate, Mannitol, Calcium Car-

*Continued on next page*

## Centrum—Cont.

bonate, Stearic Acid, Starch, Magnesium Oxide, Ascorbic Acid (Vit. C), Microcrystalline Cellulose, dl-Alpha Tocopheryl Acetate (Vit. E), Gelatin. **Contains less than 2% of the following:** Acacia, Ascorbyl Palmitate, Aspartame,** Beta Carotene, Biotin, Butylated Hydroxytoluene, Calcium Pantothenate, Carbonyl Iron, Carrageenan, Chromic Chloride, Citric Acid, Cupric Oxide, Cyanocobalamin (Vit. B₁₂), Ergocalciferol (Vit. D), Folic Acid, Glucose, Guar Gum, Lactose, Magnesium Stearate, Malic Acid, Maltodextrin, Manganese Sulfate, Mono- and Di-glycerides, Natural and Artificial Flavors, Niacinamide, Phytonadione (Vit. K), Potassium Iodide, Potassium Sorbate, Pregelatinized Starch, Purified Water, Pyridoxine Hydrochloride (Vit. B₆), Riboflavin (Vit. B₂), Silicon Dioxide, Sodium Ascorbate, Sodium Benzoate, Sodium Citrate, Sodium Molybdate, Sodium Silicoaluminate, Sorbic Acid, Thiamine Mononitrate (Vit. B₁), Tocopherol, Tribasic Calcium Phosphate, Vanillin, Vitamin A Acetate (Vit. A), Yellow 6 Aluminum Lake, Zinc Oxide. **May also contain less than 2% of the following:** Fructose. **CONTAINS ASPARTAME.**

**\*\*PHENYLKETONURICS: CONTAINS PHENYLALANINE.**

**Suggested Use:**
**Centrum Adults**—One tablet daily with food. Not formulated for use in children.
**Centrum Chewable**
Adults and children 9 years of age and older—Chew 1 tablet daily with food.

**Warnings:** Accidental overdose of iron-containing products is a leading cause of fatal poisoning in children under 6. Keep this product out of reach of children. In case of accidental overdose, call a doctor or poison control center immediately.
As with any supplement, if you are pregnant or nursing a baby, contact your healthcare professional.
Bottle sealed with printed foil under cap. Do not use if foil is torn.

**How Supplied:** Light peach, engraved CENTRUM C1.
Bottles of 50, 130, 180, 250, 360 tablets
Chewables, Bottles of 50 tablets
Storage: Store at room temperature. Keep bottle tightly closed.

---

## CENTRUM KIDS COMPLETE
**Rugrats®**
**Chewable Multivitamin Supplement (Orange, Cherry, Fruit Punch)**

**Supplement Facts:**
[See table above]

**Ingredients:** Sucrose, Dibasic Calcium Phosphate, Mannitol, Calcium Carbonate, Stearic Acid, Magnesium Oxide, Ascorbic Acid (Vit. C), Microcrystalline Cellulose, Pregelatinized Starch, dl-Al-

| Serving Size: | | ½ Tablet | 1 Tablet |
|---|---|---|---|
| **Amount Per Serving:** | | % DV for Children 2 and 3 Years (1/2 Tablet) | % DV for Adults and Children 4 Years and Older (1 Tablet) |
| Total Carbohydrate <1g | | * | <1%+ |
| Vitamin A 5000 IU (20% as Beta Carotene) | | 100% | 100% |
| Vitamin C 60 mg | | 75% | 100% |
| Vitamin D 400 IU | | 50% | 100% |
| Vitamin E 30 IU | | 150% | 100% |
| Vitamin K 10 mcg | | * | 13% |
| Thiamin 1.5 mg | | 107% | 100% |
| Riboflavin 1.7 mg | | 106% | 100% |
| Niacin 20 mg | | 111% | 100% |
| Vitamin B₆ 2 mg | | 143% | 100% |
| Folic Acid 400 mcg | | 100% | 100% |
| Vitamin B₁₂ 6 mcg | | 100% | 100% |
| Biotin 45 mcg | | 15% | 15% |
| Pantothenic Acid 10 mg | | 100% | 100% |
| Calcium 108 mg | | 7% | 11% |
| Iron 18 mg | | 90% | 100% |
| Phosphorus 50 mg | | 3% | 5% |
| Iodine 150 mcg | | 107% | 100% |
| Magnesium 40 mg | | 10% | 10% |
| Zinc 15 mg | | 94% | 100% |
| Copper 2 mg | | 100% | 100% |
| Manganese 1 mg | | * | 50% |
| Chromium 20 mcg | | * | 17% |
| Molybdenum 20 mcg | | * | 27% |

*Daily Value (%DV) not established.
+Percent Daily Values based on a 2,000 calorie diet.

pha Tocopheryl Acetate (Vit. E), Gelatin. **Contains less than 2% of the following:** Acacia, Ascorbyl Palmitate, Aspartame**, Beta Carotene, Biotin, Butylated Hydroxytoluene, Calcium Pantothenate, Carbonyl Iron, Carrageenan, Chromic Chloride, Citric Acid, Cupric Oxide, Cyanocobalamin (Vit. B₁₂), Ergocalciferol (Vit. D), FD&C Blue 2 Aluminum Lake, FD&C Red 40 Aluminum Lake, FD&C Yellow 6 Aluminum Lake, Folic Acid, Glucose, Guar Gum, Lactose, Magnesium Stearate, Malic Acid, Maltodextrin, Manganese Sulfate, Mono and Diglycerides, Natural and Artificial Flavors, Niacinamide, Phytonadione (Vit. K), Potassium Iodide, Potassium Sorbate, Purified Water, Pyridoxine Hydrochloride (Vit. B₆), Riboflavin (Vit. B₂), Silicon Dioxide, Sodium Ascorbate, Sodium Benzoate, Sodium Citrate, Sodium Molybdate, Sodium Silicoaluminate, Sorbic Acid, Starch, Thiamine Mononitrate (Vit. B₁), Tocopherol, Tribasic Calcium Phosphate, Vanillin, Vitamin A Acetate (Vit. A), Zinc Oxide. **May also contain less than 2% of the following:** Fructose. **CONTAINS ASPARTAME.**
**\*\* PHENYLKETONURICS: CONTAINS PHENYLALANINE.**

**Suggested Use:** Children 2 and 3 years of age, chew approximately ½ tablet daily with food. Adults and children 4 years of age and older, chew 1 tablet daily with food. Not formulated for use in children less than 2 years of age.
Bottle sealed with printed foil under cap. Do not use if foil is torn.

**Warnings:** Accidental overdose of iron-containing products is a leading cause of

fatal poisoning in children under 6. Keep this product out of reach of children. In case of accidental overdose, call a doctor or poison control center immediately.
**CONTAINS ASPARTAME.**
**\*\* PHENYLKETONURICS: CONTAINS PHENYLALANINE.**

**Storage:** Store at room temperature. Keep bottle tightly closed.

**How Supplied:** Assorted Flavors—Uncoated Tablet—Bottle of 60 tablets
**Also available as: Centrum® Kids™ + Extra C** (250 mg); and as: **Centrum® Kids™ + Extra Calcium** (200 mg).
Marketed by: Whitehall-Robins Healthcare, Madison, NJ 07940

---

## CENTRUM® PERFORMANCE COMPLETE MULTIVITAMIN-MULTIMINERAL SUPPLEMENT Tablets

**Supplement Facts**
Serving Size 1 Tablet

| Each Tablet Contains | %DV |
|---|---|
| Vitamin A 5000 IU (20% as Beta Carotene) | 100% |
| Vitamin C 120 mg | 200% |
| Vitamin D 400 IU | 100% |
| Vitamin E 60 IU | 200% |
| Vitamin K 25 mcg | 31% |

| | |
|---|---|
| Thiamin 4.5 mg | 300% |
| Riboflavin 5.1 mg | 300% |
| Niacin 40 mg | 200% |
| Vitamin $B_6$ 6 mg | 300% |
| Folic Acid 400 mcg | 100% |
| Vitamin $B_{12}$ 18 mcg | 300% |
| Biotin 40 mcg | 13% |
| Pantothenic Acid 10 mg | 100% |
| Calcium 100 mg | 10% |
| Iron 18 mg | 100% |
| Phosphorus 48 mg | 5% |
| Iodine 150 mcg | 100% |
| Magnesium 40 mg | 10% |
| Zinc 15 mg | 100% |
| Selenium 70 mcg | 100% |
| Copper 2 mg | 100% |
| Manganese 4 mg | 200% |
| Chromium 120 mcg | 100% |
| Molybdenum 75 mcg | 100% |
| Chloride 72 mg | 2% |
| Potassium 80 mg | 2% |
| Ginseng Root (Panax ginseng) 50 mg Standardized Extract | * |
| Ginkgo Biloba Leaf (Ginkgo biloba) 60 mg Standardized Extract | * |
| Boron 60 mcg | * |
| Nickel 5 mcg | * |
| Silicon 4 mg | * |
| Tin 10 mcg | * |
| Vanadium 10 mcg | * |

*Daily Value (%DV) not established.

**Ingredients:** Dibasic Calcium Phosphate, Potassium Chloride, Ascorbic Acid (Vit. C), Microcrystalline Cellulose, Calcium Carbonate, dl-Alpha Tocopheryl Acetate (Vit. E), Magnesium Oxide, Ginkgo Biloba Leaf (*Ginkgo biloba*) Standardized Extract, Gelatin, Ginseng Root (*Panax ginseng*) Standardized Extract, Ferrous Fumarate, Niacinamide, Crospovidone, Starch, Zinc Oxide, Calcium Pantothenate, Silicon Dioxide, Manganese Sulfate, Pyridoxine Hydrochloride (Vit $B_6$), Riboflavin (Vit. $B_2$), Thiamin Mononitrate (Vit. $B_1$), Cupric Oxide, Vitamin A Acetate, Beta Carotene, Chromium Chloride, Folic Acid, Potassium Iodide, Sodium Selenate, Sodium Molybdate, Boron, Biotin, Phytonadione (Vit K1), Sodium Metavanadate, Nickelous Sulfate, Stannous Chloride, Cyanocobalamin (Vit. $B_{12}$), Ergocalciferol (Vit. $D_2$). Contains less than 2% of the following: Acacia Gum, Ascorbyl Palmitate, Butylated Hydroxytoluene (BHT), Citric Acid, dl-Alpha Tocopherol (Vit. E), FD&C Red No. 40 Aluminum Lake, FD&C Yellow No. 6 Aluminum Lake, Glucose, Hydroxypropyl Methylcellulose, Lactose, Magnesium Stearate, Polyethylene Glycol, Polysorbate 80, Potassium Sorbate, Sodium Aluminum Silicate, Sodium Ascorbate, Sodium Benzoate, Sodium Citrate, Sorbic Acid, Sucrose, Titanium Dioxide, Tribasic Calcium Phosphate, Water. May also contain Maltodextrin.

**Suggested Use:** Adults—One tablet daily with food. Not formulated for use in children.

**Warning:** Accidental overdose of iron-containing products is a leading cause of fatal poisoning in children under 6. Keep this product out of reach of children. In case of accidental overdose, call a doctor or poison control center immediately.

**Precaution:** As with any supplement, if you are taking a prescription medication, or if you are pregnant or nursing a baby, contact your physician before using this product.
Store at room temperature. Keep bottle tightly closed. Bottle sealed with printed foil under cap. Do not use if foil is torn.

**How Supplied:** Bottles of 45, 75, 120, & 180 Tablets.

---

## CENTRUM® SILVER®
**Multivitamin/Multimineral Dietary Supplement for Adults 50+ From A to Zinc®**

---

**Supplement Facts**
**Serving Size 1 Tablet**

| Each Tablet Contains | %DV |
|---|---|
| Vitamin A 5000 IU (20% as Beta Carotene) | 100% |
| Vitamin C 60 mg | 100% |
| Vitamin D 400 IU | 100% |
| Vitamin E 45 IU | 150% |
| Vitamin K 10 mcg | 12% |
| Thiamin 1.5 mg | 100% |
| Riboflavin 1.7 mg | 100% |
| Niacin 20 mg | 100% |
| Vitamin $B_6$ 3 mg | 150% |
| Folic Acid 400 mcg | 100% |
| Vitamin $B_{12}$ 25 mcg | 417% |
| Biotin 30 mcg | 10% |
| Pantothenic Acid 10 mg | 100% |
| Calcium 200 mg | 20% |
| Phosphorus 20 mg | 2% |
| Iodine 150 mcg | 100% |
| Magnesium 100 mg | 25% |
| Zinc 15 mg | 100% |
| Copper 2 mg | 100% |
| Potassium 80 mg | 2% |
| Selenium 20 mcg | 29% |
| Manganese 2 mg | 100% |
| Chromium 150 mcg | 125% |
| Molybdenum 75 mcg | 100% |
| Chloride 72 mg | 2% |

| | |
|---|---|
| Nickel 5 mcg | * |
| Silicon 2 mg | * |
| Vanadium 10 mcg | * |
| Boron 150 mcg | * |
| Lutein 250 mcg | * |

*Daily Value (% DV) not established.

**Recommended Intake:**
Adults, 1 tablet daily with food. Not formulated for use in children.

**Warnings: Keep out of the reach of children.** As with any supplement, if you are pregnant or nursing a baby, contact your healthcare professional.

**Ingredients:** Calcium Carbonate, Magnesium Oxide, Potassium Chloride, Microcrystalline Cellulose, Dibasic Calcium Phosphate, Ascorbic Acid (Vit. C), Starch, dl-Alpha Tocopheryl Acetate (Vit. E), Gelatin, Crospovidone, Niacinamide, Zinc Oxide, Calcium Pantothenate, Silicon Dioxide, Manganese Sulfate, Pyridoxine Hydrochloride (Vit. $B_6$), Cupric Oxide, Vitamin A Acetate (Vit. A), Riboflavin (Vit. $B_2$), Thiamin Mononitrate (Vit. $B_1$), Chromium Chloride, Beta Carotene, Folic Acid, Lutein, Sodium Molybdate, Potassium Iodide, Borates, Sodium Selenate, Nickelous Sulfate, Biotin, Cyanocobalamin (Vit. $B_{12}$), Sodium Metavanadate, Phytonadione (Vit. K), Ergocalciferol (Vit. D). **Contains less than 2% of the following:** Acacia Gum, Ascorbyl Palmitate, Butylated Hydroxytoluene (BHT), Calcium Stearate, Citric Acid, dl-Alpha Tocopherol, FD&C Blue No. 2 Aluminum Lake, FD&C Red No. 40 Aluminum Lake, FD&C Yellow No. 6 Aluminum Lake, Hydroxypropyl Methylcellulose, Magnesium Stearate, Polysorbate 80, Potassium Sorbate, Sodium Aluminum Silicate, Sodium Ascorbate, Sodium Benzoate, Sodium Citrate, Sorbic Acid, Sucrose, Titanium Dioxide, Triethyl Citrate. **May also contain:** Lactose.

**How Supplied:** Bottles of 60, 100, 150, and 220 tablets
Storage: Store at Room Temperature. Keep bottle tightly closed. Bottle is sealed with printed foil under cap. Do not use if foil is torn.

---

**UNKNOWN DRUG?**
Consult the
Product Identification Guide
(Gray Pages)
for full-color photos of
leading over-the-counter
medications

## Legacy for Life™
P.O. BOX 410376
MELBOURNE, FL 32941-0376

**Direct Inquiries to:**
1.800.557.8477
www.legacyforlife.net

## BIOCHOICE
## BIOCHOICE IMMUNE[26]
## BIOCHOICE IMMUNE SUPPORT

**Description:** BioChoice® products contain hyperimmune egg powder, pure egg product derived from hens hyperimmunized with >26 inactivated enteric pathogens of human origin. (Organisms such as: *Shigella, Staphylococcus, Escherichia coli, Salmonella, Pseudomonas, Klebsiella pneumoniae, Haemophilis,* and *Streptococcus* are included in the inoculum.)

**Clinical Background:** Upon oral administration, BioChoice's specific immunoglobulins and immunomodulatory factors are passively transferred. BioChoice Immune[26] and Immune Support modulate autoimmune responses, plus support and balance:
• Cardiovascular function
• Healthy cholesterol levels
• A vital circulatory system
• A fully functional digestive tract
• Flexible and healthy joints
• Energy levels

**How Supplied:** BioChoice is available as BioChoice Immune[26], hyperimmune egg in powder and capsule form, and as BioChoice Immune Support, hyperimmune egg enriched with minerals and 100% of the daily value of more than 13 essential vitamins.

**Precautions:** Those with known allergies to eggs should consult with a health practitioner before consuming this product.
Note: BioChoice is not intended to diagnose, treat, cure, or prevent any disease. These statements have not been evaluated by the Food and Drug Administration.

*Shown in Product Identification Guide, page 509*

---

**FACED WITH AN Rx SIDE EFFECT?**
Turn to the Companion Drug Index for products that provide symptomatic relief.

---

## Mannatech, Inc.
600 S. ROYAL LANE
SUITE 200
COPPELL, TX 75019

**For Medical Professional Inquiries Contact:**
Kia Gary, RN LNCC
(972) 471-8189
Kgary@mannatech.com

**Direct Inquiries to:**
Customer Service
(972) 471-8111

**Product Information:**
**www.mannatech.com**

**Ingredient Information:**
www.glycoscience.com

## AMBROTOSE®
**A Glyconutritional Dietary Supplement**

**Supplement Facts:**
**Ambrotose® powder:**
**Serving Size 0.44 g (approx. ¼ teaspoon)**
**Powder canister: 100g or 50g**

| Amount Per Serving | % Daily Value |
|---|---|
| 0.44g | * |

* Daily Values not established.

**Ambrotose® capsules:**
**Serving Size: two capsules**
**Capsules per container: 60**

| Amount Per Serving | % Daily Value |
|---|---|
| 2 capsules | * |

* Daily Values not established.

**Ambrotose® with Lecithin capsules:**
**Ambrotose® with Lecithin Supplement Facts:**
**Serving Size: two capsules**
**Capsules per container: 60**

| Amount Per Serving | % Daily Value |
|---|---|
| 1–2 capsules | * |

* Daily Values not established.

**Ingredients:**
**Ambrotose® Powder**
(patent pending)
Arabinogalactan (Larix decidua) (gum), Rice starch, Aloe vera extract, (inner leaf gel)- Manapol® powder, Ghatti (Anogeissus latifolia)(gum), Glucosamine HCl, Tragacanth (Astragalus Gummifer) (gum).
**Ambrotose® capsules**
(patent pending)
Arabinogalactan (Larix decidua) (gum), Rice starch, Aloe vera extract, (inner leaf gel)- Manapol® powder, Ghatti (Anogeissus latifolia) (gum), Tragacanth (Astragalus gummifer) (gum).
**Ambrotose® with Lecithin capsules**
(patent pending)
Arabinogalactan (Larix decidua) (gum), Rice starch, Aloe vera extract, (inner leaf gel) - Manapol® powder, Ghatti (Anogeissus latifolia) (gum), Tragacanth (Astragalus gummifer) (gum).
Other ingredients: Calcium, lecithin powder
**For additional information on ingredients, visit www.glycoscience.com**

**Use:** Ambrotose complex is a proprietary formula designed to help provide saccharides used in glycoconjugate synthesis to promote cellular communication and immune support.** Consumers who are healthy may notice improved concentration, more energy, better sleep, improved athletic performance, and a greater sense of well-being.

**Directions:** The recommended intake of Ambrotose powder is ¼ teaspoon two times a day; the recommended intake of Ambrotose capsules or Ambrotose with Lecithin is two capsules three times a day. If desired, you may begin by taking less than the recommended intake. If well tolerated, you may gradually increase to the recommended intake. As a blend of plant saccharides, Ambrotose complex is safe in amounts well in excess of the label recommendations. Children between the ages of 12 and 48 months with growth/nutritional problems (failure to thrive) have been given 1 tablespoon a day of Ambrotose powder for 3 months with no adverse effects. Individuals have reported taking as much as 10 tablespoons of Ambrotose powder (approx. 50 grams) each day for several months with no adverse effects. The amount needed by each individual may vary with time, age, genetic makeup, metabolic rate, and activities, stress level, current dietary intake, and health challenges of the moment. A health care professional experienced with use of Ambrotose complex may be helpful.

**Warning:** Anyone who is taking medication may wish to advise his/her physician. One teaspoon of Ambrotose powder (equivalent to 12 Ambrotose capsules) contains the amount of glucose equivalent to 1/25 teaspoon of sucrose (table sugar)

**KEEP BOTTLE TIGHTLY CLOSED.**
**STORE IN A COOL, DRY PLACE.**

**How Supplied:** Bottle of 3.50 oz (100g) powder. Bottle of 1.75 oz (50g) powder. Bottle of 60 (150mg) capsules.

** This statement has not been evaluated by the Food and Drug Administration. This product is not intended to diagnose, treat, cure or prevent any disease.

Mannatech Inc.
600 S. Royal Lane, Suite 200
Coppell, Texas 75019
www.mannatech.com
*Shown in Product Identification
Guide, page 509*

---

## PHYTALOE® with Ambrotose® Complex
### A Dietary Supplement of Dried Fruits and Vegetables

**Supplement Facts:**

**Serving size: 1 capsule or ¼ teaspoon**
**Capsules per container: 60 capsules**
**Powder canister: 3.5 oz. (100g)**

|  | Amount Per Serving | % Daily Value |
|---|---|---|
| PhytAloe | 490mg | * |
| Ambrotose complex | 50mg | * |

Brocolli, Brussels sprout, cabbage, carrot, cauliflower, garlic, kale, onion, tomato, turnip, papaya, pineapple. Ambrotose complex, naturally occurring plant polysaccharides including freeze-dried Aloe vera (inner leaf gel extract) – Manapol® powder.

*Percent Daily Values not established.

**Other Ingredients:** Magnesium stearate. This product contains no sugar, starch, preservatives, synthetic colorants or chemical stabilizers.

**Use:** PhytAloe is a blend of dehydrated fruits and vegetables in combination with Ambrotose complex for immune system support.** PhytAloe contains no synthetic additives and is supplied as powder and as capsules.

**Directions:** The recommended intake of PhytAloe powder is ¼ teaspoon twice a day; the recommended intake of PhytAloe capsules is one capsule twice a day.

**Warnings:** If any one of the fruits or vegetables in PhytAloe has caused stomach upset or any other adverse reaction in the past, start below the recommended amount and gradually increase to the recommended intake as tolerated.
**KEEP BOTTLE TIGHTLY CLOSED.**
**STORE IN A COOL, DRY PLACE.**

**How Supplied:** Bottle of 60 capsules. Bottle of 3.5 oz (100g) powder.

** This statement has not been evaluated by the Food and Drug Administration. This product is not intended to diagnose, treat, cure or prevent any disease.

*Shown in Product Identification
Guide, page 509*

---

## PLUS with Ambrotose® Complex
### Dietary Supplement Caplets

**Supplement Facts:**
**Serving Size - 1 Caplet**

|  | Amount Per Serving | % Daily Value |
|---|---|---|
| Iron | 1mg | 5 |
| Wild Yam (root) | 200mg | * |
| Standardized for Phytosterols | 25mg | |
| L-Glutamic acid | 200mg | * |
| L-Glycine | 200mg | * |
| L-Lysine | 200mg | * |
| L-Arginine | 100mg | * |
| Beta Sitosterol | 25mg | * |
| Ambrotose® Complex (patent pending) | 2.5mg | * |

Naturally occurring plant polysaccharides including freeze-dried Aloe vera inner gel extract-Manapol® powder.

**Other Ingredients:** Microcrystalline cellulose, silicon dioxide, croscarmellose sodium, magnesium stearate, titanium dioxide coating.

*Daily value not established.

**For additional information on ingredients, visit www.glycoscience.com**

**Use:** PLUS caplets provide nutrients to help support the endocrine system's production and balance of hormones.** A well-functioning endocrine system works in harmony with the body's immune system, helps support the efficient metabolism of fat, and supports natural recovery from physical or emotional stress.** The functional components of PLUS caplets are wild yam extract, amino acids, and beta sitosterol. PLUS caplets contain no hormones.

**Directions:** The recommended intake of PLUS caplets is three caplets per day. Start with one caplet a day for a week, gradually increasing to two then three a day. As with all dietary supplements, pay attention to how you feel as you increase intake of PLUS.

**Warning:** After an extensive review of the literature, no documented evidence was found linking the ingredients in PLUS caplets with any form of human cancer or with any problems associated with pregnancy. However, as with all supplements, you should consult your health care professional if you are pregnant.
**KEEP BOTTLE TIGHTLY CLOSED.**
**STORE IN A COOL, DRY PLACE.**

**How Supplied:** Bottle of 90 caplets.

** This statement has not been evaluated by the Food and Drug Administration. This product is not intended to diagnose, treat, cure or prevent any disease.

*Shown in Product Identification
Guide, page 509*

---

## Matol Botanical International Ltd.
**290 LABROSSE AVENUE
POINTE-CLAIRE, QUEBEC,
CANADA, H9R 6R6**

**Direct Inquiries to:**
Ph: (800) 363-3890
website: www.matol.com

### BIOMUNE OSF™ PLUS
**Dietary supplement for immune system support**

**Description:** Biomune OSF™ Plus is an immune system support product for all ages. Biomune OSF™ Plus is a combination of a special extract of antigen infused colostrum and whey with the herb Astragalus. The exclusive colostrum/whey extract (Ai/E¹⁰™) is prepared using a patented and proprietary process unique to the nutritional industry. Astragalus is a traditional Chinese herb that is known for its immune enhancing properties. Clinical studies show that Biomune OSF™ Plus is effective in consistently and dramatically increasing Natural Killer cell activity. Medical research has shown that low NK cell activity is present in most illness. A double blind study with antigen infused dialyzable bovine colostrum/whey shows its effectiveness as an immune system modulator.

**Summary of clinical studies:**
**The Use of Dialyzable Bovine Colostrum/Whey Extract in Conjunction with a Holistic Treatment Model for Natural Killer Cell Stimulation in Chronic Illness by Jesse A. Stoff, MD**
This clinical study consists of 107 patients with an average treatment time of 13.2 months. The average initial Natural Killer (NK) cell activity was 18 Lytic Units (LU) and the average final NK cell activity was 246 LU. All patients in the study greatly improved, went into remission or recovered.
Conclusions: The Study Group demonstrated that increased NK activity paralleled restored resistance to illness and recovery from illness.
**An Examination of Immune Response Modulation in Humans by Antigen Infused Dialyzable Bovine Colostrum/Whey Extract Utilizing a Double Blind Study by Jesse A. Stoff, MD.**
This study provides double blind evidence that the cytokines, peptide neurohormones and other informational molecules in Antigen Infused Dialyzable Bovine Colostrum/Whey Extract modulate and normalize immune function. Further, Antigen Infused Dialyzable Bovine Colostrum/Whey Extract demonstrates its effectiveness as a Biological Immune Response Modulator for increasing the protective functions of the immune system.

*Continued on next page*

## Biomune OSF Plus—Cont.

Both studies are available from Matol Botanical International Ltd. upon request.

**Use:** Dietary Supplement

**Directions for Use:** Take one capsule daily for maintenance and one or two capsules every 2–3 hours when additional immune support is needed. The product can be taken daily for maintenance or as above for extended periods of time. There is no known toxicity.

**How Supplied:** One bottle contains 30 capsules.

*Shown in Product Identification Guide, page 509*

---

## Mayor Pharmaceutical Laboratories

**2401 S. 24TH ST.
PHOENIX, AZ 85034**

**Direct Inquiries to:**
Medical Director
(602) 244-8899

www.vitamist.com

### VITAMIST® Intra-Oral Spray
[vĭt '-ə-mĭst]
**Nutraceuticals/Dietary Supplements**

**Description:** VitaMist® products are patented, intra-oral sprays for the delivery of vitamins, minerals, and other nutritional supplements, directly into the oral cavity. A 55 microliter spray delivers high concentrations of nutrients directly onto the mouth's sensitive tissue. The buccal mucosa transfers the nutrients into the bloodstream. (U.S. Patent 4,525,341—Foreign patents issued and pending.)

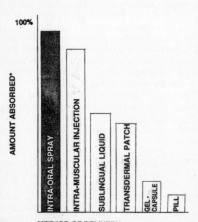

METHOD OF DELIVERY

*Representative of the product class.

**Benefits:**
- Spray supplementation provides an absorption rate approximately nine times greater than that of pills.
- Once the formula is sprayed into the mouth, the nutrients reach the bloodstream within minutes.
- No fillers or binders are added; the body receives only pure ingredients.
- An alternative method of supplementation for those that cannot take pills, or simply do not enjoy swallowing pills.
- Convenient administration; no water needed.

**Product Overview: Multiple:** vitamins and minerals in three separate formulations: adult, children's, and prenatal.
**C+Zinc:** with vitamin E and the amino acids L-lysine and glycine.
**B12:** contains 1000% of the US RDI of vitamin B12.
**Stress:** herbal formula with B vitamins.
**St. John's Wort:** St. John's wort extract with vitamin B12, ginkgo biloba, kava kava and folic acid.
**E+Selenium:** contains vitamin E and selenomethionine.
**Anti-Oxidant:** with vitamins A, C, E, niacin, folate, and beta-carotene.
**VitaSight®:** with vitamins A, C and E, beta-carotene, zinc, selenium, bilberry, lutein, and ginkgo biloba.
**Colloidal Minerals:** more than 70 trace and essential minerals from natural sources.
**Smoke-Less™:** herbal combination with additional nutrients designed to reduce cravings.
**PMS and LadyMate:** supplementation for the nutritional needs of pre-menstrual syndrome.
**Folacin:** vitamins B6 and B12 added to folate (folic acid).
**Slender-Mist®:** dietary snack supplements containing a combination of B vitamins, hydroxy-citric acid, L-carnitine and chromium. Four different flavors.
**Blue-Green Sea Spray:** spirulina extract, additional omega 3 fatty acids from flaxseed oil, and vitamin E.
**Re-Leaf:** a blend of more than 10 herbs that are recommended for minor discomfort, anxiety, and stress.
**Osteo-CalMag:** herbal supplement with additional vitamin D, calcium and magnesium.
**Pine Bark and Grape Seed:** powerful proanthocyanidins (anti-oxidants) from natural sources, with additional B vitamins.
**1-Before, 2-During, 3-After:** three performance sprays designed for the needs of physical activity.
**CardioCare™:** with vitamins C and E, the amino acids L-lysine and L-proline, coenzyme Q10 and additional herbal extracts.
**Melatonin:** a natural hormone that is effective in re-establishing sleep patterns.
**DHEA:** dehydroepiandrosterone in both men's and women's formulations.
**Revitalizer®:** high levels of B vitamins, as well as vitamins A and E, the amino acids L-cysteine and glycine, and selenium.

**GinkgoMist™:** with ginkgo biloba, vitamin B12, acetyl-L-carnitine, choline, inositol, phosphatidylserine and niacin.
**ArthriFlex™:** with chondroitin sulfate, glucosamine sulfate, vitamins C and D, calcium, manganese, boron and dong quai.
**VitaMotion-S™:** dimenhydrinate with ginger and vitamin B6.
**Echinacea + G:** combination of echinacea, goldenseal and garlic extracts, together with honey and lemon.
**Ex. O:** powerful blend of cayenne and peppermint with additional herbs recommended for allergy control.

**How Supplied:** VitaMist dietary supplements are supplied in sealed containers fitted with a natural pump. Each container provides a 30-day supply.

**Recommended Dosage:** Two sprays, four times per day, for a total dosage of eight sprays per day.

---

## McNeil Consumer and Specialty Pharmaceuticals

**Division of McNeil-PPC, Inc.
FORT WASHINGTON, PA 19034**

**Direct Inquiries to:**
Consumer Relationship Center
Fort Washington, PA 19034
(215) 273-7000

### AFLEXA™ Glucosamine Tablets

**Description:** Aflexa is a dietary supplement containing glucosamine, a natural building block of healthy cartilage. Each *AFLEXA™ Tablet* contains 300 mg glucosamine sulfate and 200 mg glucosamine hydrochloride.

**Actions:** Taken daily, *AFLEXA™* offers a number of valuable benefits:
- Helps maintain lubricating fluid in joints*
- Promotes joint flexibility and range of motion*
- Provides a natural building block of healthy cartilage*
- Promotes comfortable joint function*

**Uses:** *AFLEXA™* is intended to help maintain healthy cartilage in people whose joints may be affected by the natural aging process.

**Precautions:** **Do not use if you are allergic to shellfish.** If you are pregnant or breast-feeding, ask your doctor before use. Use only as directed. Keep out of reach of children.

**Directions:** Take one tablet three times a day. Benefits may begin within 2–4 weeks of daily use.

**Ingredients:** GLUCOSAMINE SULFATE, GLUCOSAMINE HYDROCHLORIDE, CELLULOSE, HYDROXYPRO-

PYL METHYLCELLULOSE, POLY-ETHYLENE GLYCOL, SILICON DIOXIDE, PROPYLENE GLYCOL, CROSPOVIDONE, HYDROXYPROPYL CELLULOSE, TITANIUM DIOXIDE, MAGNESIUM STEARATE, POLYSOR-BATE 80, POVIDONE.

**How Supplied:** *AFLEXA*™ is available in bottles of 50 and 110.
Store at room temperature.
DO NOT USE IF CARTON IS OPENED OR IF NECK WRAP OR FOIL INNER SEAL IS BROKEN OR MISSING.

---

* **These Statements Have Not Been Evaluated By The Food & Drug Administration. This Product Is Not Intended To Diagnose, Treat, Cure Or Prevent Any Disease.**

---

*Shown in Product Identification Guide, page 510*

---

**LACTAID® Original Strength Caplets**
(lactase enzyme)

**LACTAID® Extra Strength Caplets**
(lactase enzyme)

**LACTAID® Ultra Caplets and Chewable Tablets**
(lactase enzyme)

**Description:** Each serving size (3 caplets) of *LACTAID® Original Strength* contains 9000 FCC (Food Chemical Codex) units of lactase enzyme (derived from *Aspergillus oryzae*).
Each serving size (2 caplets) of *LACTAID® Extra Strength* contains 9000 FCC units of lactase enzyme (derived from *Aspergillus oryzae*).
Each serving size (1 caplet) of *LACTAID® Ultra Caplet* contains 9000 FCC units of lactase enzyme (derived from *Aspergillus oryzae*).
Each serving size (1 tablet) of *LACTAID® Ultra Chewable Tablet* contains 9000 FCC units of lactase enzyme (derived from *Aspergillus oryzae*).
*LACTAID®* is the original lactase dietary supplement that makes milk and dairy foods more digestible. *LACTAID®* lactase enzyme hydrolyzes lactose into two digestible simple sugars: glucose and galactose. *LACTAID® Caplets/ Chewable Tablets* are taken orally for *in vivo* hydrolysis of lactose.

**Actions:** *LACTAID® Caplets/ Chewable Tablets* work to naturally replenish lactase enzyme that aids in dairy food digestion. Lactase enzyme hydrolyzes lactose sugar (a double sugar) into its simple sugar components, glucose and galactose.

**Uses:** Lactaid contains a natural enzyme that helps your body break down lactose, the complex sugar found in dairy foods. If not properly digested, lactose can cause gas, bloating, cramps or diarrhea.*

*This statement has not been evaluated by the Food and Drug Administration. This product is not intended to diagnose, treat, cure, or prevent any disease.

**Directions:    Original Strength:** Swallow or chew 3 caplets with the first bite of dairy food. For best results, you may have to adjust the number of caplets up or down. **Extra Strength:** Swallow or chew 2 caplets with first bite of dairy food. For best results, you may have to adjust the number of caplets up or down. **Ultra Caplets:** Swallow 1 caplet with the first bite of dairy food. If you suffer from severe digestive discomfort, you may have to take more than one caplet, but no more than two at a time. **Ultra Chewables:** Chew and swallow 1 chewable tablet with your first bite of dairy food. If you suffer from severe digestive discomfort, you may have to take more than one tablet but no more than two at a time. Don't be discouraged if at first Lactaid does not work to your satisfaction. Because the degree of enzyme deficiency naturally varies from person to person and from food to food, you may have to adjust the number of caplets/ chewable tablets up or down to find your own level of comfort. Since Lactaid Caplets/Chewable Tablets work only on the food as you eat it, use them every time you enjoy dairy foods.

**Warnings:  Consult your doctor** if you experience any symptoms which are unusual or seem unrelated to the condition for which you took this product. **Do not use if carton is open or if printed plastic neckwrap is broken or if single serve packet is open.**
*LACTAID® Ultra Chewable Tablets:* Contains Phenylalanine 0.49 mg/tablet

**Ingredients:** *LACTAID® Original Strength Caplets:* Lactase Enzyme (9000 FCC Lactase units/3 caplets), Mannitol, Cellulose, Dextrose, Sodium Citrate, Magnesium Stearate.
*LACTAID® Extra Strength Caplets:* Lactase Enzyme (9000 FCC Lactase units/2 caplets), Mannitol, Cellulose, Dextrose, Sodium Citrate, Magnesium Stearate.
*LACTAID® Ultra Caplets:* Lactase Enzyme (9000 FCC Lactase units/Caplet), Cellulose, Dextrose, Sodium Citrate, Magnesium Stearate, Colloidal Silicon Dioxide.    *LACTAID®    Ultra Chewable Tablets:* Lactase Enzyme (9000 FCC Lactase units/tablet), Mannitol, Cellulose, Sodium Citrate, Dextrose, Magnesium Stearate, Flavor, Citric Acid, Acesulfame K, Aspartame.

**How Supplied:** *LACTAID® Original Strength Caplets* are available in bottles of 120 count. Store at or below room temperature (below 77°F) but do not refrigerate. Keep away from heat. *LACTAID® Extra Strength Caplets* are available in bottles of 50 count. Store at or below room temerature (below 77°F) but do not refrigerate. Keep away from heat. *LACTAID® Ultra Caplets* are available

in single serve packets in 12, 32, 60 and 90 count packages. Store at or below 86°F. Keep away from heat. *LACTAID® Ultra Chewable Tablets* are available in single serve packets of 12, 32 and 60 counts. Store at or below room temperature (below 77°F), but do not refrigerate. Keep away from heat and moisture. *LACTAID® Caplets* and *LACTAID® Ultra Chewable Tablets* are certified kosher from the Orthodox Union.
Also available: 70% lactose-reduced Lactaid Milk and 100% lactose-reduced Lactaid Milk.
*Shown in Product Identification Guide, page 510*

---

**PROBIOTICA**
**Daily Dietary Supplement**
**(Lactobacillus reuteri)**

**Description:** Each Probiotica Tablet contains 100 million cells of Lactobacillus reuteri.

**Actions:** Probiotica is intended to help people maintain gastrointestinal balance and promotes digestive function.* Probiotica helps maintain digestive health and balance by delivering "friendly" bacteria to the digestive system.*
Taken daily, Probiotica offers many healthful benefits:
• Provides natural support for digestive health and function.*
• Helps maintain a healthy balance of bacteria in the digestive system.*
• Promotes digestive functioning and gastrointestinal health.*

---

* These statements have not been evaluated by the Food & Drug Administration. This product is not intended to diagnose, treat, cure or prevent any disease.

---

**Uses:** Probiotica is a dietary supplement containing Lactobacillus reuteri, a naturally occurring healthful bacteria that promotes digestive health, balance, and function.* Helps maintain a healthy balance of "friendly" bacteria in the digestive tract.*

**Precautions:** If you are pregnant or nursing a baby, ask your doctor before use. This product is not intended for use in children under the age of 2 years. Keep out of reach of children.

**Directions:** Take one tablet per day. Chew thoroughly before swallowing. Store in a cool, dry place. Use only as directed.

**Ingredients:** Lactobacillus reuteri, mannitol, xylitol, lactulose, mono- and diglycerides, malic acid, natural lemon flavor, zein (corn protein), riboflavin phosphate (for color).

**How Supplied:** Bottles of 60.
*Shown in Product Identification Guide, page 511*

# Mission Pharmacal Company

**10999 IH 10 WEST
SUITE 1000
SAN ANTONIO, TX 78230-1355**

**Direct Inquiries to:**
PO Box 786099
San Antonio, TX 78278-6099
TOLL FREE: (800) 292-7364
(210) 696-8400
FAX: (210) 696-6010
**For Medical Information Contact:**
**In Emergencies:**
George Alexandrides
(830) 249-9822
FAX: (830) 816-2545

## CITRACAL® Ⓤ
*[sit'ra-cal]*
**Ultradense® Calcium Citrate Dietary Supplement**

**Ingredients:** Calcium (as Ultradense® calcium citrate) 200 mg, polyethylene glycol, croscarmellose sodium, hydroxypropyl methylcellulose, color added, magnesium silicate, magnesium stearate.

**Sensitive Patients:** CITRACAL® contains no wheat, barley, yeast or rye; is sugar, dairy and gluten free and contains no artificial colors.

**Directions:** Take 1 to 2 tablets twice daily or as recommended by a physician, pharmacist or health professional.

**Warning:** Keep out of reach of children.

**How Supplied:** CITRACAL® is supplied as white, rectangular (nearly oval), coated tablets in bottles of 100 UPC 0178-0800-01, and bottles of 200 UPC 0178-0800-20.
Store at room temperature.
Ⓤ=Kosher Parvae approved by Orthodox Union.

## CITRACAL® 250 MG + D
*[sit'ra-cal]*
**Ultradense® Calcium Citrate-Vitamin D Dietary Supplement**

**Ingredients:** Each tablet contains: calcium (as Ultradense® calcium citrate) 250 mg., polyethylene glycol, citric acid, microcrystalline cellulose, hydroxypropyl methylcellulose, croscarmellose sodium, color added, magnesium silicate, magnesium stearate vitamin $D_3$ (62.5 IU).

**How Supplied:** CITRACAL® 250 MG + D is available in bottles of 150 tablets, UPC 0178-0837-15.

## CITRACAL® Caplets + D
*[sit'ra-cal]*
**Ultradense® Calcium Citrate-Vitamin D Dietary Supplement**

CITRACAL® Caplets + D are supplied in an ultra-dense caplet formulation, each containing Vitamin $D_3$ (as cholescalciferol) 200 IU, and Calcium (as Ultradense® calcium citrate) 315 mg.

**Ingredients:** calcium citrate, polyethylene glycol, croscarmellose sodium, hydroxypropyl methylcellulose, color added, magnesium silicate, magnesium stearate, vitamin $D_3$.

**Directions:** Take 1 to 2 caplets two times daily or as recommended by a physician, pharmacist or health professional.

**Warning:** Keep out of reach of children.

**How Supplied:** CITRACAL® Caplets + D are available in bottles of 60 UPC 0178-0815-60, and bottles of 120 UPC 0178-0815-12.
Store at room temperature.

## CITRACAL® LIQUITAB® Ⓤ
*[sit'ra-cal]*
**Effervescent Calcium Citrate Dietary Supplement**

**Ingredients:** CITRACAL® LIQUITAB® is supplied as effervescent tablets each containing calcium (as calcium citrate) 500 mg, adipic acid, citric acid, sodium saccharin, artificial orange flavor, cellulose gum, aspartame.
**Phenylketonurics: Contains phenylalanine. Use of this product may be hazardous to your health. This product contains saccharin which has been determined to cause cancer in laboratory animals.**

**Directions:** Take 1 tablet dissolved in a glass of water, one to two times daily, or as recommended by a physician, pharmacist or health professional.

**Warning:** Keep out of reach of children.

**How Supplied:** CITRACAL® LIQUITAB® is available in bottles of 30 tablets. UPC 0178-0811-30.
Store at room temperature.
Ⓤ=Kosher Parvae approved by Orthodox Union.

## CITRACAL® PLUS
*[sit'ra-cal]*
**Ultradense® calcium citrate-Vitamin D-multimineral dietary supplement**

**Ingredients:** Each tablet contains: calcium (as Ultradense® calcium citrate) 250 mg., polyethylene glycol, magnesium oxide, povidone, croscarmellose sodium, hydroxypropyl methylcellulose, color added, pyridoxine hydrochloride, zinc oxide, sodium borate, manganese gluconate, copper gluconate, magnesium stearate, magnesium silicate, maltodextrin, vitamin $D_3$ (125 IU).

**How Supplied:** CITRACAL® PLUS is available in bottles of 150 tablets, UPC 0178-0825-15.

# Novartis Consumer Health, Inc.

**200 KIMBALL DRIVE
PARSIPPANY, NJ 07054-0622**

**Direct Product Inquiries to:**
Consumer & Professional Affairs
(800) 452-0051
Fax: (800) 635-2801
**Or write to above address.**

## BENEFIBER® Fiber Supplement

*Benefiber® is a 100% natural fiber, that can be mixed with almost anything. It's taste free, grit-free, and will never thicken. So it won't alter the taste or texture of foods or non-carbonated beverages. It can be used in coffee, pudding, soup, or whatever is desired. From the makers of ex-lax®.*

**Supplement Facts:**
**Serving Size: 1 tbsp (4g)**
**(makes 4 fl oz prepared)**

**Servings Per Container: 14, 24, 42, 80**

| Amount Per Serving | %DV |
|---|---|
| Calories 20 | |
| Total Carbohydrate 4g | 1%* |
|   Dietary Fiber 3g | 12%* |
|   Soluble Fiber 3g | † |
| Sodium 20mg | 1% |

*Percent Daily Values (DV) are based on a 2,000 calorie diet.
†Daily Value not established.

**Ingredients:** Partially Hydrolyzed Guar Gum (A 100% natural fiber).
Guar Gum is derived from the seed of the cluster bean.
Ⓤ 100% Natural Fiber–Sugar Free

**Directions for use:** Stir 1 tablespoon (tbsp) of Benefiber into at least 4 oz. of any beverage or soft food (hot or cold). Use 8 oz. if using 2 tbsp. Stir until dissolved.

| Age | Dosage |
|---|---|
| 12 yrs. to adult | 1–2 tbsp up to 3 times daily* |
| 7 to 11 yrs. | 1/2–1 tbsp up to 3 times daily** |
| Under 6 yrs. | Ask your doctor |

tbsp=tablespoon
* Not to exceed 5 tbsp per day.
**Not to exceed 2.5 tbsp per day.

Not recommended for carbonated beverages.

Store at controlled room temperature 20–25°C (68–77°F). Protect from moisture.

Use within 6 months of opening.

Keep out of reach of children.

If you are pregnant or nursing a baby, ask a health professional before use.

**Tamper Evident Feature:** Do not use if printed bottle inner seal is broken or missing or if sealed packet is broken or torn.

**How Supplied:**

- 24 serving cannister = 3.4 oz/96 g
- 42 serving cannister = 6 oz/168 g
- 80 serving cannister = 11.3 oz/320 g
- Box of 14 Ct. individual packets = 2 oz/56 g

Packaged by weight, not volume. Contents may settle during shipping and handling.

**Benefiber® guarantees your satisfaction or your money back.**

**Questions?** Call **1-800-452-0051** 24 hours a day, 7 days a week or visit us at **www.benefiber.com** for recipe ideas and additional information.

Manufactured for and Distributed by:

**Novartis Consumer Health, Inc.**

Parsippany, NJ 07054–0622

©2002

*Shown in Product Identification Guide, page 514*

---

## MAALOX® DS SOFTCHEWS

**Calcium Supplement**

**Cherry and Chocolate Flavors**

**Description:** For relief of Occasional Heartburn* and/or calcium supplementation.

**Supplement Facts:**

---

**Cherry Flavor:**

**Serving Size: 1 Chew**

| Amount Per Serving | | %DV** |
|---|---|---|
| Calories | 20 | |
| Calories from Fat | 5 | |
| Total Fat | 0 | <1% |
| Total Carbohydrates | 4g | 1% |
| Sugars | 3g | + |
| Calcium | 400mg | 40% |
| Sodium | 15mg | <1% |

---

**Chocolate Flavor:**

**Serving Size: 1 Chew**

| Amount Per Serving | | %DV** |
|---|---|---|
| Calories | 20 | |
| Calories from Fat | 5 | |
| Total Fat | 0.6g | <1% |
| Total Carbohydrates | 4g | 1% |
| Sugars | 3g | + |
| Calcium | 400mg | 40% |
| Sodium | 15mg | <1% |

**Percent Daily Values (DV) are based on a 2,000 calorie diet.
+ Daily Value not established.

**Ingredients:**

**Cherry Flavor:** Corn Syrup, High Fructose Corn Syrup, Calcium Carbonate, Sweetened Condensed Skim Milk, Sugar, Water, High Oleic Sunflower Oil, Glycerol Monostearate, Salt, Dextrin, Natural and Artificial Flavors, FD&C Red #40, Acacia, Lecithin, FD&C Red #40 Lake, FD&C Blue #1 Lake, Caramel, Tocopherol Excipient, FD&C Yellow #6 Lake.

**Chocolate Flavor:** Corn Syrup, High Fructose Corn Syrup, Calcium Carbonate, Sweetened Condensed Skim Milk, Sugar, Water, High Oleic Sunflower Oil, Chocolate Liquor, Cocoa (Processed with Alkali), Glycerol Monostearate, Salt, Artificial Flavor, Soy Lecithin.

**Warnings:** FOR ADULTS ONLY. Keep out of reach of children. Consult your health professional before using if you are pregnant or nursing a baby. Ask a doctor before use if you are taking a prescription drug. This product may interact with certain prescription drugs. Do not use for relief of heartburn for more than two weeks.

Store at controlled room temperature 20–25°C (68–77°F).

Avoid extreme heat.

**Calcium Supplement Information:**

Builds and maintains strong healthy bones*

May reduce the risk of osteoporosis

IMPORTANT INFORMATION ON OSTEOPOROSIS: Regular exercise and a healthy diet with enough calcium helps teen and young adult white and Asian women maintain good bone health and may reduce their high risk of osteoporosis later in life. Adequate calcium intake is important, but daily intakes above 2,000 mg are not likely to provide any additional benefit.

**Directions:**

**Calcium Supplement:** Take 1 Chew 3 times a day, preferably with meals.

**For relief of occasional heartburn:* Take 1 to 2 Chews up to 7 Chews a day.

**How Supplied:** Bottles of 30 chews

**Questions?** call **1-800-452-0051** 24 hours a day, 7 days a week.

---

*These statements have not been evaluated by the Food and Drug Administration. This product is not intended to diagnose, treat, cure or prevent any disease.

---

Distributed by:

**Novartis Consumer Health, Inc.**

Parsippany, NJ 07054-0622

©2001

*Shown in Product Identification Guide, page 515*

---

## SLOW FE®

**Slow Release Iron Tablets**

**Description:** SLOW FE supplies ferrous sulfate for the treatment of iron deficiency and iron deficiency anemia with a significant reduction in the incidence of the common side effects of oral iron preparations. The wax matrix delivery system of SLOW FE is designed to maximize the release of ferrous sulfate in the duodenum and the jejunum where it is best tolerated and absorbed. SLOW FE has been clinically shown to be associated with a lower incidence of constipation, diarrhea and abdominal discomfort when compared to an immediate release iron tablet[1] and a leading sustained release iron capsule.[2]

**Formula:** Each tablet contains: Active Ingredient: 160 mg. dried ferrous sulfate USP, equivalent to 50 mg. elemental iron. Inactive Ingredients: cetostearyl alcohol, FD&C Blue No. 2 aluminum lake, hydroxypropyl methylcellulose, lactose, magnesium stearate, polysorbate 80, talc, titanium dioxide, yellow iron oxide.

**Dosage:** ADULTS—one or two tablets daily or as recommended by a physician. A maximum of four tablets daily may be taken. CHILDREN—one tablet daily. Tablets must be swallowed whole.

---

**Warning:** Accidental overdose of iron-containing products is a leading cause of fatal poisoning in children under 6. Keep this product out of reach of children. In case of accidental overdose, call a doctor or poison control center immediately.

---

**Warning:** The treatment of any anemic condition should be under the advice and supervision of a physician. As oral iron products interfere with absorption of oral tetracycline antibiotics, these products should not be taken within two hours of each other. As with any drug, if you are pregnant or nursing a baby, seek the advice of a health professional before using this product.

Blister packaged for your protection. Do not use if individual seals are broken.

**How Supplied:** Child-resistant blister packages of 30, 60, and 90 ct.

Store At Controlled Room Temperature 20°–25°C (68°–77°F). Protect From Moisture.

Tablets made in Great Britain

**Novartis Consumer Health, Inc.**

Parsippany, NJ 07054-0622

**References**

1. Brock C et al. Adverse effects of iron supplementation: A comparative trial of a wax-matrix iron preparation and conventional ferrous sulfate tablets. *Clin Ther.* 1985; 7:568-573.
2. Brock C, Curry H. Comparative inci-

*Continued on next page*

---

*Information on Novartis Consumer Health, Inc., products appearing on these pages is effective as of November 2001.*

## Slow Fe—Cont.

dence of side effects of a wax-matrix and a sustained-release iron preparation. *Clin Ther.* 1985; 7:492-496.
*Shown in Product Identification Guide, page 515*

---

## SLOW FE® WITH FOLIC ACID
(Slow Release Iron, Folic Acid)
**Dietary Supplement**

**Description:** Slow Fe + Folic Acid delivers 47.5 mg. elemental iron as ferrous sulfate plus 380 mcg. folic acid using the unique wax matrix delivery system described above (for SLOW FE® Slow Release Iron Tablets).
Provides women of childbearing potential with the daily target level of folic acid to reduce the risk of neural tube birth defects. These birth defects are rare, but serious, and occur within 28 days of conception, often before a woman knows she's pregnant.

**Formula:** Each tablet contains: 47.5 mg. elemental iron as ferrous sulfate and 380 mcg. folic acid.
**Other Ingredients:** lactose, hydroxypropyl methylcellulose, talc, magnesium stearate, cetostearyl alcohol, polysorbate 80, titanium dioxide, yellow iron oxide.

**Dosage:** ADULTS—One or two tablets once a day or as recommended by a physician. A maximum of two tablets daily may be taken. CHILDREN UNDER 12—Consult a physician. Tablets must be swallowed whole.

**Warning:** The treatment of any anemic condition should be under the advice and supervision of a physician. As oral iron products interfere with absorption of oral tetracycline antibiotics, these products should not be taken within two hours of each other. Intake of folic acid from all sources should be limited to 1000 mcg. per day to prevent the masking of Vitamin $B_{12}$ deficiencies. Should you become pregnant while using this product, consult a physician as soon as possible about good prenatal care and the continued use of this product. If you are already pregnant or nursing a baby, seek the advice of a health care professional before using this product.

---

**Warning:** Accidental overdose of iron-containing products is a leading cause of fatal poisoning in children under 6. Keep this product out of reach of children. In case of accidental overdose, call a doctor or poison control center immediately.

---

**How Supplied:** Blister packages of 20 supplied in Child-Resistant packaging. Store at controlled room temperature 20–25°C (68°–77°F). Protect from moisture.
Tablets made in Great Britain

---

Novartis Consumer Health, Inc.
*Shown in Product Identification Guide, page 515*

---

## The Procter & Gamble Company
P. O. BOX 559
CINCINNATI, OH 45201

---

**Direct Inquiries to:**
Consumer Relations
(800) 832–3064

---

## METAMUCIL®
### DIETARY FIBER SUPPLEMENT
[met uh-mū sil]
**(psyllium husk)**
*Also see Metamucil Fiber Laxative in Nonprescription Drugs section*

**Description:** Metamucil contains psyllium husk (from the plant *Plantago ovata*), a concentrated source of soluble fiber which can be used to increase one's dietary fiber intake. When used as part of a diet low in saturated fat and cholesterol, 7g per day of soluble fiber from psyllium husk (the amount in 3 doses of Metamucil) may reduce the risk of heart disease by lowering cholesterol. Each dose contains approximately 3.4 grams of psyllium husk (or 2.4 grams of soluble fiber). A listing of ingredients and nutrition information is available in the listing of Metamucil Fiber Laxative in the Nonprescription Drug section. Metamucil Smooth Texture Sugar-Free Regular Flavor contains no sugar and no artificial sweeteners. Metamucil Smooth Texture Sugar-Free Orange Flavor contains aspartame (phenylalanine content of 25 mg per dose). Metamucil powdered products are gluten-free.

**Uses:** Metamucil Dietary Fiber Supplement can be used as a concentrated source of soluble fiber to increase the dietary intake of fiber. Diets low in saturated fat and cholesterol that include 7 grams of soluble fiber per day from psyllium husk, as in Metamucil, may reduce the risk of heart disease by lowering cholesterol. One adult dose of Metamucil has 2.4 grams of this soluble fiber. Consult a doctor if you are considering use of this product as part of a cholesterol-lowering program.

**Warnings:** Read entire Drug Facts section in listing for Metamucil Fiber Laxative in the Nonprescription Drug section.

**Directions:** Adults 12 yrs. & older: 1 dose in 8 oz of liquid *3 times daily*. Under 12 yrs.: Consult a doctor. See mixing directions in Drug Facts in listing for Metamucil Fiber Laxative in the Nonprescription Drug section.
NOTICE: Mix this product with at least 8 oz (a full glass) of liquid. Taking

without enough liquid may cause choking. Do not take if you have difficulty swallowing.
**For listing of ingredients and nutritional information for Metamucil Dietary Fiber Supplement, and for laxative indications and directions for use, see Metamucil Fiber Laxative in the Nonprescription Drug section.**
Notice to Health Care Professionals: To minimize the potential for allergic reaction, health care professionals who frequently dispense powdered psyllium products should avoid inhaling airborne dust while dispensing these products. Handling and Dispensing: To minimize generating airborne dust, spoon product from the canister into a glass according to label directions.

**How Supplied:** Powder: canisters and cartons of single-dose packets. For complete ingredients and sizes for each version, see Metamucil Table 1, page 745, Nonprescription Drug section.
**Questions? 1-800-983-4237**
*Shown in Product Identification Guide, page 522*

---

## Rexall Sundown
**6111 BROKEN SOUND PKWY**
**BOCA RATON, FL 33487**

---

**Direct Inquiries to:**
1-888-VITAHELP (848-2435)
www.osteobiflex.com

---

## OSTEO BI-*FLEX*®
**Double Strength**
**Glucosamine 500 mg**
**Chondroitin 400 mg**
**Dietary Supplement**
**Caplets**

**Helps rebuild cartilage & Lubricate joints***

**Description:** Osteo Bi-*Flex* is a nutritional combination of ingredients that helps rebuild cartilage and lubricate joints. Osteo Bi-*Flex* Double Strength formula provides the full daily dose of glucosamine (1500 mg) and chondroitin (1200 mg) in three, easy-to-swallow caplets.
Glucosamine is an amino monosaccharide and chondroitin is a polysaccharide, both of which occur naturally in the body. They play an important role in the production, repair and maintenance of healthy cartilage and connective tissue. Osteo Bi-*Flex* Double Strength formula provides an important nutritional approach for healthy joints and cartilage.

**Supplement Facts:**
Serving Size 3 Caplets

| Amount Per Serving | % Daily Value |
|---|---|
| Total Carbohydrate 2 g | 1%† |
| Dietary Fiber <1 g | 3%† |
| Sodium 100 mg | 4% |

Glucosamine HCl 1.5 g (1500 mg) ††
Chondroitin Sulfate 1.2 g (1200 mg) ††

---

†Percent Daily Values are based on a 2,000 calorie diet.
††Daily Value not established.

**Other Ingredients:** Red beet juice powder (color), crospovidone, magnesium stearate, microcrystalline cellulose, silica.

**Caution:** If you are allergic to shellfish, please consult your health care professional before taking this product. STORE IN A COOL, DRY PLACE. KEEP OUT OF THE REACH OF CHILDREN.

**Directions:**
**FOR ADULT USE: TAKE 3 CAPLETS PER DAY WITH FOOD.**

**How Supplied:** Bottle of 50, 110 or 150 easy-to-swallow caplets.

**Questions?** Visit us at osteobiflex.com or call toll free **1-800-VITAHELP (848-2435).**

Produced under **USP** Good Manufacturing Practices.

---

*These statements have not been evaluated by the Food and Drug Administration. This product is not intended to diagnose, treat, cure or prevent any disease.

---

Manufactured for Distribution by:
REXALL SUNDOWN, INC.
Boca Raton, FL 33487 USA
*Shown in Product Identification Guide, page 523*

---

**OSTEO BI-*FLEX*®**
**Patent-Pending Triple Strength**
**Glucosamine 750 mg**
**Chondroitin 600 mg**
**Dietary Supplement**
**Caplets**

**Helps rebuild cartilage &**
**Lubricate joints***

**Description:** Osteo Bi-*Flex* is a nutritional combination of ingredients that helps rebuild cartilage and lubricate joints. Osteo Bi-*Flex* Triple Strength complex is an exclusive, patent-pending formula. Just two easy-to-swallow caplets provide the full daily dose of glucosamine (1500 mg) and chondroitin (1200 mg).
Glucosamine is an amino monosaccharide and chondroitin is a polysaccharide, both of which occur naturally in the body. They play an important role in the production, repair and maintenance of healthy cartilage and connective tissue. The patent-pending Osteo Bi-*Flex* Triple Strength complex provides an important nutritional approach for healthy joints and cartilage.

---

**Supplement Facts:**
Serving Size 2 Caplets

| Amount Per Serving | % Daily Value |
|---|---|
| Total Carbohydrate 2 g | 1%† |
| Dietary Fiber <1 g | 3%† |
| Sodium 100 mg | 4% |
| Glucosamine HCl 1.5 g (1500 mg) | †† |
| Chondroitin Sulfate 1.2 g (1200 mg) | †† |

†Percent Daily Values are based on a 2,000 calorie diet.
††Daily Value not established.

**Other Ingredients:** Red beet juice powder (color), crospovidone, magnesium stearate, microcrystalline cellulose, silica.

**Caution:** If you are allergic to shellfish, please consult your health care professional before taking this product. STORE IN A COOL, DRY PLACE. KEEP OUT OF THE REACH OF CHILDREN.

**Directions:**
**FOR ADULT USE: TAKE 2 CAPLETS PER DAY WITH FOOD (THROUGHOUT THE DAY OR ALL AT ONCE).**

**How Supplied:** Bottle of 40, 80 or 120 easy-to-swallow caplets.

**Questions?** Visit us at osteobiflex.com or call toll free **1-888-VITAHELP (848-2435).**

Produced under **USP** Good Manufacturing Practices.

---

*These statements have not been evaluated by the Food and Drug Administration. This product is not intended to diagnose, treat, cure or prevent any disease.

---

Manufactured for Distribution by:
Rexall Sundown. Inc.
Boca Raton, FL 33487 USA
*Shown in Product Identification Guide, page 523*

---

## Sigma-Tau HealthScience, Inc.

**A division of Sigma-Tau HealthScience, S.p.A.**
**800 SOUTH FREDERICK AVE., SUITE 102**
**GAITHERSBURG, MARYLAND 20877**

**Direct Medical Inquiries to:**
Toll Free: 1 (877) PROXEED (776–9333)
Or: (301) 948–5450
Fax: (301) 948–5452
Email: proxeedinfo@ST-HS.com

**Direct Product Orders to:**
Toll Free: 1 (877) PROXEED (776–9333)
Web: www.proxeed.com

---

**PROXEED™**
[*prok'•seed*]
**Dietary Supplement**
**Promotes optimum sperm quality***

**Description:** PROXEED is a dietary supplement specifically formulated to optimize sperm quality. Sperm quality refers to motility, rapid linear progression, count, concentration and morphology.*

**Suggested Use:** To optimize sperm quality.*

**Active Ingredients:** Levocarnitine (L-carnitine) fumarate, fructose, acetyl-L-carnitine HCl, citric acid.
L-carnitine is a component of both seminal plasma and sperm cells. Because it plays a critical role in carbohydrate and fatty acid metabolism, L-carnitine is essential for optimal sperm maturation and motility.[1–3] L-carnitine also plays a critical role in cell membrane function.[4–5]
Fructose is one of the major energy-yielding substrates present in seminal fluid.[6]*
Acetyl-L-carnitine is the acetyl ester of L-carnitine and occurs naturally in the body. Acetyl-L-carnitine, also a major component of sperm cells, serves as a readily available substrate for cellular metabolism[7–9] and is important for sperm maturation and motility.[6–7,10] In addition, it plays a crucial role in maintaining cell membrane stabilization and function.
Citric acid is a key intermediate in the Kreb's Cycle.*

**Inactive Ingredients:** mannitol, polyethylene glycol, artificial flavorings, povidone, silicon dioxide.

**Supplement Facts:**
Serving Size 1 Packet
Servings Per Container 30

| | Amount Per Packet | % Daily Value |
|---|---|---|
| Calories | 10 | <1%* |
| Total Carbohydrates | 2g | <1%* |
| Sugars | 2g | ‡ |
| L-carnitine fumarate | 1g | ‡ |
| Acetyl-L-carnitine HCl | 0.5g | ‡ |

* Percent Daily Values based on a 2,000 calorie diet.
‡ Daily Value not established.

**Clinical Findings*:** Among healthy couples taking longer than expected to conceive, poor sperm quality is a contributing factor for nearly 40% of all cases.[7] PROXEED'S primary ingredients are L-carnitine fumarate and acetyl-L-carnitine HCl. In 12 clinical trials, levocar-

*Continued on next page*

## Proxeed—Cont.

nitine and acetyl-L-carnitine have been proven to provide the nutritional support needed for sperm's production of energy and optimum sperm quality.[2–3,7,10,12–19] Supplementation with the ingredients in PROXEED significantly improved percent motile sperm.[2–3,10,12–19]

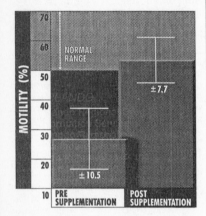

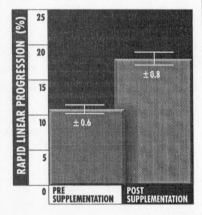

Mean (± SD) percent motile sperm was normalized after 3 months of supplementation with L-carnitine.[2] [p-not reported]*

Mean (± SEM) percent rapid linear progression showed a greater than 61.1% improvement after 4 months of supplementation with L-carnitine.[10] [p>0.001]* [See figure at top of next column]

Mean (±SEM) sperm count increased 14.7% after 4 months of supplementation with L-carnitine.[10] [p <0.001]*

Mean (± SEM) sperm concentration improved after 4 months of supplementation with L-carnitine.[10] [p <0.001]* There has been only limited data on whether the ingredients in PROXEED have a measurable effect on sperm morphology.

**Bioavailability/Pharmacokinetics:*** L-carnitine and acetyl-L-carnitine have oral bioavailabilities of between 5 and 15% in healthy adults. Clinical studies

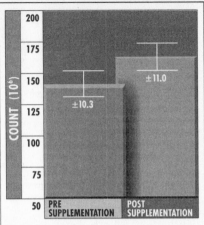

have shown that oral doses of 3 g per day (total) of carnitines are appropriate to optimize sperm quality.[2,10,15,19] The oral half-lives of L-carnitine and acetyl-L-carnitine are approximately 3–4 hours. As a result, the total daily dose should be divided b.i.d., and spaced 8 or more hours apart to maintain elevated blood levels of L-carnitine and acetyl-L-carnitine.

**Precautions:** As with all supplements, please keep this product out of the reach of children, and consult with your physician before use if you are taking any medications.

**Contraindications*:** Any known hypersensitivity or allergy to any of the ingredients in the PROXEED formula.

**Drug Interactions:** None known.

**Side Effects:*** There were no known side effects reported in the clinical trials involving the ingredients of PROXEED. Since its introduction in 1999, the primary reported side effect (<1%) has been mild gastrointestinal complaints such as upset stomach, heartburn, flatulence and loose stools.

**Dosage & Administration:** Take two packets of PROXEED per day, one packet in the morning and one packet in the evening. Mix each packet with at least 4 ounces (120 ml) of juice or other beverage. Patients who miss a dose should continue with the next dose. Double dosing is not necessary.

PROXEED is designed for long-term administration. Initial results may be seen in as few as three months, however, PROXEED should be taken for at least six months for optimal results. PROXEED should be taken for as long as attempting to conceive.* [See figure at top of next column]

On average, sperm require 74 days to mature, and up to 20 additional days to become capable of fertilization. Therefore, improvements in sperm quality while taking PROXEED will happen gradually over time.*

**How Supplied:** PROXEED is available in single dose packets packaged 30 per box. PROXEED's powder formulation

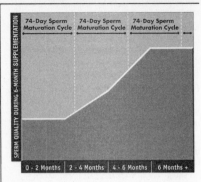

allows for the necessary ingredients in the amounts shown to be effective in clinical trials.

To order PROXEED, and for additional information, call toll-free 1-877-PROXEED (1-877-776-9333) or visit our website at www.proxeed.com.

**References:**
1. Jeulin C, Lewin LM. Role of free L-carnitine and acetyl-L-carnitine in post-gonadal maturation of mammalian spermatozoa. Hum Reprod Update 1996;2(2):87–102.
2. Vitali G, Parente R, Melotti C. Carnitine supplementation in human idiopathic asthenospermia: clinical results. Drugs Exp Clin Res 1995;21(4):157–9.
3. Loumbakis P, Anezinis P, Evangeliou A, Delakas D, Sbyrakis N, Cranidis A. Effect of L-carnitine in patients with asthenospermia. Eur Urol 1996;30(S2):255. Abstract 954.
4. Arduini A, Tyurin V, Tyurina Y, et al. Carnitine dependent long-chain acyl-transferase, an essential component of the membrane's secondary antioxidant response system in human red cells. Life Chem Rep 1994;12:49–54.
5. Virmani MA, Biselli R, Spadoni A, Rossi S, Corsico N, Calvani M, Fattorossi A, De Simone C, Arrigoni-Martelli E. Protective actions of L-carnitine and acetyl-L-carnitine on the neurotoxicity evoked by mitochondrial uncoupling or inhibitors. Pharmacol Res 1995;32(6):383-9.
6. Golan R, Shalev DP, Wasserzug O, Weissenburg R, Lewin LM. Influence of various substrates on the acetyl-carnitine: carnitine ratio in motile and immotile human spermatozoa. J Reprod Fertil 1986 Sep;78(1):287–293.
7. Moncada ML, Vicari E, Cimino C, Calogero AE, Mongioi A, D'Agata R. Effect of acetylcarnitine treatment in oligoasthenospermic patients. Acta Eur Fertil 1992;23(5):221–224.
8. Bartellini M, Canaie D, Izzo PL, Giorgi PM, Meschini P, Menchini-Fabris GF. L-carnitine and acetylcarnitine in human sperm with normal and reduced motility. Acta Europaea Fertilitatis 1987 Jan;18(1):29–31.
9. Kohengkul S, Tanphaichitr V, Muangmun V, Tanphaichitr N. Lev-

els of L-carnitine and L-0-acetylcarnitine in normal and infertile human semen: a lower level of L-0-acetylcarnitine in infertile semen. Fertil Steril 1977 Dec;28(12):1333–6.

10. Costa M, Canale D, Filicori MD, Iddio S, Lenzi A. L-carnitine in idiopathic asthenozoospermia: a multicenter study. Andrologia 1994 May;26(3):155–9.

11. Infante JP, Huszagh VA. Secondary carnitine deficiency and impaired docosahexaenoic (22:6n-3) acid synthesis: a common denominator in the pathophysiology of diseases of oxidative phosphorylation and beta-oxidation. FEBS Lett 2000;468(1):1–5.

12. Campaniello E, Petrarolo N, Meriggiola MC, Valdiserri A, Pareschi A, Ucci N, Flamigni C, Filicori M. Carnitine administration in asthenospermia [abstract]. In: IV Int Congress Andrology; 1989 May; Firenze. p. 14–18(5).

13. Muller-Tyl E, Lohninger A, Fischl F, Legenstein E, Staniek H, Kaiser E. Effects of carnitine on sperm count and motility. Fertilitat 1988; 4(1):1–4.

14. Micic S, Mladenovic I, Genbacev O. Does L-carnitine administered in vivo improve sperm motility? ARTA 1995;7:127–30.

15. Micic S. Effects of L-carnitine on sperm motility and number in infertile men [abstract]. In: 16th World Congress on Fertility and Sterility; 1998 Oct 4; San Francisco (CA).

16. Vicari, E. Effectiveness of short-term anti-oxidant high-dose therapy on IVF program outcome in infertile male patients with previous excessive sperm radical oxygen species production persistent even following antimicrobials administered for epididymitis: preliminary results. In: Ambrosini A, Melis GB, Dallapria S, Dessole S, editors. Infertility and assisted reproductive technology: from research to therapy. Bologna: Monduzzi Editore; 1997. p. 93–7.

17. Vicari E, Cerri L, Cataldo T, Lauretta M, Barone N, Laurenti A, Sidotti G. Effectiveness of single and combined antioxidant therapy in patients with astheno-necrozoospermia from non-bacterial epididymitis: effects after acetyl-L-carnitine or levocarnitine [abstract]. In: Italian Andrology Association, 12th National Conference; 1999 Jun 9–12; Copanello (CZ), Italty.

18. Vicari E, Cataldo T, Cerri L, Lauretta M, Laurenti A, Cannizzaro M. Production of oxygen free radicals in varicocele: pre- and post-treatment evaluation and observations after pharmacological trial [abstract]. In: Italian Andrology Association, 12th National Conference; 1999 Jun 9–12; Copanello (CZ), Italy.

19. Micic S, Lalic N, Bojanic N, Nale DJ. Carnitine therapy of oligospermic men [abstract]. In: J Androl 25th Annual Meeting program and abstracts; 2000 May 7–11; Boston: American Society of Andrology; 2000. p. 68. Abstract no. 135.

pxd-pi-12 ©2001 8/01

*Sigma-Tau HealthScience, Inc.*
*a division of Sigma-Tau*
*HealthScience S.p.A.*
*Gaithersburg, Maryland 20877*

---

* These statements have not been evaluated by the Food and Drug Administration. This product is not intended to diagnose, treat, cure or prevent any disease.

*Shown in Product Identification Guide, page 524*

---

# Sunpower Nutraceutical Inc.

**8850 RESEARCH DRIVE
IRVINE, CA 92618**

**Direct Inquiries to:**
Ph: (949) 833-8899

## PRODUCT LISTING

**Descriptions:** Sunpower Nutraceutical System combined vitamins, minerals, special formulated herbs, Pycnogenol® and proprietary Traditional Chinese Medicines (TCM) from S.P. Pharmaceutical Inc. (S.P.) which manufactured at GMP facility and under FDA Act and U.S. Pharmacopeia quality, purity and potency standards.

Time-released, Double-layered tablets are made by advanced manufacturing techniques which allows nutrients to be released slowly for better absorption during digestion.

**Sunpower Product Overview:**

**Sun Liver™:** contains vitamins, minerals, Pycnogenol® and S.P. Pro-Liver Formula to help to fight free radical damage, and provide nutrients essential for healthy liver function.

**Sun Cardio™:** contains CoQ10, OPC, Ginkgo Biloba, Red Wine Extract and S.P. Pro-Cardio Formula to help maintain normal cardiovascular system.

**Power Circulation™:** contains Ginkgo Biloba, Barley Grass, Lecithin and S.P. Pro-Circulation Formula to help maintain a healthy blood circulatory system.

**Sun Joint™:** contains Glucosamine, Chondroitin, Wild Yam, Bee Propolis and S.P. Pro-Connection Formula to provide essential nutrients for bone, joint, ligament and cartilage function.

**Power Lasting™:** contains Yohimbe, Damiana, Saw Palmetto, Pumpkin Seed, Sarsaparilla Root, and S.P. Pro-Long Formula to help maintain normal kidney and sexual function and enhance endurance.

**Sun Beauty™ 1:** Formulated for women ages 14–28 contains Alfalfa, St. John's Wort, Cranberry, Royal Jelly, and S.P. Beauty I Formula to help establish

---

healthy hormonal rhythms and basic immunity.

**Sun Beauty™ 2:** Formulated for women ages 29–42 contains Alfalfa, Selenium, Green Tea, Uva Ursi Leaves, Cranberry, and S.P. Beauty II Formula to support and balance a woman's vitality and healthy immunity during the menstrual cycle.

**Sun Beauty™ 3:** Formulated for women ages over 43 contains chromium, Burdock Root, Fo-Ti, Black Cohoshe, Red Clover, Chaste Tree Berries, and S.P. Beauty III Formula to support general well-being during menopause and post-menopause.

---

# Unither Pharma Incorporated

**1110 SPRING STREET
SILVER SPRING, MD 20910**

**Direct Inquiries to:**
321-779-1441

## HEARTBAR® PLUS
**60 gram bar (or drink mix)
6 grams of L-Arginine
Medical Food**

**Description:**
Bars contains over 10 g of soy protein. Represents 2 carbohydrate exchanges. Replaces 12 L-arginine tablets (500 mg per tablet).
[See table at top of next page]

**Directions: Symptomatic or high-risk population:** One HeartBar Plus daily
**At-risk population:** One HeartBar Plus daily

**Ingredients:** Toasted soy pieces, rice syrup, fructose, soy protein isolate, L-arginine hydrochloride, high fructose corn syrup, raisins, cookie pieces (wheat flour, sugar, canola oil, salt, sodium bicarbonate), natural and artificial flavor, maltodextrin, oat fiber, ethylcellulose, soy lecithin, soy isoflavones extract, modified food starch, partially hydrolyzed tapioca starch, sucralose, ascorbic acid, niacinamide, cellulose, alpha-tocopherol acetate, salt, pyridoxine hydrochloride, carrageonan, folic acid, vitamin B12.

**How Supplied:** Available in Vanilla, Peanut Butter, Cranberry, Vanilla Chocolate Coated, Peanut Butter Chocolate Coated, Cranberry Yogurt Coated, low calorie Orange Drink Mix.

Distributed by Unither Pharma
A United Therapeutics Company
1110 Spring St.
Silver Spring, MD 20910

*Continued on next page*

**Supplement Facts:**
**Nutrition Facts:**
Serving Size 1 Bar (60g)
Servings 8
Calories 220
  Fat Calories 25

*Percent Daily Values (DV) are based on a 2,000 calorie diet

| Amount/Serving | %DV* | Amount/Serving | %DV* |
|---|---|---|---|
| **Total Fat** 3g | 5% | **Total Carb.** 33g | 11% |
|   Saturated Fat 0.5g | 3% |   Fiber 2g | 8% |
| **Cholesterol** 0mg | 0% |   Sugars 18g | |
| **Sodium** 125mg | 5% | **Protein** 16g | |
| **Potassium** 190 mg | 5% | | |

Vitamin C 100% • Calcium 4% • Iron 10% • Vitamin E 30%
Niacin 90% • Vitamin B6 100% • Folate 50% • Vitamin B12 15%
Not a significant source of vitamin A.                  ©D

---

## HEARTBAR® PLUS ORANGE DRINK

**Description:**

Contains 50 mg of soy isoflavones. Replaces 12 L-arginine tablets (500 mg per tablet).

**Supplement Facts:**
**Nutrition Facts:**
Serving Size 1 Packet (15g)
Servings Per Container 8

**Amount Per Serving**
Calories 60

|  | % Daily Value* |
|---|---|
| **Total Fat** 0g | 0% |
| **Sodium** 0mg | 0% |
| **Total Carbohydrate** 9g | 3% |
| **Protein** 0g | |

Vitamin A 15% • Vitamin C 100%
Vitamin E 30% • Niacin 90%
Vitamin B6 100% • Folate 50%
Vitamin B12 15%

Not a significant source of calories from fat, saturated fat, cholesterol, dietary fibers, sugars, calcium, and iron.

---

*Percent Daily Values are based on a 2,000 calorie diet.

---

**Directions:** Add 1 packet of Heart-Bar® *Plus* Orange Drink mix to 8 oz of water. Stir or blend until completely dissolved.

**Ingredients:** L-arginine, citric acid, natural flavor, maltodextrin, soy isoflavones extract, beta carotene added for color, ascorbic acid, sucralose, alpha tocopherol acetate, niacinamide, pyridoxine hydrochloride, folic acid, vitamin B12.

Unither Pharma

United Therapeutics Company

1110 Spring Street

Silver Spring, MD 20910

## Wellness International Network, Ltd.

**5800 DEMOCRACY DRIVE
PLANO, TX 75024**

**Direct Inquiries to:**
Product Coordinator
(972) 312-1100
FAX: (972) 943-5250

## BIOLEAN®
### Herbal & Amino Acid Dietary Supplement

**Uses:** BIOLEAN® is a unique combination of Chinese herbal extracts and pharmaceutical-grade amino acids specifically designed to help raise overall health, participate in individual life extension programs, and enhance athletic performance. It has been shown to be extremely effective in promoting the healthy loss of excess body fat while helping to maintain lean body mass and potent energy levels. BIOLEAN, when used as a daily nutritional supplement, has also been shown to stimulate immune function in individuals with blunted sympathetic nervous systems, especially overweight and obese persons. It acts as a positive stimulator to immune functions involved in protection from environmental and dietary carcinogens. Components in BIOLEAN are known to cause fat loss through thermogenic activity and altered fuel metabolism resulting from sympathomimetic response to stimulation of beta receptors in adipose and muscle cells. The positive immune response, though not completely understood, is at least partially attributable to beta stimulation in adipocytes and the adaptogenic and tonifying activity of certain of the herbal extracts. This has been demonstrated in their long history of use in traditional Chinese herbal medicine as well as current scientific research which points to, among other possibilities, the extremely potent antioxidant properties found in some of the component plants, most notably in Green Tea and Schizandrae extracts. BIOLEAN may increase athletic performance and endurance through three pathways: 1) increased oxygen uptake in the lungs as a result of expanding bronchial passages; 2) enhanced mental acuity and response resulting from sympathetic nervous system stimulus; and 3) increasing the employment of fatty acids as fuel in muscle mitochondria while simultaneously sparing muscle glycogen and nitrogen.

The herbal extracts in BIOLEAN are produced in a unique and exclusive process which is proprietary to this product. Instead of creating extracts based on a set quantity of one particular active within many which may be present in any particular plant, BIOLEAN components are concentrated to maintain the natural and complete spectrum of biologically active factors, in the same ratio presented by the unprocessed plant.

**Directions:** AM Serving – Adults take one capsule and two tablets with low calorie food. PM Serving – Adults may take one tablet with low calorie food. If using BIOLEAN dietary supplement for the first time, limit daily intake to one capsule and one tablet on days one and two, and one capsule and two tablets on day three. Needs vary with each individual. This product has a maximum of 25mg concentrated ephedrine group alkaloids per serving in the form of herbal extracts.

**Warnings:** Not for use by children under the age of 18. If you are pregnant or nursing, if you have heart disease, thyroid disease, diabetes, high blood pressure, depression or other psychiatric condition, glaucoma, difficulty urinating, prostate enlargement, or seizure disorder, if you are using a monoamine oxidase inhibitor (MAOI) or any other prescription drug or over-the-counter drug containing ephedrine, pseudoephedrine or phenylpropanolamine (ingredients found in certain allergy, asthma, cough/cold and weight control products), consult a health professional before using this product. Exceeding recommended serving may cause serious adverse effects. Taking this product with other stimulants such as caffeine may cause serious side effects. Discontinue use and call a health professional immediately if you experience rapid heartbeat, dizziness, severe headache, shortness of breath, or other similar symptoms. Phenylketonurics: Contains phenylalanine. The maximum recommended daily dosage of ephedrine for a healthy, human adult is 100 mg, for not more than 12 weeks.

**Ingredients:** Calcium, Ephedra Alkaloids (as ma haung), Caffeine (as green tea leaf), Schizandrae berry, Rehmannia root, Hawthorne berry, Jujube seed, Alisma root, Angelicae dahuricae root, Epemidium, Poria Cocos, Rhizoma rhei, Stephania root, Angelicae sinensis root, Codonopsis root, Euconium bark, Notoginseng root, L-phenylalanine, L-tyrosine, L-carnitine, Cellulose, Stearic acid, Starch, Sodium lauryl sulfate, Hydroxypropyl cellulose, Magnesium stearate, Crosscarmelose sodium and Silicon dioxide.

**How Supplied:** One box contains 28 packets (28 daily servings), with one capsule and three tablets per packet.

---

## BIOLEAN Accelerator™
### Herbal & Amino Acid Formulation

**Uses:** BIOLEAN Accelerator™ is a unique combination of Chinese herbal extracts and pharmaceutical grade amino acids specifically designed to complement both BIOLEAN® and BIOLEAN Free® by extending and accelerating their actions. BIOLEAN and BIOLEAN Free are, in the traditional view of Chinese herbal medicine, strong Yang blends. This means that they are energy or heat-producing at their core. The addition of the amino acids and certain of the herbal components lends a very definite restorative or Yin element, as well. BIOLEAN Accelerator is a strong Yin herbal formula, intended to augment the lesser replenishing Yin elements of the other two herbal and amino acid supplements. Though the physiological actions of many herbs are complex and not totally understood, the formula in BIOLEAN Accelerator extends the adaptogenic, thermogenic, restorative and detoxifying results experienced with BIOLEAN and BIOLEAN Free, with an emphasis on the restorative and adaptogenic effects. The herbal formula is a combination of tonifiers traditionally used in China for the lungs, liver and kidneys.

**Directions:** For maximum effectiveness, use in conjunction with original BIOLEAN or BIOLEAN Free. (Do not consume BIOLEAN and BIOLEAN Free on the same day.) Take one tablet in the morning with original BIOLEAN or BIOLEAN Free. BIOLEAN Accelerator™ may also be taken in the afternoon with or without additional BIOLEAN or BIOLEAN Free if desired. Maximum absorption will be attained if taken with low-calorie food.

**Warnings:** Phenylketonurics: Contains Phenylalanine. Not for use by children. Consult your physician before using this product if you are taking appetite suppressing drugs or antidepressants, or if you are pregnant or lactating. If symptoms of allergy develop, discontinue use.

**Ingredients:** Each tablet contains 250 mg. herbal mix (Microcrystalline Cellulose Black Sesame Seed, Raw Chinese Foxglove Root, Chinese Wolfberry Fruit, Achyranthes Root, Cornelian Cherry Fruit, Chinese Yam, Eclipta Herb, Rose Hips, Privet Fruit, Mulberry Fruit-Spike, Polygonati Rhizome, Cooked Chinese Foxglove Root, Poria Co-

cos, Cuscuta Seed, Foxnut Seed, Alisma Rhizome, Moutan Bark, Phellodendron Bark, Anemarrhena Rhizome, Schisandra Berry, Royal Jelly), L-Tyrosine, L-Phenylalanine, Calcium Carbonate, Calcium Phosphate Dibasic, Partially Hydrogenated Vegetable Oil, Hydroxypropyl Cellulose, Croscarmelose Sodium, Magnesium Stearate, Silicon Dioxide and Sodium Lauryl Sulfate.

**How Supplied:** One bottle contains 56 tablets.

---

## BIOLEAN Free®
### Herbal & Amino Acid Dietary Supplement

**Uses:** BIOLEAN Free® is a strategic blend of herbs, spices, vitamins, minerals and amino acids specifically formulated to enhance fat utilization and energy production through various metabolic pathways. It has been shown to reduce body fat through its thermogenic effects and to enhance both physical and mental performance.

Thermogenesis refers to the body's ability to convert substrates such as proteins, fats and carbohydrates into heat energy. This is carried out most efficiently in the Brown Adipose Tissue of our body which uses fatty acids as its preferred fuel. Other fat cells, namely White Adipose Tissue, are concerned primarily with the storage of fat rather than its conversion to energy. The thermogenic pathway is complex and relies upon a series of reactions to occur. BIOLEAN Free utilizes many compounds which act at various locations in this pathway to ensure the maximum efficiency of the thermogenic process. Quebracho is one of these very special compounds. This South American plant contains quebrachine, aspidiospermine and other alkaloids that possess the ability to block alpha-2 adrenergic receptors in the body. This produces an enhanced sympathetic nervous system effect which, in turn, increases lipolysis (fat breakdown) within fat cells. The fatty acids released by this process can then be transported into the mitochondria to be used as a fuel. Ginger, cinnamon, horseradish, turmeric, cayenne and mustard are spices that stimulate thermogenesis in different ways. Some stimulate lipid mobilization in adipose tissue; others raise the resting metabolic rate; and some increase cAMP levels by inducing more beta receptors on fat cells and by increasing the concentration of adenylate cyclase. cAMP increases the breakdown of triglycerides to free fatty acids which are later used as fuel by the mitochondria in the cell. Methylxanthines (such as those found in green tea and yerba maté) also increase cAMP levels, but do this by inhibiting the enzyme, phosphodiesterase. These compounds have been noted to increase mental alertness, improve vitality, satisfy the

appetite and increase energy. In addition to its methylxanthine content, green tea has recently been shown to possess strong antioxidant properties. Yerba maté is a plant that has been shown to produce the positive effects above without causing the insomnia seen with other methylxanthine-containing plants (such as coffee and kola nut). BIOLEAN Free also contains vitamin B-3 (niacin), vitamin B-6 (pyridoxine), chromium and vanadium, which aid in the proper metabolism of fats, proteins and carbohydrates. L-tyrosine also aids in metabolism and promotes satiety through hypothalamic release of CCK. Methionine is a precursor of L-carnitine which aids in the transport of fatty acids into the mitochondria for thermogenesis. Other herbs have been utilized in BIOLEAN Free. Ginseng and ho shou wu possess adaptogenic properties. Adaptogens help the body adapt to physiological and environmental stresses. Ginseng accomplishes this through its stabilizing effect on the hypothalamic-pituitary-adrenal-sympathetic nervous system. It can mediate an increased adrenal response to stress.

Ho shou wu has a stabilizing effect on the endocrine system and has restorative properties. It is also an antioxidant with a high flavonoid content. *Centella asiatica* contains asiaticoside and has been shown to increase activity levels and ease the body's ability to overcome fatigue when taken with ginseng and cayenne. Individually, *centella* has been shown to increase memory and mental acuity in studies abroad. Uva ursi contains the glycoside arbutin and promotes urinary health and body strength through its purifying effects. Ginkgo biloba is a tree whose leaves have been used for centuries as an herbal medicine. It contains flavonoids and is therefore a strong antioxidant. It reduces the tendency of platelets to stick together by inhibiting Platelet Activating Factor. It has been shown to increase blood flow to the heart, brain and other organs.

**Directions:** Adults (18 years and older) may take 4 tablets in the mid to late morning with a low-calorie food. Needs may vary with each individual. Some persons may require less than 4 caplets, or may prefer taking 3 tablets mid morning and 1 additional tablet mid afternoon to achieve optimum results. Do not exceed recommended daily amounts. It is recommended that you drink at least eight glasses of water daily.

**Warnings:** Not for use by children, pregnant women or lactating women. Consult your physician before using this product if you are taking appetite suppressing drugs or cardiovascular medication. Consult your physician if you have hypertension, heart disease, arrhythmias, prostatic hypertrophy, glaucoma, liver disease, renal disease or diabetes. Do not use if you have hyperthyroidism,

*Continued on next page*

## Biolean Free—Cont.

psychosis, Parkinson's Disease, or are taking Monoamine oxidase inhibitors. BIOLEAN Free should not be taken on the same day as original BIOLEAN®. It is recommended that you minimize your caffeine intake while consuming this product. If allergic symptoms develop, discontinue use. Store in a cool, dry place. Keep out of reach of children.

**Ingredients:** Niacin (as niacinamide), Vitamin B6 (as pyridoxine HCl), Chromium (as chromium Chelavite® dinicotinate glycinate), Potassium (as potassium citrate), Green tea leaf extract, Yerba mate leaf extract, Korean ginseng root extract, Uva ursi leaf, Guarana seed, Quebracho bark extract, Gotu kola leaf, Ceylon cinnamon bark, Chinese horseradish root, Jamaican ginger root, Turmeric rhizome, Nigerian cayenne pepper, English mustard seed, Ho shou wu root, Ginkgo biloba leaf, L-Tyrosine, DL-Methionine, Vanadium, Dicalcium phosphate, Cellulose, Cellulose gum, Vegetable stearic acid, Silica, Vegetable magnesium stearate and vegetable resin glaze.

**How Supplied:** One box contains 28 packets, four tablets per packet.

---

## BIOLEAN LipoTrim™
### All-Natural Dietary Supplement

**Uses:** LipoTrim™ is a highly active, synergistic combination of garcinia cambogia extract and chromium polynicotinate specifically created for use with the other products in the BIOLEAN® System. The method of action is by inhibition of lipogenesis and regulation of blood glucose levels. Serum glucose derived from dietary carbohydrates and not immediately converted to energy or glycogen tends to be converted into fat stores and cholesterol. In individuals with excess body fat stores or slow basal metabolism, this tendency is thought to be higher. The garcinia cambogia extract present in LipoTrim is verified by HPLC analysis to be no less that 50%(-) hydroxycitrate (HCA). HCA inhibits ATP-citrate lyase which retards Acetyl CoA synthesis, severely restricting conversion of excess glucose into fatty acids and cholesterol. Animal studies have shown a post-meal fatty acid synthesis reduction of 40–80% for an 8–12 hour period. When glucose to fat/cholesterol conversion is retarded, glycogen conversion continues, increasing liver stores and causing satiety signals to be sent to the brain resulting in appetite suppression. In situations of intense physical exercise, increased glycogen stores have been shown to result in enhanced endurance and recovery. By restricting the activity of insulin, chromium has been shown to exhibit a regulating effect on blood glucose levels thus extending the benefits of HCA.

**Directions:** As a dietary supplement, take one capsule three times daily, 30 minutes before each meal. LipoTrim should be used in conjunction with a healthy diet and exercise plan.

**Warnings:** Do not consume if you are pregnant or lactating. Not for use by young children. Consult your physician before using this product if your diet consists of less than 1,000 calories per day.

**Ingredients:** Garcinia Cambogia (as CitriMax™* supplying naturally occuring hydroxycitrate), Chromium Polynicotinate (as Chromemate®* supplying elemental chromium).

**How Supplied:** One bottle contains 84, easy-to-swallow capsules.

---

*CitriMax™ is a trademark of InterHealth.
ChromeMate® is a registered trademark of InterHealth.

---

## FOOD FOR THOUGHT™
### Choline-Enriched Nutritional Drink

**Uses:** By utilizing scientifically established "smart nutrients," Food For Thought™ is a great-tasting citrus beverage ideal for work, school or anytime peak mental performance is desired.

Choline, a member of the B-complex family, is determined to be one of the few substances that possesses the ability to penetrate the blood-brain barrier—a protectant of the brain from the onslaught of chemicals taken into the body each day—and go directly into the brain cells to produce acetylcholine.

The most abundant neurotransmitter in the body, acetylcholine is the primary neurotransmitter between neurons and muscles. It is vital because of its role in motor behavior (muscular movement) and memory. Acetylcholine helps control muscle tone, learning, and primitive drives and emotions, while also controlling the release of the pituitary hormone vasopressin—which is involved in learning and in the regulation of urine output. Studies show that low levels of acetylcholine can contribute to lack of concentration and forgetfulness, and may interfere with sleep patterns.

Food For Thought further enhances its effectiveness through the utilization of essential vitamins—required for promoting the synthesis of brain neurotransmitters—with a unique blend of minerals. The brain uses vitamins B3 (niacin) and B6 (pyridoxine), to convert the amino acid L-tryptophan into the mood- and sleep-regulating neurotransmitter serotonin, while vitamins B1 (thiamin), B5 (pantothenic acid), B6 (pyridoxine), and C and the minerals zinc and calcium are required for the production of acetylcholine.

**Directions:** Add 6 ounces of chilled water or fruit juice to one packet of mix. Stir briskly. Consume 1–2 times per day. Keep in a cool, dry place. For maximum results, combine this product with one serving of Winrgy™.

**Warnings:** Not for use by children, pregnant or lactating women. Persons taking medications should seek medical advice before taking this product. Persons with ulcers or a history of ulcers should consult their physician before using a choline supplement. Do not consume more than four servings per day. Avoid the use of antacids containing aluminum with this product.

**Ingredients:** Carbohydrates, Sugars, Vitamin C (as ascorbic acid), Vitamin E (as alpha tocopherol acetate), Thiamin (as thiamin mononitrate), Riboflavin, Niacin (as niacinamide), Vitamin B6 (as pyridoxine hydrochloride), Vitamin B12 (as cyanocobalamin), Pantothenic Acid (as calcium pantothenate), Calcium (as calcium pantothenate), Zinc (as zinc gluconate), Copper (as copper gluconate), Chromium (as chromium aspartate), Choline (as choline bitartrate), Glycine, Lysine (as L-lysine hydrochloride), Fructose, Natural Flavors, Silicon Dioxide and Magnesium Gluconate.

**How Supplied:** One box contains 28 packets of drink mix. Serving size equals one packet.

---

## DHEA Plus™
### Pharmaceutical-Grade Formulation

**Uses:** By utilizing the latest and most advanced breakthrough applications in age management, DHEA Plus™ uniquely combines dehydroepiandrosterone (DHEA), Bioperine® and ginkgo biloba leaf to safely and effectively aid the body.

These age management factors are mainly attributed to the properties of DHEA, a natural substance obtained from the barbasco root, also known as Mexican Wild Yam, which is synthesized in a pharmaceutical laboratory to be utilized for specific health applications. Once supplemental DHEA is orally consumed, it is quickly absorbed into the bloodstream through the intestines and binds to a sulfate compound which creates DHEA-S. DHEA-S is the ultimate substance for which the body uses to manufacture hormones. Natural DHEA levels, abundant in the bloodstream and present at an even higher level in the tissues of the brain, are known to decline with age in both sexes. Scientific research proves that adequate levels of DHEA in the body can actually slow the aging process. Further studies have shown that it often prevents, improves and, many times, reverses conditions such as cancer, heart disease, memory loss, obesity and osteoporosis.

Bioperine, a pure piperine extract, enhances the body's natural thermogenic activity and is another important ingredient in DHEA Plus. Thermogenesis is the metabolic process that generates energy at the cellular level. While thermogenesis plays an integral role in our body's ability to properly utilize daily foods and nutrients in the body, it also sets in motion the mechanisms that lead to digestion and subsequent gastrointestinal absorption.

Known for possessing antioxidant activity, or flavonoid effects, ginkgo biloba proves to decrease platelet aggregation and increase vasodilation which appears to extend blood flow to the peripheral arteries and the brain. Some improvement in cognitive abilities has been noted as well as inhibition of lipid peroxidation, thereby stabilizing the cell wall against free-radical attack.

**Directions:** Adults take one capsule daily with food.

**Warnings:** This product should only be consumed by adults and is not intended for use by children. Do not consume if you are pregnant or lactating. Consult your physician before using this product if you are taking prescription medications. Persons with a history of prostate cancer should seek medical advice before using this product.

**Ingredients:** Dihydroxyepiandrosterone (DHEA), Ginkgo Biloba leaf, Bioperine, Calcium Phosphate Dibasic, Partially Hydrogenated Vegetable Oil, Talc, Magnesium Stearate, Silicon Dioxide and Croscarmellose Sodium.

**How Supplied:** One bottle contains 60 capsules.

*Bioperine is a registered trademark of Sabinsa Corporation.

---

## MASS APPEAL™
### Amino Acid & Mineral Workout Supplement

**Uses:** Utilizing natural compounds which mimic the beneficial effects of anabolic steroids, Mass Appeal™ is specifically formulated to enhance athletic performance without the harmful side effects of steroids.

Among Mass Appeal's scientifically researched and proven ingredients is creatine, a naturally occurring substance which functions as a storage molecule for high-energy phosphate – the ultimate source of muscular energy known as adenosine triphosphate, or ATP. More than 95 percent of the body's total amount of creatine is contained within the muscles, with type II muscle fibers (fibers that generate large amounts of force) possessing greater initial levels and higher rates of utilization. Unlike other artificial aids used to enhance performance, creatine monohydrate saturates the muscle cells and causes a muscle "cell volumizing" effect by beneficially forcing water molecules inside the muscle cell. This promotes an increase in muscle growth by helping muscles form new proteins faster while slowing down the destructive breakdown of muscle cells during exercise. Studies show that creatine loading not only improves per-

formance during short-duration, high intensity and intermittent exercises, but it accelerates energy recovery and reduces muscle fatigue by reducing lactic acid build-up as well.

Found in high concentrations within muscle cells and proteins throughout the body, the branched chain amino acids (BCAAs) L-leucine, L-valine and L-isoleucine are also incorporated into Mass Appeal's scientifically engineered formulation. BCAAs increase protein synthesis and can be oxidized inside muscle cells as ATP, a protein-sparing effect which indirectly increases anabolism by reducing the muscle's need to burn its own proteins during bodybuilding or strenuous exercise. When dietary intake of these amino acids is inadequate, muscle protein is broken down into its individual amino acid constituents and utilized in other essential metabolic reactions within the body. Through supplementation, the catabolic breakdown of muscle can be minimized and the muscle tissue preserved.

Alpha-ketoglutaric acid and the amino acid L-glutamine also protect against muscle catabolism by assisting muscle protein synthesis and preserving the body's natural stores of glutamine in the muscle.

Another major contributor to the Mass Appeal™ formulation is the amino acid inosine. By increasing hemoglobin's affinity for binding oxygen within red blood cells, inosine supplementation enables red blood cells to carry more oxygen as they travel from the lungs to the muscles.

Vanadyl sulfate, known for its vasodilator effects, has been shown to markedly increase the blood flow to muscle cells. Researchers also believe that this mineral not only contributes to increased efficiency in the metabolic pathways controlled by the body's insulin, but also triggers certain glucose transporters much in the same way insulin does. This results in increased glucose transport into the muscle tissue, increased glycogen storage, and decreases the breakdown of muscle protein as an energy source.

**Directions:** Adults (18 years and older) may take a loading dose of 3 packets in the morning and 2 packets in the late afternoon for one week. This dose may be repeated every three months. Following one week of the loading dose, begin the maintenance dose of 1 packet daily two hours after exercise. Needs may vary with each individual.

For individuals desiring enhanced effects, increase the loading dose to 3 to 4 packets, three times per day (morning, afternoon and evening). Following one week of this enhanced loading dose, begin the enhanced maintenance dose of 2 packets in the morning and 2 packets in the late afternoon. It is recommended that one maintain a low-fat, high-protein diet; drink at least eight glasses of water per day; and engage in 30 to 60 minutes

of aerobic and anaerobic exercise three to four times per week. For optimal effects, take in conjunction with Phyto-Vite®, Pro-Xtreme™ and Sure2Endure™.

**Warning:** Not for use by children, pregnant women or lactating women. Consult your physician before using this product if you have any medical conditions. Do not take if you have kidney disease, muscle disease or are on a protein-restricted diet. Discontinue immediately if allergic symptoms develop. Keep out of the reach of children. Store in a cool, dry place.

**Ingredients:** Creatine Monohydrate, Inosine (phosphate-bonded), L-leucine, L-valine, L-isoleucine, Alpha-Ketoglutaric acid, KIC (calcium keto-isocaproate), L-glutamine, Vanadyl Sulfate, Dicalcium phosphate, Microcrystalline Cellulose, Stearic Acid, Croscarmellose Sodium, Silica, Magnesium Stearate and film coating (hydroxypropyl methylcellulose, hydroxypropyl cellulose, polyethylene glycol, titanium dioxide and propylene glycol).

**How Supplied:** One box contains 28 packets, four tablets per packet.

---

## PRO-XTREME™
### Dietary Supplement

**Uses:** The need for protein in the human diet has been increasingly studied, especially in the last decade. As a result of this research, several factors regarding the optimal daily requirements and sources of protein have become very clear. Even the current government published RDIs, which are based solely on minimal needs for survival, have increased to .6–.8 grams per kilogram of body weight per day.

Current clinical findings however indicate that an RDI necessary to maintain optimum health for even a sedentary adult are closer to double that. Circumstances including illness, fat-loss diets, regular exercise, accelerated adolescent growth, or chronic mental or emotional stress indicate requirements 2–3 times that. Competitive or strength athletes, post surgical patients or any situation causing wasting disease such as chemotherapy, HIV, burn trauma or radiation therapy can increase the metabolic need for protein by a factor of up to 6 times the official government RDIs.

Furthermore, these figures represent protein which has been absorbed and made available to the tissues of the body and *not* merely that which has been consumed. This is a distinction current clinical research has recognized as *critical* to proper understanding of the need for protein in the human diet.

Before protein can be absorbed and utilized it must first be digested. Following digestion the free amino acids and di and

*Continued on next page*

## Pro-Xtreme—Cont.

tripeptides that result from protein breakdown are absorbed at the surface of the small intestine. The process of digestion and absorption requires several steps and is most efficient in the upper portion or proximal section of the jejunum (small intestine). In order for absorption of dietary protein to occur, it must first be reduced from larger oligo and polypeptides to di and tripeptides, the smallest protein fragments consisting of only two or three peptide-bonded amino acids, and free amino acids. Di and tripeptides have been clearly shown to be preferential over free forms. This process must occur fast enough and at a rate high enough to take advantage of the proximal transporters, those that specialize in di and tripeptides and which are in abundance only in this short section of upper intestinal bowel. Once protein has passed this lumenal area, relatively no further protein breakdown or absorption occurs. The balance moves on relatively unchanged into the colon, where it is definitely a negative health factor causing minimal gas and gastrointestinal distress, and when experienced chronically, can lead to colon disease and malignancy. It is now generally believed to be the number one factor responsible for the world's highest rate of colon cancer experienced in the U.S.

Pro-Xtreme™ is specifically engineered based on a new profile for protein in optimum human metabolism arising from these new clinical findings. With an exceptionally high di and tripeptide content of 40 percent, Pro-Xtreme™ not only promotes increased nitrogen retention—thereby minimizing the negative effects of increased protein intake or reduced caloric intake—but it works in harmony with natural gastrointestinal activity to produce maximum absorption as well.

Because of the fat content and the density of the bolus, meals containing tissue-source protein are released from the stomach and travel through the intestines at a rate which is naturally slower and more conducive to efficient digestion and absorption. The problems begin when too much tissue protein is consumed or the process of digestion and absorption is incomplete. It is estimated that at best only 30–35% of the protein consumed in an average protein-containing meal is absorbed allowing the balance of now detrimental undigested protein to pass into the colon.

In the case of liquid protein supplements, the problem is one not only of excessive amounts of protein being consumed but also the speed at which the bolus travels throughout the jejunum. Liquid meals, especially those with insufficient soluble fiber, have decreased transit time, leaving less time for digestion and absorption. Consequently, even in individuals with normal gastrointestinal function, liquid forms of whole proteins generally result in equally incomplete and oftentimes less absorption than their tissue food counterparts.

Pro-Xtreme™ utilizes sequentially hydrolyzed whey protein isolates of the highest quality to insure complete and rapid absorption of the highest levels of essential and branched-chain amino acids (BCAAs) in the preferred smallest peptide bonded form. These features, coupled with its industry-leading lowest average molecular weight, soluble-fiber content and delicious vanilla-cappuccino flavor, offer a primary source of protein that may be used any time a protein supplement is desired.

The combination and sequencing of amino acids in whey protein also results in increased tissue storage of glutathione, a stable tripeptide whose antioxidant activity is known to improve immune function. And, although whey protein naturally contains 5 to 7 percent of glutamine, the formula for Pro-Xtreme™ incorporates additional gram amounts of L-glutamine to its list of highly evolved ingredients as well. This extra step is designed to promote anticatabolic effects in skeletal muscle while focusing on gastrointestinal and immune function improvement. Glutamine and the critical BCAA leucine are deemed indispensable for the healthy functioning of other tissues and metabolic processes. By maintaining a rich supply of BCAAs, Pro-Xtreme™ proves protein sparing within muscle and offers the highest biological value possible.

Pro-Xtreme™ is formulated specifically for use with the other products in the BI-OLEAN® System.

**Directions:** Add 1 packet (40 grams) Pro-Xtreme™ to 1 cup (8 ounces) cold water and stir. There is no need for blending or shaking. Pro-Xtreme™ may also be mixed with lowfat or nonfat milk, milk substitutes or blended with ice for a delicious and nourishing dessert.

**Warning:** Phenylketonurics: Contains phenylalanine.

**Ingredients:** Calcium, Iron, Magnesium, Chloride, Sodium, Potassium, Branched Chain Amino Acid Proprietary Blend, Glutamic Acid (as whey protein hydrolysate & L-glutamine), Leucine, Aspartic Acid, Lysine, Threonine, Isoleucine, Proline, Valine, Alanine, Serine, Cysteine, Phenylalanine, Tyrosine, Arginine, Methionine, Glycine, Histidine, Tryptophan, Maltodextrin, Natural & Artificial Flavorings, Fructose, Cocoa, Salt and Sucralose.

**How Supplied:** One box contains 14 packets. Serving size equals one packet.

---

## SATIETE®
### Herbal and Amino Acid Supplement

**Uses:** With its synergistic blend of herbs and amino acids, Satiete® addresses many of today's health concerns by ensuring maximum nutritional support.

One such ingredient is 5-HTP (5-Hydroxytryptophan). 5-HTP is an amino acid derivative and the immediate precursor to serotonin, a neurotransmitter involved in regulating mood, sleep, appetite, energy level and sensitivity to pain. Like drugs known as selective serotonin reuptake inhibitors (SSRI's), 5-HTP enhances the activity of serotonin, a hormone produced by the brain that is involved in mood, sleep, and appetite. Low levels of serotonin are associated with depression, anxiety, and sleep disorders. SSRI's prevent the brain cells from using up serotonin too quickly, thereby causing a deficiency. 5-HTP increases the cell's production of serotonin, which boosts serotonin levels.

L-5-HTP is a standardized extract of Griffonia simplicifolia (containing greater than 95% anhydrous 5-HTP), and the focus of an ABC *Prime Time Live* report that aired on June 17, 1998. The news segment explored claims that 5-HTP can help alleviate the effects of a variety of conditions, including depression, anxiety, insomnia, and obesity.

The diverse physiological functions of serotonin in the body include actions as a neurotransmitter, a regulator of smooth muscle function in the cardiovascular and gastrointestinal system, and a regulator of platelet function. Serotonin is involved in numerous central nervous system actions such as regulating mood, sleep and appetite. In the gastrointestinal system, serotonin stimulates gastric motility. Serotonin also stimulates platelet aggregation.

As a precursor to serotonin, 5-HTP helps to normalize serotonin activity in the body. Considerable research has been conducted regarding the activity of 5-HTP. Some of the clinical studies are summarized below:

**Mood**—Dysregulation of serotonin metabolism in the central nervous system has been shown to affect mood. 5-HTP helps to normalize serotonin levels and, thereby, positively affect mood. In a double-blind study using objective assessments of mood, researchers in Zurich reported significant improvements in mood with 5-HTP. Likewise, in a double-blind, multi-center study in Germany, researchers reported significant improvements in both objective and self-assessment indices of mood.

**Sleep**—Many studies have shown that depletion of serotonin results in insomnia, which is reversed by administration of 5-HTP. Likewise, Soulairac and Lambinet reported that 100 mg of 5-HTP resulted in significant improvement for people who complained of trouble sleeping. Futhermore, serotonin is metabolized to the hormone melatonin, which is known to help regulate the sleep cycle; by increasing serotonin levels with 5-HTP, melatonin levels are also increased.

**Appetite**—Food intake is thought to suppress appetite through the production of serotonin from the amino acid tryptophan. Because it is an intermediary in the conversion process of tryptophan to serotonin, 5-HTP may reduce appetite in a similar manner as food intake, but without the calories. In a recent double-blind placebo-controlled study, subjects taking 5-HTP lost significant weight compared to control subjects. A reduction in carbohydrate intake and early satiety were seen in the 5-HTP group.

Another key ingredient in the Satiete formulation is Gymnema sylvestre, whose active ingredient "gymnemic acid" affects the taste buds in the oral cavity as the acid prevents the taste buds from being activated by any sugar molecules in the food; and the absorptive surface of the intestines where the acid prevents the intestine from absorbing sugar molecules. Practically speaking, this creates a reduced appetite for sweet tasting food, as well as reducing the metabolic effect of sugar by reducing its digestion in the intestines thus reducing the blood sugar level. In experimental and clinical trials, Gymnema sylvestre has been successful in treating both insulin-dependent and non-insulin dependent diabetics without reducing the blood sugar level to below the normal blood sugar levels, an effect seen with the use of insulin oral hypoglycemic sulphony lurea compounds. Due to its non-toxic nature and sweetness-suppression activity, Gymnema sylvestre can play a role in treating conditions caused by excessive sugar intake. Not only may diabetics benefit from it, conditions like obesity, hypoglycemia, anemia and osteoporosis can also be treated using Gymnema sylvestre.

Vanadyl sulfate, because of its insulin-like properties and its ability to improve cell responsiveness, is being used by progressive alternative physicians and natural healers to treat diabetes. Studies show that vanadyl is very effective in normalizing blood sugar levels and controlling conditions such as insulin resistance, or Type II diabetes.

Magnesium, malic acid and St. John's Wort are also combined in Satiete's proven formulation. Magnesium is a key mineral cofactor for many anaerobic as well as aerobic reactions that generate energy, and has an oxygen-sparing effect. It is essential for the cell's mitochondria "powerhouses" to function normally, being involved in both the production and utilization of ATP.

Malic Acid has an oxygen-sparing effect and there are a number of indications that malic acid is a very critical molecule in controlling mitochondrial function. Malate is a source of energy from the Krebs cycle and is the only metabolite of the cycle which falls in concentration during exhaustive physical activity. Depletion of malate has also been linked to physical exhaustion. By giving malic acid and magnesium as dietary supplements, flexibility to use aerobic and anaerobic energy sources can be enhanced and energy production can be boosted. Lab studies show that many patients with fibromyalgia (or with chronic fatigue) have low magnesium levels. Magnesium supplementation enhances the treatment of both conditions. Its benefits appear to result, at least in part, from its positive impact on serotonin function.

Combining 5-HTP with St. John's Wort Extract (0.3% hypericin context), malic acid, and magnesium, is part of an overall fibromyalgia treatment plan providing excellent results, due in large measure to its improvement of sleep quality and mood.

**Directions:** Start by taking one hypoallergenic tablet three times per day 30 to 60 minutes before meals. If needed after two weeks of use, increase the dosage to two tablets, three times per day. Do not exceed nine tablets daily without medical supervision.

**Warning:** If you are taking MAO inhibitor drugs, tricyclic antidepressants, SSRI antidepressants (Prozac, Paxil, Zoloft) or prescription diet drugs, do not take this product without medical supervision. If you suffer from liver or kidney disease, serious gastrointestinal disorders or carcinoid syndrome, do not take this product without medical supervision. If gastrointestinal upset develops and persists, reduce dosage, take only with large meals or discontinue use. As with any product, pregnant or lactating women should first consult their doctor.

**Ingredients:** Thiamin (as thiamin HCl), Riboflavin, Niacin (as niacinamide), Vitamin B6 (as pyridoxine HCl), Folic Acid, Vitamin B12 (as cyanocobalamin), Magnesium (as magnesium oxide), Malic Acid, St. John's Wort herb extract, Griffonia Simplicifolia seed extract, Gymnema Sylvestris Leaf, Ginkgo Biloba leaf extract, Vanadyl Sulfate, Adenoside Triphosphate (ATP), Ribonucleic Acid (RNA), Microcrystalline Cellulose, Stearic Acid, Croscarmellose Sodium, Magnesium Stearate, Silicon Dioxide, Ethylcellulose and Hydroxypropylcellulose.

**How Supplied:** One bottle contains 84 tablets.

---

## STEPHAN Clarity™
### Nutritional Supplement

**Uses:** STEPHAN Clarity™, designed for use by both men and women, contains selected tissue proteins in the form of nutrients important to memory and concentration.

This is achieved by utilizing such ingredients as lecithin and glutamic acid. Lecithin is a popular supplement widely embraced for the treatment and prevention of memory loss. Known for properties that have been scientifically proven to increase the firing of neurons in the nervous system, glutamic acid is an amino acid which influences the body by serving as brain fuel. It also metabolizes sugars and fats, as well as detoxifies.

Ginkgo biloba, a third primary ingredient in STEPHAN Clarity™, is a special additive which increases the flow of blood to the brain and is noted for improving concentration and learning ability. Recently, a study published in the *Journal of the American Medical Association* demonstrated that ginkgo biloba extract improves mental performance in dementias for individuals with Alzheimer's disease and multi-infarct dementia. It was also reported to stabilize and – in 20% of the cases – improve the subjects' functioning for periods of six months to a year.

Together with the support of carefully selected vitamins, minerals, amino acids, and herbs, STEPHAN Clarity™ is a natural and effective way to better one's health.

**Directions:** Take one to two capsules per day.

**Warnings:** Phenylketonurics: Contains Phenylalanine.

**Ingredients:** Vitamin A (as acetate), Vitamin C (as ascorbic acid), Vitamin D (as cholecalciferol), Vitamin E (as DL-alpha tocopheryl acetate), Thiamin (as thiamin HCl), Riboflavin, Niacin (as niacinamide), Vitamin B6 (as pyridoxine HCl), Folic Acid, Vitamin B12 (as cyanocobalamin), Biotin, Pantothenic Acid (as D-calcium pantothenic acid), Lecithin, Bee Pollen, Glutamic Acid (as L-glutamic acid), Ribonucleic Acid (RNA), Ginkgo Biloba 8:1 extract (leaf), Aspartic Acid (as L-aspartic acid) Leucine (as L-leucine), Arginine (as L-arginine), Lysine (as L-lysine), Phenylalanine (as L-phenylalanine), Serine (as L-serine), Proline (as L-proline), Valine (as L-valine), Isoleucine (as L-isoleucine), Alanine (as L-alanine), Glycine (as L-glycine), Threonine (as L-threonine), Tyrosine (as L-tyrosine), Histidine (as L-histidine), Methionine (as L-methionine), Adenosine Triphosphate Cysteine (as L-cysteine), Talc, Ethylcellulose and Silicon Dioxide.

**How Supplied:** One bottle contains 60 easy-to-swallow capsules.

---

## STEPHAN™ Elasticity®
### Nutritional Supplement

**Uses:** A nutritional food supplement for men and women, STEPHAN™ Elasticity® contains a scientifically balanced mixture of specific tissue proteins established as important for skin tone and texture.

Utilizing such scientifically respected ingredients as vitamin A and selenium, STEPHAN Elasticity is also supported by various other vitamins, minerals and amino acids dedicated to epidermal appearance.

Due to its antioxidant properties, vitamin A has been dubbed the "skin vitamin." It is commonly used as a means of preventing premature aging of the skin. In addition, synthetic derivatives of vitamin A are often used to treat acne and psoriasis.

*Continued on next page*

## Stephan Elasticity—Cont.

Selenium is also considered beneficial to the skin. It was recently reported that low blood selenium in the context of low blood vitamin A increases the risk for certain types of skin cancer.

**Directions:** Take one to two capsules per day.

**Warning:** Accidental overdose of iron-containing products is a leading cause of fatal poisoning in children under 6. Keep this product out of the reach of children. In case of accidental overdose, call a doctor or poison control center immediately. Phenylketonurics: Contains Phenylalanine.

**Ingredients:** Vitamin A (as acetate), Vitamin C (as ascorbic acid), Vitamin E (as DL-alpha tocopheryl acetate), Calcium (as calcium amino acid chelate), Iron (as iron amino acid chelate), Magnesium (as magnesium amino acid chelate), Zinc (as zinc amino acid chelate), Selenium (as selenium acid chelate), Manganese (as manganese amino acid chelate), Chromium (as chromium amino acid chelate), Horsetail (Equisetum arvense), Fucus Vesiculosus, Glutamic Acid (as L-glutamic acid), Ribonucleic Acid (RNA), Aspartic Acid (as L-aspartic acid), Leucine (as L-leucine), Arginine (as L-arginine HCl), Lysine (as Lysine HCl), Serine (as L-serine), Phenylalanine (as L-phenylalanine), Proline (as L-proline), Valine (as L-valine), Isoleucine (as L-isoleucine), Alanine (as L-alanine), Glycine (as L-glycine), Threonine (as L-threonine), Tyrosine (as L-tyrosine), Histidine (as L-histidine), Methionine (as L-methionine), Adenosine Triphosphate, Cysteine (as L-cysteine HCl), Talc, Ethylcellulose, Food Glaze and Silicon Dioxide.

**How Supplied:** One bottle contains 60 easy-to-swallow capsules.

---

## STEPHAN Elixir®
### Nutritional Supplement

**Uses:** Formulated with an exclusive blend of specific proteins, STEPHAN Elixir® is ideal for both men and women. These tissue proteins are supported by vitamins, minerals, amino acids and herbs recognized as important for general health and well-being.

Among the scientifically researched and proven ingredients utilized in STEPHAN Elixir are vitamin E and cysteine. Vitamin E protects against the ravages of aging in several ways. It is essential for the normal functioning of the body and is especially important for normal neurological functions in humans. It also serves as a potent antioxidant and has been dubbed the body's "first line of defense" against free-radical attack by helping to guard against free radicals, the type of cellular damage that has been linked to the initiation of cancer and heart disease.

Cysteine has also been found to inactivate free radicals and thus protect and preserve the cells. This sulfur-containing amino acid is a precursor of glutathione, a tripeptide, that is claimed to safeguard the body against various toxins and pollutants, therefore extending the life span.

**Directions:** Take one to two capsules per day.

**Warnings:** Accidental overdose of iron-containing products is a leading cause of fatal poisoning in children under 6. Keep this product out of the reach of children. In case of accidental overdose, call a doctor or poison control center immediately. Phenylketonurics: Contains phenylalanine.

**Ingredients:** Vitamin A (as vitamin A acetate), Vitamin C (as ascorbic acid), Vitamin D (as cholecalciferol), Vitamin E (as D-alpha tocopheryl acetate), Thiamin (as thiamin HCl), Riboflavin, Niacin (as niacinamide), Vitamin B6 (as pyridoxine HCl), Folic Acid, Vitamin B12 (as cyanocobalamin), Biotin, Pantothenic Acid (as D-calcium pantothenate), Calcium (as D-calcium pantothenate), Iron (as amino acid chelate), Zinc (as zinc amino acid chelate), Selenium (as selenium amino acid chelate), Bee Pollen, Glutamic Acid (as isolated soy protein), Citric Acid, Ginkgo Biloba 4:1 extract (leaf), Malic Acid, Yeast (RNA), Aspartic Acid, Leucine, Arginine, Lysine, Phenylalanine, Serine, Proline, Valine, Isoleucine, Alanine, Glycine, Threonine, Tyrosine, Histidine, Methionine, Cysteine, Tryptophan, Adenosine Triphosphate, Ribonucleic Acid (RNA), Starch, Talc and Silicon Dioxide.

**How Supplied:** One bottle contains 60 easy-to-swallow capsules.

---

## STEPHAN Essential®
### Nutritional Supplement

**Uses:** STEPHAN Essential® is a nutritional food supplement which contains specific tissue proteins supported by vitamins, minerals, herbs and amino acids that are proactive to cardiovascular and circulatory management. L-carnitine, vitamin E and linoleic acid are only some of these very important components.

Scientifically researched and a major contributor to the effects of STEPHAN Essential, L-carnitine is necessary for the transport of long-chain fatty acids into the mitochondria, the metabolic furnaces of the cells. These fatty acids prove a major source for the production of energy in the heart and skeletal muscles, structures that are particularly vulnerable to L-carnitine deficiency. Appropriate levels of L-carnitine in the body have been shown to protect against cardiovascular disease, muscle disease, diabetes and kidney disease.

While vitamin E has proven beneficial in serving to boost the immune system and protect against cardiovascular disease, it has also been established as an important therapy for disorders related to neurologic symptoms. Omega 3–Oil, another important addition to STEPHAN Essential, can lower serum cholesterol levels and decrease platelet stickiness, proving beneficial in the prevention of coronary heart disease.

STEPHAN Essential may be consumed by both men and women.

**Directions:** Take one to two capsules per day.

**Warnings:** Phenylketonurics: Contains Phenylalanine.

**Ingredients:** Vitamin E (as D-alpha tocopheryl succinate), Magnesium (as magnesium amino acid chelate), Selenium (as selenium amino acid chelate), Bee Pollen, Carnitine (as L-carnitine bitartrate), Fish Oil (as omega 3 fatty acids), Glutamic Acid, Yeast (RNA), Aspartic Acid, Leucine, Arginine, Lysine, Phenylalanine, Serine, Proline, Valine, Isoleucine, Alanine, Glycine, Threonine, Tyrosine, Histidine, Adenosine Triphosphate, Methionine, Cysteine, Tryptophan, Talc and Silicon Dioxide.

**How Supplied:** One bottle contains 60 easy-to-swallow capsules.

---

## STEPHAN Feminine®
### Nutritional Supplement

**Uses:** Specifically designed for women, STEPHAN Feminine® contains selected tissue proteins supported by vitamins, minerals and amino acids regarded as important to the ever-changing female body. This is achieved through such scientifically researched ingredients as magnesium and boron.

STEPHAN Feminine utilizes magnesium as an important ingredient responsible for regulating the flow of calcium between cells. Studies reveal that women with high-calcium diets report fewer PMS symptoms including less irritability and depression, as well as fewer headaches, backaches and cramps. Magnesium thus ensures individuals are receiving maximum benefits from calcium intake.

Researchers also report many promising results on the effects of dietary boron. Conclusions show that supplementary boron markedly reduces the excretion of both calcium and magnesium while increasing production of an active form of estrogen and testosterone.

**Directions:** Take one to two capsules per day.

**Warnings:** Phenylketonurics: Contains Phenylalanine.

**Ingredients:** Vitamin E (as DL-alpha tocopheryl acetate), Selenium (as selenium amino acid chelate), Magnesium Oxide, Glutamic Acid, Ribonucleic Acid (RNA), Aspartic Acid, Leucine, Arginine, Lysine, Phenylalanine, Serine, Proline,

Valine, Isoleucine, Alanine, Glycine, Threonine, Tyrosine, Histidine, Methionine, Cysteine, Tryptophan, Adenosine Triphosphate, Boron (as boron amino acid chelate), Talc and Silicon Dioxide.

**How Supplied:** One bottle contains 60 easy-to-swallow capsules.

---

## STEPHAN™ Flexibility®
### Nutritional Supplement

**Uses:** A nutritional supplement for both men and women, STEPHAN™ Flexibility® is rich with exclusive proteins which are supported by vitamins, minerals and amino acids recognized as beneficial to the health of joint and soft tissues.

Glycine, an amino acid, is one very significant ingredient utilized in STEPHAN Flexibility. In a pilot study investigating the possibility of glycine's effect on spastic control, a 25% improvement was noted on subjects with chronic multiple sclerosis. Furthermore, all patients benefited to some degree, and no toxicity or other adverse side effects were noted.

Another important amino acid in STEPHAN Flexibility is L-histidine. Reports suggest that supplementary L-histidine may actually boost the activity of suppressor T cells. Because rheumatoid arthritis is one of the many autoimmune diseases in which T-cell activity is subnormal, these conclusions lend further support that L-histidine may prove beneficial in its treatment.

Vitamin E can also be found in STEPHAN Flexibility because of its ability to relieve muscular cramps. According to one popular study, supplemental vitamin E caused remarkable relief from persistent nocturnal leg and foot cramps in 82% of the 125 patients tested.

**Directions:** Take one to two capsules per day.

**Warnings:** Phenylketonurics: Contains Phenylalanine.

**Ingredients:** Vitamin A (as vitamin A palmitate), Vitamin C (as ascorbic acid), Vitamin D (as cholecalciferol), Vitamin E (as DL-alpha tocopheryl acetate), Thiamin (as thiamin HCl), Riboflavin, Niacin (as niacinamide), Vitamin B6, (as pyridoxine HCl), Folic Acid, Vitamin B12 (as cyanocobalamin), Biotin, Pantothenic Acid (as D-calcium pantothenate), Calcium (as calcium amino acid chelate), Zinc (as zinc amino acid chelate), Selenium (as selenium amino acid chelate), Glutamic Acid (as L-glutamic acid), Ribonucleic Acid (RNA), Aspartic Acid (as L-aspartic acid), Leucine (as L-leucine), Arginine (as L-arginine), Lysine (as L-lysine), Bee Pollen, Phenylalanine (as L-phenylalanine), Serine (as L-serine), Proline (as L-proline), Valine (as L-valine), Isoleucine (as L-isoleucine), Alanine (as L-alanine), Glycine (as L-glycine), Threonine (as L-threonine), Tyrosine (as L-tyrosine), Histidine (as L-histidine), Methionine (as L-methionine), Adenoside Triphosphate, Boron (as boron amino acid chelate), Cysteine (as L-cysteine), Talc, Whey, Magnesium Stearate, Silicon Dioxide and Cellulose.

**How Supplied:** One bottle contains 60 easy-to-swallow capsules.

---

## STEPHAN Lovpil™
### Nutritional Supplement

**Uses:** STEPHAN Lovpil™ is a nutritional food supplement for men and women of all ages that is formulated with vitamins, minerals, herbs, amino acids and selected proteins recognized as important for general health and sexual vitality.

Damiana, typically thought of as an aphrodisiac by those who are familiar with its effects, is an important ingredient utilized in STEPHAN Lovpil. A major herbal remedy in Mexican medical folklore, damiana is often used for the treatment of both impotency and sterility. However, its proven stimulating properties of male virility and libido make it an ideal addition to STEPHAN Lovpil's formulation.

A number of scientific studies have shown a direct relationship between low sperm count and diets deficient in arginine. Well established as being significant to normal sperm production, arginine is, therefore, an important contributor to STEPHAN Lovpil.

A third imperative ingredient is vitamin C. Scientific studies have uncovered that ascorbic acid may actually protect human sperm from oxidative DNA damage, which could in turn help prevent birth defects.

**Directions:** Take one to two capsules per day.

**Warnings:** Phenylketonurics: Contains Phenylalanine.

**Ingredients:** Vitamin A (as vitamin A acetate), Vitamin C (as ascorbic acid), Vitamin D (as cholecalciferol), Folic Acid, Vitamin B12 (as cyanocobalamin), Calcium (as calcium carbonate), Zinc (as zinc amino acid chelate), Selenium (as selenomethionine), Manganese (as manganese amino acid chelate), Damiana (leaf), Isolated Soybean Protein, Ribonucleic Acid (RNA), Adenosine Triphosphate, Talc, Magnesium Stearate and Silicon Dioxide.

**How Supplied:** One bottle contains 60 easy-to-swallow capsules.

---

## STEPHAN Masculine®
### Nutritional Supplement

**Uses:** A nutritional food supplement formulated for the adult male, STEPHAN Masculine® contains a special blend of nutrients with vitamins, minerals, herbs and amino acids.

Scientifically researched ingredients have been carefully selected to help ensure STEPHAN Masculine's effectiveness. Zinc is one such ingredient. Proven to be closely interrelated with the male sex hormone, testosterone, zinc deficiency often results in regression of the male sex glands, decreased sexual interest, mental lethargy, emotional problems and even poor appetite. It has been found that in males with only a mild zinc deficiency, zinc supplementation was accompanied by increased sperm count and plasma testosterone.

**Directions:** Take one to two capsules per day.

**Ingredients:** Calcium (as calcium carbonate), Magnesium (as magnesium amino acid chelate), Zinc (as zinc amino acid chelate), Histidine (as L-histidine), Bee Pollen, Parsley (leaf), Ribonucleic Acid (RNA), Adenosine Triphosphate Talc and Magnesium Stearate.

**How Supplied:** One bottle contains 60 easy-to-swallow capsules.

---

## PHYTO-VITE®
### Advanced Antioxidant, Vitamin and Mineral Supplement

**Uses:** Phyto-Vite® is a state-of-the-art nutritional supplement providing chelated minerals, vitamins and a diverse group of antioxidants. It was formulated to meet the nutritional needs of our society where studies estimate only 9% consume foods in the quantities necessary to protect against the oxidative damage caused by free radicals.

The antioxidant coverage provided by Phyto-Vite is both comprehensive and diverse. First, it includes optimal amounts of vitamins A, C, and E as well as the pro-vitamins alpha and beta carotene. Vitamin A, in addition to its antioxidant capabilities, is also felt to improve immune function, protein synthesis, RNA synthesis and steroid hormone synthesis. In this product, vitamin A is derived from two sources: retinyl palmitate and lemongrass. Additional vitamin A activity is provided by the alpha and beta carotene found in *Dunaliella salina*. These carotenoids are strong antioxidants in their own right; however, they can also be converted to vitamin A. This occurs only when the body is deficient in this vitamin. Consequently, vitamin A toxicity cannot be caused by alpha or beta carotene. Vitamin C has long been associated with wound healing, collagen formation, and maintaining the structural integrity of capillaries, cartilage, dentine and bone. Its antioxidant effects are felt to play a major role in the prevention of cardiovascular disease and some cancers. Phyto-Vite utilizes esterified vitamin C which has been shown to provide a quicker uptake and a decreased rate of excretion when compared

*Continued on next page*

## Phyto-Vite—Cont.

with conventional vitamin C. This allows for higher, more sustained levels of this vitamin in the body. Phyto-Vite also contains 400 I.U. of vitamin E, from natural sources. The antioxidant effects of vitamin E have been shown to stabilize cell membranes, increase HDL cholesterol, and decrease platelet aggregation.

Many flavonoids are incorporated into Phyto-Vite. These substances possess antioxidant activity themselves and also potentiate the effects of vitamins C and E. This later effect is produced by decreasing the degradation of vitamin C and E into inactive metabolites. Ginkgo biloba has flavonoid activity as well as other significant effects. Among these are a decrease in platelet aggregation and an increase in vasodilation which appears to increase blood flow to the peripheral arteries and the brain. Some improvement in cognitive abilities has been noted. It also helps to inhibit lipid peroxidation, thereby stabilizing the cell wall against free radical attack.

A phytonutrient blend has been incorporated into Phyto-Vite to further enhance its antioxidant effects. Phytonutrient is a term given to the thousands of chemical compounds found in fruits and vegetables. Some of these compounds, including sulforaphane in broccoli and isothiocyanate in cabbage, have been shown to inhibit cancer in laboratory animals and human cell cultures. Others have shown great promise in aiding the cardiovascular system. Currently, much research is ongoing to isolate and identify more of these compounds, but it has already been clearly established that phytonutrients work best when the entire plant source is used rather than just the isolated compound. The phytonutrients found in Phyto-Vite are obtained from alfalfa (lutein), broccoli (indoles), cabbage (isothiocyanates), cayenne (capsanthin and capsorubin), green onion (thioallyl compounds), parsley (chlorophyll), spirulina (gamma linolenic acid), tomato (lycopene), soy isoflavones (genistein, lecithin and daidzein), aged garlic concentrate, and Pure-Gar-A-8000™ (allicin).

The antioxidant minerals copper, zinc, manganese and selenium have also been incorporated into Phyto-Vite. These minerals have been chelated via a patented process in which the mineral is wrapped within an amino acid. Once inside the body, the minerals can then be utilized in the millions of metabolic reactions that take place in the body. With this process, overall mineral absorption can approach 95% instead of the 5 to 10% absorption seen with other mineral supplements.

Phyto-Vite also provides two antioxidant enzymes (catalase and peroxidase). These help to reduce the body's free radical burden by neutralizing free radicals in the pharynx or stomach.

There are three other features that make Phyto-Vite unique among supplements. First, a small amount of canola oil was included to aid in the proper absorption of fat soluble vitamins, even on an empty stomach. Canola oil also provides essential fatty acids. Second, the product is formed into prolonged-release tablets which allow flexibility in dosing frequency. It can be taken all at once or staggered throughout the day. Dissolution testing has been performed to insure that the product will dissolve properly. Lastly, Phyto-Vite tablets are covered with a Betacoat™. This is a beta carotene coating that is designed to provide antioxidant coverage to the tablet itself. This helps to protect the integrity and activity of the product.

**Directions:** As a dietary supplement take six tablets per day with eight ounces of liquid. Tablets may be taken all at once or staggered throughout the day.

**Warnings:** If pregnant or lactating, consult physician before using. Accidental overdose of iron-containing products is a leading cause of fatal poisoning in children under 6. Keep this product out of reach of children. In case of accidental overdose, call a doctor or poison control center immediately. This hypoallergenic formula is free of dairy, yeast, wheat, sugar, starch, animal products, dyes, preservatives, artificial flavors and pesticide residues.

**Ingredients:** Vitamin A (as retinyl palmitate and 80% as beta-carotene and mixed carotenoids from D. salina algae), Vitamin C (as calcium ascorbate), Vitamin D (as cholecalciferol), Vitamin E (as D-alpha-tocopheryl succinate), Vitamin K (as phylloquinone), Thiamin (as thiamin mononitrate), Riboflavin, Niacin (as niacinamide), Vitamin B6 (as pyridoxine HCl), Folate (as folic acid), Vitamin B12 (as cyanocobalamin), Biotin, Pantothenic Acid (as D-calcium pantothenate), Calcium (as dicalcium phosphate, calcium carbonate, citrate and lactate), Iron (as Ferrochel® iron bisglycinate), Phosphorus (as dicalcium phosphate), Iodine [from kelp (Ascophyllum nodosum)], Magnesium (as magnesium oxide, magnesium amino acid chelate and magnesium citrate), Zinc (as zinc Chelazome® glycinate), Selenium (as L-selenomethionine), Copper (as copper Chelazome glycinate), Manganese (as manganese Chelazome glycinate), Chromium (as chromium Chelavite® glycinate), Potassium (as potassium citrate), Alfalfa leaf, Aged garlic bulb concentrate, Pur-Gar® A-10,000 odorless garlic bulb, Soy protein isolate, Broccoli floret, Cabbage leaf, Cayenne pepper fruit, Green onion bulb, Parsley leaf, Tomato, Spirulina algae, Canola oil concentrate, Citrus bioflavonoid complex, Rutin and quercetin dihydrate, Choline (as choline bitartrate), Inositol, PABA, Ginkgo biloba leaf standardized extract (24% ginkgo flavone glycosides and 6% terpene lactones), Bilberry fruit standardized extract (25% antihocyanosides), Catalase enzymes,

Grape seed proanthocyanidins, Red grape skin extract (14–18% total polyphenols), Boron (as boron citrate), Microcrystalline cellulose, stearic acid, silica, magnesium stearate, croscarmellose sodium and pharmaceutical glaze with vanillin.

**How Supplied:** One bottle contains 180 Betacoat™ tablets.

## STEPHAN Protector® Nutritional Supplement

**Uses:** STEPHAN Protector® is a nutritional food supplement that combines specific proteins, vitamins, minerals and amino acids recognized as important for the health of areas associated with the human immune system.

Among these specially selected and scientifically researched ingredients are astragalus, kelp and arginine. Known for its strengthening effects of both the immune and digestive systems, astragalus can be combined with other herbs to increase phagocytosis, interferon production and the number of macrophages. It, in combination, enhances T-cell transformation and functions as an adaptogen to relieve stress-induced immune system suppression.

Research clearly indicates that kelp supplies dozens of important nutrients for improved cardiovascular health and is used to balance the thyroid gland. Arginine stimulates the thymus gland and promotes production of lymphocytes, crucial for immunity, in that gland. The arginine lymphocytes are not only produced in better quantity, but they have also proven more active and effective in fighting illness.

STEPHAN Protector may be used by men and women of all ages.

**Directions:** Take one to two capsules per day.

**Warnings:** Phenylketonurics: Contains Phenylalanine.

**Ingredients:** Bee Pollen, Astragalus, Kelp, Glutamic Acid, Ribonucleic Acid, Aspartic Acid, Leucine, Arginine, Lysine, Phenylalanine, Serine, Proline, Valine, Isoleucine, Alanine, Glycine, Threonine, Tyrosine, Histidine, Methionine, Cysteine, Tryptophan Adenosine Triphosphate, Cellulose, Talc, Magnesium Stearate and Silicon Dioxide.

**How Supplied:** One bottle contains 60 easy-to-swallow capsules.

## STEPHAN Relief® Nutritional Supplement

**Uses:** Designed for both men and women, STEPHAN Relief® has been formulated with a special combination of nutrients, vitamins, minerals, amino acids and herbs which are recognized as important to the digestive and excretory systems.

Parsley, one of the ingredients found in STEPHAN Relief and a member of the carrot family, can be used as a carminative and an aid to digestion. While the root has a mild diuretic property, parsley has also been reported, in large doses, to lower blood pressure.

A second important ingredient in STEPHAN Relief is psyllium. This gel-forming fiber is used in many bulk laxatives to promote bowel regularity. In recent years, because of its ability to lower cholesterol, psyllium has gained widespread popularity and can be found in some ready-to-eat cereals.

**Directions:** Take one to two capsules per day.

**Ingredients:** Pantothenic Acid (as D-calcium pantothenate), Fucus Vesiculosus 5:1 extract (leaf), Parsley 4:1 extract (leaf), Plantago Ovata Seed (psyllium), Isoleucine (as L-isoleucine), Leucine (as L-leucine), Valine (as L-valine), Bee Pollen, Ribonucleic Acid (RNA), Adenosine Triphosphate, Ethylcellulose, Talc and Silicon Dioxide.

**How Supplied:** One bottle contains 60 easy-to-swallow capsules.

---

## SLEEP-TITE™
### Herbal Sleep Aid

**Uses:** Sleep-Tite™ is a non-addicting herbal sleep aid formulated to promote a deeper, more restorative sleep without the use of pharmaceutically synthesized hormones. With the body's overall health, and proper functioning, dependent upon efficient sleep patterns in order to achieve cellular, organ, tissue and emotional repair, this powerful tool's primary function is to rejuvenate and restore by assisting the body in initiating and maintaining sleep.

Sleep-Tite is a blend of 10 highly effective, all-natural herbs. California poppy, passion flower, valerian, kava kava and skullcap have been used for centuries as a remedy for insomnia because of their calming effects and ability to relieve muscle tension. Hops and celery seed produce a generalized calming effect and are especially helpful for indigestion, gastrointestinal and smooth muscle relaxation. Chamomile also has a relaxing effect on the body and the gastrointestinal tract, but with the added benefit of producing anti-inflammatory effects on joints. Feverfew has been used as a treatment for fever, migraines and arthritic complaints dating back to ancient Greece. A study published in *Lancet* demonstrated that feverfew inhibited the body's production of prostaglandin and serotonin. These biochemicals can cause inflammation, fever and the vasoactive response that triggers migraine headaches.

By utilizing this unique blend of herbs to aid in the effective initiation and maintenance of sleep patterns, Sleep-Tite can

be consumed by adults, thereby promoting physical and emotional well-being in a safe, active manner.

**Directions:** Adults (18 years and older) may take two Sleep-Tite caplets approximately 30 to 60 minutes prior to bedtime. Needs may vary with each individual. Some persons may require less than two caplets to achieve optimum results. Do not exceed recommended nightly amounts.

**Warnings:** Not for use by children, pregnant women or lactating women. Consult your physician before using this product if you have any medical condition or are taking antidepressant, sedative or hypnotic medications. Do not take this product if using Monoamine Oxidase (M.A.O.) Inhibitors. This product may cause drowsiness and should not be taken with alcohol or while operating a vehicle or other machinery. If allergic symptoms develop, discontinue use. Store in a cool, dry place. Keep out of reach of children.

**Ingredients:** European Valerian Root 4:1 extract, Celery Seed 4:1 extract, Hops Strobile 4:1 extract, Passion Flower 4:1 extract (whole plant), California Poppy 5:1 extract (aerial parts), Chamomile Flower 5:1 extract, Chinese Fu Ling 5:1 extract (Poria Cocos), Kava Kava Root 5:1 extract, Feverfew 5:1 extract (aerial parts), Skullcap (aerial parts), Dicalcium Phosphate, Microcrystalline Cellulose, Croscarmellose Sodium, Stearic Acid, Silica, Magnesium Stearate and Sugar Coat (calcium sulfate, sucrose, kaolin, talc, gelatin, shellac, titanium dioxide, anise oil, beeswax and carnauba wax).

**How Supplied:** One box contains 28 packets. Two caplets per packet.

---

## STEPHAN Tranquility™
### Nutritional Supplement

**Uses:** Designed for both men and women, STEPHAN Tranquility™ is a nutritional food supplement which contains a blend of vitamins, minerals and amino acids recognized as important to areas involved in stress management.

Myo-Inositol is among these specially researched ingredients. It has long been claimed to lower blood concentrations of triglycerides and cholesterol, as well as to generally protect against cardiovascular disease. In addition, Myo-Inositol intake can influence the phosphatidylinositol levels in the membranes of brain cells. Compounds derived from this process could conceivably have some beneficial effect on insomnia and anxiety proving a safer alternative than most to treat these common problems.

Another key ingredient used in STEPHAN Tranquility is valerian root, a folk remedy used throughout the years for several disorders including insomnia, hysteria, palpitations, nervousness and menstrual problems. Valerian root con-

tains valepotriates which are said to be the source of its sedative effects. Studies reveal that valeranon, an essential oil component of this herb, produces a pronounced smooth-muscle effect on the intestine.

**Directions:** Take one to two capsules per day.

**Warnings:** Phenylketonurics: Contains Phenylalanine.

**Ingredients:** Vitamin A (as vitamin A palmitate), Vitamin C (as ascorbic acid), Vitamin D (as cholecalciferol), Vitamin E (as DL-alpha tocopheryl acetate), Thiamin (as thiamin HCI), Riboflavin, Niacin (as niacinamide), Vitamin B6 (as pyridoxine HCI), Folic Acid, Vitamin B12 (as cyanocobalamin), Biotin, Pantothenic Acid (as D-calcium pantothenate), Calcium (as calcium amino acid chelate), Magnesium (as magnesium amino acid chelate), Glutamic Acid, Choline Bitartrate, Inositol, Lecithin, Ribonucleic Acid (RNA), Valerian root 4:1 extract (Valerian officianalis), Aspartic Acid, Leucine, Arginine, Lysine, Phenylalanine, Serine, Proline, Valine, Isoleucine, Alanine, Glycine, Threonine, Tyrosine, Histidine, Methionine, Adenosine Triphosphate, Cysteine, Talc, Silicon Dioxide and Hydroxypropyl Cellulose.

**How Supplied:** One bottle contains 60 easy-to-swallow capsules.

---

## SURE2ENDURE™
### Herbal, Vitamin & Mineral Workout Supplement

**Uses:** Attaining peak physical and athletic performance can be an elusive and time-consuming endeavor. It requires a conditioning process whereby the body's endurance, stamina and ability to recover are enhanced. Sure2Endure™ is formulated to aid in this process through an innovative blend of herbs, vitamins and minerals.

Among these specially selected ingredients is ciwujia (*Radix Acanthopanax senticosus*). Used in traditional Chinese medicine for almost 1,700 years to treat fatigue and boost the immune system, ciwujia has been shown to improve overall performance in aerobic exercise, endurance activities and weight lifting without any stimulant effects. According to a recent study, ciwujia increases fat metabolism during exercise by shifting toward the use of fat as an energy source instead of carbohydrates. In addition, the caffeine-free herb improves endurance by reducing lactic acid build-up in the muscles. This process delays the muscle fatigue which often leads to muscle pain and cramps.

Sure2Endure™ also provides antioxidant coverage and enzyme cofactors. Vitamins C and E address the otherwise high levels of free radicals generated

*Continued on next page*

## Sure2Endure—Cont.

from the oxidation of fuel substrates during exercise, while vitamins B1 (thiamin), B2 (riboflavin), B6 (pyridoxine), and B12 (cyanocobalamin) aid in proper carbohydrate metabolism and serve as cofactors in numerous biochemical reactions in the body. Ciwujia has been credited with antioxidant properties as well. Since tissue stress and damage are often the result of strenuous exercise, it is important to maintain proper integrity and recovery of connective tissue. Glucosamine, one of the basic constituents making up joint cartilage, is another special additive to Sure2Endure™. This substance enhances the synthesis of cartilage cells and protects against destructive enzymes. It stabilizes cell membranes and intercellular collagen thereby protecting cartilage during rest, exercise and recovery.

The anti-inflammatory activities of bromelain and boswellia further prove beneficial to the health of joint and soft tissues.

**Directions:** Adults (18 years and older) take 3 tablets one hour prior to exercise. Needs may vary with each individual. For optimum performance, use in conjunction with BIOLEAN® or BIOLEAN Free® one hour before exercise. PhytoVite® may be taken with this product to maximize the antioxidant effect necessary with exercise. Pro-Xtreme™ and Mass Appeal™ may also be consumed for maximum effectiveness.

**Warning:** Not for use by children, pregnant women or lactating women. Consult your physician before using this product if you have any medical conditions. Discontinue immediately if allergic symptoms develop. Keep out of the reach of children. Store in a cool, dry place.

**Ingredients:** Vitamin C (as ascorbic acid), Vitamin E (as d-alpha tocopheryl succinate), Thiamin (as thiamin mononitrate), Riboflavin, Vitamin B6 (as pyridoxine hydrochloride), Vitamin B12 (as cyanocobalamin), Chromium (as patented Chelavite® chromium dinicotinate glycinate), Ciwujia root standardized extract (0.8% eleutherosides) (Acanthopanax senticosus), Magnesium L-aspartate, Potassium L-aspartate, Boswellia Serrata standardized extract (40% boswellic acids (as gum resins), Bromelain (600 GDU/g), Glucosamine hydrochloride, Dicalcium Phosphate, Microcrystalline Cellulose, Croscarmellose Sodium, Stearic Acid, Silica, Magnesium Stearate and Sugar Coat (calcium sulfate, sucrose, kaolin, talc, gelatin, shellac, titanium dioxide, wintergreen oil, FD&C yellow #5, FD&C blue #1, beeswax and carnauba wax).

**How Supplied:** One box contains 28 packets, three tablets per packet.

---

## WINRGY™
**Nutritional Drink with Vitamin C**

**Uses:** Through nutrients in the diet, nerves are able to send signals throughout the body called neurotransmitters. One such neurotransmitter, noradrenaline, provides individuals with the necessary alertness and energy required in day-to-day activity. A unique blend of vitamins and minerals important to the creation of noradrenaline has been incorporated into Winrgy™, making it a delicious, nutritional alternative to coffee and cola.

Studies reveal that vitamin B2 (riboflavin) helps the body release energy from protein, carbohydrates and fat, while vitamin B12 (cobalamin) is given to combat fatigue and alleviate neurological problems, including weakness and memory loss. Another important component of Winrgy, vitamin B3 (niacin), works with both thiamin and riboflavin in the metabolism of carbohydrates and is essential for providing energy for cell tissue growth. Niacin has also proven to dilate blood vessels and thereby increase the blood flow to various organs of the body, sometimes resulting in a blush of the skin and a healthy sense of warmth. Unlike caffeine, Winrgy offers the raw materials necessary to continue the production of noradrenaline and is ideal for anytime performance is required.

**Directions:** Add 6 ounces of chilled water or fruit juice to one packet of mix. Stir briskly. Consume 1–2 times per day. Keep in a cool, dry place. For maximum results, combine this product with one serving size of Food For Thought.™

**Warnings:** Phenylketonurics: Contains Phenylalanine. Not for use by children, pregnant or lactating women. Persons taking medications should seek medical advice before taking this product. Do not consume more than four servings per day. Avoid the use of antacids containing aluminum with this product.

**Ingredients:** Vitamin C (as ascorbic acid), Vitamin E (as alpha tocopherol acetate), Thiamin (as thiamin mononitrate), Riboflavin, Niacin (as niacinamide), Vitamin B6 (as pyridoxine hydrochloride, Folic Acid, Vitamin B12, Pantothenic Acid (as calcium pantothenate), Zinc (as zinc gluconate), Copper (as copper gluconate), Manganese (as manganese aspartate), Chromium (as chromium aspartate), Potassium (as potassium aspartate), Phenylalanine (as L-phenylalanine), Taurine, Glycine, Caffeine, Fructose, Natural Flavor, Citric Acid and Silicon Dioxide.

**How Supplied:** One box contains 28 packets. Serving size equals one packet.

---

# YOUNGEVITY
# THE ANTI-AGING CO.
**3227 SKYLANE DRIVE**
**DALLAS, TEXAS 75006**

**Direct Inquiries to:**
Website: www.youngevity.com
eMail:　　asd@youngevity.com
Corporate Fax: 972-404-3067
Corporate Tel: 972-239-6864 ext. 108

OUR ANTI-AGING, LIFE-CHANGING PRODUCTS ARE MANUFACTURED TO PHARMACEUTICAL STANDARDS

**The Anti-Aging Daily Premium Pak:** contains 60 Packets. Each Packet contains: 3 Capsules of Daily Premium Multiple, 1 Capsule of Super Anti-Oxidant Complex, 1 Capsule of Super Cell Protector, 1 Soft Gel Capsule of EFA Complex

---

**Serving Size: 1 Packet (7 Capsules & 1 Soft Gel Capsule)**
**Servings Per Container: 60**

| Amount Per Serving | | | % Daily Value* |
|---|---|---|---|
| Vitamin A (as beta carotene, retinyl acetate, mixed carotenoids) | 11250 | I.U. | 225% |
| Vitamin C (as ascorbic acid, calcium ascorbate) | 360 | mg | 600% |
| Vitamin D (as cholecalciferol) | 417 | I.U. | 104% |
| Vitamin E (as d-alpha tocopheryl acetate) | 130 | I.U. | 433% |
| Vitamin B1 (as thiamine mononitrate) | 12 | mg | 800% |
| Vitamin B2 (as riboflavin) | 12 | mg | 706% |
| Vitamin B3 (as niacinamide) | 20 | mg | 100% |
| Vitamin B6 (as pyridoxine hydrochloride) | 12 | mg | 600% |
| Vitamin B9 (as folic acid) | 400 | mcg | 100% |
| Vitamin B12 (as cyanocobalamin) | 6 | mcg | 100% |
| Vitamin H (as biotin) | 150 | mcg | 50% |
| Vitamin B5 (as d-calcium pantothenate) | 12 | mg | 120% |
| Calcium (as amino acid chelate, carbonate, di-calcium phosphate, ascorbate) | 202 | mg | 203% |
| Iron (as amino acid chelate) | 9 | mg | 50% |
| Phosphorus (as di-calcium phosphate) | 40 | mg | 4% |
| Iodine (as potassium iodide) | 75 | mcg | 50% |
| Magnesium (as magnesium oxide, amino acid chelate) | 74 | mg | 18% |
| Zinc (as amino acid chelate) | 8 | mg | 50% |
| Selenium (as amino acid chelate) | 10 | mcg | 14% |
| Copper (as amino acid chelate) | 1 | mg | 50% |
| Manganese (as amino acid chelate) | 1 | mg | 50% |
| Chromium (as amino acid chelate) | 75 | mcg | 63% |
| Molybdenum (as amino acid chelate) | 10 | mcg | 13% |

*Continued on next page*

**Serving Size: 1 Packet (7 Capsules & 1 Soft Gel Capsule)**
**Servings Per Container: 60** *(cont.)*

| Amount Per Serving | | | % Daily Value* |
|---|---|---|---|
| PATENTED ANTI-AGING MIRACLEMINERALS THE VILCABAMBA MINERAL ESSENCE<sup>fi</sup> PROPRIETARYBLEND—Potassium,**Calcium, Magnesium, Zinc, Chromium, Selenium, Iron, Copper, Molybdenum, Vanadium, Iodine, Cobalt, Manganese | 285 | mg | ** |
| Organic Flaxseed Oil | 205 | mg | ** |
| Omega-3 (from evening primrose oil, borage oil, organic flaxseed oil, marine lipid oil) | 154 | mg | ** |
| Omega-6 (from evening primrose oil, borage oil, organic flaxseed oil, marine lipid oil) | 128 | mg | ** |
| Evening Primrose Oil | 100 | mg | ** |
| Borage Oil | 100 | mg | ** |
| Marine Lipid Oil | 95 | mg | ** |
| Grape Seed Extract (standardized to provide 68.45mg proanthocyanidins) *(Vitis vinifera)* (seed) | 72 | mg | ** |
| Omega-9 (from evening primrose oil, borage oil, organic flaxseed oil, marine lipid oil) | 59 | mg | ** |
| Rose Hips *(Rosa Canina)*(fruit) | 46 | mg | ** |
| Broccoli *(Brassica oleracea v. botrytis)* (florets) | 38 | mg | ** |
| Garlic *(Allium sativum)*(clove) | 38 | mg | ** |
| Barley Grass *(Hordeum vulgare)* (young grass) | 35 | mg | ** |
| Beet Juice Powder *(Beta vulgaris)* (root) | 35 | mg | ** |
| Carrot Powder *(Daucus carota)*(fresh carrots) | 35 | mg | ** |
| Papaya *(Carrica papaya)*(leaf) | 35 | mg | ** |
| Pineapple Extract *(Ananas comosus)* (fruit) | 35 | mg | ** |
| Wheat Grass *(Triticum aestivum)* (organic) | 35 | mg | ** |
| Apple Pectin *(Malus sylvestris)* (organic) | 26 | mg | ** |
| Hesperidin Complex | 25 | mg | ** |
| Rutin *(Sophora japonica)* | 25 | mg | ** |
| Quercetin | 25 | mg | ** |
| Alpha Lipoic Acid | 22 | mg | ** |
| Plant Enzyme Blend | 20 | mg | ** |
| Lactobacillus Acidophilus | 20 | mg | ** |
| Parsley *(Petroselinum crispum)* (aerial parts) | 20 | mg | ** |
| Hawthorn *(Crataegus oxycantha)* (berry & leaf) | 15 | mg | ** |
| Milk Thistle Extract (standardized to provide 12mg silymarin) *(Silyburn marianum)* (fruit) | 15 | mg | ** |
| Curcuminoids (from tumeric extract) *(Curcuma longa)* (rhizome) | 15 | mg | ** |
| Horsetail *(Equisetum majus)*(aerial parts) | 11 | mg | ** |
| Carnitine (as acetyl l-carnitine) | 10 | mg | ** |
| CoEnzyme Q10 | 5 | mg | ** |
| Potassium (as amino acid chelate, potassium iodide) | 10 | mg | ** |
| Alfalfa *(Medicajo sativa)*(leaf & stem) | 3 | mg | ** |
| Ginkgo Biloba Extract (standardized to provide .72mg flavonglycosides and .18mg terpenes) *(Ginkgo biloba)*(leaf) | 3 | mg | ** |
| Kelp *(Laminaria spp.)* | 3 | mg | ** |
| Licorice Root *(Glycyrrhiza glabra)* (rhizome & root) | 3 | mg | ** |
| Citrus Bioflavanoid Complex | 2 | mg | ** |
| Soy Isoflavones *(Glycine max)*(seed) | 2 | mg | ** |
| Lycopene (from tomato extract) *(Lycopersicum esculentum)* (fruit) | 1 | mg | ** |
| Boron (as amino acid chelate) | 80 | mcg | ** |

---

* Percent Daily Values are based on a 2,000 calorie diet
** Daily Value Not Established
Contains less than 2% of the Daily Value of these Nutrients

with CoQ10, 1 Capsule of Concentrated Fruits & Vegetables and 1 Capsule of Bone Building Formula. The strongest, most complete, multi-vitamin, multi-mineral and herbal supplement on the market.

**Every Capsule Contains Our Patented Anti-Aging Miracle Minerals:** Proprietary Blend: Potassium, Calcium, Magnesium, Zinc, Chromium, Selenium, Iron, Copper, Molybdenum, Vanadium, Iodine, Cobalt and Manganese.

## ANTI-AGING DAILY PREMIUM PAK
**The Ultimate Anti-Aging Program**

**Each Packet Contains:**
**DAILY PREMIUM MULTIPLE**
**3 Capsules in Packet**
28 Anti-Aging Proprietary Complex Anti-Oxidants, Synergistic Vitamins, Synergistic Herbs & Digestive Enzymes
**SUPER ANTI-OXIDANT COMPLEX**
**1 Capsule in Packet**
**SUPER ANTI-OXIDANT CELL PRTCTR**
**1 Capsule in Packet**
Grape Seed Extract
1 Super Anti-Oxidant Cell Protector
11 Anti-Oxidant Actives
**ESSENTIAL FATTY ACIDS COMPLEX WITH CoQ10**
**1 Soft Gel Capsule in Packet**
Flaxseed, Evening Primrose, Borage, Marine Lipids, Omega-3, 6 and 9 Fatty Acids, CoQ10
**FRUITS & VEGETABLES**
**1 Capsule in Packet**
Live Food Enzymes
7 Anti-Aging Green Foods
8 Anti-Aging Fruits & Bio-Factors
6 Anti-Aging Live Plant Enzymes
**BONE BUILDING FORMULA**
**1 Capsule in Packet**
Building and Maintaining Bone Mass
4 Bone Building Structural Minerals:
3 Anti-Aging Activators
**Supplement Facts:**
[See table on bottom of previous page and top of page]
Other Ingredients: Gelatin, glycerin, water, yellow beeswax, rice flour, microcrystalline cellulose, magnesium stearate (vegetable source), silicon dioxide.

**Directions:** Take 2–3 Paks Daily, one after each meal
**How Supplied:** 30 or 60 Paks Per Box

# DRUG INFORMATION CENTERS

For additional information on overdosage, adverse reactions, drug interactions, and any other medication problem, specialized drug information centers are strategically located throughout the nation. Use the directory that follows to find the center nearest you. Listings are alphabetical by state and city.

## ALABAMA

### BIRMINGHAM
**Drug Information Service**
**University of Alabama**
**Hospital**
619 S. 20th St.
1720 Jefferson Tower
Birmingham, AL 35249-6860
Mon.-Fri. 8 AM-5 PM
    205-934-2162
Fax: 205-934-3501
www.health.uab.edu/pharmacy

**Global Drug**
**Information Center**
**Samford University**
**McWhorter School**
**of Pharmacy**
800 Lakeshore Dr.
Birmingham, AL 35229-7027
Mon.-Fri. 8 AM-4:30 PM
    205-726-2659
Fax: 205-726-4012
www.samford.edu.schools/
pharmacy/dic/index.html

### HUNTSVILLE
**Huntsville Hospital Drug**
**Information Center**
101 Sivley Rd.
Huntsville, AL 35801
Mon.-Fri. 8 AM-5 PM
    256-517-8288
Fax: 256-517-6558

## ARIZONA

### TUCSON
**Arizona Poison and Drug**
**Information Center**
**Arizona Health**
**Sciences Center**
**University Medical Center**
1501 N. Campbell Ave.
Room 1156
Tucson, AZ 85724
7 days/week, 24 hours
    520-626-6016
    800-362-0101 (AZ)
Fax: 520-626-2720
www.pharmacy.arizona.edu

## ARKANSAS

### LITTLE ROCK
**Arkansas Poison and Drug**
**Information Center**
4301 West Markham St.,
Slot 522-2
Little Rock, AK 72205
7 days/week, 24 hours
    501-686-5540
    **(for healthcare**
    **professionals only)**
    800-228-1233 (AK)
    **(for healthcare**
    **professionals only)**
    800-376-4766 (AK)
    **(for general public)**
Fax: 501-686-7357

## CALIFORNIA

### LOS ANGELES
**Los Angeles Regional**
**Drug Information Center**
**LAC & USC Medical Center**
1200 N. State St.
Room 2218
Los Angeles, CA 90033
Mon.-Fri. 8 AM-4:30 PM
    323-226-7741
Fax: 323-226-4194

### MARTINEZ
**Drug Information Service**
**VA Northern California**
**Health Care System**
Pharmacy Service 119
150 Muir Rd.
Martinez, CA 94553
Mon.-Fri. 8 PM-4:30 PM
    925-372-2167
Fax: 925-372-2169
cherie.dillon@med.va.gov

### SAN DIEGO
**Drug Information Center**
**U.S. Naval Hospital**
34800 Bob Wilson Dr.
San Diego, CA 92134-5000
Mon.-Fri. 8 AM-4 PM
    619-532-8417
Fax: 619-352-5898

**Drug Information Service**
**University of California**
**San Diego Medical Center**
135 Dickinson St.
Mailing address:
200 West Arbor Drive
MC 8925
San Diego, CA 92103-8925
Mon.-Fri. 9 AM-5 PM
    900-288-8273
Fax: 858-715-6323

### SAN FRANCISCO
**Drug Information Analysis**
**Service**
**University of California,**
**San Francisco**
521 Parnassus Ave.,
Room C152
San Francisco, CA 94143-
    0622
Mon.-Fri. 9 AM-4:30 PM
    415-502-9540
    **(for healthcare**
    **professionals only)**
Fax: 415-502-0792
E-mail: DIAS@itsa.ucsf.edu

### STANFORD
**Drug Information Center**
**University of California**
**Stanford Hospital and**
**Clinics**
300 Pasteur Dr.
Room H-0301
Stanford, CA 94305
Mon.-Fri. 8 AM-4 PM
    650-723-6422
Fax: 650-725-5028

## COLORADO

### DENVER
**Rocky Mountain Poison**
**and Drug Consultation**
**Center**
1001 Yosemite St.
Denver, CO 80230
7 days/week, 24 hours
    303-893-3784
    **(For Denver County**
    **residents only)**
Fax: 303-739-1119

**Drug Information Center**
**University of Colorado**
**Health Science Center**
**School of Pharmacy**
4200 E. 9th Ave., Box C239
Denver, CO 80262
Mon.-Fri. 8:30 AM-4:30 PM
    303-315-8489
Fax: 303-315-3353

## CONNECTICUT

### FARMINGTON
**Drug Information Service**
**University of Connecticut**
**Health Center**
263 Farmington Ave.
Farmington, CT 06030
Mon.-Fri. 7 AM-4 PM
    860-679-2783
Fax: 860-679-1231
wnelson@nso.uchc.edu

### HARTFORD
**Drug Information Center**
**Hartford Hospital**
P.O. Box 5037
80 Seymour St.
Hartford, CT 06102
Mon.-Fri. 8:30 AM-5 PM
    860-545-2221
    860-545-2961
    (After 5 PM)
Fax: 860-545-4371
www.harthosp.org

### NEW HAVEN
**Drug Information Center**
**Yale-New Haven Hospital**
20 York St.
New Haven, CT 06504
Mon.-Fri. 9 AM-5 PM
    203-688-2248
Fax: 203-688-3691
www.ynhh.com

## DISTRICT OF COLUMBIA

**Drug Information Service**
**Howard University Hospital**
Room BB06
2041 Georgia Ave. NW
Washington, DC 20060
Mon.-Fri. 8 AM-4 PM
　　202-865-1325
　　202-865-7413
Fax: 202-865-7410

## FLORIDA

*GAINESVILLE*
**Drug Information &**
**Pharmacy Resource**
**Center**
**SHANDS Hospital at**
**University of Florida**
P.O. Box 100316
Gainesville, FL 32610-0316
Mon.-Fri. 9 AM-5 PM
　　352-265-0408
　　**(for healthcare**
　　**professionals only)**
Fax: 352-338-9860
www.cop.ufl.edu/vdis

*JACKSONVILLE*
**Drug Information Service**
**SHANDS Jacksonville**
655 W. 8th St.
Jacksonville, FL 32209
Mon.-Fri. 8 AM-5 PM
　　904-244-4185
Fax: 904-244-4272
www.cop.ufl.edu/vdis

*MIAMI*
**Drug Information**
**Center (119)**
**Miami VA Medical Center**
1201 NW 16th St.
Pharmacy 119
Miami, FL 33125
Mon.-Fri. 7:00 AM-3:30 PM
　　305-324-3237
　　**(for healthcare**
　　**professionals only)**
Fax: 305-324-3394

*ORLANDO*
**Orlando Regional Drug**
**Information Service**
**Orlando Regional**
**Healthcare System**
1414 Kuhl Ave., MP 192
Orlando, FL 32806
Mon.-Fri. 8 AM-4:30 PM
　　407-841-5111,
　　ext. 8717
Fax: 407-649-1827
E-mail: druginfo@orhs.org

*TALLAHASSEE*
**Drug Information**
**Education Center**
**Florida Agricultural and**
**Mechanical University**
**College of Pharmacy**
Honor House, Room 200
Tallahassee, FL 32307
Mon.-Fri. 9 AM-5 PM
　　850-488-5239
　　850-599-3064
　　800-451-3181
Fax: 850-412-7020
www.pharmacy.samu.edu

## GEORGIA

*ATLANTA*
**Emory University Hospital**
**Dept. of Pharmaceutical**
**Services-Drug Information**
1364 Clifton Rd. NE
Atlanta, GA 30322
Mon.-Fri. 8:30 AM-5 PM
　　404-712-4640
Fax: 404-712-7577

**Drug Information Service**
**Northside Hospital**
1000 Johnson Ferry Rd. NE
Atlanta, GA 30342
Mon.-Fri. 9 AM-4 PM
　　404-851-8676
　　(GA only)
Fax: 404-851-8682

*AUGUSTA*
**Drug Information Center**
**Medical College of Georgia**
**Hospital and Clinic**
BI2101
1120 15th St.
Augusta, GA 30912
Mon.-Fri. 8:30 AM-5 PM
　　706-721-2887
Fax: 706-721-3827

*COLUMBUS*
**Columbus Regional Drug**
**Information Center**
710 Center St.
Columbus, GA 31902
Mon.-Fri. 8 AM-5 PM
　　706-571-1934
　　**(for healthcare**
　　**professionals only)**
Fax: 706-571-1625

## IDAHO

*POCATELLO*
**Drug Information Center**
**Idaho State University**
**School of Pharmacy**
Campus Box 8092
Pocatello, ID 83209
Mon.-Thur. 8:30 AM-5 PM
Fri. 8:30 AM-2:30 PM
　　208-282-4689
　　800-334-7139 (ID only)
Fax: 208-282-3003
http://rx.isu.edu/services_
contacts/idis/

## ILLINOIS

*CHICAGO*
**Drug Information Center**
**Northwestern Memorial**
**Hospital**
251 E. Huron
Feinberg LC-700B
Chicago, IL 60611
Mon.-Fri. 8 AM-5 PM
　　312-926-7573
Fax: 312-926-7956

**Drug Information Services**
**University of Chicago**
5841 S. Maryland Ave.
MC 0010
Chicago, IL 60637
Mon.-Fri. 8 AM-5 PM
　　773-702-1388
Fax: 773-702-6631

**Drug Information Center**
**University of Illinois at**
**Chicago**
833 S. Wood St.
Chicago, IL 60612
Mon.-Fri. 8 AM-4 PM
　　312-996-0209
Fax: 312-996-0448
www.uic.edu/pharmacy/
services/di/index.html

*HARVEY*
**Drug Information Center**
**Ingalls Memorial Hospital**
1 Ingalls Dr.
Harvey, IL 60426
Mon.-Fri. 8 AM-4:30 PM
　　708-915-4430
Fax: 708-915-3108

*HINES*
**Drug Information Service**
**Hines Veterans**
**Administration Hospital**
Pharmacy Services MC119
P.O. Box 5000
Hines, IL 60141-5000
Mon.-Fri. 8 AM-4:30 PM
　　708-202-8387,
　　ext. 23780
Fax: 708-202-2675

*PARK RIDGE*
**Drug Information Center**
**Lutheran General Hospital**
1775 Dempster St.
Park Ridge, IL 60068
Mon.-Fri. 7:30 AM-4 PM
　　847-723-8128
　　**(for healthcare**
　　**professionals only)**
Fax: 847-723-2326

## INDIANA

*INDIANAPOLIS*
**Drug Information Center**
**St. Vincent Hospital**
**and Health Services**
2001 W. 86th St.
Indianapolis, IN 46260
Mon.-Fri. 8 AM-4 PM
　　317-338-3200
　　**(for healthcare**
　　**professionals only)**
Fax: 317-338-3041

**Drug Information Service**
**Clarian Health Partners**
Pharmacy Department I-65
at 21st
Room CG04
Indianapolis, IN 46202
Mon.-Fri. 8:30 AM-4:30 PM
　　317-962-1750
Fax: 317-962-1756

*MUNCIE*
**Drug Information Center**
**Ball Memorial Hospital**
2401 University Ave.
Muncie, IN 47303
7 days/week, 24 hours
　　765-747-3035
Fax: 765-751-2522
E-mail:
kwolfe@chs.cami3.com

## IOWA

*DES MOINES*
**Regional Drug**
**Information Center**
**Mercy Medical Center-**
**Des Moines**
1111 Sixth Ave.
Des Moines, IA 50314
Mon.-Fri. 8 AM-4:30 PM
　　515-247-3286
　　(answered 7 days,
　　24 hours)
Fax: 515-247-3966

## IOWA CITY

**Drug Information Center**
**University of Iowa**
**Hospitals and Clinics**
200 Hawkins Dr.
Iowa City, IA 52242
Mon.-Fri. 8 AM-4:30 PM
   319-356-2600
   **(for healthcare**
   **professionals only)**
Fax: 319-384-8840

# KANSAS

## KANSAS CITY

**Drug Information Center**
**University of Kansas**
**Medical Center**
3901 Rainbow Blvd.
Kansas City, KS 66160
Mon.-Fri. 8:30 AM-6 PM
   913-588-2328
   **(for healthcare**
   **professionals only)**
Fax: 913-588-2350
E-mail: druginfo@kumc.edu

# KENTUCKY

## LEXINGTON

**Drug Information Center**
**Chandler Medical Center**
**College of Pharmacy**
**University of Kentucky**
800 Rose St., C-117
Lexington, KY 40536-0293
Mon.-Fri. 8 AM-5 PM
   859-323-5320
Fax: 859-323-2049
E-mail:
cqwhit1@pop.uky.edu

# LOUISIANA

## MONROE

**Louisiana Drug and Poison**
**Information Center**
**University of Louisiana at**
**Monroe College of**
**Pharmacy**
Monroe, LA 71209-6430
Mon.-Fri. 8 AM-4:30 PM
   318-342-1710
Fax: 318-342-1744
E-mail: pyross@ulm.edu

## NEW ORLEANS

**Xavier University Drug**
**Information Center**
**Tulane University**
**Hospital and Clinic**
Box HC12
1415 Tulane Ave.
New Orleans, LA 70112
Mon.-Fri. 9 AM-5 PM
   504-588-5670
Fax: 504-588-5862
E-mail:
mharris6@tulane.edu

# MARYLAND

## ANDREWS AFB

**Drug Information Services**
89 MDTS/SGQP
1050 W. Perimeter Rd.
Suite D1-119
Andrews AFB, MD 20762-
       6660
Mon.-Fri. 7:30 AM-5 PM
   240-857-4565
Fax: 240-857-8892

## ANNAPOLIS

**The Anne Arundel**
**Medical Center**
**Dept. of Pharmacy**
64 Franklin St.
Annapolis, MD 21401
7 days/week, 24 hours
   410-267-1126
   410-267-1000
   (switchboard)
Fax: 410-267-1628
www.aahs.org

## BALTIMORE

**Drug Information Service**
**Johns Hopkins Hospital**
600 N. Wolfe St.,
Halsted 503
Baltimore, MD 21287-6180
Mon.-Fri. 8:30 AM-5 PM
   410-955-6348
Fax: 410-955-8283

**Drug Information Service**
**University of Maryland**
**School of Pharmacy**
Pharmacy Hall Room 762
20 North Pine St.
Baltimore, MD 21201
Mon.-Fri. 8:30 AM-5 PM
   410-706-7568
Fax: 410-706-0754
www.pharmacy.umaryland.
edu/umdi

## BETHESDA

**Drug Information Service**
**National Institutes of**
**Health**
Building 10, Room 1S-259
10 Center Dr. (MSC1196)
Bethesda, MD 20892-1196
Mon.-Fri. 8:30 AM-5 PM
   301-496-2407
Fax: 301-496-0210
www.cc.nih.gov/phar

## EASTON

**Drug Information**
**Pharmacy Dept.**
**Memorial Hospital**
219 S. Washington St.
Easton, MD 21601
Mon.-Fri. 7 AM-Midnight
Sat.-Sun. 7 AM-5:30 PM
   410-822-1000,
   ext. 5645
Fax: 410-820-9489

# MASSACHUSETTS

## BOSTON

**Drug Information Services**
**Brigham and Women's**
**Hospital**
75 Frances St.
Boston, MA 02115
Mon.-Fri. 7 AM-3:30 PM
   617-732-7166
Fax: 617-732-7497

**Drug Information Center**
**New England Medical**
**Center Pharmacy**
750 Washington St.
Box 420
Boston, MA 02111
Mon.-Fri. 9 AM-5 PM
   617-636-8985
Fax: 617-636-4567

## WORCESTER

**Drug Information Center**
**UMass Memorial**
**Healthcare Hospital**
55 Lake Ave. North
Worcester, MA 01655
Mon.-Fri. 8:30 AM-5 PM
   508-856-3456
   508-856-2775
   (24 hour)
Fax: 508-856-1850

# MICHIGAN

## ANN ARBOR

**Drug Information and**
**Pharmacy Services**
**University of Michigan**
**Medical Center**
1500 East Medical
Center Dr.
UHB2 D301 Box 0008
Ann Arbor, MI 48109-0008
Mon.-Fri. 8 AM-5 PM
   734-936-8200
   734-936-8251
Fax: 734-936-7027
www.phar.med.umich.
edu/public

## DETROIT

**Drug Information Center**
**Department of Pharmacy**
**Services**
**Detroit Receiving Hospital**
**and University Health**
**Center**
4201 St. Antoine Blvd.
Detroit, MI 48201
Mon.-Fri. 8 AM-5 PM
   313-745-4556
Fax: 313-993-2522
www.dmcpharmacy.org

## LANSING

**Drug Information Services**
**Sparrow Hospital**
1215 East Michigan Ave.
Lansing, MI 48912
7 days/week, 24 hours
   517-483-2444
Fax: 517-483-2088

## PONTIAC

**Drug Information Center**
**St. Joseph Mercy Hospital**
44405 Woodward Ave.
Pontiac, MI 48341
Mon.-Fri. 8 AM-4:30 PM
   248-858-3055
Fax: 248-858-3010

## ROYAL OAK

**Drug Information Services**
**William Beaumont Hospital**
3601 West 13 Mile Rd.
Royal Oak, MI 48073-6769
Mon.-Fri. 8 AM-4:30 PM
   248-551-4077
Fax: 248-551-3301

## SOUTHFIELD

**Drug Information Service**
**Providence Hospital**
16001 West 9 Mile Rd.
Southfield, MI 48075
Mon.-Fri. 8 AM-4 PM
   248-424-3125
Fax: 248-424-5364

# MISSISSIPPI

## JACKSON

**Drug Information Center**
**University of Mississippi**
**Medical Center**
2500 N. State St.
Jackson, MS 39216
Mon.-Fri. 8 AM-4:30 PM
   601-984-2060
Fax: 601-984-2064

## MISSOURI

### KANSAS CITY
**University of
Missouri-Kansas City
Drug Information Center**
2411 Holmes St., MG-200
Kansas City, MO 64108-
      2792
Mon.-Fri. 8 AM-5 PM
    816-235-5490
Fax: 816-235-5491
www.umkc.edu/druginfo

### SPRINGFIELD
**Drug Information Center
St. Johns Regional
Health Center**
1235 E. Cherokee St.
Springfield, MO 65804
Mon.-Fri. 7:30 AM-4:30 PM
    417-885-3488
Fax: 417-888-7788
E-mail:
tbarks@sprg.smhs.com

### ST. JOSEPH
**Drug Information Service
Heartland Hospital West**
801 Faraon St.
St. Joseph, MO 64501
Mon.-Fri. 9 AM-5:30 PM
    816-271-7582
Fax: 816-271-7590

## MONTANA

### MISSOULA
**Drug Information Service
University of Montana
School of Pharmacy and
Allied Health Sciences**
Missoula, MT 59812-1522
Mon.-Fri. 8 AM-5 PM
    406-243-5254
Fax: 406-243-5256
E-mail:
druginfo@selway.umt.edu
www.umt.edu/druginfo

## NEBRASKA

### OMAHA
**Drug Information Service
School of Pharmacy
Creighton University**
2500 California Plaza
Omaha, NE 68178
Mon.-Fri. 8:30 AM-5:00 PM
    402-280-5101
Fax: 402-280-5149
www.druginfo.creighton.
edu

## NEW JERSEY

### NEWARK
**New Jersey Poison
Information and Education
System**
201 Lyons Ave.
Newark, NJ 07112
7 days/week, 24 hours
    973-926-7443
    800-222-1222
    **(poison control)**
Fax: 973-926-0013
E-mail: bruce@ibm.net
www.njpies.org

### NEW BRUNSWICK
**Drug Information Service
Robert Wood Johnson
University Hospital**
Pharmacy Department
1 Robert Wood Johnson Pl.
New Brunswick, NJ 08901
Mon.-Fri. 8:30 AM-4:30 PM
    732-937-8842
Fax: 732-937-8584

## NEW MEXICO

### ALBUQUERQUE
**New Mexico Poison &
Drug Information Center
University of New Mexico
Health Sciences Center**
Albuquerque, NM 87131
7 days/week, 24 hours
    505-272-2222
    800-432-6866
    (NM only)
Fax: 505-272-5892

## NEW YORK

### BROOKLYN
**International Drug
Information Center
Long Island University
Arnold & Marie Schwartz
College of Pharmacy &
Health Sciences**
1 University Plaza
RM-HS509
75 Dekalb Ave.
Brooklyn, NY 11201
Mon.-Fri. 9 AM-5 PM
    718-488-1064
Fax: 718-780-4056
www.liu.edu

**Drug Information Center
Brookdale University
Hospital and Medical
Center**
1 Brookdale Plaza
Brooklyn, NY 11212
Mon.-Fri. 8 AM-4 PM
    718-240-5983
Fax: 718-240-5987

### COOPERSTOWN
**Drug Information Center
Bassett Healthcare**
1 Atwell Rd.
Cooperstown, NY 13326
7 days/week, 24 hours
    607-547-3686
Fax: 607-547-3629

### JAMAICA
**Drug Information Center
St. John's University
College of Pharmacy and
Allied Health Professions**
8000 Utopia Pkwy.
Jamaica, NY 11439
Mon.-Fri. 8:30 AM-3:30 PM
    718-990-2149
Fax: 718-990-2151
druginfo@stjohns.edu

### NEW HYDE PARK
**Drug Information Center
St. Johns University at
Long Island Jewish
Medical Center**
270-05 76th Ave.
New Hyde Park, NY 11040
Mon.-Fri. 8 AM-3 PM
    718-470-DRUG
        (3784)
Fax: 718-470-1742

### NEW YORK CITY
**Drug Information Center
Memorial Sloan-Kettering
Cancer Center**
1275 York Ave.
RM S-712
New York, NY 10021
Mon.-Fri. 9 AM-5 PM
    212-639-7552
Fax: 212-639-2171

**Drug Information Center
Mount Sinai Medical
Center**
1 Gustave Levy Pl.
New York, NY 10029
Mon.-Fri. 9 AM-5 PM
    212-241-6619
Fax: 212-348-7927

**Drug Information Service
New York Presbyterian
Hospital**
Room K04
525 E. 68th St.
New York, NY 10021
Mon.-Fri. 9 AM-5 PM
    212-746-0741
Fax: 212-746-4434

### ROCHESTER
**Finger Lakes
Poison and Drug
Information Center
University of Rochester**
601 Elmwood Ave.
Rochester, NY 14642
7 days/week, 24 hours
    716-275-3718
    716-275-3232
    (after 5 PM)
Fax: 716-244-1677

### ROCKVILLE CENTER
**Drug Information Center
Mercy Medical Center**
1000 North Village Ave.
Rockville Center, NY 11570
Mon.-Fri. 8 AM-4 PM
    516-705-1053
Fax: 516-705-1071

## NORTH CAROLINA

### BUIES CREEK
**Drug Information Center
School of Pharmacy
Campbell University**
P.O. Box 1090
Buies Creek, NC 27506
Mon.-Fri. 8:30 AM-4:30 PM
    910-893-1478
    800-760-9697,
    ext. 2701
    800-327-5467
    (NC only)
Fax: 910-893-1476
E-mail: dic@mailcenter.
campbell.edu

### CHAPEL HILL
**Drug Information Center
University of North
Carolina Hospitals**
101 Manning Dr.
Chapel Hill, NC 27514
Mon.-Fri. 8 AM-4:30 PM
    919-966-2373
Fax: 919-966-1791

### DURHAM
**Drug Information Center
Duke University Health
Systems**
DUMC Box 3089
Durham, NC 27710
Mon.-Fri. 8 AM-5 PM
    919-684-5125
Fax: 919-681-3895

*GREENVILLE*

**Eastern Carolina Drug
Information Center
Pitt County
Memorial Hospital
Dept. of Pharmacy Service**
2100 Stantonsburg Rd.
Greenville, NC 27835
Mon.-Fri. 8 AM-5 PM
    252-816-4257
Fax: 252-816-7425

*WINSTON-SALEM*

**Drug Information
Service Center
Wake-Forest University
Baptist Medical Center**
Medical Center Blvd.
Winston-Salem, NC 27157
Mon.-Fri. 8 AM-5 PM
    336-716-2037
    **(for healthcare
    professionals only)**
Fax: 336-716-2186

# OHIO

*ADA*

**Drug Information Center
Raabe College of
Pharmacy
Ohio Northern University**
Ada, OH 45810
Mon.-Fri. 9 AM-5 PM
    419-772-2307
Fax: 419-772-2289
www.onu.edu/pharmacy/
druginfo

*CINCINNATI*

**Drug Information Center
Children's Hospital
Medical Center**
3333 Burnet Ave. VP-3
Cincinnati, OH 45229
Mon.-Fri. 9 AM-5 PM
    513-636-5054
    513-636-5111
    (24 hour)
    **(for healthcare
    professionals only)**
Fax: 513-636-5069

*CLEVELAND*

**Drug Information Service
Cleveland Clinic
Foundation**
9500 Euclid Ave.
Cleveland, OH 44195
Mon.-Fri. 8:30 AM-4:30 PM
    216-444-6456
    **(for healthcare
    professionals only)**
Fax: 216-444-6157

*COLUMBUS*

**Drug Information Center
Ohio State University
Hospital
Dept. of Pharmacy**
Doan Hall 368
410 W. 10th Ave.
Columbus, OH 43210-1228
Mon.-Fri. 8 AM-4 PM
    614-293-8679
Fax: 614-293-3264

**Drug Information Center
Riverside Methodist
Hospital**
3535 Olentangy River Road
Columbus, OH 43214
Mon.-Fri. 8:30 AM-4 PM
    614-566-5425
Fax: 614-566-5447,
    614-566-5850

*TOLEDO*

**Drug Information Services
St. Vincent Mercy Medical
Center**
2213 Cherry St.
Toledo, Ohio 43608-2691
Mon.-Fri. 8 AM-4 PM
    419-251-4227
Fax: 419-251-3662
E-mail: tschampel-1
@med.ctr.osu.edu
http://rx.med.ctr.
ohio-state.edu

# OKLAHOMA

*OKLAHOMA CITY*

**Drug Information Service
Integris Health**
3300 Northwest
Expressway
Oklahoma City, OK 73112
Mon.-Fri. 8 AM-4:30 PM
    405-949-3660
Fax: 405-951-8274

**Drug Information Center
OU Medical Center
Presbyterian Tower**
700 NE 13th St.
Oklahoma City, OK 73104
Mon.-Fri. 8 AM-4:30 PM
    405-271-6226
Fax: 405-271-6281

*TULSA*

**Drug Information Center
Saint Francis Hospital**
6161 S. Yale Ave.
Tulsa, OK 74136
Mon.-Fri. 8 AM-4 PM
    918-494-6339
    **(for healthcare
    professionals only)**
Fax: 918-494-1893

# PENNSYLVANIA

*PHILADELPHIA*

**Drug Information Center
Temple University Hospital
Dept. of Pharmacy**
3401 N. Broad St.
Philadelphia, PA 19140
Mon.-Fri. 8 AM-4:30 PM
    215-707-4644
Fax: 215-707-3463

**Drug Information Service
Tenet Health System
Department of Pharmacy**
MS 451
Broad and Vine Streets
Philadelphia, PA 19102
Mon.-Fri. 8 AM-4 PM
    215-762-DRUG
        (3784)
    **(for healthcare
    professionals only)**
Fax: 215-762-7993

**Drug Information Service
Dept. of Pharmacy
Thomas Jefferson
University Hospital**
111 S. 11th St.
Philadelphia, PA 19107-5098
Mon.-Fri. 8 AM-5 PM
    215-955-8877
Fax: 215-923-3316

**University of Pennsylvania
Health System Drug
Information Service
Hospital of the University
of Pennsylvania
Department of Pharmacy**
3400 Spruce St.
Philadelphia, PA 19104
Mon.-Fri. 8:30 AM-4 PM
    215-662-2903
Fax: 215-662-4319

*PITTSBURGH*

**The Christopher and
Nicole Browett
Pharmaceutical
Information Center
Mylan School of Pharmacy
Duquesne University**
431 Mellon Hall
Pittsburgh, PA 15282
Mon.-Fri. 8 AM-4 PM
    412-396-4600
Fax: 412-396-4488

**Drug Information Center
University of Pittsburgh**
137 Victoria Hall
Pittsburgh, PA 15261
Mon.-Fri. 8:30 AM-4:30 PM
    412-624-3784
    **(for healthcare
    professionals only)**
Fax: 412-624-6350
E-mail: druginfo@msx.
upmc.edu

*UPLAND*

**Drug Information Center
Crozer-Chester Medical
Center
Dept. of Pharmacy**
1 Medical Center Blvd.
Upland, PA 19013
Mon.-Fri. 8 AM-4:30 PM
    610-447-2851
    610-447-2862
    (after hours)
    **(both numbers are
    for healthcare
    professionals only)**
Fax: 610-447-2820

*WILLIAMSPORT*

**Drug Information
Pharmacy Dept.
Susquehanna Health
System**
Rural Avenue Campus
Williamsport, PA 17701
24 hours/7 days a week
    570-321-3083
Fax: 570-321-3230

# PUERTO RICO

*PONCE*

**Centro Informacion
Medicamentos
Escuela de Medicina de
Ponce**
P.O. Box 7004
Ponce, PR 00732-7004
Mon.-Fri. 8 AM-4:30 PM
    787-259-7085
    (Spanish and English)
    787-840-2575
    (switchboard)
Fax: 787-842-0461

*SAN JUAN*

**Centro de Informacion de
Medicamentos-CIM
Escuela de Farmacia-RCM**
P.O. Box 365067
San Juan, PR 00936-5067
Mon.-Fri. 8 AM-4:30 PM
    787-758-2525,
    ext. 1516
Fax: 787-763-0196
E-mail:
cimrcm@rcm.upr.edu

## SOUTH CAROLINA

### CHARLESTON

**Drug Information Service
Medical University of
South Carolina**
150 Ashley Ave.
Rutledge Tower
Annex, Room 604
P.O. Box 250584
Charleston, SC 29425-0810
Mon.-Fri. 9 AM-5:30 PM
    843-792-3896
    800-922-5250
Fax:  843-792-5532

### COLUMBIA

**Drug Information Service
University of South
Carolina
College of Pharmacy
University of South
Carolina**
Columbia, SC 29208
Mon.-Fri. 8 AM-5 PM
    803-777-7804
Fax:  803-777-6127

### SPARTANBURG

**Drug Information Center
Spartanburg Regional
Medical Center**
101 E. Wood St.
Spartanburg, SC 29303
Mon.-Fri. 8 AM-5 PM
    864-560-6910
Fax:  864-560-7323

## TENNESSEE

### KNOXVILLE

**Drug Information Center
University of Tennessee
Medical Center at
Knoxville**
1924 Alcoa Highway
Knoxville, TN 37920-6999
Mon.-Fri. 8 AM-4:30 PM
    865-544-9124
Fax:  865-525-0326
    865-544-8242

### MEMPHIS

**South East Regional Drug
Information Center
VA Medical Center**
1030 Jefferson Ave.
Memphis, TN 38104
Mon.-Fri. 7:30 AM-4 PM
    901-523-8990,
    ext. 6720
Fax:  901-577-7306

**Drug Information Center
University of Tennessee**
875 Monroe Ave.
Suite 116
Memphis, TN 38163
Mon.-Fri. 7 AM-5 PM
    901-448-5555
Fax:  901-448-5419
E-mail: utdic@utmem.edu

## TEXAS

### AMARILLO

**Drug Information Center
Texas Tech University
School of Pharmacy**
1300 Coulter
Amarillo, TX 79106
Mon.-Fri. 8 AM-5 PM
    806-356-4008
    **(for healthcare
    professionals only)**
Fax:  806-356-4017

### GALVESTON

**Drug Information Center
University of Texas
Medical Branch**
301 University Blvd. - G01
Galveston, TX 77555-0701
Mon.-Fri. 8 AM-5 PM
    409-772-2734
Fax:  409-747-5222

### HOUSTON

**Drug Information Center
Ben Taub General Hospital
Texas Southern
University/HCHD**
1504 Taub Loop
Houston, TX 77030
Mon.-Fri. 8 AM-5 PM
    713-873-3710
Fax:  713-873-3711

### LACKLAND A.F.B.

**Drug Information Center
Dept. of Pharmacy
Wilford Hall Medical
Center**
2200 Berquist Dr.
Suite 1
Lackland A.F.B., TX 78236
7 days/week, 24 hours
    210-292-5414
Fax:  210-292-3722

### LUBBOCK

**Drug Information and
Consultation Service**
Covenant Medical Center
3615 19th St.
Lubbock, TX 79410
Mon.-Fri. 8 AM-5 PM
    806-725-0408
Fax:  806-725-0305

### SAN ANTONIO

**Drug Information Service
University of Texas
Health Science Center
at San Antonio**
Department of
Pharmacology
7703 Floyd Curl Drive
San Antonio, TX 78229-3900
Mon.-Thur. 8 AM-5 PM
Fri. 8 AM-3 PM
    210-567-4280
Fax:  210-567-4305

### TEMPLE

**Drug Information Center
Scott and White
Memorial Hospital**
2401 S. 31st St.
Temple, TX 76508
Mon.-Fri. 8 AM-6 PM
    254-724-4636
Fax:  254-724-1731

## UTAH

### SALT LAKE CITY

**Drug Information Service
University of Utah Hospital
Dept. of Pharmacy
Services**
Room A-050
50 N. Medical Dr.
Salt Lake City, UT 84132
Mon.-Fri. 8:30 AM-4:30 PM
    801-581-2073
Fax:  801-585-6688
E-mail:
drug.info@hsc.utah.edu

## VIRGINIA

### HAMPTON

**Drug Information Service
Hampton University School
of Pharmacy**
Kittrell Hall Room 208
Hampton, VA 23668
Mon.-Fri. 8 AM-5 PM
    757-728-6687
    757-728-6693
    (drug info hotline)
Fax:  757-728-6696
E-mail: druginfo@
hamptonu.edu

## WEST VIRGINIA

### MORGANTOWN

**West Virginia Drug
Information Center
WV University-
Robert C. Byrd
Health Sciences Center**
1124 HSN, P.O. Box 9550
Morgantown, WV 26506
Mon.-Fri. 8:30 AM-5 PM
    304-293-6640
    800-352-2501 (WV)
Fax:  304-293-7672

## WYOMING

### LARAMIE

**Drug Information Center
University of Wyoming**
P.O. Box 3375
Laramie, WY 82071
Mon.-Fri. 8 AM-5 PM
    307-766-6988
Fax:  307-766-2953
E-mail: kendrag@uwyo.edu

# POISON CONTROL CENTERS

Across America there's now a single emergency phone number that automatically links callers with their regional poison control center. This new toll-free number, **800-222-1222**, is being used by every state with the exception of California, which has yet to implement the switch. A few local poison centers and the National Animal Poison Control Center (which appears at the end of the listings) are not part of this nationwide system and continue to use separate numbers.

Most of the centers listed below are certified by the American Association of Poison Control Centers.

**Certified centers are marked by an asterisk after the name**. Each has to meet certain criteria. It must, for example, serve a large geographic area; it must be open 24 hours a day and provide direct-dial or toll-free access; it must be supervised by a medical director; and it must have registered pharmacists or nurses available to answer questions from the public.

Within each state, centers are listed alphabetically by city. Telephone numbers designated "TTY" are teletype lines for the hearing-impaired. "TDD" numbers reach a telecommunication device for the deaf.

## ALABAMA

*BIRMINGHAM*

**Regional Poison Control Center, The Children's Hospital of Alabama (*)**
1600 7th Ave. South
Birmingham, AL 35233-1711
**Emergency:** 800-222-1222
Fax: 205-939-9245

*TUSCALOOSA*

**Alabama Poison Center (*)**
2503 Phoenix Dr.
Tuscaloosa, AL 35405
Business: 205-345-0600
**Emergency:** 800-222-1222
Fax: 205-343-7410

## ALASKA

*ANCHORAGE*

**Anchorage Poison Control Center, Providence Hospital**
P.O. Box 196604
3200 Providence Dr.
Anchorage, AK 99519-6604
Business: 907-562-2211, ext. 3193
**Emergency:** 800-222-1222
Fax: 907-261-3684

*(PORTLAND, OR)*

**Oregon Poison Center (*)**
**Oregon Health Sciences University**
3181 SW Sam Jackson Park Rd, CB550
Portland, OR 97201
**Emergency:** 800-222-1222
Fax: 503-494-4980

## ARIZONA

*PHOENIX*

**Samaritan Regional Poison Center (*)**
**Good Samaritan Regional Medical Center**
Ancillary 1
1111 East McDowell Rd.
Phoenix, AZ 85006
Business: 602-495-4884
**Emergency:** 800-222-1222
Fax: 602-256-7579

*TUCSON*

**Arizona Poison and Drug Information Center (*)**
**Arizona Health Sciences Center**
1501 N. Campbell Ave.
Room 1156
Tucson, AZ 85724
**Emergency:** 800-222-1222
Fax: 520-626-2720

## ARKANSAS

*LITTLE ROCK*

**Arkansas Poison and Drug Information Center**
**College of Pharmacy - UAMS**
4301 West Markham St.
Mail Slot 522
Little Rock, AR 72205-7122
Business: 501-686-6161
**Emergency:** 800-222-1222
TDD/TTY: 800-641-3805

## CALIFORNIA

*FRESNO*

**California Poison Control System-Fresno/Madera (*)**
**Valley Children's Hospital**
9300 Valley Children's Place
MB 15
Madera, CA 93638-8762
Business: 559-353-3000
**Emergency:** 800-876-4766 (CA)
TDD/TTY: 800-972-3323

*SACRAMENTO*

**California Poison Control System-Sacramento (*)**
UCDMC-HSF Room 1024
2315 Stockton Blvd.
Sacramento, CA 95817
Business: 916-227-1400
**Emergency:** 800-876-4766 (CA)
TDD/TTY: 800-972-3323
Fax: 916-227-1414

*SAN DIEGO*

**California Poison Control System-San Diego (*)**
**UCSD Medical Center**
200 West Arbor Dr.
San Diego, CA 92103-8925
**Emergency:** 800-876-4766 (CA)
TDD/TTY: 800-972-3323

*SAN FRANCISCO*

**California Poison Control System-San Francisco (*)**
UCSF Box 1369
1001 Potrero Ave., Room 1E86
San Francisco, CA 94143
**Emergency:** 800-876-4766 (CA)
TDD/TTY: 800-972-3323

## COLORADO

*DENVER*

**Rocky Mountain Poison and Drug Center (*)**
1010 Yosemite Circle
Suite 200
Denver, CO 80230-6800
Business: 303-739-1100
**Emergency:** 800-222-1222
TTY: 303-739-1127 (CO)
Fax: 303-739-1119

## CONNECTICUT

*FARMINGTON*

**Connecticut Regional Poison Control Center (*)**
**University of Connecticut Health Center**
263 Farmington Ave.
Farmington, CT 06030-5365
Business: 860-679-3056
**Emergency:** 800-222-1222
TDD/TTY: 866-218-5372
Fax: 860-679-1623

## DELAWARE

*PHILADELPHIA, PA*

**The Poison Control Center of Philadelphia (*)**
3535 Market St.
Suite 985
Philadelphia, PA 19104-3309
Business: 215-590-2003
**Emergency:** 800-222-1222
TDD/TTY: 215-590-8789
Fax: 215-590-4419

# DISTRICT OF COLUMBIA

*WASHINGTON, DC*
**National Capital
Poison Center (*)**
3201 New Mexico Ave., NW
Suite 310
Washington, DC 20016
Business:      202-362-3867
**Emergency: 800-222-1222**
TTY:           202-362-8563
Fax:           202-362-8377

# FLORIDA

*JACKSONVILLE*
**Florida Poison Information
Center-Jacksonville (*)
SHANDS Jacksonville
Medical Center**
655 West 8th St.
Jacksonville, FL 32209
**Emergency: 800-222-1222**
TDD/TTY:      800-282-3171
              (FL)
Fax:          904-244-4063

*MIAMI*
**Florida Poison Information
Center-Miami (*)
University of Miami
Department of Pediatrics
Jackson Memorial
Medical Center**
P.O. Box 016960 (R-131)
Miami, FL 33101
Business:     305-585-5253
**Emergency: 800-222-1222**
Fax:          305-545-9762

*TAMPA*
**Florida Poison
Information Center-Tampa (*)
Tampa General Hospital**
P.O. Box 1289
Tampa, FL 33601
**Emergency: 800-222-1222**
Fax:          813-253-4443

# GEORGIA

*ATLANTA*
**Georgia Poison Center (*)
Hughes Spalding
Children's Hospital, Grady
Health System**
80 Butler St., SE
P.O. Box 26066
Atlanta, GA 30335-3801
**Emergency: 800-222-1222**
TDD:          404-616-9287
Fax:          404-616-6657

# HAWAII

*HONOLULU*
**Hawaii Poison Center**
1319 Punahou St.
Honolulu, HI 96826
**Emergency: 800-222-1222**
Fax:          808-535-7922

# IDAHO

*(DENVER, CO)*
**Rocky Mountain Poison
& Drug Center (*)**
1010 Yosemite Circle,
Suite 200
Denver, CO 80230-6800
**Emergency: 800-222-1222**
TTY:          303-739-1127
              (ID)
Fax:          303-739-1119

# ILLINOIS

*CHICAGO*
**Illinois Poison Center (*)**
222 South Riverside Plaza
Suite 1900
Chicago, IL 60606
Business:     312-906-6136
**Emergency: 800-222-1222**
TDD/TTY:      312-906-6185
Fax:          312-803-5400

# INDIANA

*INDIANAPOLIS*
**Indiana Poison Center (*)
Methodist Hospital
Clarian Health Partners**
I-65 at 21st St.
P.O. Box 1367
Indianapolis, IN 46206-1367
**Emergency: 800-222-1222**
TTY:          317-962-2336
Fax:          317-962-2337

# IOWA

*SIOUX CITY*
**Iowa Statewide Poison
Control Center
St. Luke's Regional
Medical Center**
2720 Stone Park Blvd.
Sioux City, IA 51104
Business:     712-279-3710
**Emergency: 800-222-1222**
Fax:          712-234-8775

# KANSAS

*KANSAS CITY*
**Mid-America Poison
Control Center,
University of Kansas
Medical Center**
3901 Rainbow Blvd.
Room B-400
Kansas City, KS 66160-7231
Business &    913-588-6638
**Emergency: 800-222-1222**
TDD:          913-588-6639
Fax:          913-588-2350

*TOPEKA*
**Stormont-Vail Regional
Medical Center
Poison Control Center**
1500 S.W. 10th
Topeka, KS 66604-1353
Business:     785-354-6106
**Emergency: 800-222-1222**
              800-332-6633
              (KS)
Fax:          785-354-5004

# KENTUCKY

*LOUISVILLE*
**Kentucky Regional
Poison Center (*)**
Medical Towers South
Suite 572
234 East Gray St.
Louisville, KY 40202
Business:     502-629-7264
**Emergency: 800-222-1222**
              502-589-8222
Fax:          502-629-7277

# LOUISIANA

*MONROE*
**Louisiana Drug and Poison
Information Center (*)
University of Louisiana at
Monroe College of
Pharmacy**
Sugar Hall
Monroe, LA 71209-6430
Business:     318-342-1710
**Emergency: 800-222-1222**
Fax:          318-342-1744

# MAINE

*PORTLAND*
**Maine Poison Center
Maine Medical Center**
22 Bramhall St.
Portland, ME 04102
**Emergency: 800-222-1222**
TDD/TTY:      207-871-2879
              877-299-4447
              (ME)
Fax:          207-871-6226

# MARYLAND

*BALTIMORE*
**Maryland Poison Center (*)
University of Maryland at
Baltimore
School of Pharmacy**
20 North Pine St., PH 772
Baltimore, MD 21201
Business:     410-706-7604
**Emergency: 800-222-1222**
TDD:          410-706-1858
Fax:          410-706-7184

# MASSACHUSETTS

*BOSTON*
**Regional Center for Poison
Control and Prevention (*)**
300 Longwood Ave.
Boston, MA 02115
**Emergency: 800-222-1222**
TDD/TTY:      888-244-5313
Fax:          617-738-0032

# MICHIGAN

*DETROIT*
**Regional Poison
Control Center (*)
Children's Hospital of
Michigan**
4160 John R. Harper
Professional Office Bldg.
Suite 616
Detroit, MI 48201
Business:     313-745-5335
**Emergency: 800-222-1222**
TDD/TTY:      800-356-3232
Fax:          313-745-5493

*GRAND RAPIDS*

**DeVos Children's Hospital Regional Poison Center (\*)**
100 Michigan St., NE
Grand Rapids, MI 49503
Business: 616-774-7851
Emergency: 800-222-1222
TDD/TTY: 800-356-3232
Fax: 616-774-7204

## MINNESOTA

*MINNEAPOLIS*

**Hennepin Regional Poison Center (\*) Hennepin County Medical Center**
701 Park Ave.
Minneapolis, MN 55415
Business: 612-347-3144
Emergency: 800-222-1222
TTY: 612-904-4691
Fax: 612-904-4289

## MISSISSIPPI

*HATTIESBURG*

**Poison Center, Forrest General Hospital**
P. O. Box 16389
400 South 28th Ave.
Hattiesburg, MS 39404
Emergency: 601-288-2199
Fax: 601-288-2125

*JACKSON*

**Mississippi Regional Poison Control Center, University of Mississippi Medical Center**
2500 North State St.
Jackson, MS 39216
Business: 601-984-1675
Emergency: 800-222-1222
Fax: 601-984-1676

## MISSOURI

*ST. LOUIS*

**Cardinal Glennon Children's Hospital Regional Poison Center (\*)**
1465 South Grand Blvd.
St. Louis, MO 63104
Emergency: 800-222-1222
TTY: 314-577-5336
Fax: 314-577-5355

## MONTANA

*(DENVER, CO)*

**Rocky Mountain Poison and Drug Center (\*)**
1010 Yosemite Circle
Suite 200
Denver, CO 80230-6800
Emergency: 800-222-1222
Fax: 303-739-1119

## NEBRASKA

*OMAHA*

**The Poison Center (\*) Children's Hospital**
8200 Dodge St.
Omaha, NE 68114
Emergency: 800-222-1222

## NEVADA

*(DENVER, CO)*

**Rocky Mountain Poison and Drug Center (\*)**
1010 Yosemite Circle
Suite 200
Denver, CO 80230-6800
Emergency: 800-222-1222
Fax: 303-739-1119

## NEW HAMPSHIRE

*LEBANON*

**New Hampshire Poison Information Center, Dartmouth-Hitchcock Medical Center**
1 Medical Center Dr.
Lebanon, NH 03756
Emergency: 800-222-1222
Fax: 603-650-8986

## NEW JERSEY

*NEWARK*

**New Jersey Poison Information and Education System (\*)**
201 Lyons Ave.
Newark, NJ 07112
Business: 973-926-7443
Emergency: 800-222-1222
TDD/TTY: 973-926-8008
Fax: 973-926-0013

## NEW MEXICO

*ALBUQUERQUE*

**New Mexico Poison and Drug Information Center (\*) University of New Mexico**
Health Science Center
Library, Room 130
Albuquerque, NM 87131-1076
Emergency: 800-222-1222
Fax: 505-272-5892

## NEW YORK

*BUFFALO*

**Western New York Regional Poison Control Center (\*) Children's Hospital of Buffalo**
219 Bryant St.
Buffalo, NY 14222
Business: 716-878-7657
Emergency: 800-222-1222

*MINEOLA*

**Long Island Regional Poison and Drug Information Center (\*) Winthrop University Hospital**
259 First St.
Mineola, NY 11501
Emergency: 800-222-1222
TDD: 516-747-3323
(Nassau)
516-924-8811
(Suffolk)
Fax: 516-739-2070

*NEW YORK CITY*

**New York City Poison Control Center (\*) NYC Dept. of Health**
455 First Ave., Room 123
New York, NY 10016
Business: 212-447-8152
Emergency: 800-222-1222
(English) 212-340-4494
212-POISONS
(212-764-7667)

Emergency: 212-VENENOS
(Spanish) (212-836-3667)
TDD: 212-689-9014
Fax: 212-447-8223

## ROCHESTER (italic)

*ROCHESTER*

**Finger Lakes Regional Poison and Drug Information Center (\*) University of Rochester Medical Center**
601 Elmwood Ave.
Box 321
Rochester, NY 14642
Business: 716-273-4155
Emergency: 800-222-1222
TTY: 716-273-3854
Fax: 716-244-1677

*SLEEPY HOLLOW*

**Hudson Valley Regional Poison Center, Phelps Memorial Hospital Center**
701 N. Broadway
Sleepy Hollow, NY 10591
Emergency: 914-366-3030
800-222-1222
Fax: 914-366-1400

*SYRACUSE*

**Central New York Poison Center (\*) SUNY Health Science Center**
750 East Adams St.
Syracuse, NY 13210
Business: 315-464-7078
Emergency: 800-222-1222
Fax: 315-464-7077

## NORTH CAROLINA

*CHARLOTTE*

**Carolinas Poison Center (\*) Carolinas Medical Center**
5000 Airport Center Pkwy.
Suite B
Charlotte, NC 28208
Business: 704-395-3795
Emergency: 800-222-1222

## NORTH DAKOTA

*FARGO*

**North Dakota Poison Information Center, Meritcare Medical Center**
720 4th St. North
Fargo, ND 58122
Business: 701-234-6062
Emergency: 800-222-1222
Fax: 701-234-5090

# OHIO

## CINCINNATI

**Cincinnati Drug and Poison Information Center (\*)
Regional Poison Control System**
3333 Burnet Ave.
Vernon Place, 3rd Floor
Cincinnati, OH 45229
Emergency: 513-558-5111
800-222-1222
TDD/TTY: 800-253-7955
Fax: 513-636-5069

## CLEVELAND

**Greater Cleveland Poison Control Center**
11100 Euclid Ave.
Cleveland, OH 44106-6010
Emergency: 216-231-4455
800-222-1222
Fax: 216-844-3242

## COLUMBUS

**Central Ohio Poison Center (\*)**
700 Children's Dr.
Room L032
Columbus, OH 43205-2696
Business: 614-722-2635
Emergency: 614-228-1323
800-222-1222
937-222-2227
(Dayton Region)
TTY: 614-228-2272
Fax: 614-228-2672

## TOLEDO

**Poison Information Center of Northwest Ohio Medical College of Ohio Hospital**
3000 Arlington Ave.
Toledo, OH 43614
Emergency: 419-383-3897
800-222-1222
Fax: 419-383-6066

# OKLAHOMA

## OKLAHOMA CITY

**Oklahoma Poison Control Center,
University of Oklahoma**
940 Northeast 13th St.
Room 3512
Oklahoma City, OK 73104
Business: 405-271-5062
Emergency: 800-222-1222
TDD: 405-271-1122
Fax: 405-271-1816

# OREGON

## PORTLAND

**Oregon Poison Center (\*)
Oregon Health Sciences University**
3181 S.W. Sam Jackson Park Rd. CB 550
Portland, OR 97201
Emergency: 800-222-1222
Fax: 503-494-4980

# PENNSYLVANIA

## HERSHEY

**Central Pennsylvania Poison Center (\*)
Pennsylvania State University
Milton S. Hershey Medical Center**
500 University Dr.
MC H043, P.O. Box 850
Hershey, PA 17033-0850
Emergency: 800-222-1222
717-531-6111
TTY: 717-531-8335
Fax: 717-531-6932

## PHILADELPHIA

**The Poison Control Center (\*)**
3535 Market St., Suite 985
Philadelphia, PA 19104-3309
Business: 215-590-2003
Emergency: 800-222-1222
TDD/TTY: 215-590-8789
Fax: 215-590-4419

## PITTSBURGH

**Pittsburgh Poison Center (\*)
Children's Hospital of Pittsburgh**
3705 Fifth Ave.
Pittsburgh, PA 15213
Business: 412-692-5600
Emergency: 800-222-1222
Fax: 412-692-7497

# PUERTO RICO

## SANTURCE

**San Jorge Children's Hospital Poison Center**
258 San Jorge St.
Santurce, PR 00912
Emergency: 787-726-5674

# RHODE ISLAND

**(BOSTON, MA)**

**Regional Center for Poison Control and Prevention (\*)**
300 Longwood Ave.
Boston, MA 02115
Emergency: 800-222-1222
TDD/TTY: 888-244-5313
Fax: 617-738-0032

# SOUTH CAROLINA

## COLUMBIA

**Palmetto Poison Center, College of Pharmacy, University of South Carolina**
Columbia, SC 29208
Business: 803-777-7909
Emergency: 800-222-1222
Fax: 803-777-6127

# SOUTH DAKOTA

**(FARGO, ND)**

**North Dakota Poison Information Center Meritcare Medical Center**
720 4th St. North
Fargo, ND 58122
Business: 701-234-6062
Emergency: 701-234-5575
800-732-2200
(SD, MN, ND)
Fax: 701-234-5090

**(MINNEAPOLIS, MN)**

**Hennepin Regional Poison Center (\*) Hennepin County Medical Center**
701 Park Ave.
Minneapolis, MN 55415
Business: 612-347-3144
Emergency: 800-222-1222
TTY: 612-904-4691
Fax: 612-904-4289

# TENNESSEE

## MEMPHIS

**Southern Poison Center University of Tennessee**
875 Monroe Ave.
Suite 104
Memphis, TN 38163
Business: 901-448-6800
Emergency: 800-222-1222
Fax: 901-448-5419

## NASHVILLE

**Middle Tennessee Poison Center (\*)**
1161 21st Ave. South
501 Oxford House
Nashville, TN 37232-4632
Business: 615-936-0760
Emergency: 800-222-1222
TDD: 615-936-2047
Fax: 615-936-0756

# TEXAS

## AMARILLO

**Texas Panhandle Poison Center
Northwest Texas Hospital**
1501 S. Coulter Dr.
Amarillo, TX 79106
Emergency: 800-222-1222

## DALLAS

**North Texas Poison Center (\*)
Texas Poison Center Network
Parkland Health and Hospital System**
5201 Harry Hines Blvd.
P.O. Box 35926
Dallas, TX 75235
Business: 214-589-0911
Emergency: 800-222-1222
Fax: 214-590-5008

## EL PASO

**West Texas Regional Poison Center (\*)
Thomason Hospital**
4815 Alameda Ave.
El Paso, TX 79905
Business 915-534-3800
Emergency: 800-222-1222

## GALVESTON

**Southeast Texas Poison Center (\*)
The University of Texas Medical Branch**
3112 Trauma Bldg.
301 University Ave.
Galveston, TX 77555-1175
Business: 409-766-4403
Emergency: 800-222-1222
TDD/TTY: 800-764-7661
(TX)
Fax: 409-772-3917

## SAN ANTONIO

**South Texas
Poison Center (\*)
The University of Texas
Health Science Center–
San Antonio**
7703 Floyd Curl Dr.,
MC 7849
San Antonio, TX 78229-3900
**Emergency:** 800-222-1222
TDD/TTY:    800-764-7661
            (TX)
Fax:        210-567-5718

## TEMPLE

**Central Texas Poison
Center (\*)
Scott & White Memorial
Hospital**
2401 South 31st St.
Temple, TX 76508
**Emergency:** 800-222-1222
Fax:        254-724-1731

# UTAH

## SALT LAKE CITY

**Utah Poison Control
Center (\*)**
410 Chipeta Way
Suite 230
Salt Lake City, UT 84108
**Emergency:** 800-222-1222
Fax:        801-581-4199

# VERMONT

## BURLINGTON

**Vermont Poison Center,
Fletcher Allen Health Care**
111 Colchester Ave.
Burlington, VT 05401
Business:    802-847-2721
**Emergency:** 800-222-1222
Fax:        802-847-4802

# VIRGINIA

## CHARLOTTESVILLE

**Blue Ridge Poison
Center (\*)
University of Virginia
Health System**
PO Box 800774
Charlottesville, VA 22908-
            0774
**Emergency:** 800-222-1222
Fax:        804-971-8657

## RICHMOND

**Virginia Poison Center (\*)
Virginia Commonwealth
University**
P.O. Box 980522
Richmond, VA 23298-0522
**Emergency:** 800-222-1222
TDD/TTY:    800-828-1120
Fax:        804-828-5291

# WASHINGTON

## SEATTLE

**Washington Poison
Center (\*)**
155 NE 100th St.
Suite 400
Seattle, WA 98125-8012
Business:    206-517-2351
**Emergency:** 800-222-1222
TDD:        800-572-0638
            (WA)
            206-517-2394
Fax:        206-526-8490

# WEST VIRGINIA

## CHARLESTON

**West Virginia
Poison Center (\*)**
3110 MacCorkle Ave. SE
Charleston, WV 25304
Business:    304-347-1212
**Emergency:** 800-222-1222
Fax:        304-348-9560

# WISCONSIN

## MADISON

**Poison Control Center,
University of Wisconsin
Hospital and Clinics**
600 Highland Ave.
F6-133
Madison, WI 53792
**Emergency:** 800-815-8855

## MILWAUKEE

**Children's Hospital
of Wisconsin Poison
Center**
9000 W. Wisconsin Ave.
P.O. Box 1997,
Mail Station 677A
Milwaukee, WI 53201-1997
Business:    414-266-2000
**Emergency:** 800-222-1222
TDD/TTY:    414-266-2542
Fax:        414-266-2820

# WYOMING

*(OMAHA, NE)*
**The Poison Center (\*)
Children's Hospital**
8301 Dodge St.
Omaha, NE 68114
**Emergency:** 800-222-1222

# ASPCA/NATIONAL ANIMAL POISON CONTROL CENTER

1717 South Philo Rd.
Suite 36
Urbana, IL 61802
Business:    217-337-5030
**Emergency:** 888-426-4435
            900-680-0000
Fax:        217-337-0599

# POPULAR HERBS

Reliable information on herbal remedies is still hard to come by, yet Americans spend more than $4 billion each year on herbal products. Even more surprising are the findings from a recent *Prevention* magazine survey: Nearly 23 million consumers use herbal remedies *instead* of taking prescription medicine, and about 20 million take botanicals along with either OTC or prescription drugs.

To prepare you for those times when patients ask about the latest herbal "discovery"—as they surely will—we've compiled a quick reference of the most commonly used herbs. The information is based on the findings of the German Regulatory Authority's "Commission E"—currently the most authoritative source of information on botanical medicines. For a more thorough discussion of over 700 herbs, consult the second edition of the *PDR® for Herbal Medicines™*.

**Aloe *(Aloe vera)*.** The gel from the Aloe plant is an ancient remedy used externally for its antibacterial, antiviral, anti-inflammatory, and pain-relieving effects. It is used topically in skin moisturizers and to treat burns, wounds, psoriasis, and frostbite. While the internal use of Aloe is suggested as a treatment for several conditions including constipation, there is no evidence of its efficacy. In fact, internal use is not recommended because of the risk of serious adverse effects.

*Warning:* Aloe should not be used by pregnant or breastfeeding women, or by people with severe intestinal disorders. Aloe should not be taken with certain drugs associated with potassium loss—such as diuretics, corticosteroids, and antiarrhythmics and other heart medications—or with the herb Licorice.

**Arnica *(Arnica montana)*.** The Arnica plant is used externally for pain and inflammation due to injury, and as an anti-infectious agent. Arnica should be discontinued immediately in the event of an allergic reaction to external application. The herb should not be used on open skin wounds.

*Warning:* Although Europeans take Arnica internally to treat respiratory infections, internal use is not recommended due to the risk of serious cardiac adverse effects.

**Astragalus *(Astragalus species)*.** Astragalus, or Huang-Qi, is used to improve immune function and strengthen the cardiovascular system. Compounds in Astragalus may also have beneficial antiviral, antioxidant, memory-enhancing, and liver-protecting effects, although the nature of those effects on specific diseases has not been established.

*Warning:* The use of Astragalus must be carefully monitored by a physician due to its potentially dangerous adverse effects, particularly in people with immune disorders or those taking blood-thinning medications.

**Barberry *(Berberis vulgaris)*.** Both the fruit and root bark of the Barberry plant are used in folk medicine. The berry is a source of vitamin C, which stimulates the immune system, improves iron absorption, and protects against scurvy. The fruit's acid content has a mild diuretic effect that is thought to aid in urinary tract infections. Barberry root bark may reduce blood pressure, relieve constipation, and have some antibiotic effects.

*Warning:* Pregnant and nursing women should not use Barberry.

**Bilberry *(Vaccinium myrtillus)*.** The astringent effects of Bilberry fruit are used to treat inflammation of the mouth and throat, and both the fruit and leaves are used for diarrhea. Reports citing Bilberry as a treatment for diabetic retinopathy need further confirmation.

*Warning:* The herb should not be used with blood-thinning drugs, including aspirin.

**Black Cohosh *(Cimicifuga racemosa)*.** The hormone-modulating effects of Black Cohosh make it useful for women with menopausal symptoms and premenstrual syndrome.

*Warning:* Due to a risk of spontaneous abortion, Black Cohosh should not be used during pregnancy. The herb should not be taken with drugs that lower blood pressure.

**Butcher's Broom *(Ruscus aculeatus)*.** This herb, native to the Mediterranean regions of Europe, Africa, and western Asia, is used medicinally as a diuretic, anti-inflammatory, and for its beneficial effects on circulation. Butcher's Broom is used to relieve the discomforts of hemorrhoids, such as itching and burning, and the leg heaviness, pain, cramping, and swelling of chronic venous insufficiency.

**Cat's Claw *(Uncaria tomentosa)*.** The root of the South American Cat's Claw contains compounds that have immune-stimulating, anti-inflammatory, and anticancer effects. Although human studies have yet to be conducted, Cat's Claw is often used to treat cancer; arthritis and rheumatic disorders; and AIDS and other viral diseases.

*Warning:* Cat's Claw should not be used by pregnant or breastfeeding women, or by people with autoimmune disorders, multiple sclerosis, tuberculosis, transplant recipients, and children under 2 years of age.

**Cayenne (Capsicum annuum).** Externally, Cayenne is used to relieve the pain of muscle tension and spasm, diabetic neuropathy, and rheumatism. Cayenne is sometimes taken internally to relieve gastrointestinal disorders, although human studies have yet to confirm such uses.

*Warning:* Topical Cayenne preparations should not be used for more than two consecutive days, with a two-week break between applications. It should never be used on broken skin or near the eyes. When used internally, Cayenne preparations should not be taken with aspirin or antifungal drugs.

**Chamomile (Matricaria recutita).** Chamomile tea—which has anti-inflammatory, antispasmodic, and muscle-relaxing effects—is used to treat gastrointestinal disorders such as indigestion and gas.

*Warning:* Chamomile should not be used by pregnant women.

**Comfrey (Symphytum officinale).** This herb is applied topically as an anti-inflammatory; it is used for bruises and sprains and to promote bone healing.

*Warning:* Because of possible toxic adverse effects, Comfrey should not be taken internally. The herb is contraindicated in pregnant and breastfeeding women.

**Dandelion (Taraxacum officinale).** Dandelion, commonly used as an addition to the salad bowl, is recommended as an effective remedy for digestive and liver complaints, urinary tract infection, and as an appetite stimulant.

*Warning:* Although the herb is sometimes used for gallbladder complaints, this should only be done under a doctor's supervision. People with bile duct obstruction or stomach ulcer should not use Dandelion.

**Dong Quai (Angelica sinensis).** Dong Quai root is used in China as a women's health tonic. It is particularly used as a remedy for fibrocystic breast disease, premenstrual syndrome, painful periods, and menopausal symptoms. Dong Quai is also used in cardiovascular disease to treat high blood pressure and improve poor circulation.

*Warning:* Dong Quai should not be used by pregnant or breastfeeding women. The herb can also cause photosensitivity.

**Echinacea (Echinacea purpurea).** This species of Echinacea is a well-established immune-system stimulator; it is used to treat flu, coughs and colds, bronchitis, urinary tract infections, wounds and burns, and inflammation of the mouth and pharynx.

*Warning:* It should not be used in patients who have autoimmune disorders such as multiple sclerosis, collagen disease, AIDS, or tuberculosis. The herb is also contraindicated in patients who have diabetes and in pregnant or breastfeeding women. Echinacea should not be used with the following: anticancer agents, anti-organ rejection drugs, corticosteroids, or immunosuppressants.

**Evening Primrose (Oenothera biennis).** The anti-inflammatory compounds in Evening Primrose oil have been extensively studied, but no definitive indication has been accepted. Some herbalists consider the oil useful for treating breast pain, premenstrual syndrome, and menopausal symptoms. Capsules containing at least 500 milligrams of the oil are approved in Germany as a remedy for eczema.

*Warning:* People with seizure disorder or schizophrenia should not take Evening Primrose oil.

**Feverfew (Tanacetum parthenium).** Feverfew is used to treat migraine headaches, allergies, and arthritic and rheumatic diseases.

*Warning:* Feverfew should not be used during pregnancy or breastfeeding. It is also contraindicated in people with bleeding disorders, and in those who are taking anticoagulants, including aspirin.

**Flax (Linum usitatissimum).** Ground Flax (also known as Linseed) is used internally to relieve constipation. It is also used externally as a compress to relieve skin inflammation.

*Warning:* Flax should not be used internally in the cases of bowel or esophageal obstruction; or in the presence of gastrointestinal or esophageal inflammation.

**Fo-Ti (Polygonum multiflorum).** The Asian herb Fo-Ti is used for constipation, atherosclerosis, high cholesterol, and as an immune enhancer.

*Warning:* Because of its laxative action, the herb may cause diarrhea. Taking the unprocessed root may cause skin rash; and overdosage may cause numbness in the extremities.

**Garlic (Allium sativum).** Garlic is used as a treatment for hardening of the arteries, high blood pressure, and to reduce cholesterol levels. It may also have antibacterial and antiviral effects.

*Warning:* Garlic can cause allergic skin and respiratory reactions. It should not be used by people with bleeding disorders, or by those taking blood thinners (including aspirin) or NSAID therapy. Nursing women should also not use Garlic.

**Ginger (Zingiber officinale).** Ginger root is a treatment for motion sickness and loss of appetite. It is also indicated for nausea and vomiting associated with chemotherapy, and to help control nausea and vomiting in postoperative patients.

*Warning:* Ginger should not be used for morning sickness associated with pregnancy, or by nursing mothers. People who have gallstones or bleeding disorders should not take Ginger. The herb is also contraindicated in those taking blood thinners (including aspirin) or NSAID therapy.

**Ginkgo *(Gingko biloba).*** Ginkgo has proven useful for dementia, Alzheimer's disease, peripheral arterial occlusive disease, vertigo, and tinnitus of vascular origin.

*Warning:* Ginkgo should not be used by people who have bleeding disorders, or who are taking blood thinners (including aspirin) or NSAID therapy.

**Ginseng *(Panax ginseng).*** The Ginseng root is used for fatigue and to improve concentration and stamina. Ginseng may also have antiviral, antioxidant, and anticancer effects.

*Warning:* Caution with Ginseng is urged in people with cardiovascular disease or diabetes. People who are taking diabetes drugs, diuretics, blood thinners (including aspirin), MAO inhibitors, or NSAIDs should not take Ginseng. It should not be used during pregnancy or breastfeeding, or by those with bleeding disorders. Taking large amounts can result in Ginseng abuse syndrome, which is characterized by high blood pressure, insomnia, water retention, and muscle tension.

**Goldenseal *(Hydrastis canadensis).*** Goldenseal contains the compound berberine, which is used for gastritis, gastric ulcer, gallbladder disease, and acute diarrhea. It can be useful as an adjunct therapy in cancer treatment, and is also used to treat chronic eye infection.

*Warning:* Goldenseal should not be used by pregnant or breastfeeding women, or by people who have bleeding disorders; it should also not be combined with blood thinners (including aspirin) or NSAIDs. Use of Goldenseal for extended periods can result in digestive disorders, constipation, excitement, hallucination or delirium, and decreased vitamin B absorption. **Overdosage can result in convulsion, difficulty breathing, and paralysis.**

**Gotu Kola *(Centella asiatica).*** Gotu Kola is used internally for chronic venous insufficiency and venous hypertension. In animal and lab studies, Gotu Kola was also effective for ulcers and varicose veins. The herb is used externally to treat wounds; if a rash develops, discontinue topical use.

**Great Burnet *(Sanguisorba officinalis).*** Great Burnet may be used both externally and internally for its astringent, decongestant, and diuretic properties. Internal uses include menopausal symptoms, intestinal bladder problems, and venous disorders. It is also prepared for external use as a plaster for wounds and ulcers.

**Green Tea *(Camellia sinensis).*** Green Tea, which is rich in catechins and flavonoids, is used to help prevent cancer. The antibacterial effects of Green Tea mouthwash are useful in the prevention of dental cavities.

Keep in mind that Green Tea contains caffeine and should be used sparingly by pregnant and breastfeeding women, and by those who are caffeine-sensitive.

**Hawthorn *(Crataegus laevigata).*** Hawthorn contains several compounds that are considered beneficial to the heart. It is used for cardiac insufficiency, angina, congestive heart failure, and irregular heartbeat.

*Warning:* Hawthorn should not be used in children under 12, or in the first trimester of pregnancy. People taking Hawthorn must be carefully monitored by a physician, especially in cases where it is combined with cardiac glycosides, beta-blockers, or calcium channel blockers. Hawthorn should not be taken with cisapride. Overuse can lead to low blood pressure, irregular heartbeat, and excessive sleepiness.

**Horse Chestnut *(Aesculus hippocastanum).*** Both the seed and leaf of Horse Chestnut are used medicinally. The seed is indicated for the symptoms of chronic venous insufficiency, including pain, cramping, swelling, sensations of heaviness, and night cramping. Horse Chestnut leaf is used for venous disorders such as varicose veins, hemorrhoids, and phlebitis.

*Warning:* People taking blood thinners (including aspirin) should not use Horse Chestnut.

**Kava-kava *(Piper methysticum).*** The active compounds in Kava are lactones, which have antispasmodic, muscle-relaxing, and anticonvulsive effects; Kava can also thin the blood. The herb is used for nervousness, insomnia, tension, stress, and agitation.

*Warning:* People who are depressed should not take Kava. The herb is also contraindicated in pregnant or nursing women and in those with liver disorders. Overuse of Kava can result in skin rash or weight loss. Kava use for more than three months should be supervised by a physician. The herb should not be combined with alcohol, anti-anxiety or mood-altering drugs (including barbiturates), or levodopa.

**Licorice *(Glycyrrhiza glabra).*** The sweet root of the Licorice plant has a long history of use in traditional medicine. It contains various compounds with anti-inflammatory and other soothing effects that make it helpful as a treatment for ulcers and digestive disorders such as gastritis. It also acts as an expectorant for cough and bronchitis.

*Warning:* Licorice should not be taken with digoxin, diuretics, or medications that lower blood pressure. Licorice should also not be used in people with hepatitis and other liver disorders, kidney disease, diabetes, arrhythmias, high blood pressure, muscle cramping, low potassium levels, and pregnancy

**Ma-Huang *(Ephedra sinica).*** Ma-Huang contains compounds that alleviate bronchial constriction and is used in folk remedies as a treatment for coughs and bronchitis.

*Warning:* The adverse effects of Ma-Huang outweigh any possible benefits. The herb should not be taken by pregnant or breastfeeding women, or by people with the following: anxiety, high blood pressure, glaucoma, brain tumors, prostate disorders, adrenal tumors, cardiac arrhythmia, or thyroid disease. Ma-Huang should not be combined with caffeine, decongestants, stimulants, glaucoma medication, MAO inhibitors, anesthetics, or labor-inducing drugs. **Overdosage can result in death.**

**Milk Thistle** *(Silybum marianum).* The compounds in Milk Thistle seed have protective and regenerative effects on the liver. It is used as a treatment for liver and gallbladder disorders such as jaundice, toxic liver damage, cirrhosis of the liver, and gallbladder pain.

*Warning:* The herb should not be used with antipsychotic drugs, yohimbine, or male hormones.

**Pumpkin Seed** *(Cucurbita pepo).* Pumpkin Seed has anti-inflammatory and antioxidant properties. It is used to treat irritable bladder and symptoms of benign prostatic hyperplasia (eg, obstructed urinary flow). It does not, however, appear to relieve an enlarged prostate.

**Pygeum** *(Pygeum africanum).* Pygeum bark contains compounds that inhibit the inflammation and swelling associated with benign prostatic hyperplasia.

*Warning:* The herb should not be used by pregnant or breastfeeding women. People with stomach disorders should check with their physician before using Pygeum.

**Saw Palmetto** *(Serenoa repens).* The anti-inflammatory and testosterone-moderating effects of Saw Palmetto make it useful for treating benign prostatic hyperplalsia; the herb is used for treating irritable bladder as well.

*Warning:* Saw Palmetto should not be used by pregnant or breastfeeding women. The herb should be avoided by those who have hormone-driven cancers or a family history of such cancers. People with stomach disorders and those who are taking hormones or hormone-like drugs should check with their physician before taking it.

**St. John's Wort** *(Hypericum perforatum).* St. John's Wort is one of the better studied herbs. Various compounds in St. John's Wort have antidepressant, anti-inflammatory, and antibacterial effects. It is used internally for depression and anxiety, and externally for wounds, burns, skin inflammation, and blunt injuries.

*Warning:* St. John's Wort can cause photosensitivity if taken for too long or at high doses. It can also cause gastrointestinal discomfort and headache. Combining St. John's Wort with other antidepressant medications such as MAO inhibitors, selective serotonin reuptake inhibitors (including fluoxetine, paroxetine, sertraline, fluvoxamine, or citalopram), or nefazodone could cause "serotonin syndrome"—a condition characterized by sweating, tremor, confusion, and agitation. The herb should also not be combined with the following: antibiotics that have photosensitizing effects, cyclosporine, indinavir, combination oral contraceptives, reserpine, barbiturates, theophylline, or digoxin.

**Stinging Nettle** *(Urtica dioica).* Both the flowers and root of the Stinging Nettle plant contain beneficial compounds used in various conditions. The flower is used internally and externally for rheumatism; it is used internally for urinary tract infections and kidney and bladder stones. The root is used for irritable bladder and to help relieve symptoms of benign prostatic hyperplasia (eg, obstructed urinary flow), although it does not reduce prostate enlargement.

*Warning:* Stinging Nettle should not be used by people who suffer from fluid retention due to impaired cardiac or kidney function.

**Uva-Ursi** *(Arctostaphylos uva-ursi).* Uva-ursi is used in the treatment of urinary tract infections because of its astringent and antibacterial effects.

*Warning:* The herb should not be used by pregnant or breastfeeding women; it should also not be used in children under 12 years of age, as it could cause liver damage. Uva-ursi should not be combined with diuretics, NSAIDs, or with substances (food or medication) that promote acidity in the urine.

**Valerian** *(Valeriana officinalis).* Valerian root contains sedative compounds that are useful in nervousness and insomnia. It is recommended for many other unproven uses such as headache, anxiety disorders, premenstrual syndrome, and menopausal symptoms.

*Warning:* Patients should avoid operating motor vehicles for several hours after taking Valerian. The herb should not be used by pregnant or breastfeeding women. Valerian extract or bath oils should not be used by people suffering from skin disorders, fever, infectious disease, heart disease, or muscle tension. Valerian should not be taken with barbituates or benzodiazepenes.

**Vitex** *(Vitex agnus-castus).* Vitex (also known as Chaste Tree) is used as a treatment for premenstrual syndrome and menopausal symptoms.

*Warning:* Because of its hormonal effects, Vitex should not be used by pregnant or breastfeeding women. Occasionally, rash can occur. The herb should not be used with drugs that affect dopamine levels.

**Wild Yam** *(Dioscorea villosa).* Popular reports have led to the belief that Wild Yam is a "natural" source of the hormone progesterone. While Wild Yam is used as a constituent of artificial progesterone pharmaceutically, the body cannot complete the conversion process by itself. The herb can also be useful in treating high cholesterol.

*Warning:* Because of possible hormonal effects, pregnant and nursing women should not use Wild Yam. The herb should not be taken with estrogen-containing drugs or indomethacin.

**Yohimbe** *(Pausinystalia yohimbe).* Yohimbe is prepared pharmaceutically under the brand name Yocon and is used to treat erectile dysfunction. Compounds in Yohimbe stimulate norepinephrine, which improves blood flow to the penis. The risks, however, of unregulated ingestion of the herb are thought to outweigh the benefits. Therefore, it is recommended that Yohimbe be taken only under strict medical supervision.

*Warning:* Yohimbe should not be used by women, especially pregnant or breastfeeding women. It is also contraindicated in patients with liver or kidney disease, posttraumatic stress disorder, high blood pressure, panic disorder, or Parkinson's disease. The herb should not be taken with naltrexone, blood pressure medication, alcohol, or morphine. Patients should check with their doctor before taking Yohimbe with any OTC product.

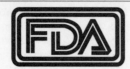

# U.S. FOOD AND DRUG ADMINISTRATION

**Professional and Consumer Information Numbers**

## Medical Product Reporting Programs

**MedWatch (24 hour service)** ...........................................................................................**800-332-1088**
*Reporting of problems with drugs, devices, biologics (except vaccines), medical foods, dietary supplements.*

**Vaccine Adverse Event Reporting System (24 hour service)** ...............................**800-822-7967**
*Reporting of vaccine-related problems.*

**Mandatory Medical Device Reporting** .........................................................................**301-827-0360**
*Reporting required from user facilities regarding device-related deaths and serious injuries.*

**Veterinary Adverse Drug Reaction Program** .............................................................**888-332-8387**
*Reporting of adverse drug events in animals.*

**Medical Advertising Information** ..................................................................................**301-827-2828**
*Inquiries from health professionals regarding product promotion.*

**USP Medication Errors** ..................................................................................................**800-233-7767**
*Reporting of medication errors or near-errors to help avoid future problems through improvement in product names and packaging.*

## Information for Health Professionals

**Center for Drugs Information Branch** ...........................................................................**301-827-4573**
*Information on human drugs including hormones.*

**Center for Biologics Office of Communication** .........................................................**301-827-2000**
*Information on biological products including vaccines and blood.*

**Center for Devices and Radiological Health** .............................................................**301-443-4190**
*Automated request for information on medical devices and radiation-emitting products.*

**Emergency Operations** ..................................................................................................**301-443-1240**
*Emergencies involving FDA-regulated products, tampering reports, and emergency Investigational New Drug requests.*

**Office of Orphan Products Development** .....................................................................**301-827-3666**
*Information on products for rare diseases.*

## General Information

**General Consumer Inquiries** .........................................................................................**888-463-6332**
*Consumer information on regulated products/issues.*

**Freedom of Information** .................................................................................................**301-827-6500**
*Requests for publicly available FDA documents.*

**Office of Public Affairs** .................................................................................................**301-827-6250**
*Interviews/press inquiries on FDA activities.*

**Center for Food Safety and Applied Nutrition** ..........................................................**888-723-3366**
*Information on food safety, seafood, dietary supplements, women's nutrition, and cosmetics.*